Clinical Research in Occupational Therapy
Fourth Edition

Clinical Research in Occupational Therapy

Fourth Edition

Franklin Stein, Ph.D., OTR/L
The University of North Dakota
Vermillion, North Dakota

Susan K. Cutler, Ph.D., NCSP
Morningside College
Sioux City, Iowa

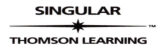

SINGULAR
™
THOMSON LEARNING

Africa • Australia • Canada • Denmark • Japan • Mexico • New Zealand • Philippines
Puerto Rico • Singapore • Spain • United Kingdom • United States

NOTICE TO THE READER

COPYRIGHT © 2000 Delmar. Singular Publishing Group is an imprint of Delmar, a division of Thomson Learning. Thomson Learning™ is a trademark used herein under license.

Printed in Canada
2 3 4 5 6 XXX 03 02 01

For more information, contact Delmar, 3 Columbia Circle, PO Box 15015, Albany, NY 12212-0515; or find us on the World Wide Web at http://www.delmar.com

Library of Congress Cataloging-in-Publication Data:
Stein, Franklin.
    Clinical research in occupational therapy / by Franklin Stein, Susan K. Cutler.—4th ed.
        p.; cm.
    Includes bibliographical references and index.
    ISBN 0-7693-0047-2 (softcover : alk. paper)
        1. Occupational therapy—Research—Methodology. I. Cutler, Susan K. II. Stein, Franklin. Clinical research in allied health and special education. III. Title.
        [DNLM: 1. Occupational Therapy. 2. Research. WB 555 S819c 2000]
    RM735.42.S74 2000
    615.8'515'072—dc21   99-086956

Contents

Preface to the Fourth Edition

The fourth edition of *Clinical Research* presents a comprehensive approach to assisting the clinician and researcher to test and validate practice. Qualitative and quantitative research models are presented, with accompanying examples from the occupational therapy literature. Good research is tied to internal and external validity, that is, the control of extraneous variables that could distort results and the ability to generalize results to clinical practice. Evidenced-based practice is based on the development of treatment protocols that can be adapted to the individual needs of the client. Research provides the clinician with the documented evidence to substantiate practice and to communicate its effectiveness to other clinicians and consumers. Without clinical research to validate practice, the clinician cannot justify the treatment methods used in occupational therapy.

The major revisions in the fourth edition include:

1. Contrasting qualitative and quantitative research models as applied to occupational therapy.
2. An expanded discussion of action research and its relevance to occupational therapy.
3. Redesign of figures and tables in a clearer format to help the prospective researcher design a feasible research proposal.
4. An example of a research proposal in occupational therapy that can serve as a model for a graduate research project, thesis, or dissertation.
5. A descriptive analysis of the most widely used tests and assessments are presented so that they can be considered by occupational therapists and other allied health practitioners in selecting an outcome measure.
6. An up-to-date reference guide of Web addresses of health care organizations and consumer groups.
7. An example of an informed consent form that can be used to obtain human subjects' approval from an Institutional Review Board (IRB).
8. Documentation methods for electronic references conforming to the American Psychological Association style.
9. A step-by-step model to help the clinical researcher through the design and implementation of a research study in occupational therapy.
10. The identification of potentially major flaws in a research study that can threaten internal and external validity.
11. An outline of the history of occupational therapy, highlighting the major landmarks affecting practice.

As with any revised edition, spelling, grammar, and typographical corrections have been made and wording, when unclear, has been improved.

At a time when there are major changes occuring in health care systems throughout the world, occupational therapists can make important contributions in preventing and treating diseases and in habilitating and restoring function through purposeful activities. We can only demonstrate our effectiveness through the results of clinical research. We hope this book will assist occupational therapists in creating evidenced-based practice for the 21st century.

Acknowledgments

First, I would like to thank the administrators and Board of Regents at the University of South Dakota for granting me a sabbatical for the fall semester, 1999, which I spent mostly in Sweden at the University of Uppsala. During the summer of 1999, Sue Cutler and I worked diligently on the revisions, which were completed in the fall. I sincerely appreciate the assistance from Ingrid Södderback and her doctoral students in Uppsala for sharpening and clarifying my thinking. My visits and lectures at the University of Örebrö, the Karolinska Institute, and Jyväskylä University in Finland challenged many concepts and my vision of research in occupational therapy. I learned immensely from these experiences. My colleagues and students at the University of South Dakota served as my support system. To my wife Jennie and family: David, Sharon, Jacqueline, and Natalie; Jessie, Chris, and Celeste; and Barbara and Craig, I appreciate your confidence in me to continue my intellectual pursuits.

Introduction

The first edition of this book was published in 1976. At that time, it was the first textbook on clinical research in the allied health professions. Since then, numerous texts have been published about research from the perspective of clinical practice in occupational therapy, physical therapy, and speech-language pathology and audiology. The current edition, the fourth, is a collaborative effort where the authors combine their expertise in occupational therapy, counseling psychology, and special education into a textbook on clinical research. In preparing this edition, we raised the question, What characterizes a good textbook in clinical research? In reviewing other textbooks and reexamining the strengths and weaknesses of this book, we came up with the following points:

1. The textbook should be well written and easily understood by undergraduate and graduate students. Complex concepts should be explained carefully and presented in a logical sequence.

2. There should be an historical perspective in the text that connects the student to other researchers who laid the foundation for clinical practice. The allied health professions and special education are a continuation of the scientific and medical revolutions that created the helping professions. As clinicians, we are dependent on the early research in anatomy and physiology, testing and measurement, medical instrumentation, clinical medicine, and environmental health. The knowledge gained in the basic sciences impact strongly on the clinical professions. As scholars, we know that current practice stands on the shoulders of the giants in basic and clinical research.

3. Within the context of the book, there should be many examples from the literature as well as hypothetical examples explaining theoretical concepts and research principles. The book should come from a pragmatic perspective that presents feasible ideas.

4. The book should be a resource for further study in related areas. References and addresses should be liberally found throughout the book to point the student in the right direction.

5. Statistical procedures should be clearly explained in a stepwise procedure. The concept underlying the statistical technique should be emphasized. Although there are a number of software programs and statistical packages, it is important for the student to understand how the statistical results are derived. The student should have a strong background in descriptive statistics before learning inferential statistics.

6. In the textbook, there should be an example of a research proposal that can serve as a model for the student researcher. The research proposal should be feasible and realistically implemented.

7. The textbook should be comprehensive and include a number of different research models that are appropriate for research in occupational therapy, physical therapy, special education, rehabilitation counseling, and other allied health fields.

8. Qualitative as well as quantitative research models should be described, with examples from the literature. Both models are appropriate and relevant. The research design is judged on its own merits as far as validity and application to clinical practice or health care.

9. The emphasis in research is in raising relevant and feasible questions. The student should be encouraged to ask

questions that generate intellectual interest and curiosity. The processes of doing research and searching the research literature are as important as reporting results. Research should be a process of discovery and intellectual excitement.

10. The student who is designing and carrying out a research study should see the relationship between one's research study and one's professional role, whether it be a clinician, administrator, educator, or researcher.

11. The research text should help the student develop a critical view of research. The student should be able to read the literature with a critical eye and carry over this knowledge to clinical practice, especially in clinical reasoning.

12. The student should have a strong appreciation of the ethical issues involved with human research. Students should be able to design an informed consent form and be able to safeguard the research subject from unnecessary psychological or physical risks.

One of the major purposes of this textbook is to link research to clinical practice. It is important within this context that the researcher raise many questions relating to clinical practice in developing a research proposal. As the student or clinical researcher works on the preparation of a research design, he or she should keep in mind the practical implications of the research study. The content of the chapters in this textbook are organized comprehensively to include all the components in research, from generating a research topic, carrying out a literature review, designing a research study, selecting a measuring instrument, statistical analysis of data, and writing a scientific paper. The textbook is organized to enable a student to write a research proposal, critically evaluate a published study, and prepare a manuscript for a refereed journal.

In writing this edition, the authors developed a conceptual model that serves as a rationale for the book.

1. The medical model underlies the clinical practice in allied health and special education. Historically, the medical model includes arriving at a diagnosis that serves as the basis of treatment. Understanding of the medical model and its historical perspective is important for clinicians in rehabilitation and special education because we work closely with physicians in a team approach. The development of educational, psychological, and sociological factors in treatment does not negate the medical model. Effective rehabilitation and habilitation depends on a holistic approach to the patient that includes the medical model and an educational-psychological approach.

2. Conceptually, we emphasize the strengths of individuals with disabilities as the basis of good treatment. In planning treatment interventions, the clinician evaluates both the strengths and weaknesses in the client and then develops with the client a goal-directed plan for achieving functional independence.

3. Good treatment means fitting the treatment procedure to the patient and not fitting the patient to a treatment method. The clinician should avoid a "Procrustean Bed" where treatment methods are advocated and generalized to all patients. Good treatment is based on the individual needs of the patient and the consideration of multiple approaches.

4. The goal of clinical research is to discover, through objective and systematic inquiry, the most effective treatment methods that can be applied to the client with a disability. Research should be driven by theory and explanation.

5. The relationship between clinical research and clinical practice is based on the premise that good treatment depends on multiple factors, including the

therapist's skill, the effectiveness of a treatment methodology, the appropriateness of the client, and environmental factors that affect treatment. Clinical research strives to understand the relationship between these factors in clinical treatment.

6. Doing research and critically evaluating the findings help the student to become an effective clinician. Because clinical practice is dependent on clinical reasoning and decision making, the effective clinician applies the scientific method in practice. The research-oriented practitioner is able to evaluate the literature and to incorporate current research findings into clinical practice.

CHAPTER

A Short History of the Scientific Method in Medicine, Rehabilitation, and Habilitation

> *Medical research on the scale to which it is developed today is a modern invention. A hundred years ago it was limited to the part-time activities of a few dozen individuals working in their private rooms (one could hardly call them laboratories) at home or in a university. Today it provides a life-time's career for thousands of medical scientists working in specially built laboratories in universities and research institutes financed by government or the pharmaceutical industry.*
> —N. Poynter, 1971, *Medicine and Man*, p. 6

Operational Learning Objectives

By the end of this chapter, the learner will

1. Define research and the primary purposes of research in occupational therapy and special education
2. Describe seven stages in the history of medicine
3. Explain the cyclical nature of medical progress
4. Recognize the important contributions of medical researchers toward the im-

provement in environmental health and clinical practice

5. Understand the importance of methodological discoveries in diagnosis, prevention, and treatment
6. Indicate the reasons for the growth of the allied health professions that are related to the rehabilitation movement
7. Explain the important stages in the development of special education
8. Identify trends in rehabilitation research

1.1 Definition and Purposes of Research in Occupational Therapy and Special Education

What is research? Research is a systematic and objective investigation as carried out by identifying a problem, stating a hypothesis or guiding question, and collecting primary data. The emerging methods of research have generated qualitative and quantitative designs. Action research, the application of research to a site-specific environment, is an outgrowth of both qualitative and quantitative research.

Research in occupational therapy and special education have many purposes, some of which are listed in the following examples:

▶ **Measure effectiveness of treatment methods, interventions, and teaching techniques.** For example, one might want to determine the effectiveness of sensory integration therapy on the academic achievement of students with a learning disability or the effectiveness of relaxation therapy on alleviating symptoms of depression.
▶ **Accountability to communicate the effectiveness of treatment methods, interventions, and teaching procedures to government agencies and funding sources.** For example, the researcher decides to publish the results of several research studies that demonstrate the effectiveness of occupational therapy with consumers with disabilities or students in a special education program.
▶ **Explore and compare different strategies for treatment and intervention.** For example, therapists might compare the effectiveness of social skills training and biofeedback in persons with schizophrenia, whereas teachers might compare the use of phonemic analysis versus whole language in teaching reading to students with dyslexia.
▶ **Help clinicians or teachers to plan action research in site-specific environment.** For example, occupational therapists col-

lect data on how to decrease the number of Medicare rejections in a specific hospital. Special educators might examine the effectiveness of small group instruction versus individual instruction in a specific program.
▶ **Enable clinicians or teachers to be better consumers of research.** For example, a clinician doing a research study in splinting can evaluate other studies in the same area. Likewise, a teacher who examines the literature for characteristics of an effective classroom may utilize the findings to improve his or her own classroom.
▶ **Develop interventions, treatment protocols, educational strategies, assessment procedures and tools, or software products that will later be evaluated for effectiveness.** For example, an occupational therapist is interested in developing a treatment protocol to reduce anxiety in individuals with depression. A teacher may want to increase the attention span in a student with attention-deficit hyperactivity disorder.
▶ **Apply research techniques to evaluate programs and facilities in meeting standards of practice.** For example, The Rehabilitation Accreditation Commission (CARF) applies research methods to evaluate a rehabilitation facility.
▶ **Reconstruct historical events to understand the basis for a current treatment.** For example, an occupational therapist will examine the historical basis for treating individuals with spinal cord injuries, whereas teachers in special education might examine reasons for the shift between various reading methods.
▶ **Examine reasons for improvement or failure of a specific treatment through a retrospective case study.** For example, a client with a diagnosis of multiple sclerosis showed remission of symptoms after a 3-month intervention. The researcher seeks to examine the variables that led to improvement.
▶ **Explore relationships between associated variables.** A clinician might want

to examine the relationship between perceptual motor skills and self-care abilities or perceptual motor skills and writing achievement.

▶ **Examine the characteristics of a homogeneous population.** For example, one might want to explore the leisure interests in individuals with disabilities.

Research in rehabilitation and habilitation is a direct result of the methodology of scientific medicine. The rehabilitation professions emerged from the scientific findings in medicine that began in the 19th and 20th centuries. In rehabilitation professions, such as occupational therapy, physical therapy, speech pathology, and audiology, the results of these findings have lead to direct application. In this chapter, we review the eight stages in scientific medicine that are the core of scientific inquiry in the rehabilitation professions. In Chapter 3, we discuss the models of research that have evolved from questions proposed by researchers.

1.2 Historical Review of Research in Medicine, Rehabilitation, and Habilitation

Before the beginnings of modern science in the latter half of the 19th century, relationships between causes and effects still retained explanations that bordered on the supernatural. Vitalism, a recurrent movement in medicine, was typified by the 18th-century physician who ascribed mysterious substances in the blood to life functions. This theory was an outcome of the prescientific thinking that gave way to the systematic and orderly explanations that we now associate with modern scientific research. The breakthrough in understanding the disease process began with the laboratory experimentation of Pasteur (1822–1895), who served as a model for the medical scientist. The impact of scientific technology in the treatment and rehabilitation of the sick and the disabled has been a re-

markable record in human progress. In only a few other areas of knowledge has man made greater strides. How and why did this happen?

The analysis of the progress in medical science, rehabilitation, and special education is divided into seven stages identified in Figure 1–1. These seven stages are progressive, interactive, and dynamic. For example, basic research in biological and chemical processes in Stage I continues to be important as evidenced by the investigations of DNA and RNA as the building blocks in protoplasm. Similarly, methodological research is in the forefront by virtue of the integration of high technology with clinical practice as demonstrated in the areas of prosthetics, transplant operations, kidney dialysis techniques, and artificial replacement of bodily organs. Medical scientists are constantly refining treatment and preventive methodologies. Immunologists who formerly sought chemicals to destroy harmful bacteria and viruses have led the way for present-day investigators searching for vaccines to prevent cancerous growths and life-threatening diseases, such as Acquired Immune Deficiency Syndrome (AIDS).

Progress in science is cyclical and cumulative. As knowledge grows, medical scientists refine their methods of research. Stages of development in medicine point to the cumulative process of obtaining knowledge and to the evolutionary process of scientific methodology and its impact on clinical practice.

1.3 Biological Description, Stage I

1.3.1 The Growth of Scientific Anatomy and Physiology

The earliest medical research started with the discovery of the physiological processes and anatomical systems of the body. Biological description: Stage I, the evolution

STAGE I	STAGE II
BIOLOGICAL DESCRIPTION	*METHODOLOGICAL*
Accurate description of anatomical structure and physiological processes, producing a basic understanding of the bodily organs and systems.	Development of instruments, procedures, and tests to produce valid and reliable methods in evaluation, diagnosis, and treatment.

STAGE III	STAGE IV	STAGE V
ETIOLOGY	*PREVENTION*	*TREATMENT*
Understanding of disease processes and cause–effect relationships, to produce a science of medicine and universal agreement in diagnosing diseases.	Development of medical technology to prevent initial onset of disease, resulting in the science of immunology and public health.	Application of treatment techniques based on a theoretical understanding of disease processes, leading to the growth of chemical intervention, antiseptic surgery, and nursing care in hospitals.

STAGE VI	STAGE VII
REHABILITATION	*HABILITATION AND SPECIAL EDUCATION/PROGRAMMING INTERVENTIONS*
Development of therapeutic techniques and restoration of maximum function for individuals with chronic disabilities, leading to the evolution of Allied Health professions.	The identification of treatments for developmental and social disabilities by applying specialized educational and psychological techniques to populations at risk.

Figure 1–1. Seven stages in the history of medicine, health, and rehabilitation. The seven stages are progressive, interactive, and dynamic.

of medical research, is outlined in Table 1–1. Knowledge of the anatomical structure of animals during the Middle Ages and the Renaissance was greatly influenced by Galen (138–201 A.D.), who experimented on lower mammals; Leonardo Da Vinci (1452–1519), who made precise drawings of human anatomy; and later by Vesalius (1514–1564), who, through careful dissection, described human anatomy. Identifying and describing the anatomical structures of the body led to increased knowledge about relationships between systems and the interrelationships of cardiovascular, respiratory, and genitourinary functions. Harvey's (1578–1657) concept of the circulation of

Table 1–1. The Emergence of the Medical Scientist: Stage 1

Medical Events	Discovery Dates	Scientists	Implications
Hippocratic writings	400–500 B.C.	Hippocrates (500 B.C.)	Provided a model for medical practitioners based on ethical and humane treatment
Systematic study of bodily processes	169–180 A.D.	Claudius Galen (129–199 A.D.)	Influenced medical practice for 1300 years, presenting an eclectic synthesis of prior knowledge
"The Canon of Medicine"	translated 1187	Avicenna (980–1037)	Significant figure of Arabic medicine whose work was dogma during the Middle Ages
"Paragranum": The four pillars of medicine: philosophy, astronomy, chemistry, and virtue	1530	Paracelsus (1493–1541)	Created the foundation for general medical practice based on a knowledge of pharmaceutical chemistry
Atlas of Anatomy "De humani corporis fabrica"	1543	Andreas Vesalius (1514–1564)	Made descriptive anatomy the basis of medicine and replaced aspects of Galen's work
Manual of Surgery	1543	Ambroise Pare (1510–1590)	Generated surgical innovations based upon accurate anatomical knowledge
Discovery of the circulation of the blood "Exercitatio"	1628	William Harvey (1578–1657)	Integrated anatomy with physiological knowledge of blood circulation
Digestive system "Experiments and Observations of Gastric Juice and the Physiology of Digestion"	1833	William Beaumont (1785–1853)	Used objective observation in discovering the process of digestion

blood, for example, led the way to an understanding of the internal environment of the body. Galen, Da Vinci, and Harvey were among the first scholars to accurately describe the human body; however, the ancient Greeks initially brought rational thought to an evaluation of health and disease. The Hippocratic writings reflect the depth of Greek thought.

1.3.2 The Hippocratic Writings

The first stage in the history of medicine was essentially clinical observation. The healer applying Hippocratic methods used himself as a measuring instrument, carefully noting what he saw, felt, smelled, and heard. He used rational thought regarding the causes and treatments of diseases based on these observations. In the ancient Greek civilization, scholars were allowed the freedom to speculate on all aspects of human life. Thus, the model for the Western physician emerged. Hippocrates, who is traditionally called the Father of Medicine, was probably representative of a number of individuals. It is more accurate to speak of the "Hippocratic writings" than to attribute all of ancient Greek medicine to one individual. The Hippocratic writings cover many areas of medicine, including ethics, disease etiology, anatomy, physiology, and treatment. These writings are not a consistent work linking theory to practice, but a compendium of clinical histories and a description of Hellenistic medicine.

We know little about Hippocrates' life, except that he lived during the 5th century B.C. in Cos, an island off the Greek mainland, and that he was a famous practitioner and teacher of medicine. The following excerpt from the Hippocratic writings, *On the Articulations* (ca. 400 B.C./1952) translated by Francis Adams, demonstrates the method of clinical observation used to diagnose a dislocation of the shoulder joint and the importance of individual differences in human anatomy:

> A dislocation may be recognized by the following symptoms: Since the parts of a man's body are proportionate to one another, as the arms and the legs, the sound should always be compared with the unsound, the unsound with the sound, not paying regard to the joints of other individuals (for one person's joints are more prominent than another's), but looking to those of the patient, to ascertain whether the sound joint be unlike the unsound. This is a proper rule, and yet it may lead to much error; and on this account it is not sufficient to know this art in theory, but also by actual practice; for many persons from pain, or from any other cause, when their joints are not dislocated, cannot put the parts into the same positions as the sound body can be put into; one ought therefore to know and be acquainted beforehand with such an attitude. But in a dislocated joint the head of the humerus appears lying much more in the armpit than it is in the sound joint; and also, above, at the top of the shoulder, the part appears hollow, and the acromion is prominent, owing to the bone of the joint having sunk into the part below; there is a source of error in this case also, as will be described and also, the elbow of the dislocated arm is farther removed from the ribs than that of the other; but by using force it may be approximated, though with considerable pain; and also they cannot with the elbow extended raise the arm to the ear, as they can the sound arm, nor

> move it about as formerly in this direction and that. These, then, are the symptoms of dislocation at the shoulder. (as cited in Hutchins, 1952, pp. 94–95).

The Hippocratic writings with their emphasis on dietetics, exercise, and natural methods were the complete holistic guide for the ancient physician.

1.3.3 Galen

Greek medicine provided the foundation for medical practice in the Western world. Galen, a product of the Roman civilization, was the next link in the chain of medicine. He was born in Pergamum, Greece, in the 2nd century A.D. when Roman civilization controlled much of the Western world. Galen was educated in philosophy, mathematics, and natural science. He learned medicine by traveling to places where the great physicians practiced. After acquiring knowledge steeped in the Hippocratic tradition, he became a doctor to the gladiators who performed in the Roman arenas. Galen became an acclaimed practitioner in Rome and later spent his time writing extensively. He is a model for the medical scientist who engages in clinical practice, teaching, and scholarly publication. Galen's genius was in his ability to integrate prior knowledge with his clinical observations of disease. Unfortunately, his writings on medicine became authoritative dogma from the Middle Ages to the time of the rebirth of scientific inquiry in the Renaissance. The following excerpt from Galen (ca. 192 A.D./1971) typifies his skill in teaching anatomy, as well as his careful methods of observation.

> Since therefore, the form of the body is assimilated to the bones, to which the nature of the other parts corresponds, I would have you first gain an exact and practical knowledge of human bones. It is not enough to study them casually or read of in a book; no, not even in mine, which some call Osteologia, others Skeletons, and yet others simply On Bones,

though I am persuaded that it excels all earlier works in accuracy, brevity, and lucidity.

Make it rather your serious endeavor not only to acquire accurate book-knowledge of each bone, but also to examine assiduously with your own eyes the human bones themselves. This is quite easy at Alexandria because the physicians there employ ocular demonstration in teaching osteology to students. For this reason, if for no other, try to visit Alexandria. But if you cannot, it is still possible to see something of human bones. I, at least, have done so often on the breaking open of a grave or tomb. Thus once a river, inundating a recent hastily made grave, broke it up, washing away the body. The flesh had putrefied, though the bones still held together in their proper relations. It was carried down a stadium (roughly 200 yards), and reaching marshy ground, drifted ashore. This skeleton was as though deliberately prepared for such elementary teaching.

If you have not the luck to see anything of this sort, dissect an ape and having removed the flesh, observe each bone with care. Choose those apes likest man with short jaws and small canines. You will find other parts also resembling man's, for they can walk and run on two feet. Those, on the other hand, like the dog-faced baboons with long snouts and large canines, far from walking or running on their hindlegs, can hardly stand upright. The more human sort have a nearly erect posture; but firstly the head of the femur fits into the socket at the hipjoint rather transversely, and secondly, of the muscles which extend downward to the knee, some go further (than in man). Both these features check and impede erectness of posture, as do the feet themselves, which have comparatively narrow heels and are deeply cleft between the toes.

I therefore maintain that the bones must be learnt either from man, or ape, or better from both, before dissecting the muscles, for those two (namely bones and muscles) form the ground-work of the other parts, the foundations, as it were, of a building. And next, study arteries, veins, and nerves. Familiarity with dissection of these will bring you to the inward

parts and so to a knowledge of the viscera, the fat, and the glands, which also you should examine separately, in detail. Such should be the order of your training. (as cited in Wightman, 1971, pp. 32–33)

1.3.4 Renaissance Medicine in the 16th and 17th Centuries

The history of medicine parallels, in many ways, the rise of Western civilization. The Middle Ages was a sterile period for the growth of new ideas and experimentation. Medical practice existed then as dogma, closely linked to practices and beliefs of the Church. Although Medieval Europe adhered to rigid doctrine, medical practice flourished in the Middle East as represented by the Arab physician, Avicenna (980–1037). With the onset of the Renaissance, scientists carried out experiments on human dissection under great risk of public denouncement and physical punishment. In spite of this, a psychological climate was established in the 16th century that allowed medical scholars and scientists to seek the truth by experimentation. Physicians made great strides in integrating laboratory observations with clinical practice.

Renaissance physicians rekindled the torch of medical science that had been stagnant for approximately 1,000 years. The scientists of the Renaissance were scholars familiar with Greek and Roman writings who questioned all knowledge and accepted little dogma. Furthermore, they reexamined the anatomical knowledge of Galen, experimented in chemistry, and sought explanations for the life processes in humans. In short, their work marked the beginning of the science of physiology.

1.3.5 Andreas Vesalius and the Refinement of Human Anatomy

The most important medical anatomist of the Renaissance was Andreas Vesalius. He was the first medical specialist in human anatomy. By critically examining the work of Galen, he realized that Galen's observations of anatomy were not based on human dissection but were descriptions of the bodily structures of monkeys, pigs, and goats. From 1537 to 1542, Vesalius worked on an anatomical atlas, *De humani corporis fabrica libri septea,* which was published in 1593. The book contained 663 folio pages. Vesalius' research on human anatomy became the basis of medical science and provided the necessary knowledge for the surgeon. The interplay between laboratory observations and clinical practice provided scholars with the data they needed for readjusting theory to practice and practice to theory. The model for obtaining anatomical knowledge in the medical sciences was forged in the 16th century.

1.3.6 Paracelsus the Medical Chemist

The next great development in medicine was in the area of physiology. Chemistry and physics are the bases of physiology. The understanding of human physiology awaited great discoveries in these areas. The first physician to apply chemistry to an understanding of biological processes was Paracelsus. He advocated using pharmaceutical agents singly or in combination to treat specific illnesses. He used sulphur, lead, antimony, mercury, iron, and copper as therapeutics. Paracelsus emphasized the relationship between practical clinical experience and scientific experimentation as evidenced in the following quotation from his work *Paragranum* written about 1528 (as cited in Wightman, 1971):

> The doctor must therefore be practiced in Experienz; and medicine is nothing but a wide, certain, Experienz, namely that every procedure is based in Experienz. And that is experientia which is correctly and truly founded. Anyone who has learnt his stuff without Experienz is a doubtful doctor.
>
> Experientia is like a judge; and whether a procedure is undertaken or not depends on its approval; wherefore Experienz ought to keep pace with science, for without science Experienz is nothing. Similar an Experiment grounded in Experienz is well founded and its further use understood. . . . Experiment divorced from science is but a matter of chance. (pp. 50–51)

1.3.7 William Harvey

The culmination of man's knowledge in physiology during the Renaissance was achieved in the publication by William Harvey in 1628. The publication *Exercitatio* described accurately for the first time the circulation of the blood. Harvey, an English physician, was trained in Padua, Italy, where Vesalius had taught human anatomy. After mastering the physiological theories of his time, he proposed questions, such as: What is the pulse? How does breathing affect the actions of the heart? How does the blood move? These questions directed Harvey's experimental procedures. First, he systematically stated a testable hypothesis on the circulation of the blood, and then he proceeded with rigorous experimental observation. He used precise measurements in recording pulse rate and the volume of blood ejected by the heart over time. He observed the movements of the heart and blood in living animals. He also analyzed the blood circulation of the fetus to support his theory. By using the scientific method, Harvey was able to discover the most vital process in human life. He did this by (a) presenting a researchable question, (b) mastering the published literature on blood flow, (c) using accurate observations, (d) being guided by predictive hypothesis, (e) using rigorous procedures for collecting data, (f) applying measurement to the process of blood flow, and (g) making a deductive analysis and conclusions.

Harvey's achievement in describing the circulation of the blood ranks with Newton's discovery of gravity as one of the greatest scientific accomplishments in the 17th century. Harvey's work at first was met with the jealousy and suspicion that many times accompanies an important discovery or change of thinking. In the first chapter from *Exercitatio* entitled "The Author's Motives for Writing" (1628/1952), Harvey explained his reasons for publishing his findings and his desire to bring objective criticism to his work.

> I have not hesitated to expose my views upon these subjects, not only in private to my friends, but also in public, in my anatomical lectures, after the manner of the Academy of old.
>
> These views as usual, pleased some more, others less; some chide and calumniated me, and laid it to me as a crime that I had dared to depart from the precepts and opinions of all anatomists; others desired further explanations of the novelties, which they said were both worthy of consideration, and might perchance be found of single use. At length, yielding to the requests of my friends, that all might be made participators in my labors, and partly moved by the envy of others, who receiving my views with uncandid minds and understanding them indifferently, have essayed to traduce me publicly. I have moved to commit these things to the press, in order that all may be enabled to form an opinion both of me and my labours. (pp. 273–274)

By the end of the 17th century, the medical scientist had emerged. At this point in history, medical practice was not at all consistent, yet there was a body of knowledge being created that served as the basis for later discoveries and practices. Medical schools were founded in Europe during the 17th century, but it was not until the latter half of the 19th century that medical education was rigorously evaluated. These discoveries occurred in a comparatively short period of intense activity from the 19th century to the present. The early research describing the human organism served as a foundation of scientific knowledge that was later expanded and incorporated into clinical practice.

1.4 Methodological Process, Stage II

1.4.1 Development of Medical Technology in the 18th and 19th Centuries

The second stage in medical research was the development of precision instruments and test procedures that enabled the medical scientist to examine and measure the internal processes in the body. Typical among early scientific inventors in medicine was Laennec (1781–1826) who, by watching children playing with hollow cylinders, invented the stethoscope. Methodological research over the centuries has brought about technological advances such as the electroencephalogram, electrocardiogram, X-Ray, procedures for urine analysis, positron emission tomography (PET), single photon emission computed tomography (SPECT), computed tomographic X-Ray (CT or CAT scan), magnetic resonance imaging (MRI), and other important instruments and procedures that have become basic tools in clinical medicine. Moreover, technology is continually being refined and updated.

Methodological research is unique in its application of industrial technology to the problems of diagnosis and treatment. Initially, the great advances in methodology coincided with the rise of the industrial revolution in the 18th century. Medical scientists who were able to apply industrial technology to medical practice found a wealth of ideas. These advances are examples of interdisciplinary research where investigators from diverse disciplines have applied their special knowledge to a specific research problem.

Norbert Wiener (1948), who proposed the theory of cybernetics, used interdisciplinary seminars as a means of generating new ideas and stimulating creative thinking. Presently, engineers are working in conjunction with medical scientists to create artificial materials and devices that can replace organs in the body. Biomedical engineering is a direct application of methodological research to medicine. Prosthetics, self-help devices, and orthotics are examples of methodological research applied to the field of rehabilitation. Table 1–2 summarizes the major methodological inventions that have impacted medical care.

Table 1–2. Methodological Advances: Stage II

Medical Events	Dates	Scientists	Implications
Clinical thermometer	1614	Santotio Santorio (1561–1636)	Physical examination in clinical medicine
Microscopical anatomy	1661	Marcello Malpighi (1628–1694)	Diagnostic studies of the blood
Clinical microscope	1695	Antony Van Leeuwenhoek (1632–1694)	Refinement of microscope
Technique of thoracic percussion	1761	Leopold Auenbrugger (1722–1809)	Diagnosis of respiratory disorders
Stethoscope	1819	Rene Laennec (1781–1826)	Diagnosis of circulatory disorders
Hypodermic syringe	1853	Alexander Wood (1817–1884)	Blood transfusions
Method for testing the quantity of sugar in urine	1848	Herman von Fehling (1811–1885)	Diagnosis of diabetes mellitus
X-Ray	1895	Wilhelm Roentgen (1845–1923)	Detection of tuberculosis, fractures, and dislocations
Ophthalmoscope	1851	Hermann von Helmholtz (1821–1894)	Detection of morbid changes in the eye
Cystoscope	1890	Max Nitze (1847–1907)	Disease of urinary system
Electrocardiograph (EKG)	1903	Willem Einthoven (1860–1927)	Coronary functioning
Electroencephalograph (EEG)	1929	Hans Berger (1873–1941)	Cerebral dysfunction
Magnetic resonance phenomena used in magnetic resonance imagery	1952	Edward M. Purcell (1905–1983) Felix Bloch (1912–1997)	Diagnostic assistance
Computed axial tomography (CAT)	1972	Allan Cormack, (1924–1998) Sir Godfrey Hounsfield (1919–)	Diagnostic assistance
Pulsed neuromagnetic resonance (NMR) and magnetic resonance imagery (MRI)	1975	Richard Ernst	Diagnostic assistance
Positron emission tomography (PET)	late 1970s	William H. Sweet Gordon Brownell	Diagnostic assistance
Single photon emission computed tomography (SPECT)	late 1970s	R. Q. Edwards D. E. Kuhl	Diagnostic assistance

1.4.2 The Practice of Medicine in the First Half of the 19th Century

The latter half of the 19th century was a golden period in the history of medicine. During this time, medical schools were given the legal authority to certify physicians. Examinations were required for anyone who practiced medicine in the United States and Europe. In England, for example, a Medical Register was established in 1858. Atwater (1973), in an article documenting the medical profession in Rochester, New York, from 1811–1860, described the current state of medical knowledge available to general practitioners. Table 1–3 contains an abstracted description of the advances in medicine made during the prior three centuries according to Atwater.

Although medicine had achieved great gains up until this period, most contagious diseases except for smallpox were untreatable. Surgeons worked at a great disadvantage without antiseptic techniques, and hospitals did not provide the care we associate with excellent nursing. Medical advances would have to wait for Pasteur, Lister, Morton, and Florence Nightingale to provide the revolutionary innovations.

1.5 Etiological Advances, Stage III

1.5.1 Medical Research in the Latter Half of the 19th Century

The third stage in medical research was the integration of physiology and pathology with the use of a reliable methodology to arrive at a diagnosis. The evolution of the *dynamic understanding of the disease process* is described in Table 1–4. During this stage, an understanding of the etiology of a disease through experimental laboratory research was used to verify cause-effect relationships. This breakthrough in treating disease on a scientific basis started with Pasteur's discovery of the germ theory. From Pasteur's work, laboratory scientists were able to investigate disease processes by identifying a specific microorganism. The age of chemotherapy was initiated. For every microorganism causing a disease (that was isolated in the laboratory), researchers sought a chemical substance harmless to the body to counteract the germ. From 1850 to 1910, the process of identifying the germ responsible for a disease and the discovery of a chemical to eliminate the germ was the basis for the rapid conquest of many communicable diseases. The elimination of many communicable diseases would not have occurred without the microscope and the laboratory techniques of microbiology and biochemistry. The technology for protecting the individual from infectious diseases was a direct result of the understanding of human physiology and cellular theory. Septic techniques for surgery were later developed by Lister (1827–1912), who was greatly influenced by the work of Pasteur, and by Semmelweis (1818–1865), an obstetrician who recognized the importance of hospital surgeons using prophylactic techniques during childbirth to prevent infection.

The knowledge of cellular activity by Virchow (1821–1902) was another line of evidence verifying the germ theory of disease. According to Virchow, the cause of disease was a result of changes at the cellular level. Virchow's cellular theory of disease compelled pathologists to use microscopes in searching for lesions and abnormalities within the cells. Metchnikoff (1845–1916) discovered phagocytosis, recognizing that white blood corpuscles in the body counteract disease. The understanding of the dynamics of disease led to the science of clinical medicine.

Physicians were then able to diagnose disease through laboratory microscope techniques, thus replacing vitalism and metaphysics as explanations for the onset of communicable disease. Probably the most important work on medical research in the 19th century was Claude Bernard's *Introduction to the Study of Experimental Medicine* published in 1895. Pasteur acknowledged

Table 1–3. Progress in Surgery, Clinical Medicine, and Public Health up until Pasteur's Formulation of the Germ Theory in 1878

Surgery	Diagnosis and Treatment	Public Health
Use of ether and chloroform as anesthetics	Use of microscope, auscultation, and stethoscope in diagnosis	Construction of municipal sewers
Setting of broken bones and reduction of dislocated joints	Dynamic understanding of anatomy and physiology	Recording of vital statistics
Removal of superficial diseased tissue and kidney stones	Isolation of patients with contagious diseases	Custodial care of people who are insane, retarded, poor, or homeless
Widespread practice of obstetrics and gynecology	Relief of local pain pharmacologically	Prevention of smallpox through vaccination

Table 1–4. Dynamic Understanding of Disease Processes: Stage III

Medical Event	Date	Scientist	Implications
Clinical physiology	1857	Claude Bernard (1813–1878)	Treatment of physiologic and metabolic disorders through pharmacology
Cell theory	1858	Rudolf Ludwig Virchow (1821–1902)	Cellular pathology as the basis of treatment
Germ theory	1878	Louis Pasteur (1822–1895)	The role of microorganisms in disease established
Bacteriology	1882	Robert Koch (1843–1910)	Treatment of bacterial infections could be controlled by the physician
Role of filterable viruses	1888	Pierre Roux (1853–1933)	Identification of viruses resulted in the search for preventative measures
Immunization process	1892	Elie Metchnikoff (1845–1916)	Understanding of the body's "phagocytosis" defense mechanisms against disease was recognized
Chemotherapy	1899	Paul Ehrlich (1854–1915)	Specific chemical compounds used to treat communicable diseases

Bernard as an important influence in his own work. Bernard's major contributions to understanding disease included physiology of digestion, neurophysiology, pharmacology, and organic chemistry. Bernard's work has had a profound influence in medical science. Concepts such as homeostasis and stress introduced by Cannon (1932) and Selye (1956) are based on Bernard's experimental findings on the internal gastrointestinal environment. Bernard, through his experimental methodology, established the future direction of medical research based on rigorous observation, repeated replication, and the acceptance or rejection of a hypothesis. "Scientific generalization must proceed from particular facts to principles" (Bernard, 1865/1957, p. 2). This simple statement is the foundation of 20th century medical research.

With a refined scientific methodology and a comprehensive theory of disease, medical researchers from about 1880 to 1910 made dramatic progress in identifying disease agents. This advance is exemplified by Koch's work in tuberculosis in 1890, von Behring's work in diphtheria in 1900, and Ehrlich's persistent search for a chemical to counteract syphilis, culminating in the discovery of the drug Salvarsan (arsphenamine) in 1910, after 606 experimental trials.

1.6 Prevention, Stage IV

1.6.1 Preventive Medicine in the 20th Century

The advances in medical research that have had the most dramatic effect in eliminating diseases can be attributed to primary prevention, including public health techniques and mass vaccinations. Public health measures, such as purification of water, elimination of human waste products, and protection against food spoilage, were used by ancient civilizations such as the Egyptians, Greeks, and Romans. When superstition prevailed over using prophylactic methods, however, as during the Middle Ages in Europe, epidemics and widespread disease occurred. Throughout the world, the potential for epidemics still exists in underdeveloped countries or in war and disaster zones where public health measures have been disregarded. The elimination of typhus, cholera, bubonic plague, polio, and smallpox in areas with access to modern medicine has been accomplished through the combination of medical advances and public health technology. Vaccination as a means of preventing disease has provided the means to control widespread epidemics that dramatically reduced populations in the past. The first physician to conceive the use of vaccinations to prevent disease was Jenner (1749–1823), who experimented with cowpox infection, a mild disease, as a means of pro-

tecting against smallpox, one of the leading causes of death in the 18th century. Jenner noted that dairymaids who contracted cowpox by milking infected cows developed a natural immunity to smallpox. This observation led him to believe that if people were deliberately infected with cowpox, they would escape the dreaded smallpox. In 1798, Jenner published his findings, which included 23 case histories of individuals inoculated with cowpox.

Initially, Jenner's work was not accepted by the medical community in England. He gradually gained recognition after his work was replicated by other physicians. Jenner's original research on vaccinations remained singularly unique until Pasteur's discovery of the germ theory about 100 years later in 1878. Jenner's method of inoculation to prevent disease was rediscovered by medical researchers who were later able to isolate pathogenic bacteria and viruses. Table 1–5 lists many of the communicable diseases that are now controlled by vaccination.

Presently, the concept of preventive medicine includes the following health procedures:

▶ Inoculation to prevent communicable diseases
▶ Environmental health to reduce atmospheric and water pollution
▶ Prenatal care to prevent birth defects
▶ Mental health community services to prevent institutionalization
▶ Family planning and population control
▶ Supervision of food handling and processing of foods to prevent botulism
▶ Prevention of industrial accidents through ergonomics
▶ Sanitary engineering to prevent typhus and cholera

Until the 20th century, physicians were able to do little for a severely ill patient. The introduction of chemotherapy, aseptic surgery, and efficient hospital care changed the course of medical practice.

Table 1–5. Control of Communicable Diseases through Immunization

Disease	Causative Agent	Medical Researcher	Discovery Date
Bubonic plague	Bacterium	S. Kitasato, Alexandre Yersin	1893–1894
Cholera	Bacterium	Robert Koch	1884
Diphtheria	Bacterium	Emil Von Behring	1890
Measles	Virus	Francesio Cenci	1901
Poliomyelitis	Virus	Jonas Salk	1954
Rabies	Virus	Louis Pasteur	1885
Rocky Mountain spotted fever	Virus	Howard Ricketts	1909
Smallpox	Virus	Edward Jenner	1796
Tuberculosis	Bacterium	Albert Calmette, Camille Guerin	1921
Typhoid fever	Bacterium	Almroth Wright	1906
Typhus	Virus	Charles Nicolle	1910
Yellow fever	Virus	Max Thieler	1936

1.7 Chemotherapy, Surgery, and Hospital Care: The Bases of Treatment, Stage V

1.7.1 Chemotherapy

As knowledge about anatomy and physiology progressed, technology was developed to improve the diagnoses of illnesses. The foundations, created to produce a body of knowledge underlying therapeutics, resulted in chemotherapy, surgery, and hospital care as the bases of modern day treatment. Although ancient civilizations, and primitive cultures existing today, have used various effective treatments, the causes of diseases and the rationale for understanding the processes were veiled in mystery. For example, rauwolfia serpentine was used in India (100 A.D.) as the "medicine of sad men" (Thornwald, 1963, p. 205) without the present understanding of the biochemical process of a tranquilizer. Ancient Egyptian doctors used mud and soil in the treatment of eye diseases. This type of "sewerage pharmacology" was not understood until 1948 when Dr. Benjamin M.

Dugger, a professor of plant physiology at the University of Wisconsin, discovered the drug aureomycin, a chemical similar to natural substances found near the Nile River. Aureomycin has been highly effective in the treatment of trachoma. For centuries, practical treatment for many disabilities, diseases, and illnesses has been applied by trial and error without an understanding of the theoretical dynamics of the disease processes. Healers, such as shamans and witch doctors, intersperse treatment with superstition, sometimes attaining positive results. The important difference between applying therapeutics in modern science and in prescientific civilizations is in the explanation of why a specific treatment cures a disease. The search for cures to diseases, beginning with the germ theory of Pasteur and continuing through Alexander Fleming's discovery of penicillin in 1928 and Selman A. Waksman's discovery of streptomycin in 1944, spurred the corporate growth of therapeutic pharmaceutics. Modern medicine is heavily dependent on the availability of various drugs to control abnormal physical conditions, such as hypertension, arteriosclerosis, blood clotting, edema, and emotional illness. Hormone therapy, uses of vitamins, and dietetics are other common methods akin to chemical therapy as forms of treatment.

1.7.2 Surgery

Surgical intervention, a second form of treatment, accounts for modern medicine's most dramatic successes, along with chemotherapy. Approximately 40,000 to 50,000 major and minor operations are performed every day in the 6,000 U.S. hospitals. A list of the most frequent surgical procedures performed in the United States is shown in Table 1–6 (Kozak & Owings, 1998). As with drug therapy, surgery was used by physicians in ancient civilizations. For example, the ancient Romans (ca. 70 B.C.–200 B.C.) used up to 200 different surgical instruments in various operations. In addition, ligature of blood vessels was performed; obstetric surgery, specifically Caesarean sec-

tion, was known; and even anesthesia was used (Marti-Ibanez, 1962).

Modern surgery as an effective and safe method was the result of two important events: the development of antiseptics by Lister in 1867, who tested the capacity of carbolic acid in preventing infection in general surgery, and the discovery of ether anesthesia as a practical method by William Morton, a dentist, in 1846.

1.7.3 Hospital Care

The third component in the development of modern treatment, parallel to chemotherapy and surgery, was the rise of hospital nursing care. Florence Nightingale's role in developing the nursing profession is legendary. Single-handedly, she aroused world public opinion about the plight of hospital patients, who were often left to die because of neglect. The story of Florence Nightingale's success is well known. During

Table 1–6. Most Frequent Surgical Procedures in the United States in 1995

Procedure	Number (in thousands)	Rate per 10,000 Population
Endoscopy of small intestine	2,383	91.2
Arteriography and angiocardiography	2,358	90.2
Extraction of lens	2,335	89.3
Endoscopy of large intestine	2,321	88.8
Insertion of prosthetic lens	1,777	68.0
Injection or infusion of therapeutic or prophylactic substance	1,745	66.8
Episiotomy with or without forceps or vacuum extraction	1,411	54.0
Cardiac catheterization	1,389	53.1
Excision or destruction of lesion	1,300	49.7
Diagnostic ultrasound	1,288	49.3
Respiratory therapy	1,132	43.3
Computerized axial tomography	1,038	39.7

Note. The information contained in this table is based on data from the *Vital and Health Statistics, Ambulatory and Inpatient Procedures in the United States, 1995*, Series 13: Data from the National Health Care Survey No. 135 by L. J. Kozak and M. F. Owings, 1998, U.S. Department of Health and Human Services, Centers for Disease Control and Prevention, National Centers for Health Statistics, p. 8. This publication is available through http://www.cdc.gov/nchswww/data/sr13_135.pdf

the Crimean War of 1854, she organized a group of nurses to tend wounded British soldiers. Her experience gave her the insight into the need for clean, efficient hospitals. Reform in hospital care became a national issue in England after the Crimean War, and social legislation was enacted to provide governmental support. Florence Nightingale also started the first school of nursing at St. Thomas' Hospital, London, in 1860. With hospital reform enacted through legislation and a nursing school started, the foundation for progress in the treatment of the hospitalized patient was established.

Below is a short outline of the historical development of hospitals as documented by Rene Sand (1952):

1. Ancient Greece, 6th Century, B.C.: A large open building was provided for the Greek physician. It comprised a waiting room, consulting room, and theater for operations and dressings.
2. Ancient Rome, 1st Century, A.D.: Sick bays were attached to the family estates of the wealthy.
3. Early Medieval Europe, 4th Century, A.D.: Early Christians established "hospitia" for travelers, abandoned children, and the sick who were traveling on their way to pilgrimages. Care was under the direction of monastic and sisterly orders.
4. Middle East, 12th Century, A.D.: Moslems in Baghdad founded the first hospitals where physicians cared for the ill. Special wards for mental illness, blindness, and leprosy were established.
5. Later Middle Ages, Europe, 5th to 14th Centuries: Hostelries under the jurisdiction of the Roman Catholic Church provided care for the sick. Brothers and sisters of the Roman Catholic Church in attached ecclesiastical hospitals provided treatment remedies, performed simple operations, and attended those with serious illnesses.
6. Renaissance Europe, 15th Century: For the first time in the Western world, phy-sicians and midwives treated the sick in hospitals. Terminal patients were segregated from the acutely ill.
7. Europe, 18th Century: Gradually hospitals began to treat emergency care patients, outpatient departments grew, and hospitals served as training facilities for medical students.
8. Europe, America, 19th Century: Nursing care was established in hospitals. Antiseptic surgery, anesthesia, and improvement in general care of the hospitalized patient were initiated.
9. Worldwide, 20th Century: The growth of specialized hospitals, regional planning, and national health services. A world movement exists in extending health care to underdeveloped countries under the auspices of the United Nations, World Health Organization (WHO).

Current medical treatment is based on the principle of healing—stopping the progression of a disease and promoting natural bodily processes. Chemotherapy, surgery, and nursing care are the three basic methods that have made medical practice effective in treating many communicable diseases and physiological disorders and anatomical defects. The limitations of medical treatment for individuals with severe chronic disabilities, such as schizophrenia, arthritis, cardiovascular disease, and cerebral vascular accident (CVA) are clearly evident. Medical treatment alone is effective only when the disease process can be narrowed down to a specific etiology. Chronic diseases present problems of multiple etiologies and treatment requiring complex solutions and interdisciplinary efforts. The search for solutions to the chronic disabilities led to the rehabilitation movement.

1.8 Rehabilitation Movement, Stage VI

The emergence of rehabilitation as a distinct entity in the health care system began only 83 years ago. The aftermath of World War I saw the beginning of the rehabilitation movement, coinciding with the need for restoring function to those who were permanently disabled. One may ask why the rehabilitation field developed at that time and not in prior periods of recovery from war. The historical factors that led to the rehabilitation movement are outlined in Table 1–7. Until the 18th century, chronic illness and permanent disability in general were not always considered medical problems. For instance, psychiatric illness and epilepsy were considered problems of morality and satanic possession. Treatment of psychiatric illness, if any, was stark, brutal, or radical. Before the rise of large institutions providing custodial care for psychiatric patients, the attitude toward chronic mental illness was at best benign neglect and at worst rejection and punishment. In a related area, birth injuries such as cerebral palsy were misunderstood by ancient cultures. Not until 1862, when W. T. Little, an English orthopedic surgeon, described the relationship between birth injury and neurological disorders, was there any dynamic understanding of this disability. Individuals with other chronic disabilities, such as arthritis, emphysema, cerebrovascular stroke, cardiovascular disease, and spinal cord injuries, were left either to the custodial care of the family or were placed into the hands of charlatans who promised miraculous cures.

1.8.1 Social Welfare and Rehabilitation

The change from custodial care to therapeutic treatment of the individual with chronic disabilities occurred at a period of time in history when social welfare had become a worldwide concern. Social Security was the forerunner in public health and medicine for the indigent with chronic disabilities. Germany, in 1883, and England, in 1897, were the first countries in Europe to enact legislation providing worker's compensation to cover disability and illness re-

sulting from occupational accidents. The progress toward social and occupational health and safety is described in Figure 1–2. Governmental financial support, resulting from national policies on health and welfare, was necessary because of the enormous hospital resources and health personnel required in the rehabilitation of individuals with disabilities. In the United States, social security legislation, first enacted in 1935, has been a major impetus for the development of the rehabilitation movement. Change in societies' attitudes toward the individual with chronic disabilities, as evidenced in the social welfare movement, has encouraged the growth of the allied health professions.

1.8.2 The Evolution of Allied Health Professions, Phase I

Three major phases in the history of rehabilitation have affected the growth of the allied health professions. The first phase occurred shortly after World War I. During this period, the need for physical and social rehabilitation of the individuals with disabilities was recognized by the medical community. Casualties from the war included individuals with lower extremity amputation, victims of poisonous gas resulting in neurological disabilities, and soldiers with psychiatric disabilities caused by shell shock. At that time, these veterans of the war needed assistance in readjusting to community living. Reconstruction workers recruited from nursing staffs were the first health personnel in rehabilitation. Immediately after World War I, the goal of rehabilitation was primarily humane and supportive to the medical treatment. There was no direct effort by the rehabilitation workers to change the course of a disability or to make the individual with disabilities more functional. During the late 1920s, rehabilitation departments were established for the first time in hospitals. The health personnel recruited to work in these departments were, on the whole, dedicated people who applied caring support and

Table 1–7. Historical Factors Leading to the Rehabilitation Movement

- Incorporation of scientific methodology into clinical medicine
- Industrialization and its impact on clinical procedures for diagnosis and treatment
- Large population of veterans with disabilities from World War I
- The availability of financial resources through Social Security and National Health Insurance schemes
- Medical specialties and the development of allied health professions
- Public acceptance that individuals with disabilities can be restored to independence through rehabilitation
- Public acceptance of individuals with disabilities in social and work situations

activity to facilitate the patient's readjustment to the community.

1.8.3 The Education and Professionalization, Phase II

The second phase of rehabilitation, during the 1930s, 1940s, and 1950s, can be identified as the *educational and professionalization* phase. Table 1–8 lists the major landmarks in physical rehabilitation. During this time, programs in colleges and universities were initiated, professional associations grew, and rehabilitation services evolved. The training of allied health specialists who had a unique combination of knowledge in the application of activities and rehabilitation techniques, understanding of medical treatment, and a background in the social sciences were considered necessary preparation for working in a hospital setting. The concepts underlying rehabilitation at that time were taken from other clinical and applied disciplines such as anatomy, physiology, nutrition, language development, psychology, clinical medicine, and education.

1.8.4 Physical Medicine and Rehabilitation

The first rehabilitation medical service in a general hospital was created in 1946, in Bellevue Hospital, New York City (Rusk, 1971). This unit served as a model for the interdisciplinary rehabilitation team. In addition, the physiatry specialty in rehabili-

tation medicine was started. Conceptually, rehabilitation was defined as restoring the individual to the highest level of cognitive, physical, economic, social, and emotional independence. This process, involving a team evaluation of the patient's functions, establishment of treatment goals and priorities, and an interdisciplinary approach to treatment, became the model for rehabilitation. This process is listed in Figure 1–3.

Parallel to the evolution of a medical rehabilitation team was the involvement of the federal and state governments in providing vocational rehabilitation services that resulted from the Vocational Rehabilitation Act of 1954. Sheltered workshops, such as Abilities Inc. in New York City, Epi-Hab in Los Angeles, Goodwill Industries, and Community Workshops in Boston, provided the vocational training component and the specialized employment placement that helped reemploy individuals with disabilities.

1.8.5 Allied Health Treatment Technologies

As the training of allied health professionals developed during the 1940s and 1950s, a treatment technology emerged, especially in physical therapy. Methods for objectively assessing muscle function were established (Daniels, Williams, & Worthingham, 1956; Kendall & Kendall, 1949). Electrodiagnosis of muscle function, measurement of range of motion, and techniques for improving

ANTIQUITY
- Manual labor and tradesmen neglected
- Occupational diseases ignored

MEDIEVAL GUILDS
- Voluntary associations formed for mutual aid protection of tradesman
- Assist worker with disabilities
- Assist in funeral expenses

SOCIETY OF ARTIFICERS
- Established apprenticeship system
- Workday regulated 12–13 hours

PROTECTION OF MINERS (16th Century)
- Ventilating machines for mines

OCCUPATIONAL MEDICINE (Established 17th Century)
- Relationship between occupation and disease investigated medically
- Prevention measures introduced—rest intervals, positioning, cleanliness, protective clothing

COMPILING OF VITAL STATISTICS ON OCCUPATIONAL DISEASE (18th Century)
- Use of medical inspectors

PROTECTION OF VULNERABLE WORKERS IN DANGEROUS TRADES (19th Century)
- Public health legislation to regulate child labor
- Work day reduced to 10 hours

WORKMEN'S COMPENSATION (1890–1910)
- Compensate workers for occupational accidents and diseases

NATIONAL WOMEN'S TRADE UNION (1920)
- Protection of women from dangerous industries

WORKER HEALTH BUREAU (Established 1927)

SOCIAL SECURITY LEGISLATION (1930s)
- Place safety and health activities within Labor Department

OCCUPATIONAL SAFETY AND HEALTH AGENCIES (Established 1970)
- On site inspections, regulations, and enforcement of laws relating to dangerous and unhealthy conditions in all industries

SCIENTIFIC INVESTIGATIONS OF PREVENTION AND TREATMENT OF OCCUPATIONAL INJURIES AND DISEASES (1980s)
- Application of ergonomics and rehabilitation of principles

FUTURE TRENDS IN OCCUPATIONAL MEDICINE
- Occupational health teams: ergonomist, occupational therapist, physician, industrial hygienist, physical therapist, safety officer, and nurse
- Investigation of physical, chemical, biological, and psychological factors in work environment that may cause or aggravate disease in individuals who are vulnerable
- Investigation of long-term effects of exposure to toxic chemicals, repetitive motion, vibration, excessive noise, extreme temperature, radiation, dust, bacteria

Figure 1–2. Progress toward social reform in occupational health and safety.

Table 1–8. Early Landmarks in Rehabilitation Movement: Stage VI

Rehabilitation Events	Dates	Contributors	Significance
First comprehensive rehabilitation	1946	Howard Rusk	Served as model for physical medicine program in a general hospital rehabilitation team approach
Physical therapy methods	1949	H. O. Kendall and F. P. Kendall	Basis for physical therapy techniques for muscle testing and patient evaluation
Retraining methods of activities of daily living	1956	Edith Buchwald Lawton	Provided functional rehabilitation methods for increasing independence
Vocational rehabilitation	1957	Lloyd H. Lofquist	Established the role of the rehabilitation counselor
Aphasia rehabilitation	1955	Martha L. Taylor and M. Marks	Provided rehabilitation techniques for speech therapy
Prosthetics	1959	M. H. Anderson et al.	Led to cooperative research by physicians, engineers, and prosthetists in the design of artificial limbs
Orthotics	1962	Muriel Zimmerman	Led to the development of self-help devices for the homemaker and worker with physical disabilities

muscle and joint action through heat, ultraviolet rays, electrical stimulation, whirlpool, and cold packs were developed through trial and error and clinical practice. These techniques were a major part of the physical therapist's treatment procedures (Downer, 1970). The need for retraining patients in activities of daily living was recognized by therapists as an important area for intervention. Lawton (1956), working with Howard Rusk at the Institute of Physical Medicine and Rehabilitation, published a manual for therapists describing methods to retrain patients to become functionally independent in their everyday activities. The need to retrain patients with aphasia to regain their use of language as the result of a stroke or brain injury led to the development of sequentially programmed techniques (Taylor & Marks, 1955).

Another important component of rehabilitation was in the area of vocational rehabilitation. Lofquist (1957), McGowan (1960), and Patterson (1958) were some of the early workers who defined the role of

the rehabilitation counselor in prevocational evaluation, special placement, and vocational training. Occupational therapy progressed as an integral part of the rehabilitation movement in a more general direction than physical therapy or speech therapy. The use of activities as treatment modalities in work, leisure, and activities of daily living was applied to a broader spectrum of disabilities. Occupational therapists worked mainly in rehabilitation departments, psychiatric state hospitals, Veteran Administration facilities, and state schools for the physically and mentally handicapped (Willard & Spackman, 1971). As the rehabilitation movement gained momentum in the 1950s, biomedical research in the replacement of limbs and joints led to the field of prosthetics. The design of component parts, fitting of the prosthesis, and gait training gave rise to another member of the physical rehabilitation team, the prosthetist (Anderson, Bechtol, & Sollars, 1959). Specialization in "rehabilitation" also occurred at a rapid rate within the fields of

CHRONIC DISABILITY	EVALUATION OF FUNCTION	TREATMENT
o Amputee	o Activities of daily living	o Chemotherapy
o Arthritis	o Ambulation	o Dietetics
o Cardiovascular	o Diet	o Nursing care
o Degenerative diseases of the CNS	o Leisure activities	o Occupational therapy
o Emphysema and pulmonary disease	o Muscular and joint function	o Orthotics
o Epilepsy	o Neurological processes	o Physical therapy
o Spinal cord injury	o Psychological factors	o Prosthetics
o Stroke	o Speech and language	o Psychological counseling
	o Vocational adjustment	o Social work
		o Speech therapy
		o Surgery
		o Vocational rehabilitation

Figure 1–3. The process of physical medicine and rehabilitation. Rehabilitation is the process of regaining skills after having lost them. After an evaluation of function, treatment can begin.

nutrition, social work, psychology, and nursing.

1.8.6 Psychiatric Rehabilitation

In comparison with physical rehabilitation techniques, psychiatric treatment has lagged behind in developing the technology to treat the individual with mental illness. The initial optimism from 1930 to 1950 that was generated by biological interventions, such as electric convulsive therapy, insulin therapy, Metrazol treatment, and psychosurgery, has faded. From the 1960s to the 1990s psychiatric treatment remained in a state of disarray. The onset of neuroleptic drugs and the community mental health movement in the 1960s led to the dismantling of large psychiatric hospitals that served as custodial "warehouses" for the patients who were chronically mentally ill.

Since the 1960s, the length of hospitalization for psychiatric patients has been reduced, but the number of individuals with mental illness living in the community and without treatment has increased. Current enlightened psychiatric treatment emphasizes early return to the community in combination with outpatient vocational rehabilitation. In many state hospitals for the mentally ill, a large percentage of patients who are elderly form a residual population from the custodial period. This population is mainly rejected, untreated, and provided mainly with maintenance care. Other individuals with mental illness are in nursing homes or left untreated in large cities as members of homeless populations.

Evaluation of psychiatric treatment still remains a fertile area for clinical researchers. Apart from descriptive observations, few comprehensive studies have analyzed treatment techniques in depth. Although many clinicians believe that what they are doing is beneficial, there is little evidence or hard data to support their claims.

Why has psychiatric rehabilitation lagged behind other areas of medical progress? First, there has been wide disagreement in identifying, diagnosing, and treating mental illness in spite of the attempt to classify it as exemplified in the *Diagnostic and Statistical Manual of Mental Disorders* (American Psychiatric Association [APA], 1994). Theorists have differed widely in their approaches in psychiatry, advocating specific treatment techniques for the broad spectrum of mental illness. Many clinical researchers have failed to recognize the individual needs of patients and the differential effects of treatment. A second reason for the lag in scientific progress in psychiatric rehabilitation is the lack of comprehensive studies. Psychiatric research has been fixed at the 19th century two-variable research stage model, which assumed a single-factor cause for mental illness. If progress in psychiatric rehabilitation is to occur, multidisciplinary efforts must investigate mental illness on a broad front, using a biopsychosocial model, rather than narrow, one-dimensional research. The promise in psychiatric rehabilitation lies in a holistic approach, the incorporation of a community mental health model relying on half-way houses, vocational programs, and support groups, with an individualized approach to evaluation, education, psychotherapy, counseling, and drug treatment.

1.8.7 Third Phase of Allied Health, 1960 to Present

This evolution leads to the present period of rehabilitation, which has been characterized by various treatment theories. Unfortunately, these theories have become so specialized that professionals in allied health fields can no longer change from one disability area to another without familiarizing themselves with a vast amount of knowledge and technology. For example, allied health professionals have specialized in diverse areas such as augmentative communication, computer technology, sensory integration therapy (SI), neurodevelopmental therapy (NDT), robotics, telemetry, cinematography, and biofeedback. These areas of rehabilitation are unique. They are interdisciplinary in nature and incorporate theories and findings from the physical and social sciences. Table 1–9 shows the rapid growth of the allied health professions from 1950 to the present.

The extraordinary growth of the allied health professions in the last 50 years is apparent if one examines the percentage increase in the number of active practitioners and the number of professional schools. In comparison with the United States' population increase from 150 million in 1949 to 210 million in 1972, one would have expected the professions to increase about 40%. We find, however, that professions such as occupational therapy and physical therapy increased 300% during the same period. The number of radiologic technologists increased 685%, registered nurses increased 149%, and physicians increased 58% during this period. On the other hand, the smallest increases were in the numbers of chiropractic, osteopathy, optometry, and pharmacy professionals. The growth of the allied health professions has continued into the 1980s and 1990s with forecasts of continued growth into the 21st century.

Another indication of the rapid expansion of the allied health professions is the emergence of new fields that did not exist 40 years ago. *The Occupational Outlook Handbook* (1951) did not include many allied health professions, which appeared in later editions, starting with 1972 (see Table 1–10).

1.8.8 Rehabilitation Research Trends (1950–1975)

Goldberg (1974), in an analysis of rehabilitation research, identified 10 areas that are related to clinical practice.

Table 1–9. The Growth of Health Profession, 1950 to 1996

Health Specialty	Postsecondary Training (Years)	Active Practitioners				
		1950	1972	1980	1992	1996
Chiropractor	6–8	14,000	16,000	23,000	46,000	44,000
Dentist	6–8	75,300	105,000	126,000	183,000	162,000
Dietitian and nutritionists	5	15,000	33,000	N.A.	50,000	158,000
Occupational therapist	4–5	2,300	7,500	19,000	40,000	57,000
Optometrist	6	17,000	18,700	23,000	31,000	41,000
Pharmacist	5–6	100,000	131,000	141,000	163,000	172,000
Physical therapist	4–5	4,500	18,000	34,000	90,000	115,000
Physician	8–15	200,000	316,500	405,000	556,000	560,000
Physician assistant[a]	2–5	—	303	9,222	22,305	64,000
Podiatrist	6–8	6,400	7,300	12,000	14,700	11,000
Psychologist	5–9	10,000	57,000	106,000	144,000	143,000
Registered nurse	3–5	300,500	750,000	1,105,000	1,835,000	1,971,000
Respiratory therapist	2–4	—	17,000	—	74,000	82,000
Speech-language pathologist and audiologist	6	2,000	27,000	40,000	73,000	87,000
Social worker	6	100,000	185,000	345,000	484,000	585,000

Note. The information contained in this table is based on data from U.S. Department Labor, *Occupational Outlook Handbook* (1951, 1974–1975, 1982–1983, 1992–1993, 1994–1995, 1998–1999). Available at: http://stats.bls.gov/search/oco_s.asp and from information obtained from professional societies.

[a]Physician assistant programs were started in 1967.

▶ **Program Evaluation:** the assessment of the effectiveness of a clinical program in reaching stated objectives or meeting a list of criteria

▶ **Management:** the study of factors related to health manpower, cost effectiveness, and comprehensive planning in providing health care to those in need of services

▶ **Dissemination:** the process of communicating research findings over a wide area, including to professional and lay persons

▶ **Involvement of Consumer Groups:** the identification of research problems

▶ **Chronic Severe Disability:** functional problems as a major focus of research in rehabilitation

▶ **Social Problems:** alcoholism, adult crime, drug addiction, and juvenile delinquency as areas included under health-related problems instead of correctional problems

▶ **Functional Assessment Methods:** targeted to the individuals with severe disabilities who are in supported employment and working at home

▶ **Need for Follow-Up and Follow-Along Research:** evaluation of the continuity of care

▶ **Rehabilitation Utilization:** incorporation of rehabilitation research in clinical practices

▶ **Rehabilitation Engineering:** interdisciplinary research in solving practical rehabilitation problems especially in the

Table I–10. The Growth of Health Professions of Technologists and Assistants, 1972–1996

Health Field	1972	1986	1990	1996
Dental hygienist	17,000	87,000	97,000	133,000
Electrocardiograph technician	10,000	18,000	16,000	15,000
Electroencephalograph technician	3,500	5,900	6,700	64,000
Medical record technician	8,000	40,000	—	87,000
Nuclear medicine technologist	—	9,700	10,000	13,000
Occupational therapy assistant	6,000	9,000[a]	9,600	16,000
Physical therapy assistant	10,000	12,000[a]	45,000	84,000
Radiology technologist	55,000	115,000	149,000	174,000
Respiratory therapist	17,000	56,000	60,000	82,000
Surgical technician	25,000	37,000	38,000	49,000

Note. Data in this table are taken from the U.S. Department of Labor, *Occupational Outlook Handbook* (1972–1973, 1988–1989, 1992–1993, 1998–1999). Available at: http://stats.bls.gov/ocohome.htm

[a]Projections are based on estimates from the professional association.

fields of prosthetics, orthotics, communication, mobility, and independent living.

These trends continue to have an impact on current rehabilitation research in the 1990s. From the initial emphasis on the physical restoration of the individual, researchers are now turning to the more complex chronic social problems that are associated with poverty, substandard housing, undernourishment, alienation, and addiction. Evidence is present that severe chronic disabilities, such as polio, tuberculosis, stroke, emphysema, and coronary thrombosis, can be alleviated or reduced through public health immunization programs, balanced nutrition, exercise regimes, and self-monitoring of symptoms. The cost of preventing chronic illnesses is much less than the cost of rehabilitation. Primary, secondary, and tertiary prevention have begun to make an impact in the work of allied health professionals. Research has an important part in justifying the efficacy of treatment intervention, either in restoring function or preventing chronic disability.

Current trends in rehabilitation research are listed in Table 1–11.

1.9 Habilitation and Special Education, Stage VII

The success of the rehabilitation movement led to the field of habilitation, which goes beyond the medical model. While the medical model traditionally relies on etiology, diagnosis, and treatment, habilitation includes the integration of psychological, sociological, and educational fields of knowledge emphasizing research in developmental theory and educational technology. Rehabilitation is traditionally defined as the restoration of function and the maximization of abilities in individuals with chronic disabilities. In contrast, habilitation is defined as the development of functions and capabilities in individuals with disabilities occurring at birth, during childhood, or during a traumatic incident (e.g., traumatic brain injury, posttraumatic stress). The process of habilitation is presented in Figure 1–4. The

Table 1–11. Current Trends in Rehabilitation Research (1999)

- Development of standardized (norm-referenced and criterion-referenced) outcome measures that have acceptable coefficients of reliability and validity
- Evaluation of treatment techniques using prospective designs
- Operational definitions of treatment methods that can be replicated in clinical practice
- Controlled observation of normal developmental landmarks that serve as reference points for populations with disabilities
- Fundamental investigations of the biopsychosocial nature of disease and underlying dynamics
- Survey of the perceptions of patients with chronic disabilities toward their disability and their evaluation of treatment techniques
- The incorporation of high technology instrumentation in evaluation and treatment, such as microcomputers, cinematography, and psychophysiological measures
- Qualitative research and action research methods

child with mental retardation, the individual who is congenitally blind or deaf, the child born with a missing limb or with cerebral palsy, the child with autism, and the child who is extremely disadvantaged have needs that are different from adults who acquired a physical disability. Helping the child develop independence, coping skills, and physical and mental capabilities to adapt to societal demands requires specialized techniques. The child who is developmentally delayed, unlike the adult with a disability, has not lost a capacity or skill that requires remedial education, sensory retraining, or vocational readjustment. Instead, the child with a disability needs special education, sensorimotor-language training, occupational preparation, and training for activities of daily living basic to the habilitation process. Special education services, available for individuals with special needs, have been developed to provide training and instruction in functional skills necessary for independent living and self-support. What were the early historical precursors to the field of habilitation?

1.9.1 Initial Concern for Those With Disabilities

Although prior to the 20th century some services were available for individuals

with disabilities, these services were minimal, generally no more than custodial care and assistance through the efforts of religious orders and voluntary charities. The earliest report of attempts to treat and educate the blind was the establishment of a hospital in 1260 (Hallahan & Kauffman, 1993; Juul, 1981). Rousseau (1712–1779), a philosopher and theorist, petitioned in his treatise "Emile" for the study of children directly rather than using what was known about adults and applying that knowledge to children. "Nature intends that children shall be children before they are men. . . . Treat your pupil as his age demands" (Rousseau, 1762/1883, pp. 52, 54).

During the mid 1800s, Jacob Rodreques Pereire (1715–1780), a Spanish medical doctor living in France, developed an oral method to teach individuals with severe hearing loss to read and speak. At the same time, a Frenchman, Abbé de l'Epée (1712–1789) developed a manual sign language for "deaf-mutes." "The natural language of the Deaf and Dumb is the language of signs; nature and their different wants are their only tutors in it: and they have no other language as long as they have no further instructors" (Epée, 1784/1820, as cited in Lane, 1976, p. 79).

Sicard (1742–1833), a French medical doctor influential in the education of the

CHILDHOOD DISABILITIES RELATED TO GENETIC, EMBRYOLOGIC OR TRAUMA INJURY	EVALUATION OF FUNCTION	EDUCATIONAL AND TREATMENT TECHNIQUES
▸ Attention-Deficit Hyperactivity Disorder (ADHD)	▸ Academic	▸ Augmentative communication
▸ Autism	▸ Activities of daily living (ADL)	▸ Braille
▸ Blindness	▸ Intellectual	▸ Computer- and robotics-assisted treatment
▸ Cerebral palsy	▸ Leisure interests	▸ Individualized learning
▸ Childhood amputee	▸ Neuromuscular	▸ Medical treatment
▸ Dyslexia	▸ Psychosocial	▸ Motor therapy
▸ Fetal alcohol syndrome	▸ Sensory	▸ Psychological counseling
▸ Hearing impaired	▸ Neuropsychological	▸ Self-care skills
▸ Juvenile arthritis	▸ Prevocational	▸ Sensorimotor training
▸ Learning disabilities		▸ Sign language
▸ Mental retardation		▸ Speech and language therapy
▸ Orthopedic impairments		▸ Vocational development
▸ Pervasive developmental disabilities		
▸ Traumatic brain injury		

Figure 1–4. The process of habilitation, or development of function. Children with special needs are evaluated and then taught using appropriate educational and treatment techniques.

"deaf-mutes" expanded Epée's methods, producing a way to teach "deaf-mutes" to read and write:

> [Epée] saw that the deaf-mute expressed his physical needs without instruction; that one could, with the same signs, communicate to him the expression of the same needs and could indicate the things that one wanted to designate: these were the first words of a new language which this great man has enriched, to the astonishment of all of Europe. (Sicard, 1795, as cited in Lane, 1976, p. 79)

1.9.2 Itard's Influence

The earliest reported case of enlightened intervention with children identified as being mentally retarded was Jean-Marc Gaspard Itard's (1774–1838) work with Victor, "the wild boy of Aveyron" (Lane, 1976). Victor (ca. 1785–1828), who emerged from the forests of Aveyron between 1797 and 1800, was thought to have been abandoned by his parents as an infant or young child. Itard, a young physician, was assigned the responsibility to teach Victor. Itard applied methods developed earlier by Epée and Sicard. These methods included breaking up each task into small segments and using techniques that had been successful for "deaf-mutes." In this way, Itard believed that he could teach Victor to be social and use language (Lane, 1976; Winnie, 1912). After 6 years, even though Itard considered his work a failure, Victor had developed some social skills and could read a few words. On the other hand, Itard's work with Victor inspired him to further his methods for teaching "deaf-mutes":

> The child, who was called the wild boy of Aveyron, did not receive from my intensive care all the advantages that I had hoped. But the many observations that I could make and the techniques of instruction inspired by the inflexibility of his organs were not entirely fruitless, and I later found a more suitable application for

> them with some of our children whose mutism is the result of obstacles that are more easily overcome. (Itard, 1825, as cited in Lane, 1976, p. 185)

Several authors in education (Forness & Kavale, 1984; Hunt & Marshall, 1994) have recognized the significant contribution of Itard's work with Victor to present-day methods used in special education classes. In his effort to teach Victor, Itard developed methods that encompassed multiple senses (auditory, visual, kinesthetic) and demonstrated that individual instruction could be successful. Eduardo Séquin (1812–1880), a student of Itard, advanced these methods. He opened the first school for the "intellectually deficient" in 1837 and demonstrated that they could be systematically trained and educated. Finally, as a physician involved in the education and treatment of individuals with disabilities, Itard played a significant part in the development of educational and treatment services for individuals with disabilities (Forness & Kavale). Initially, the emphasis of special education relied on a medical model using etiology, symptomology, differential diagnosis, and specialized treatment. This resulted in an educational system based on classification and segregation, rather than a system based on community participation and mainstreaming in general education. It is notable that Itard's work using a single case study has lead to the development of general methods for teaching children with disabilities (Kirk & Gallagher, 1989).

1.9.3 Montessori's Contribution to Special Education

The following quote is from Marie Montessori who, as a physician and teacher, established the basis for special education in Italy at the end of the 19th century. "In this method the lesson corresponds to an experiment, the more fully the teacher is acquainted with the methods of experimental psychology, the better will she understand how to give the lesson" (Montessori, 1912, p. 107).

Montessori advocated that the special education teacher of the mentally retarded should use observation and experimentation in sequencing pedagogical activities. Montessori, who acknowledges the influence of Itard and Séquin, was a forerunner in the movement to provide special education methods through perceptual-motor training to the child with disabilities. These materials and methods were based on concrete, three-dimensional manipulatives (hands-on activities) that allowed exploration and learning through discovery. Today these methods are used with populations of typical children and children with special needs (Shea & Bauer, 1994).

Theoretically, Montessori's method changed the direction of treatment from a medical model to a model based on education, psychology, and child development. This approach was not limited to the child with mental retardation. For example, Louis Braille, who was blind, developed a system of reading for the blind over a period from 1825 to 1852 (Illingworth, 1910). This method of teaching was the basis of special education for the blind in the early 1900s. Analogous to Braille as a method for teaching the blind was sign language for the deaf, devised by Abbé de l'Epée around 1755 (Winnie, 1912). The oral method was later practiced in Germany by Heinicke and Hill, who felt that speech development in the deaf child should parallel normal speech development (Winnie, 1912). Because of the complexity in educating blind and deaf children, special schools that segregated them from the public schools were founded. The significance of the Montessori method for those with mental retardation, of the Braille system for the blind, and of sign language for the deaf is that these methods compensate for the child's inability to learn in a typical classroom. They are specific, technological advances designed to help the child to learn. These methods have allowed special education to be effective for children who are blind, deaf, or mentally retarded.

1.9.4 Services in the United States

Séquin's contribution to the education of individuals with disabilities extended to the United States. Through the efforts of Samuel Gridley Howe, Séquin immigrated to the United States in 1848 where he shared his knowledge of educational methods for teaching individuals with mental retardation. He was later instrumental in founding the American Association on Mental Deficiency (AAMD), an association that continues to further the understanding of mental retardation (Lane, 1976).

In the United States, Reverend Thomas Gallaudet, Horace Mann, and Samuel Gridley Howe were pioneers in the early development of special schools for children with disabilities. In 1817, in Hartford Connecticut, Gallaudet, assisted by Clerc, a "deaf-mute" trained by Sicard, founded the first residential school for the deaf (Lane, 1976). This outstanding school still exists. Gallaudet University, located in Washington, D.C., is the only liberal arts college established for students with hearing impairments. The university was founded by Gallaudet's grandson in 1864 (Lane, 1976). In 1829, Howe opened the Perkins Institute at Watertown, Massachusetts, a residential school for students with visual impairments. This school is well known because Anne Sullivan, teacher of Helen Keller, was trained there. Fernald State School, the first institution for individuals with mental retardation, was opened in 1848, with the Commonwealth of Massachusetts assuming full financial responsibility (Sigmon, 1987). In addition to Séquin and his work in mental retardation, individuals such as Louis Braille and Alexander Graham Bell, who was instrumental in the amplification of sound for the hearing impaired, greatly influenced the teaching methods used in these early institutions (Kirk & Gallagher, 1989).

A major change in educational practices in the United States occurred when individual states mandated compulsory education between 1852 and 1918. Although some students with disabilities were taught in the general education program, the degree of severity in these individuals resulted in the creation of residential institutions, segregated day schools, and special classes. The first special education day school in the United States, the Horace Mann School, was opened in 1868 in Roxbury, Massachusetts. New Jersey, in 1911, was the first state to mandate programs for students with disabilities (Sigmon, 1987). Individuals confined to wheelchairs or with severe disabilities continued to be excluded from public schools until the 1960s and 1970s. The right for children with disabilities to be educated in a public school was mandated by court decisions such as *Pennsylvania Association of Retarded Citizens (PARC) v. Pennsylvania* (1971) and *Mills v. Board of Education, Washington, D.C.* (1971). Decisions from these judicial cases supported the position that individuals with disabilities were entitled to a free and appropriate public education (FAPE) regardless of the degree of severity or educational need (Turnbull, 1998).

1.9.5 Special Education and Testing

In 1905, Alfred Binet (1857–1911), a French psychologist, was commissioned by the French Government to provide a useful assessment tool that would identify those children who needed special techniques to learn. Binet began working to develop methods of assessing intelligence in 1886. His first book, published at that time, was entitled *Psychologie du Raissonnement (The Psychology of Reasoning; 1899/1912)*. This was the beginning of intelligence testing as we know it today. (More information regarding Binet and the development of intelligence tests can be found in the chapter on testing in the discussion on intelligence testing.) In the United States, Lewis Terman

(1877–1956) and Henry Herbert Goddard (1866–1957), strongly influenced by Binet, continued the development of intelligence tests. Both believed that intelligence was inherited, stable, and did not change over time. A student's failure in the general education curriculum was explained by his or her inadequate intellectual level, not by methods of teaching or environmental factors. As a result, in the first half of the 20th century, institutionalization and segregation of those individuals with severe intellectual deficits and physical disabilities became the norm. It was not until the 1960s when there was a major push toward normalization (Wolfensberger, 1972) and deinstitutionalization that individuals with mental retardation and physical impairments were returned to the community and local school programs.

Historically, the habilitation of those with mild mental retardation, blindness, and deafness has been more successful than the habilitation of individuals with brain damage, autism, or social deprivation. One reason for these differences has been in the specialized educational curricula that have been developed to compensate for the child's disability. Methods for educating students with brain damage, autism, or social deprivation were slower to develop.

During the latter half of the 19th century and the beginnings of the 20th century, physicians such as James Hinshelwood (1917) and Samuel T. Orton (1879–1948) used adult models to understand reasons for learning difficulties in children who were not deaf, blind, or mentally retarded. Both clinicians developed a multisensory method for teaching reading. Later, their ideas were expanded by special educators. The methods developed are still used today in many classrooms (Mercer, 1983).

The aftermath of World War I was another turning point in the development of educational programs for individuals with brain injuries. Kurt Goldstein (1878–1965), in his experimental work with soldiers who had sustained head injuries during battle, contributed much to the understanding of the consequences of brain damage. His work inspired Alfred Strauss and Heinz Werner (Strauss & Werner, 1943) to study children with brain damage during the 1930s and 1940s at Wayne County Training School in Michigan. Their findings led to the identification of a group of children with brain damage. Although these children appeared to be mentally retarded, the cause of the retardation was not genetic. Moreover, their behavioral characteristics were similar to the symptoms displayed by soldiers with brain injuries, such as perseveration, distractibility, inattention, and memory problems (Mercer, 1983). In their classic book, *Psychopathology and Education of the Brain-Injured Child,* Strauss and Lehtinen (1947) described symptoms and behaviors of the child with brain injury and justified special education methods for teaching this group of children. Prior to the published works by Strauss and collaborators (Strauss & Kephart, 1940; Strauss & Lehtinen, 1947; Strauss & Werner, 1941; Werner & Strauss, 1941), treatment for the child with brain damage was undifferentiated. Strauss and Lehtinen (1947) described the problem as follows: "The response of the brain-injured child to the school situation is frequently inadequate, conspicuously disturbing, and persistently troublesome" (p. 127).

A. R. Luria (1961) and L. Vygotsky (1934/ 1961), Russian neuropsychologists, were influential in the understanding of brain functioning and language development. Luria believed that the brain was made up of three functional units: the brainstem, involved with arousal and attention; the posterior portion, involved with taking in and processing of sensory information; and the anterior portion, implicated in planning, monitoring, and verifying one's performance. Luria and Vygotsky postulated that the development of language played an important part in one's ability to organize tasks involving planning, self-monitoring, and self-regulating. Individuals with brain damage who no longer use language for organization manifest extreme difficulties in

self-regulatory and self-monitoring activities. Likewise, children who do not use language for organization do not develop self-regulation or planning skills. These ideas of Luria and Vygotsky have influenced the way we teach all students in developmentally appropriate early-childhood classes.

Until recently, children with autism faced an even more uncertain future because of the lack of effective methods to compensate for their disability. For example, Bettelheim (1967) described the initial reaction to the orthogenic school and the problems of communication in an 11-year-old girl with autism:

> At first what little speech she had consisted of very rare, simple, highly selective and only whispered echolalia. For example, when we asked her if she wanted some candy she would merely echo "can-dy." She would say "no" but never "yes". . . . It was not our language she used, but a private one of her own. (p. 162)

Currently, programs such as TEACCH (Treatment and Education of Autistic Children and Communication Handicapped Children) at the University of North Carolina in Chapel Hill provide expertise and technical assistance in diagnosis and treatment to teachers and parents of students with autism (Edwards & Bristol, 1991).

As with the child with brain damage or autism, the socially disadvantaged child has been an enigma in the classroom. Gordon (1968) characterized the child who is socially disadvantaged as unprepared for a normal educational experience. He wrote: "As a consequence, these children show in school disproportionately high rates of social maladjustment, behavioral disturbance, physical disability, academic retardation and mental subnormality" (p. 6). Many of the children formerly characterized as socially disadvantaged are now diagnosed with Attention Deficit-Hyperactivity Disorder (ADHD).

In 1963, at the first national meeting of what later became the Association for Children with Learning Disabilities (now named the Learning Disabilities Association), the term *learning disabilities* was identified by Samuel A. Kirk (1963):

> Recently I have used the term "learning disabilities" to describe a group of children who have disorders in development, in language, speech, reading, and associated communication skills needed for social interaction. In this group I do not include children who have sensory handicaps such as blindness or deafness, because we have methods of managing and training the deaf and the blind. I also exclude from this group children who have generalized mental retardation. (p. 3)

Another impetus for the development of appropriate educational programs for individuals with disabilities was the formation of various organizations, such as the March of Dimes, National Easter Seal Society, and United Cerebral Palsy, designed to provide community-based services. Although these organizations originally provided resources for equipment and medical care for children with disabilities, parents of these children became politically proactive in obtaining rehabilitation hospitals and clinics, special education programs, community services, and barrier-free environments. These organizations have been instrumental in the development of support groups for families and in the publication and distribution of educational materials on prevention and treatment of disabilities.

Compared with children who have disabilities that cause severe problems in communication and learning, children with physical impairment who have normal language and sensory functions present different problems in habilitation. Physical barriers present problems in architectural design. Emotional and social adjustment are affected by the self-concept of children with disabilities, as well as by their feelings of competence. Other chronic disabilities of childhood such as juvenile arthritis, ulcerative colitis, childhood diabetes, heart defects, and epilepsy profoundly affect the child's development and require adaptive or specialized treatment methods.

1.9.6 Recent Trends in Services for Individuals With Disabilities

Since the passing of Section 504 of the Rehabilitation Act in 1973, the Education for the Handicapped Act (EHA; Public Law 94-142) in 1974, the reauthorization and amendment of EHA as Public Law 99-457, the passing of the Americans with Disabilities Act (1990), the reauthorization and amendment of EHA as Public Law 101-456, also known as Individuals with Disabilities Education Act (IDEA) in 1990, and the Individuals with Disabilities Education Act Amendments of 1997 (IDEA; P.L. 105-17) programs for students with special needs have grown by leaps and bounds. For example, in 1976–1977, approximately 3.5 million students were served in special education. By 1987–1988, this number had risen to 4.1 million, and by 1996–1997, there were 5.2 million (U.S. Department of Education, 1998). Approximately 7,000 occupational therapists were employed by the schools during the 1995–1996 school year, and approximately 600 openings were available. Treatment and educational services are provided by public schools for any student from birth to age 21 who is at risk or is disabled. In addition, a continuum of services are available that range from consulting with the general education teacher about a student's needs, to providing an intense, restrictive residential setting for a student. Augmentative communication, life-skills training, and assistive technology are provided to the student when needed (Meyen & Skrtic, 1988).

During the 1950s, 1960s, and 1970s, services for students with special needs were available primarily in residential institutions, special day schools, or special classes that were often physically isolated and segregated from the mainstreamed students. The concept of least restrictive environment, delineated in EHA (P.L. 94–142), states that each student will be educated in the program that allows him or her to be educated with his or her own peers to the maximum extent possible. Efficacy studies showed that special classes are ineffective for students with mild disabilities (Dunn, 1968; Epps & Tindall, 1987; Haynes & Jenkins, 1986); however, students with special needs continued to be educated outside the mainstreamed population. Madeline Will (1986), the Assistant Secretary of Education, strongly recommended that students with mild disabilities be returned to general education. She argued that general educators should take more responsibility for teaching these students. This position, originally called the Regular Education Initiative, is now known as the General Education Initiative. Some individuals, such as Sailor (1991) and Stainback and Stainback (1992) have proposed total inclusion, that is, placement of all students, regardless of their educational needs, into their home schools and into the regular classroom. Others (Vergason & Anderegg, 1992) have encouraged a range of inclusiveness, with each student's placement based on individual needs and related to specific long-term goals. This latter stance appears to be more in accord with the concept of Least Restrictive Environment (LRE) as stated in IDEA. Preservice preparation programs are being restructured to enable general educators, special educators, occupational therapists, physical therapists, speech-language pathologists, school psychologists, and audiologists to participate in collaborative efforts. If the current trend continues, students with mild or moderate disabilities will be served within the general education curriculum, with adaptation as needed. Students with severe disabilities may continue to receive educational services in special class placements, especially when the educational needs include self-care skills and independent living skills.

Although much has been achieved in the development of programs and services for those individuals with special needs, there is much more to accomplish. We are only

beginning to understand how to remediate and improve cognitive deficits. Augmentative communication and the use of technology in education and training are still in the infancy stage of development. Although increased medical technology has made it possible to keep infants and patients with severe disabilities alive, we have only just begun to develop educational and training needs for these individuals.

Habilitation is the latest frontier in health research. Much research remains to develop the knowledge and technology that will facilitate growth and learning in the child with disabilities. The progress that has been made is the result of the persistent efforts of investigators devoting a lifetime of work to specific problems.

1.10 Research and the Future of Health Care

What are the future directions and goals of health care? The physician, an individual educated in the arts and science of healing, historically has been the primary health practitioner. At first, education of the physician was "at the foot of a master;" later, formal training permitted one to legally practice medicine. It is only in the last 100 years that medicine has become a science with reliable and valid methods. The science of modern medicine began with Claude Bernard and Louis Pasteur, who provided the research methods and theory of disease that underlie clinical practice. Progress has been dramatic since the late 1800s, culminating with the elimination of many major diseases through vaccination, chemotherapy, surgery, and effective hospital care. Preventive medicine is now the cornerstone of health maintenance. At the beginning of the 21st century, researchers are mobilizing their efforts to discover means to prevent premature deaths from heart disease, stroke, cancer, arthritis, emphysema, and AIDS. Ironically, chronic disabilities continue to persist as people live longer.

As new diseases emerge (e.g., ebola virus), they present new challenges for medical researchers.

A second trend in medical progress is toward self-regulation of health care through education and monitoring of bodily symptoms. The individual's understanding of one's own anatomical, physiological, and psychological makeup through public health education continues to play an increasingly important role. Present trends have included wellness as part of the curriculum. Educating the public toward an understanding of the relationship between mind and body is an example of the wellness movement. The trend toward self-regulation in health will lead to more responsibility for one's own well-being in preventing illness through activities such as exercise, stress management, diet, and complementary medicines. Scientific research will explore the effectiveness of these methods.

Another trend in health care is the growth of specialized health professions. Up until 1920, the doctor and the nurse were the main health care providers. More than 100 health-related professions now exist. These new positions, such as cardiovascular technologist, respiratory therapist, nuclear medicine technologist, sanitarian, and public health educator, are the result of progress made in medical technology and the advancement of public health methods. New professions will continue to emerge from advanced technology. As research refines the diagnosis and treatment of illness,

there will be a parallel growth in specialized health professions.

The medical practice of the future may well be dominated by machines that monitor physiological changes; control the heart rate; stimulate nerves, muscle, and skin; replace bodily organs; and, in general, receive and transmit information to and from the body (Longmore, 1970). These medical machines will be designed to adapt to the internal organism of the body. Computers connected to the machines will be programmed to interpret accurately the information received. This relationship is shown in Table 1–12.

Another trend in rehabilitation medicine is the merging of technology in assisting individuals with disabilities. For many years, professionals in rehabilitation have recognized the need to develop devices and apparati to help individuals with disabilities maximize their independence and functional activities. The growth of the fields of orthotics (braces and splints), self-help devices, prosthetics (design of artificial limbs), and assistive technology is a direct result of this vision. Methodological research in health care is an example of interdisciplinary cooperation between scientists. Biomedical engineering, which emerged as a complex multidisciplinary field incorporating medicine, engineering, psychology, economics, computer technology, law, sociology, and the environmental sciences, has grown rapidly in the last 50 years. Rushmer (1972), a researcher at the Center

Table 1–12. Computer Application in Diagnosis and Treatment

Bodily Processes	Machine Monitoring	Computer Diagnosis
Circulatory	Electrocardiogram	
Gastrointestinal	Electroencephalogram	Aids health
Neurophysiological	Respirator	professionals in diagnosis and
Genitourinary	Magnetic resonance imagery (MRI)	prescription of
Skeletal-muscular	Computerized axial tomography (CT-Scan)	treatment
Respiration		

for Bioengineering, University of Washington, Seattle, was one of the first to describe the interaction of these multidisciplines. Table 1–13 is adapted from his description.

The merging of medicine with the social sciences to find solutions to the complex problems of mental illness, alcoholism, drug addiction, and criminology is inevi-

table. Interdisciplinary approaches to prevention and rehabilitation will result in the merging of the physical and social sciences. The study of the relationship between psychology and physiology and the immune system has lead to the field of psychoneuroimmuniology. The relationship of poverty, alienation, malaise, and hopelessness

Table 1–13. The Current Scope of Biomedical Engineering: Potential Areas of Interaction Between Life Sciences and Engineering

Applied Bioengineering			
Technological Development	**Therapeutic Techniques**	**Health Care System**	**Environmental Engineering**
Research Tools • physical measure • chemical composition • microscopy • isotope	Occupational therapy Physical therapy Radiation therapy Respiratory treatments Special education Speech-language therapy Surgical instruments	Organization Medical economics Long-range planning	*Pollution* • air • water • noise • solid waste • food Human fertility Population control
Clinical Interventions • audiology • cardiology • gastrointestinal • genitourinal • musculoskeletal • neurology • respiratory	*Monitoring* • intensive care • surgical, postop • coronary care • ward supervision	*Methods* *Improvements* • support functions • service functions • nursing • facilities design • medical care • community care • independent living	
Diagnostic data • automation • chemistry • microbiology • pathology • multiphasic screening	*Artificial organs* • sensory aids • heart–lung machine • artificial kidneys • artificial extremities: arms, legs	*Operations research* • optimization of laboratories • support functions • personnel • processing • scheduling	*Aerospace* • environment control • closed ecological systems • physiological adaptation
Computer applications • data processing • analysis • retrieval • diagnosis	*Transplants* • liver • heart • blood vessels • kidneys	*Cost benefit analysis* • cost accounting • evaluation of results • beneficial economy	Underwater compression effects Heat conservation Communication

Source: Adapted from *Medical Engineering: Projections for Health Care Delivery,* (p. 13), by R. F. Rushmer, 1972, New York: Academic Press. Copyright 1994 by Academic Press.

(which are social variables) to the onset of disease, self-destruction, and social aggression have attracted the attention of health researchers who work closely with social scientists.

The controversy in the United States during the 1990s regarding the creation of a national health care system was influenced by the health consumer's concern about being denied the right to choose a health plan. The rise of health maintenance organizations (HMOs) and managed care in the 1990s brought attention to the issue of quality health care.

Currently, health care is dominated by a biomedical model in which prescriptive drugs have dominated treatment. The overprescribing of drugs such as Prozac®, Ritalin®, Tagamet®, and the overuse of drugs such as ibuprofen® by the general public have led many health care consumers to alternative medicines. It is hoped that research will resolve the conflict between the biomedical model and alternative medicine, promoting a holistic approach to health care.

A delicate balance between governmental intervention and the respect for the sanctity and privacy of the individual must be maintained. The right of every individual to the very best health care should be among the most important priorities for every nation. In evaluating and treating clients, occupational therapy and special education should be guided by the application of sound research. In the following chapters, the methods and procedures intrinsic to scientific research applied to occupational therapy and special education are presented.

In 1998, the World Health Organization examined the international health trends. This report can be obtained at http://www.who.int/whr/1998/factse.htm and is reproduced in the following chart.

FIFTY FACTS FROM THE WORLD HEALTH REPORT 1998
GLOBAL HEALTH SITUATION AND TRENDS 1955–2025
(reproduced from http://www.who.int/whr/1998/factse.htm)

Population

1. The global population was 2.8 billion in 1955 and is 5.8 billion now. It will increase by nearly 80 million people a year to reach about 8 billion by the year 2025.
2. In 1955, 68% of the global population lived in rural areas and 32% in urban areas. In 1995 the ratio was 55% rural and 45% urban; by 2025 it will be 41% rural and 59% urban.
3. Every day in 1997, about 365,000 babies were born, and about 140,000 people died, giving a natural increase of about 220,000 people a day.
4. Today's population is made up of 613 million children under 5; 1.7 billion children and adolescents aged 5–19; 3.1 billion adults aged 20–64; and 390 million over 65.
5. The proportion of older people requiring support from adults of working age will increase from 10.5% in 1955 and 12.3% in 1995 to 17.2% in 2025.
6. In 1955, there were 12 people aged over 65 for every 100 aged under 20. By 1995, the old/young ratio was 16/100; by 2025 it will be 31/100.
7. The proportion of young people under 20 years will fall from 40% now to 32% of the total population by 2025, despite reaching 2.6 billion—an actual increase of 252 million.

continued

8. The number of people aged over 65 will rise from 390 million now to 800 million by 2025—reaching 10% of the total population.
9. By 2025, increases of up to 300% of the older population are expected in many developing countries, especially in Latin America and Asia.
10. Globally, the population of children under 5 will grow by just 0.25% annually between 1995–2025, while the population over 65 years will grow by 2.6%.
11. The average number of babies per woman of child-bearing age was 5.0 in 1955, falling to 2.9 in 1995 and reaching 2.3 in 2025. While only 3 countries were below the population replacement level of 2.1 babies in 1955, there will be 102 such countries by 2025.

Life expectancy
12. Average life expectancy at birth in 1955 was just 48 years; in 1995 it was 65 years; in 2025 it will reach 73 years.
13. By the year 2025, it is expected that no country will have a life expectancy of less than 50 years.
14. More than 50 million people live today in countries with a life expectancy of less than 45 years.
15. Over 5 billion people in 120 countries today have life expectancy of more than 60 years.
16. About 300 million people live in 16 countries where life expectancy actually decreased between 1975–1995.
17. Many thousands of people born this year will live through the 21st century and see the advent of the 22nd century. For example, while there were only 200 centenarians in France in 1950, by the year 2050, the number is projected to reach 150,000—a 750-fold increase in 100 years.

Age structure of deaths
18. In 1955, 40% of all deaths were among children under 5 years, 10% were in 5–19 year-olds, 28% were among adults aged 20–64, and 21% were among the over-65s.
19. In 1995, only 21% of all deaths were among the under-5s, 7% among those 5–19, 29% among those 20–64, and 43% among the over-65s.
20. By 2025, 8% of all deaths will be in the under-5s, 3% among 5–19 year-olds, 27% among 20–64 year-olds and 63% among the over-65s.

Leading causes of global deaths
21. In 1997, of a global total of 52.2 million deaths, 17.3 million were due to infectious and parasitic diseases; 15.3 million were due to circulatory diseases; 6.2 million were due to cancer; 2.9 million were due to respiratory diseases, mainly chronic obstructive pulmonary disease; and 3.6 million were due to perinatal conditions.
22. Leading causes of death from infectious diseases were acute lower respiratory infections (3.7 million), tuberculosis (2.9 million), diarrhoea (2.5 million), HIV/AIDS (2.3 million) and malaria (1.5–2.7 million).
23. Most deaths from circulatory diseases were coronary heart disease (7.2 million), cerebrovascular disease (4.6 million), other heart diseases (3 million).
24. Leading causes of death from cancers were those of the lung (1.1 million), stomach (765,000), colon and rectum (525,000) liver, (505,000), and breast (385,000).

Health of infants and small children

25. Spectacular progress in reducing under 5 mortality achieved in the last few decades is projected to continue. There were about 10 million such deaths in 1997 compared to 21 million in 1955.

26. The infant mortality rate per 1,000 live births was 148 in 1955; 59 in 1995; and is projected to be 29 in 2025. The under-5 mortality rates per 1,000 live births for the same years are 210, 78, and 37 respectively.

27. By 2025 there will still be 5 million deaths among children under five—97% of them in the developing world, and most of them due to infectious diseases such as pneumonia and diarrhoea, combined with malnutrition.

28. There are still 24 million low-birth weight babies born every year. They are more likely to die early, and those who survive may suffer illness, stunted growth or even problems into adult life.

29. In 1995, 27% (168 million) of all children under 5 were underweight. Mortality rates are 5 times higher among severely underweight children than those of normal weight.

30. About 50% of deaths among children under 5 are associated with malnutrition.

31. At least two million a year of the under-five deaths could be prevented by existing vaccines. Most of the rest are preventable by other means.

Health of older children and adolescents

32. One of the biggest 21st century hazards to children will be the continuing spread of HIV/AIDS. In 1997, 590,000 children age under 15 became infected with HIV. The disease could reverse some of the major gains in child health in the last 50 years.

33. The transition from childhood to adulthood will be marked for many in the coming years by such potentially deadly "rites of passage" as violence, delinquency, drugs, alcohol, motor accidents and sexual hazards such as HIV and other sexually transmitted diseases. Those growing up in poor urban areas are more likely to be most at risk.

34. The number of young women aged 15–19 will increase from 251 million in 1995 to 307 million in 2025.

35. In 1995, young women aged 15–19 gave birth to 17 million babies. Because of population increase, that number is expected to drop only to 16 million in 2025. Pregnancy and childbirth in adolescence pose higher risks for both mother and child.

Health of adults

36. Infectious diseases will still dominate in developing countries. As the economies of these countries grow, non-communicable diseases will become more prevalent. This will be due largely to the adoption of "western" lifestyles and their accompanying risk factors—smoking, high-fat diet, obesity and lack of exercise.

37. In developed countries, non-communicable diseases will remain dominant. Heart disease and stroke have declined as causes of death in recent decades, while death rates from some cancers have risen.

38. About 1.8 million adults died of AIDS in 1997 and the annual death toll is likely to continue to rise for some years.

continued

39. Diabetes cases in adults will more than double globally from 143 million in 1997 to 300 million by 2025 largely because of dietary and other lifestyle factors.
40. Cancer will remain one of the leading causes of death worldwide. Only one-third of all cancers can be cured by earlier detection combined with effective treatment.
41. By 2025 the risk of cancer will continue to increase in developing countries, with stable if not declining rates in industrialized countries.
42. Cases and deaths of lung cancer and colon or rectal cancer will increase, largely due to smoking and unhealthy diet respectively. Lung cancer deaths among women will rise in virtually all industrialized countries, but stomach cancer will become less common generally, mainly because of improved food conservation, dietary changes and declining related infection.
43. Cervical cancer is expected to decrease further in industrialized countries due to screening. The incidence is almost four times greater in the developing world. The possible advent of a vaccine would greatly benefit both the developed and developing countries.
44. Liver cancer will decrease because of the results of current and future immunization against the hepatitis B virus in many countries.
45. In general, more than 15 million adults aged 20–64 are dying every year. Most of these deaths are premature and preventable.
46. Among the premature deaths are those of 585,000 young women who die each year in pregnancy or childbirth. Most of these deaths are preventable. Where women have many pregnancies the risk of related death over the course of a lifetime is compounded. While the risk in Europe is just one in 1,400, in Asia it is one in 65, and in Africa, one in 16.

Health of older people
47. Cancer and heart disease are more related to the 70–75 age group than any other; people over 75 become more prone to impairments of hearing, vision, mobility and mental function.
48. Over 80% of circulatory disease deaths occur in people over 65. Worldwide, circulatory disease is the leading cause of death and disability in people over 65 years.
49. Data from France and the United States show breast cancer on average deprives women of at least 10 years of life expectancy, while prostate cancer reduces male average life expectancy by only one year.
50. The risk of developing dementia rises steeply with age in people over 60 years. Women are more likely to suffer than men because of their greater longevity.

CHAPTER

The Scientific Method and Research Models

> *This fusion of art and science has pushed medical knowledge to the point where persons doing research are aware that human beings should be studied in their day-to-day environments as well as in the laboratory and the clinic, and in psychosocial as well as biophysical perspective, if we are to understand fully the conditions and processes of both health and disease.*
>
> —L. W. Simmons and H. G. Wolff, 1954,
> *Social Science in Medicine*, p. 5

Operational Learning Objectives

By the end of this chapter, the learner will

1. Define the following terms:
   - ▶ research
   - ▶ theory
   - ▶ scientific method
   - ▶ independent and dependent variable
   - ▶ associational or statistical relationship
   - ▶ hypothesis
2. Give examples of common fallacies in scientific thinking
3. Outline and analyze the components of a research article
4. Identify overall objectives of the researcher
5. Contrast the nomothetic and idiographic methods of scientific inquiry
6. Compare and contrast research models
7. Compare and contrast quantitative, qualitative, and action research

2.1 Science, Research, and Theory

The concept of the scientific method was first introduced by the Greeks, who proposed that knowledge is enacted by a hypothesis that leads to observation and logical reasoning (Northrop, 1931). The scientific method ensures an empirical view of the world. In general, the scientific method can be summarized in four steps:

1. A hypothesis that is testable is proposed.
2. Objective observations are collected.
3. Results are analyzed in an unbiased manner.
4. Conclusions proposed are based on the results of the study and previous knowledge.

The dictionary definition of *research* is "the diligent and systematic inquiry, or investigation into a subject in order to discuss facts or principles" (Barnhard, 1948). *Science* is defined as the "systematic, objective study of empirical phenomena and the resultant bodies of knowledge" (Gould & Kolb, 1964). Research and science are almost identical in definition; both imply systematic objective inquiry resulting in knowledge. Scientific *theory,* on the other hand, is a comprehensive explanation of empirical data. Theory predicts what will be observed through research. A theory represents a *deductive* system of understanding the world. It predicts laws in nature that form consistent cause-effect relationships. Theories are developed by considering the underlying processes, linking an observed cause with an effect.

For example, when medical scientists investigated the relationship between a specific bacteria and the cause of a disease, a theory was proposed to explain this relationship. The theory served as the *underlying explanation,* that is, the link between the *independent variable* (presumed cause) and *dependent variable* (presumed effect). This relationship is schematically diagrammed next (Gould & Kolb, 1964):

INDEPENDENT VARIABLE	UNDERLYING EXPLANATION	DEPENDENT VARIABLE
Cause	**Process**	**Effect**
Germ	Germ Theory	Disease

2.1.1 Theory Building

Theory building is a key part of research. Many assumed cause-effect relationships instead may be actuality *associational* or *statistical relationships* where a direct one-to-one ratio between cause and effect does not exist. Instances of associational relationships are those phenomena in nature that may occur together, such as precipitation in India and an increased birth rate, or solar activity and wars. By proposing a theory, a researcher seeks to explain the direct relationship between observed causes and effects. Theory building is a way of distinguishing those relationships that are interdependent. Theories may also be developed by scientists who have systematically collected data. Generally, scientific theories generate research and predict relationships between variables.

2.1.2 Characteristics of a Theory

A theory is defined "as a set of interrelated constructs (concepts), definitions and propositions that present a systematic view of phenomena by specifying relations among variables, with the purpose of explaining and predicting phenomena" (Kerlinger, 1986, p. 9). In general, scientific theories are characterized by certain assumptions:

▶ *Technical vocabulary, language, or terms are generated by a theory.* For example, Piaget, in developing a theory of cognitive development, introduced the terms *assimilation, accommodation,* and *differentiation.* Theorists now use these terms in child development to explain how a child thinks. Freud, in introducing the theory of psychoanalysis, gave new meaning to familiar terms such as *ego, id, super ego, unconscious, libido,* and *catharsis.* These terms lose their ordinary connotations and take on the precise meanings of the theorist.

▶ *Natural phenomena or behavior can be explained by a theory.* For example, Darwin's theory of evolution was shaped by his observations of animal behavior and the examination of fossils. He formulated a theory from years of painstaking field observation. The pieces of evidence he amassed on animal and plant evolution were mosaics that he put together like a picture puzzle to form a comprehensive theory. His research expeditions were guided by questions that sought to explain the wide variations in animal behavior that he observed in his travel expeditions to South America.

▶ *A theory is a tentative set of beliefs that can be verified by scientific research.* Pasteur, in 1863, proposed the germ theory after proving that the processes of putrefaction and fermentation were caused by microorganisms. In 1880, Koch built on the work of Pasteur by completing scientific laboratory investigation of tuberculosis and cholera, thus demonstrating the validity of the germ theory.

▶ *A theory predicts events that can be simulated in the laboratory or observed under controlled conditions.* The theory of genetic determinacy predicts that a child born with a chromosomal deficit such as Down syndrome will become mentally retarded. An infant is diagnosed with Down syndrome when an extra chromosome 21 is detected through genetic screening.

▶ *A theory allows a researcher to interpret results and to form conclusions.* Lorenz, an ethnologist who received the Nobel Prize in Medicine, studied instinctive behavior patterns and proposed a theory of aggression. This theory seeks to explain the presence of conflicts and wars throughout human history.

▶ *A theory generates knowledge and leads to the development of further theories.* Gesell's theory of development predicted that normal human growth is based on sequential, hierarchical stages that unfold at critical ages. Other theorists, such as Erikson (eight stages of psychosocial development), Kohlberg (theory of moral reasoning), and Brofenbrenner (theory of ecological systems), were greatly influenced by Gesell's works in the 1920s.

▶ *A theory can be completely or partially true or completely or partially false.* When Freud proposed the psychoanalytic theory at the turn of the 19th century, many of his colleagues completely rejected his work as unsubstantiated and based on clinical speculation. Psychoanalysis was later incorporated into psychiatric treatment programs, especially in the United States, from the beginning of the 20th century until about 1960 when criticism started to appear in the professional journals. Many parts of Freud's theory, such as the terms he defined, are widely used in many studies of psychotherapy. Is psychoanalysis a valid theory of behavior? This question is still unresolved.

For clinical research, theories are a critical component in a study. To paraphrase Kurt Lewin (1939), nothing is so practical as a good theory. A scientific theory implies that phenomena or events in the world can be explained in a logical or rational way. Theories are the engines for scientific research that encompass an inductive system of knowledge. Data, which are collections of facts or information, result from research and, in turn, can eventually generate scientific laws. The systematic collection of data entails procedures for the review of previous results, the selection of research subjects, and the use of measuring instruments.

The relationship between theories and laws are diagramed in Figure 2–1. In all scientific research, the objectivity of the investigator is the most crucial variable. How a clinician or special educator gains knowledge is often through the process of

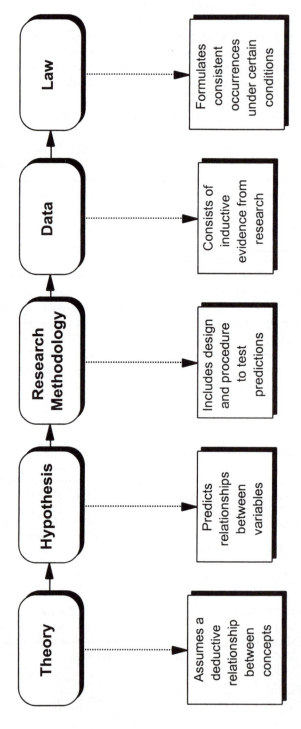

Figure 2–1. Relationship between theory and law. A theory can become a law only through accurate and systematic research.

constructivism. Proponents of this paradigm of learning (constructivism) believe that a person gains knowledge through relating a personal experience to what he or she already knows. Constructivism is learner-driven rather than teacher-initiated. A person can construct his or her knowledge base in a number of ways. Figure 2–2 describes major factors that promote constructivism.

2.2 Fallacies Related to Research

Before the development of scientific research at the turn of the century, our knowledge of medicine rested on a combination of trial and error methodology and deductive reasoning based on *a priori* assumptions. Fallacies growing out of the acceptance of invalid methods of treatment were common during times of superstition, such as in the Dark Ages in Europe and in primitive societies. These fallacies are incorrect arguments that are psychologically persuasive and, in some societies, continue to influence health practices. For example,

contemporary practitioners who treat patients with methods that have no theoretical foundation act as if there were data supporting their methods. Some clinicians advocate a particular treatment method or drug based on the fallacious premise that a disease is highly prevalent, and therefore, any treatment is better than no treatment. Also, explanations by "authorities in the field" are used to support therapeutic applications. In the past, experimentation with radical procedures, such as the use of psychosurgery with psychiatric patients, was rationalized as relevant to treatment merely because the patients were severely psychotic and considered hopeless. Or, to cite another fallacy, people refuse to accept data linking smoking to lung cancer and heart disease because they assume it cannot happen to them, but only to other persons. A knowledge of the more common fallacies is helpful to analyze objectively the validity of published studies. Copi (1953) proposed common fallacies that can occur in scientific research. These fallacies and others applied to health research and clinical practice are listed here.

CONSTRUCTING A KNOWLEDGE BASE

APPEAL TO AUTHORITY

- Read a journal article
- Read a textbook
- Attend a workshop or in-service
- Take a specialized class
- Consult with an expert

DEDUCTIVE/PHILOSOPHICAL REASONING

- Develop a theoretical model based on experience or personal observation

SCIENTIFIC METHOD

- Meta-analysis to examine statistical significance of studies related to the subject
- Test theory through a research study

EMPIRICAL APPLICATION

- Apply newly gained knowledge to clinical practice or classroom technique
- Action research

Figure 2–2. Factors that promote constructivism or the construction of one's knowledge base.

2.2.1 Irrelevant Conclusion

This fallacy is evident when an investigator intends to establish a particular conclusion by shifting his argument to another conclusion. For example, a clinician seeks support for a treatment method for patients with arthritis by arguing that arthritis is a crippling disease affecting millions of individuals. The fallacy in this argument is that the clinician proposes the acceptance of a treatment method based on the irrelevant fact that a specific disease is widespread. In this case, the specific treatment method that is introduced requires objective data to support its use irrespective of the pressing need to help patients with arthritis. Another example of this fallacy in research is the use of unreliable or invalid tests because no other tests for measuring a specific variable exist. For example, a test written in English is given to a speaker whose first language is Navajo because there are no tests written in Navajo. Results obtained are questionable and probably invalid. If a test is invalid or unreliable, it should not be used to measure function.

2.2.2 Appeal to Authority

It is fallacious for a researcher to accept the opinions of respected scientists on the sole basis of their reputation but without any supporting data. For example, in recognizing an authority's knowledge of nutrition, an investigator may use his or her opinions to support a position that megavitamins are an effective treatment for patients with schizophrenia. The authority on nutrition may not have any research data to support or negate this position. A respected authority's personal opinion is not valid scientific evidence. Researchers who appeal to authorities as supporting evidence fail to separate a scientist's previous reputation from his current opinion. In an age of specialization, scientists are no longer encyclopedists who are knowledgeable in all areas. The intensive study required for excellence

in one area makes it almost impossible to have expertise even in related areas. When a researcher uses greatly respected scientists' opinions as supporting evidence, especially outside their area of competence, he or she is committing the fallacy of appeal to authority.

2.2.3 False Cause

This fallacy is common in societies where superstition and ignorance of cause and effect exist. Curing diseases through the laying on of hands, special amulets, or magical words are examples of the use of false cause by faith healers. It is also common in nonexperimental research where correlational relationships are observed. For example, it may be noted that a full moon is associated with an increase in admissions to psychiatric hospitals. The relationship between the full moon and insanity is then fallaciously transposed to the conclusion that a full moon causes insanity. A cause-and-effect relationship is not established by correlational data.

In the absence of valid causes of a disease, simple and reductive explanations often are accepted. For example, a researcher investigating a complex variable, such as a learning disability, may accept prima facie evidence that the learning disability is caused by hyperactivity. The researcher bases this conclusion on correlational evidence that children with a learning disability are also hyperactive. The fallaciousness of the argument is illustrated in Figure 2–3.

In this hypothetical example, not all individuals with ADHD have a learning disability, although a large number of individuals with a learning disability do have ADHD. Nonetheless, there is no evidence to support the conclusion that ADHD causes a learning disability or that a learning disability causes ADHD. The very nature of a complex variable presupposes multiple causes and interactional effects among variables.

Another example of false cause in clinical practice is observing the effectiveness of a treatment method without adequately ex-

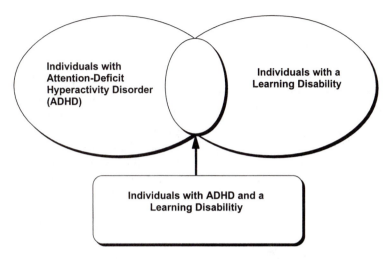

Figure 2–3. The diagram depicts the fallacy of the argument that all individuals with attention-deficit hyperactivity disorder (ADHD) are learning disabled. In fact, there are two populations: individuals with ADHD and those with learning disabilities. A few of the individuals have both conditions.

plaining the direct effect of treatment on improvement. Even though a treatment method is associated sequentially with improvement, it does not logically follow that it alone changed the condition of the patient. There may be other factors in a patient's experience or in the research conditions that could have contributed to a patient's or subject's improvement. These potential factors, which could affect the result of an experiment, must be controlled before a researcher can conclude that a specific treatment affects improvement. For example, the *placebo effect* (or "dummy treatment") is widely recognized in drug research as a change in a condition brought about seemingly by a drug but in reality by the power of suggestion that is attached to a drug. The *Hawthorne effect* is another example of a camouflaged relationship between cause and effect. In the Hawthorne effect, the change in behavior is produced by the attention of the researcher or clinician to the subjects or patients rather than solely by the specific treatment method applied. False cause is a fallacy based on traditional thinking or superstition and without supporting research evidence.

2.2.4 Ambiguity

The lack of rigor in operationally defining terms and variables used in research produces the fallacy of ambiguity. When researchers compare outcome studies of wellness, perception, functional capacity, or weight loss, false conclusions may result if their comparisons fail to acknowledge the differences in defining and measuring these variables. Wellness can be defined in multiple ways and is measured by various tests and outcome measures. How the researcher defines and measures wellness will affect the conclusions and comparisons made. When a researcher states that there is a direct relationship between healthy living and wellness, one must denote how these variables were operationally defined. Otherwise one may be operating on a simplistic and false basis that fails to take into consideration the various ways of operationally defining wellness.

For the purpose of explanation, let us examine a hypothetical example of ambiguity as shown in Table 2–1. In this example, if the researcher did not state how these two variables—healthy living and wellness—

Table 2–1. Operationally Defining Ambiguous Terms

Presumed Cause: Healthy Living	Presumed Effect (outcome measures): Wellness
1. Balanced diet	1. Trips to a physician
2. Adequate exercise	2. Self-report
3. Reduction of stress	3. Findings from a
4. Positive interpersonal	physical examination
relationship	4. Standardized test of
	wellness

are operationally defined, then there is no basis for comparing the results. In actuality, there are many different studies measuring the relationship between these two abstract variables. For example, in one study the researcher could examine the effects of nutrition on the four outcome measures; in another study, exercise could be substituted for nutrition. Each of these presumed causes and effects will need to be elaborated on further so that another researcher can replicate the study.

Complex abstract variables that are investigated by researchers must be operationally defined; that is, the measuring instrument or procedure must be clearly identified before studies can be compared and conclusions proposed. Ambiguity is an example of comparing "apples with oranges." For example, an investigator decides to use diet therapy as an *independent variable* (presumed cause) and weight reduction as the *dependent variable* (presumed effect); however, the specific method employed in diet therapy and the method used in measuring weight reduction are the variables that are, in fact, being investigated, not diet therapy or weight reduction per se. Clearly, operationally defining variables is important in eliminating the fallacy of ambiguity.

2.2.5 Generalization

Much of scientific research involves collecting group data from a representative sample of a target population. Group data represent the average of all individual scores. Also, the data imply a range of scores from high to low on specific measured variables. The fallacy of generalization occurs when a researcher applies group data to a specific individual subject. For example, a researcher collects evidence of a statistically significant relationship between the absence of epilepsy and the occurrence of schizophrenia. The researcher concludes this from a study of seizures in which there were fewer individuals with epilepsy among patients with schizophrenia compared to the general population. The statistics are based on probability factors, not on a one-to-one relationship, however. The investigator can conclude only that there are fewer individuals with epilepsy in a population of individuals also exhibiting schizophrenia than in the general population, but not that every individual with epilepsy will not become schizophrenic nor that every individual with schizophrenia will not be epileptic. Nor can one conclude that if epilepsy is produced through electric shock, schizophrenia can be prevented or treated. This is a fallacy where group data describing a population is generalized to every individual in the population. Group data cannot be applied to individuals whenever probability statistics do not approach 100%. The error variance in probability makes it impossible to make predictions about the specific individual from group data. One can only describe the general characteristics of groups, not the individual subjects that comprise the group. From probability statistics we can describe groups of patients, students, hospitals, or schools, but we are unable to predict the individual case with any complete certainty.

Another example of generalization fallacy is in the selection of students based on entry examinations, such as the Scholastic Aptitude Test or Graduate Record Examination. For example, a researcher interested in predicting academic success in an occupational therapy program may find a positive correlation of $r = .73$ between aptitude test scores and grade point averages. This is not a perfect correlation, however, and it indicates only that many students with high aptitude test scores will attain relatively high grade point averages. If a program director has to predict a specific individual's success or failure, the data cannot support complete accuracy. In fact, the chances of error in predicting a specific individual's grade point average are high, although there may be accuracy in predicting a group's success in a program.

An example of the fallacy of generalization applied to clinical treatment is the *"Procrustean bed."* In this case, clinicians who advocate a specific treatment method apply this method as a panacea to all patients regardless of individual differences. The clinician falsely applies the treatment method as a cure-all. Good treatment implies fitting the best available treatment method to the individual based on his or her needs rather than fitting the patient to the treatment.

In spite of the strong arguments used to convince researchers and clinicians to accept the findings of a study or the efficacy of a treatment method, the fallacies of irrelevant conclusion, appeal to authority, false cause, ambiguity, and generalization must be recognized by consumers of research as totally unacceptable means of advancing knowledge. The following discussion includes positive guidelines for analyzing the research process and the qualities of the researcher.

2.3 Critical Analysis of the Research Process

How is a research study judged to be either adequate or valid? How does one analyze the components of research and detect the biases of the investigator, the limitations of the design, and the deficiencies of the sampling procedure? The consumer of research must critically evaluate the methodology of a study before fully accepting the results and conclusions. Many times, the results of

a study are reported in the media without evaluating the methodology. The results of research can play a prominent role in supporting or negating a particular theory or social action. Governmental policies affecting funding patterns and priorities of social programs are influenced by the results of research studies. For example, continued funding of the children's television program *Sesame Street* is dependent on data that support the position that the program has educational value. Early childhood programs such as Head Start, manpower retraining, state mental health systems, and graduate training programs in occupational therapy professions are examples where evaluation research is used to justify federal grant support. The unfortunate policy of "benign neglect" toward minority groups during the latter half of the 1960s and the 1970s was a result of government-sponsored research that supported the discontinuance of many antipoverty programs. When research is used as evidence to initiate or discontinue social programs, there is an obvious need to evaluate methodology before accepting or rejecting the conclusions. Research is not acceptable merely on the basis of social appeal, no matter how noble the conclusions. Political considerations are one of the abuses of research that confront investigators of controversial social issues, such as community health programs or family planning.

In spite of the diversity in content and the differences in application to treatment, all research has a common methodological format. When a researcher poses a question, the process of research is initiated. The question generates a search of the literature, predictions of results, and a controlled objective procedure for collecting data. Background questions are generated by an investigator to help lead into specific research questions. This is a way of helping students to discover research topics of interest to them and to narrow a research study to feasible dimensions.

Raising background questions is a "brainstorming" tactic to lead one into a review of the literature. The student or clinical investigator is encouraged to list as many basic questions as possible to initiate a study. For example, if the goal of a clinical research is to determine the most effective treatment methods for children with traumatic brain injury (TBI), the background questions related to TBI would include:

▶ How is TBI operationally defined?
▶ What are the diagnostic tests to identify TBI?
▶ What is the prevalence and incidence rates of TBI?
▶ What are the most common treatment methods for children with TBI?
▶ What are the research data supporting treatment interventions for TBI?
▶ What are outcome measures used to measure treatment effectiveness?
▶ What is the typical course of the disability?
▶ What is the prognosis of TBI?
▶ How can vocational rehabilitation be used to treat individuals with TBI?
▶ How are functional capacity evaluations applied?

The investigator uses a literature review to answer some of these background questions. This process enables the investigator to become familiar with the research literature and to begin narrowing the study. In general, research is a process of systematically accumulating knowledge. What has been done previously is incorporated into current research. Background questions generate the research process and set in motion the beginning stages of completing a research study. Figure 2–4 describes this process.

The following outline of a research study is based on the scientific method. It is a systematic and objective way to investigate a topic.

I. A *Title* includes variables investigated, populations studied, and generalizable settings.
II. An *Abstract* is usually between 150 and 300 words, contains one or two sentences from each section of the research study, and summarizes the findings and recommendations for further research.
III. The *Problem* includes the research questions examined and the stated need and significance of the study.
IV. A *Literature Review* contains the findings of related studies that are obtained through a systematic search.
V. *Stated Hypotheses* include the operationally defined variables and research predictions.
VI. A *Methodology* section includes procedures for selecting subjects, screening criteria, measuring instruments, data collection procedures, a plan for statistical analysis, and the obtaining of human ethics approval.
VII. *Results* include objective findings that are statistically analyzed and organized into tables, charts, and graphs.
VIII. *Discussion, Conclusions, and Recommendations* include the significance of the findings related to previous research and the implications for further investigations.

Each of the subsections can be analyzed by posing specific questions relating to the objectivity of the investigator and the validity of the methods. For example:

I. Title
   1. Does the title of the study clearly define what was actually done by the investigator, or does it refer only to a segment of the study?
   2. Can the results of the study be generalized to the population identified by the title?
   3. Are the variables stated in the title identifiable and unambiguous?
II. Abstract
   1. Are the number of words between 150 and 300?
   2. Does the abstract include the highlights from each section of the study?

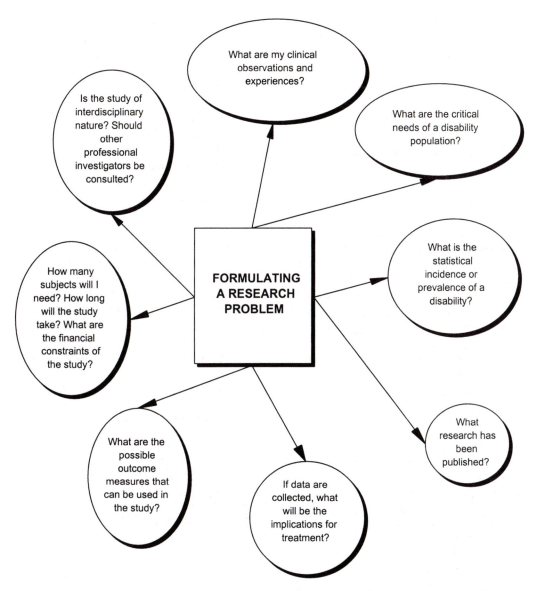

Figure 2–4. Raising basic questions, such as those in this figure, lead to a review of the literature as the beginning of a research study.

3. Does the abstract summarize the findings or results of the study?
4. Are implications or recommendations for further research summarized?

III. The Problem or Research Question
  1. Are the purposes or objectives of the study stated clearly?
  2. Are the research questions clearly identified?

3. Is the study justified in relation to social need, significance, or potential contribution to occupational therapy or special education?
4. Are statistics used to support the incidence and prevalence of a disability or to justify the investigation?
5. What is the relationship of the study to occupational therapy or special education?

6. Does the study have a potential significant contribution to evaluation methods, treatment techniques, student training, or program administration?
7. Are the projected results of the study practical so they can be implemented into practice?
8. Is the researcher being objective in selecting a specific problem for investigation, or is there evidence that personal biases will affect the results?

IV. Literature Review
1. What data collection methods did the investigator use in systematically reviewing the literature?
2. Are there theoretical assumptions that are unstated but are tacitly accepted?
3. What major areas were reviewed?
4. Was the literature search exhaustive in regard to the research problem?
5. Did the investigator separate subjective opinions and untested theories from research findings?
6. Was the investigator objective in listing results from studies that refute the stated hypotheses as well as those studies that support the hypotheses?
7. How were previous studies reported? Did the investigator describe the number and characteristics of subjects and tests used when reporting the results of studies?
8. Are references up to date?
9. Did the researcher review a wide range of journals related to the research topic?

V. Stated Hypotheses
1. Are independent and dependent variables identifiable?
2. Are variables operationally defined?
3. Did the investigator present guiding questions?
4. Were hypotheses generated from a review of the literature, and did the investigator cite previous findings?
5. Were the hypotheses stated in null form or directionally?

VI. Research Methodology
1. How were the subjects selected for the study: randomly, convenience sample, or volunteers?
2. Were screening criteria used in selecting a representative sample?
3. Were subjects a representative sample for a specified target population?
4. How were the measuring instruments selected?
5. Did the investigator state the reliability and validity of measuring instruments?
6. Do the measuring instruments have a test manual including standardized procedures for data collection and scoring?
7. How did researcher inform subjects of risks and benefits of study?
8. Can the research study be replicated?
9. Did the investigator carefully outline the procedure for data collection?

VII. Results
1. What statistical techniques were used in analyzing the data?
2. How were the results reported?
3. At what level of statistical significance were results accepted?
4. Were limitations of the study presented?

VIII. Discussion, Conclusions, and Recommendations
1. Were the findings incorporated with previous literature?
2. Were conclusions justified from reported results?
3. Is researcher bias evident in interpreting results or "rationalizing away" results?
4. Were there unforeseen events that influenced results?
5. Are results omitted that contradict the hypothesis?
6. Is further research indicated?

2.4 Qualities of a Researcher

What are the qualities of a researcher? Scholars analyzing the process of research consider that the attitudes and integrity of the researcher are sometimes more important than the rigor of the methodology and the veneer of scientism. The following has been enlarged from Gee's (1950) discussion of the qualities of a researcher.

2.4.1 Dissonance

The researcher feels uncomfortable with an aspect of the world and the problem serves as the energizer for action. Research is perceived as problem oriented. Semmelweis's concern over the large number of maternal deaths after pregnancy and Salk's experimenting with a vaccine to prevent polio are two examples of medical researchers who were motivated by dissonance. Investigators starting with a problem such as delinquency, malnutrition, AIDS, cancer, or homelessness are energized and moved to action by the amount of pain, anxiety, and degradation that a problem produces in society and arouses public empathy.

2.4.2 Objectivity

This quality enables an investigator to follow the data where it takes one instead of arriving at a conclusion first and then collecting data to support personal biases. Objectivity many times leads to accidental discoveries made through serendipity and happenstance. The researcher is open to accepting whatever the data reveal. Accidental discoveries of major significance are numerous in the history of science and technology: Bell's discovery of the telephone; Edison's stumbling upon the phonograph; Goodyear's accidentally inventing a process to vulcanize rubber; Roentgen's noticing chemical changes on paper, which led to the invention of the X-ray; and Fleming's discovery of penicillin.

2.4.3 Perseverance

The scientist's persistence and dedication to an area of research is prominent in medicine. The history of medical research is filled with researchers such as the Curies,

who devoted their entire professional lives to uncovering the properties of radium. Perseverance and persistence are necessary qualities if a researcher wants to uncover ample evidence before publishing findings. The pressure on the contemporary researcher to rush to publish results discourages persistent and painstaking efforts to accumulate overwhelming evidence. The tendency to release findings prematurely, such as in pharmaceutics, has led to medical calamities such as the effects of the drug Thalidomide on fetal development. The need still remains for the researcher to persevere in the face of the pressure to publish.

2.4.4 Intellectual Curiosity

The scientist pursues a topic not only for the practical benefits that may result from the study, but because of the desire to know. Basic research is ordinarily carried out because of the intellectual curiosity of the investigator. The basic research that produced the breakthrough in understanding the anatomy and physiology of humans came about because of Renaissance scientists' need to know. How does the body function? What are the basic processes in cell division? What is the basic chemistry of living protoplasm? Questions regarding the essential nature of the universe and matter can be answered only by research conducted by individuals with intellectual curiosity. The researcher who earnestly seeks knowledge is likely to be diligent and persevere in attaining some significant goal.

2.4.5 Self-Criticism

The investigator pursuing an area of interest needs to evaluate work critically by redesigning problems, reworking hypotheses, and initiating new methods for collecting data. The ability to examine one's work critically is important in preventing stagnation. Research involves a continual process of questioning, of obtaining evidence, and requestioning. The data from research serve as feedback for the reformulation of hypotheses only if the researcher is able to criticize oneself objectively.

2.4.6 Creativity

Being creative does not necessarily mean being novel or different. The creative researcher juxtaposes different ideas and integrates previous knowledge with contemporary issues. The qualities of risk, innovation, and independence are aspects of creativity. At odds with creativity are conformity and the need to please others while denying one's own ideas. Creativity may be a necessary quality in the researcher who desires more than fulfilling the needs of a corporate body or serving as a data collector for someone else's mission. Formulation and planning a research design is a creative act. The process of identifying a research problem and designing an objective method to test a hypothesis demands a creative quality.

2.4.7 Integrity

The researcher represents an attitude of mind. In applied health and educational fields, the researcher must be guided by ethical principles that involve a respect for the rights of participants and the honesty to bide by one's own research design and report data as found. The researcher who is engaging in human research is ethically bound not to abuse participants. The demand by social action groups and consumer advocates for formalized regulations in regard to the use of human subjects—especially in institutional environments such as prisons, psychiatric centers, chronic disease hospitals, and state schools for individuals with retardation—reflects the past abuses in human research. An informed consent contract between researcher and subject must be included in every research design. The contract shall include the following considerations:

1. The exact procedure to be carried out must be explained in language that is understandable to the participants. Jar-
gon and technical terms should be avoided.
2. The possible physical and psychological side effects in the study and the steps taken by the researcher to prevent harm to the participants should be stated.
3. The participant's time commitment in the study, procedures involved, and place of study should be clearly stated.
4. If the participants are mentally or physically incompetent or under age, then legal guardians or parents should be asked to provide written consent for the participants' inclusion in a study.
5. If the researcher requires that the purposes of the study not be revealed to the participants, then the researcher should explain this openly to the participants.
6. The researcher should not use coercion through any means that imply social disapproval or by penalizing the participants for not participating in the study.
7. If participants are paid for participation in an experiment, it should be based on work and time considerations, not as a camouflaged attempt to disguise the risks involved in being a participant or as an inducement to vulnerable individuals.
8. The findings of the research are to be treated as confidential; an individual participant's data should not be identified. Ongoing research data should be stored in a locked cabinet.

No research is so important that it disregards the rights of participants. The practices during World War II by the Nazis who engaged in human research without any regard for human rights is an extreme example of the abuse of research done with fanaticism and conformity to political goals. A researcher's integrity should be within the confines of an ethical code that must go beyond the mere search for data. Research with human subjects is not a pure or amoral theoretical activity.

Integrity in research also involves honesty in abiding by a research design and in reporting data accurately. Many times overzealous researchers are eager to present a theory of treatment or technological advance without having conclusive evidence. The pressure to present significant or dramatic findings sometimes is a result of the ego needs of the researcher. Unfortunately, it may become more important for the researcher to gain personal distinction than to report one's data honestly. The scientific community frequently has witnessed personality struggles in which rival researchers engaged competitively while striving for national recognition (Watson, 1968). The research in heart transplants, cancer, and DNA have been marked by personality conflicts.

2.4.8 Replication

Scientific research does not exist in a vacuum, nor is it usually the product of a single individual. When researchers investigate something, they typically build on the work of others. Even the giants of science, such as Newton, Einstein, Pasteur, and Edison, were vitally aware of previous research findings in the literature. Replication means that the researcher is able to repeat an experiment that was reported previously. The researcher who initially carries through an experiment must be able to describe the methodology in sufficient detail to allow other researchers to repeat the experiment. Research is not a mysterious activity carefully guarded and left to mystics. It is an open activity in which a scientific community of scholars engages. Without replication, knowledge would be stagnant, as in the Dark Ages when researchers carefully hid their methods of alchemy and magic. In clinical research, it is vital that investigators share their findings with the clinical community and also receive feedback from clinicians who undertake pilot studies of new practices and treatments.

2.5 Nomothetic Versus Idiographic Methods

One of the most important goals in scientific research is prediction. Whether it is the prediction that a drug will cause certain beneficial effects in the body or that a surgical operation will improve the functioning of a bodily organ, the scientific investigator seeks to discover relationships that may be universally true. The search for general laws in nature is defined as a *nomothetic* approach to science. However, the individual is affected by numerous idiosyncratic factors, such as physiological, emotional, and social influences, that are complex, unique, and sometimes unpredictable. The *idiographic* approach to science pertains to the intensive study of individuals within their own particular genetic milieu and environment. The nomothetic approach tends to be quantitative research, while qualitative research is generally used with idiographic approaches.

2.5.1 Nomothetic Approach to Science

If we assume that every individual's behavior can be predicted, then we ascribe to a nomothetic approach; as scientists, we seek general laws that can predict behavior. Behavior modification and operant conditioning assume that individuals are operating under general laws of nature, especially defined as reward and punishment (Skinner, 1953). The precursors of behaviorism were the logical positivists who theorized that all meaningful scientific propositions are derived from experience and can be expressed in quantifiable physicalistic language (Spence, 1948). This concept of physicalism has tried to incorporate empirical methods of collecting data into the social sciences. The technology of the logical positivists in social science is based on empirical methods of experimental control and objective observation. The major limitation of a nomothetic approach to social science is in the inability to operationally define and measure social variables such as motivation, interests, attitudes, emotions, and thinking. Behaviorism and scientific empiricism apply a psycho-physiological model; historically, the major contributions of behaviorism to social science has been by investigators such as Pavlov (1927) in classical conditioning, Wolpe (1969) in desensitization experiments, and Miller (1969) in biofeedback and conditioning experiments of the autonomic nervous systems of the body.

2.5.2 Idiographic Approach to Science

Psychoanalysis, phenomenology, Gestalt psychology, and the humanistic movement in the social sciences are examples of idiographic approaches. The subjective nature of experience and the uniqueness of the individual are, in these approaches, the vantage points for investigations. Social scientists use the case study approach in trying to understand the dynamic forces that influence an individual's behavior. The individual is perceived as an active agent interacting with the world continuously and always in the process of change. Gestalt investigations are concerned with the perceptual processes and individual differences among people and within a humanistic framework (Perls, 1969). These idiographic approaches to scientific knowledge assume that prediction in human beings is limited to the single individual, as no two individuals share the same genetic background, physiological makeup, or psychological experiences.

How does an understanding of these two approaches, nomothetic and idiographic, affect our understanding of research in occupational therapy and special education? In the nomothetic approach, we assume that general laws control human behavior and physiological responses. For example, in medicine, when an individual is treated with a drug for a specific illness, the physician assumes this patient will react as other individuals do to the same drug. Treatment is presented in relation to the illness, not in relation to the specific individual. Researchers investigating cause-and-effect relationships frequently assume a nomothetic approach. By contrast, with the idiographic approach, the clinician evaluates the patient by considering individual differences and idiosyncratic traits and treats by pre-

scribing a specific regimen. Case studies, single-subject design, and naturalistic observations are the methods used in idiographic approaches.

The history of medicine, occupational therapy, rehabilitation, and special education contains many examples of both approaches. In analyzing a research study or designing an experiment, either a nomothetic (quantitative) or idiographic (qualitative) approach may be appropriate.

2.6 Types of Inquiry

There are two categories of scientific inquiry: retrospective and prospective. Each has its own advantages and disadvantages (Hill, 1971).

Retrospective research examines data or events from an historical viewpoint. For example, the investigator may be interested in the causes of multiple sclerosis or the evolution of multisensory teaching. In both cases, the investigation includes the analysis of sequential events leading to the current understanding of disease, events, or methodology. In correlational research, the investigator examines the relationship between two variables or two groups. For example, one might examine the relationship between perceptual abilities and intelligence. In retrospective designs, the investigator does not establish a cause-effect relationship.

Prospective research, on the other hand, predicts the effect of the independent variable on the dependent variable, thereby establishing a cause-effect relationship. In experimental prospective designs, the research manipulates the independent variable and observes its effect on the dependent variable. For example, in a study examining the effects of aquatic therapy on the reduction of symptoms in individuals with multiple sclerosis, the researcher provides aquatic therapy to an experimental group and compares it to a control group in which no aquatic therapy is provided.

The prospective design is also used in longitudinal research where a researcher examines the effects of a variable over time. For example, studies of the effects of prenatal exposure to cocaine on academic success are underway (Delaney-Black et al., 1998; Richardson, 1998).

"The advantages and disadvantages of the two approaches are these" (Hill, 1971, p. 48):

▶ In a prospective method, the sample is more easily defined and may be more representative of a target population than in the retrospective design.
▶ Extraneous variables are more easily controlled in an experimental prospective design.
▶ In a longitudinal prospective design, such as in the Framingham Study, individuals can be followed up over a long period of time to determine the impact of risk factors.
▶ In a retrospective design, the subjects can be identified as a convenient sample and events or variables contributing to the condition can be studied in depth.
▶ One disadvantage of a retrospective design is that cause-effect cannot be determined by the results of the research; rather, a statistical or correlational relationship can be established and used as the basis for a prospective experimental design.

2.7 Models of Research

Research is defined as objective systematic investigation. The process of designing a research study is one of the most creative acts in science. In this process, the researcher can generate new knowledge, synthesize findings from different studies, and develop new theories by being innovative. The research design is an outline of the systematic plan for collecting data. From this outline, the investigator develops a plan of action. Table 2–2 describes the steps involved in designing a research study, and Figure 2–5 gives an example.

The diversity of research designs in occupational therapy and special education is characterized by problem-based research. These studies might include the following: (a) evaluating the efficacy of a treatment method in occupational therapy, (b) surveying the attitudes of a population of individuals with spinal cord injury, (c) carrying out an organizational case study of a sheltered workshop for adults, (d) constructing a rating scale to evaluate student teachers or interns, or (e) correlating a relationship between perceptual skills and academic ability. In each of these research examples, a method of data collection serves as the "skeleton" for the study. The research approach chosen is a decision based on the purposes of the study and the data collection methods available to the investigator. Approaches to research may include qualitative or quantitative analysis, action research, or a combination of any of these. Table 2–3 describes these approaches.

Research models appropriate to problems in occupational therapy, rehabilitation, and habilitation are summarized in Table 2–4 and described in Chapters 3 and 4. These models were identified by analyzing the methods used in the important landmark studies in the biological and social sciences and in the Allied Health and Rehabilitation literature.

Research is not limited to one methodology. Investigators who carry out an unbiased research plan and collect objective data are engaging in research whether they wear a white coat in a laboratory or do historical research in a library. In practice, some investigators combine both qualitative and quantitative research models. For example, the same study may involve constructing an instrument for measuring clinical effectiveness and then carrying out an experimental design. Another frequently used research methodology is to survey two populations (survey research models) and then compare differences between the two samples (correlational research model).

The diversity of research models available for the multiple problems of a disability is illustrated by the varied approaches in investigating the aging process. For example,

Table 2–2. Steps in Formulating a Feasible Question in Qualitative, Quantitative, and Action Research

Step	Tasks	Rationale	Example
1	List numerous questions about topics in which the clinician, teacher, or student is interested.	Allows the investigator to select areas of interest and locate relevant studies.	What are the most effective treatment methods for treating spasticity?
2	Locate a secondary source, such as a text or review article.	Enables the researcher to have an overview of the topic and provides a means for locating research articles.	A recent (within the last 5 years) textbook or review article on cerebral palsy.
3	Do a mini-literature review using primary sources (e.g., research articles).	Investigator becomes familiar with the current research in the area of interest.	A current (within the last 3 years) research article on treatment of spasticity.
4	Identify an expert in the field.	This expert can serve as an informal consultant for locating resources, identifying additional aspects, and narrowing the research.	A clinician or special educator who has worked with children with cerebral palsy.
5	Narrow the research topic.	When a research topic is too broad, the researcher has difficulty operationally defining the variables or generalizing the results.	Is neurodevelopmental treatment (NDT) more effective than sensory integration (SI) therapy in reducing spasticity in children with cerebral palsy?
6	Determine the feasibility of the research question.	The ability to do the research is dependent on several factors, such as the availability of participants, time elements, costs of the study, or the ability to control extraneous variables.	NDT and SI are used with children with cerebral palsy in a children's care facility.

amyloid has been identified hypothetically as a protein that, when accumulating in the body, may be a factor in accelerating the general process of aging. The relationship between amyloid and aging can be analyzed from many perspectives by using more than one research model. For instance, an experimental design using animal research is one possibility (Flood & Morley, 1998). Here the investigator can form two animal groups, one receiving amyloid injections and the other as a control. The results of this hypothetical design could yield empirical data regarding the direct relationship between amyloid and aging in mammals.

Another design applying a correlational model could be created by testing retrospectively the relationship between explicit memory with Alzheimer's disease as compared to control subjects without impairment (Fleischman & Gabriele, 1998). A methodologist may be interested in devising an instrument for detecting the presence of amyloid in the bloodstream (Ronald and Nancy Reagan Research Institute of the Alzheimer's Association and the National Institute on Aging Working Group, 1998). A retrospective clinical case study of Alzheimer's and the examination of neurological changes is another research possibility (Fukutani et al., 1997). An examination of

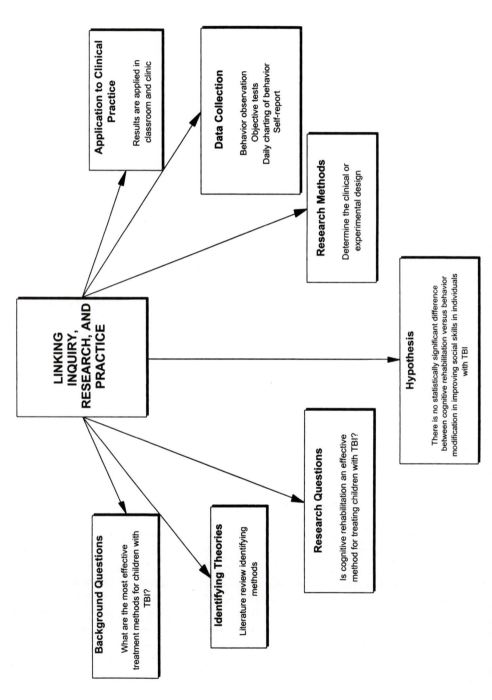

Figure 2–5. Relationship between scientific inquiry, theory, research, and clinical practice. This relationship is pictured using an example of research in traumatic brain injury (TBI).

Table 2–3. Comparison of Quantitative and Qualitative Research Methods

	Quantitative	*Qualitative*
Definition	Empirical method that is based on hypothesis testing and control and measurement of variables within a value-free framework	Study of people and events in a natural setting to make sense of and obtain meaning from the phenomena observed and experienced, emphasizing a value-laden nature of inquiry (Denzin & Lincoln, 1994a)
Underlying assumptions	Reality is based on natural laws that predict outcome (nomothetic). Variables are operationalized and the relationships between the variables can be measured. The hypothesis is stated before data collection occurs. In experimental design, the investigator manipulates the independent variable(s), and measures the dependent variable(s). Standardized tests or procedures are used to collect data. The researcher assumes an objective, unbiased attitude toward participants. Representative samples of a target population are obtained through random sampling.	Reality is based on the subjective interpretation of the study (idiographic approach). Variables are difficult to measure because of the complexity and interconnectedness. Analysis of data collection is heuristic and ends with grounded theory. Variables emerge as the researcher collects and analyzes subjective data. Researcher as an interviewer serves as the instrument for collecting data. The researcher interacts on a personal, subjective level with the participants. A "snowballing effect" is used to obtain a convenience sample of the target population.
Models for conducting research	Experimental Correlational Methodological Evaluation Heuristic Case study (prospective) Survey (assessment)	Case study (retrospective or prospective) Phenomenology Biographical or historiography Ethnography Grounded theory or heuristic Survey (interview)
Techniques of data collection	Structured forced-choice questionnaire and surveys Standardized tests or procedures (performance or paper and pencil) Frequency count or interval recording Rate of response Triangulation	Structured and unstructured interviews Case studies Observation Diaries, journals, and personal experiences Introspection Interactional and visual texts Archival records Field notes Triangulation
Analysis of data	Application of descriptive and inferential statistics to test hypothesis or guiding question	Content analysis to develop naturalistic generalizations (e.g., themes, meanings, theories

Note: Adapted from "Introduction: Entering the Field of Qualitative Research," by N. K. Denzin and Y. S. Lincoln, 1994. In N. K. Denzin & Y. S. Lincoln (Eds.), *Handbook of Qualitative Research* (pp. 1–17). Thousand Oaks, CA: Sage. Copyright 1994 by Sage. *Becoming Qualitative Researchers: An Introduction,* by C. Glesne and A. Peshkin, 1992, New York: Longman. Copyright 1992 by Longman. *Nursing and Health Care Research; A Skills-Based Introduction* (2nd ed.), by C. Clifford, 1990, London: Prentice-Hall. Copyright 1990 by Prentice-Hall. *Qualitative Inquiry and Research Design: Choosing Among Five Traditions,* by J. W. Creswell, 1998, Thousand Oaks, CA: Sage. Copyright 1998 by Sage.

Table 2–4. Research Models

Research Models	Tasks of Researcher	Significance
Quantitative Models		
Experimental (group or case study)	Direct manipulation of independent variables and examination of effects in highly controlled settings	Determine empirically the effectiveness of treatment or classroom procedures
Methodological	Construction of a measuring instrument, curriculum, or therapeutic procedures/approaches	Innovative methods or procedures, including technology
Correlational (retrospective design)	Test of the relationships between nonmanipulated variables	Identifying factors that are presumed to have an associational relationship
Qualitative Models		
Observation (Child development, ethnography, descriptive case study)	In-depth study of individuals, groups, or systems	Identify underlying dynamics in individuals or groups or organizational models of practice to affect change
Historical	Investigation of past events through primary sources (e.g., interviews, documents)	Reconstruction of past events to understand contemporary problems
Either Quantitative or Qualitative		
Evaluation	Critical analysis of health care delivery systems and educational programs	Objective and/or qualitative assessment of the effectiveness of systems and treatment programs
Heuristic and operations	Discovery of possible causative factors in chronic disabilities, analysis of time, space, and cost factors	Generate further research by identifying significant variables
Longitudinal (prospective studies)	Follow-up studies to determine the effectiveness of a treatment technique or the effects of variable on maturation	Determine long-term effects of variables (e.g., genetic, environment, and intervention)
Survey	Study of the characteristics of homogeneous populations	Description of general factors that characterize a group

the relationship between diet and the precursors to amyloid would add another dimension to data collection (Howland et al., 1998).

The research models employed by investigators imply certain hypotheses in generating data collection procedures. Research investigations into specific problems can take place from many perspectives. A knowledge of specific research models en-

ables the investigator to attack problems from more than one dimension. Table 2–5 demonstrates how several research models can be applied to a multifaceted investigation of the aging process.

2.7.1 Action Research

Another application to the scientific method is action research. Action research developed

Table 2–5. Relationship Between Research Models: Aging Example

Experimental or Prospective:	Use of laboratory animals (induce aging or retard aging) and study of physiological variables
Methodological:	Construct tests and instruments to measure neuropsychological aspects of aging
Evaluation:	Evaluate the effectiveness of an independent living facility for individuals who are elderly to increase quality of life
Heuristic:	Discover the underlying factors related to premature aging, such as in progeria
Correlational or retrospective:	Compare individuals who have retired and who are active in the community with comparable individuals who are inactive
Qualitative case study:	Use a case study analysis of an individual who is older expressing feelings of hopelessness
Survey:	Identify the life styles of a homogeneous group of individuals who are elderly living in their own homes
Historical:	Document through a study of federal legislation a society's changing attitudes toward individuals who have Alzheimer's disease

out of Dewey's (1933) concept of learning by doing through creative problem solving. Lewin's (1939) field theory in which he examined the forces in the environment that impacted on the individual is the theoretical foundation for action research. Action research is defined as a problem-oriented investigation that is applied in site-specific environments such as an industry, school, classroom, hospital, clinic, or home setting. In action research, the teacher or clinician, as the researcher, applies quantitative and qualitative research methods to specific problems originating out of a curriculum, treatment program, or ergonomic situation.

Where can action research be applied? Action research can be applied in the following ways:

▶ Within the school setting, when there is concern about overall achievement, teachers or occupational therapists may use action research to develop ways of changing or modifying the curriculum to allow all students to benefit from instruction.

▶ When occupational therapists and special education teachers work collabora-

tively to develop methods for students with developmental disabilities to become more functionally independent in self-care tasks, they may use action research. For example, they examine the effectiveness of teaching work adjustment skills to a student who has a goal of local employment. The success of the student may possibly enable this method to be applied to another student in the same school or may lead to a revision of the method.

▶ An occupational therapist fabricates a splint in a hand therapy clinic for patients who have had carpel tunnel release surgery. Using action research, the occupational therapist seeks to devise a splint that keeps the wrist in a neutral position and facilities the healing process.

▶ In a psychosocial setting, the occupational therapist designs strategies to help patients with a diagnosis of depression to be self-motivated and to self-regulate their symptoms. Action research is used to enable the therapist to select the most effective strategies.

▶ Within the home, an occupational therapist uses action research to modify the home environment so that an individual with a stroke is able to be independent. The occupational therapist considers accessibility, kitchen adaptations, placement for furniture and electronic equipment to enable an individual to be functional.

Characteristics of action research

▶ Action research occurs in a local, naturalistic setting, sometimes referred to as site-based.
▶ Research may be applied to a setting (e.g., school, organization, hospital, or home), to a classroom or clinic, or to a single individual (e.g., single-subject design).
▶ The results of the research are usually not generalized outside of the specific setting.
▶ Quantitative and qualitative research methods can be applied to the investigation. For example, use of standardized tests, observational methods, and statistical analysis may be used to examine the effectiveness of the program.
▶ Occupational therapists and teachers act as the participant-observer by planning the research, collecting data, and analyzing and interpreting the results. The research is designed and conducted in the teachers' or therapists' own setting as a means of improving one's teaching, therapy, or ergonomic adaptations.
▶ Problem-solving methods are used to generate possible solutions. For example, a therapist working in a long-term care facility may be looking for ways to increase the morale among staff, or a teacher may be looking for better ways to teach students with ADHD.

Possible outcomes of action research for occupational therapists

▶ Students in special education who are receiving services either in a pull-out program (i.e., where students leave the general education classroom to go into a special classroom) or in the general education program will benefit as changes are made in their individualized program because of the outcome of the action research.
▶ Occupational therapists and special educators work together to modify the program for a student who is having difficulty with handwriting. The special educator and the therapist will look at building up the size of the pencil to make it easier to grasp, use of a neutral position and pincer grip for handwriting, perceptual motor activities to increase performance, methods for improving posture, or changes of furniture to improve ergonomic adaptations.
▶ Students with developmental disabilities will be taught how to be more independent in activities of daily living (ADLs) within the community.
▶ Within occupational therapy, results of action research will enable individuals with spinal cord injuries to become employable in a local community.
▶ The occupational therapist will devise methods to decrease carpel tunnel syndrome in individuals working in a meat-packing plant.
▶ Occupational therapists working with an individual with depression will develop strategies for sleep hygiene to enable him or her to sleep better.

2.7.2 Scholarly Models not Based on the Scientific Method

These research models are not the only methods of organizing knowledge. A theoretical paper in which a scientist integrates and synthesizes knowledge by creating a conceptual model and a position paper in which a health practitioner advocates a governmental policy such as National Health Insurance are both examples of nonresearch that are scholarly and original. The important difference between research and a scholarly essay or exposition is that in research the investigator formulates a problem first and then objectively collects data related to the problem. In a nonresearch scholarly article, the investigator presents a position or theory and then cites evidence in its support. Another scholarly model is a case study in which a clinician describes a disease process or a treatment technique with a specific individual. Because this model is case-specific, the author does not usually attempt to control variables or generalize the information to another situation. A review paper can also be a model of scholarly work. In this paper, the author integrates studies to generate a body of knowledge. A summary of scholarly nonresearch articles are described in Table 2–6.

For the last 100 years, the scientific method has generated many research mod-els. Although for many years research generally was limited to those who did not teach or conduct therapy, there is a need for clinicians and teachers to apply evidence-based practice in their everyday work. Qualitative and quantitative methods can be applied within one's own setting through action research, while scholarly papers can be written through a review of articles in the literature. It is incumbent on those of us in the clinical and teaching fields to use an evidence-based practice model to establish the efficacy of our practices.

Table 2–6. Scholarly Nonresearch Articles in Health Care and Special Education

Scholarly Article	Tasks of Writer	Significance
Position paper	Advocate reforms of health care or educational systems, legislation, ethics of research, standards of practice	Presentation of policy statements and editorials
Theoretical exposition	Explain relationships between variables and predict outcomes	Logical explanation in natural or social science using deductive reasoning
Case study presentation*	Present chronological history of an individual, such as one's course of illness, or treatment effectiveness	Sequential description of disease process or treatment in an individual
Review Paper	Integrate and synthesize published research	Exploration of current state of knowledge in specified field

*A case study can be used as a research model in both qualitative and quantitative research.

CHAPTER

Quantitative Research Models

> *The clinical trial is a carefully, and ethically, designed experiment with the aim of answering some precisely framed question. In its most rigorous form it demands equivalent groups of patients concurrently treated in different ways.*
> —Sir A. B. Hill, 1971, *Principles of Medical Statistics*, p. 273

Operational Learning Objectives

By the end of this chapter, the learner will
1. Define quantitative research
2. Define key terms in quantitative research methods
3. Critically analyze examples of research from the occupational therapy and special education literature
4. Identify types of quantitative research

Quantitative research is an empirical method that is based on hypothesis testing and control and measurement of variables within a value-free framework. Empiricism is defined as gaining data through the senses that are observable, objective, and verifiable. An example of empirical data is measuring hand strength with a dynometer. Another example is measuring the rate of words per minute that a student reads. Empirical data must be operationally defined so that it can be reproduced by another investigator. In quantitative research, the investigator begins with a hypothesis that predicts the results of the investigation. Some key terms used in quantitative research are described in Table 3–1.

3.1 Factors in Quantitative Research Models

The following factors are the sine qua non of quantitative research models.

▶ *A justification and rationale for the research:* This includes a justification for the research based on the significance of the research. For example, a researcher justifies the need for research in spinal cord injury by describing the number of individuals who incur such an injury and by the cost of the injury. In special education, a teacher may justify the examination of different ways to work with students with autism based on the increasing incidence of this population.

Table 3–1. Key Definitions in Quantitative Research

Control group	a group selected to compare with the experimental group. This group may be a nonintervention group with no treatment, or it may receive a different treatment method. For example, the researcher may wish to determine the effects of splinting on reducing carpal tunnel syndrome and may introduce exercise in the control group.
Dependent variable	in clinical research, the treatment effect or outcome resulting from the intervention of the independent variable. For example, the dependent variable in a study of sensory integration therapy could be a reduction of tactile defensiveness in children.
Empirical data	data based on controlled observation that is observable, measured, verified, and replicated.
Evidence-based practice	use of contemporary research findings as the basis for clinical reasoning in selecting the most effective treatment method.
Experimental group	a group that is manipulated by the researcher. For example, the experimental group could receive heart-rate biofeedback or relaxation therapy or handwriting instruction. The treatment represents the independent variable in experimental research.
External validity	the degree to which results can be generalized to a target population. External validity depends on the representativeness of a sample and the rigor of the experiment. Replication of a study producing consistent results increases the external validity.
Extraneous variable	a variable not manipulated by the researcher but that can potentially affect the results of a study. Extraneous variables can include such factors as gender, intelligence, severity of disability, or socioeconomic status. These variables, if they are uncontrolled, can threaten the internal validity of a study.
Hypothesis	a statement that predicts results and is testable by a systematic methodology. An hypothesis can be either null or directional. An example of a stated hypothesis is: "There is a statistically significant difference in reducing spasticity in children with cerebral palsy when using neurodevelopmental treatment as compared to splinting." or "There is a statistically significant difference in reading achievement when using a phonetic method when compared to whole language."
Independent variable	a variable manipulated by the researcher. In clinical research it represents the treatment method, such as aquatic therapy, progressive relaxation, or phonemic awareness.

► *An extensive review of literature:* The researcher identifies and analyzes previous research related to the topic of study. For example, a researcher examining animal-assisted therapy would search the databases for previous studies.

► *Operational definitions of research variables:* The researcher must operationally define each of the variables being examined. These variables include the treatment intervention, the outcome measures, the participants, and the setting where the experiment takes place.

► *Identification of extraneous variables that could confound the results:* The investigator tries to control the static variables, such as gender, age, socioeconomic status, ethnicity, and handedness.

► *Statement of hypothesis or guiding question:* Prior to collecting data, the researcher predicts or hypothesizes the results of the study.

► *An objective, unbiased method for collecting data:* A research design that can be reproduced is developed by the investigator.

► *Separate sections for results and discussion:* After the data are collected, the investigator designs tables, figures, and graphs to depict the results in an objective manner. A discussion of the results is more subjective and allows the investigator to speculate on the implications of the study.

► *Limitations of the study and recommendations for further research:* The researcher

Table 3–1. *(continued)*

Internal validity	the degree of rigor in an experiment in controlling for extraneous variables and error variance. Potential threats to internal validity have been identified as extraneous historical factors, maturation, instrumentation, and lack of random sampling. Internal validity is an indication of the trustworthiness of the results. Well-designed studies with good control of variables that can potentially distort the results have high internal validity. The quality of a research study is increased by eliminating the threats to internal validity.
Null hypothesis	a statement by the researcher that predicts no statistically significant difference or relationship between variables. For example, a clinical researcher states, "There is no statistically significant difference between a prescriptive aerobic exercise and Prozac® in reducing clinical depression."
Operational definition of a variable	specific measure, observation, or criteria that defines a variable. For example, activities of daily living (ADL) skills may be defined as the score obtained on the Barthel Index. An operational definition is important in replicating a study or in evaluating a group of studies using a method such as through a meta-analysis.
Pre-post group design with control group	classical experimental design where the investigator compares the results obtained by both groups.
Random sampling	an unbiased portion of a target population selected by chance, such as through random numbers.
Reliability	a measure of the consistency of a test instrument. For example, on a test with high reliability, one would expect approximately the same results on two different administrations when there is no change in subject.
Replicability	the ability to repeat an experiement or scientific procedure. The purpose is to strengthen generalizability of the findings and to ensure external validity.
Treatment protocol	the operational definition of the independent variable or treatment method. The treatment protocol should have enough detail so that it can be replicated. One purpose of designing a treatment protocol is to evaluate its effectiveness.
Validity	as pertaining to measurement, the degree to which a test or measuring instrument actually measures what it purports to measure.

acknowledges limitations in the methodology or uncontrolled variables that could affect the results and makes recommendations that could improve future studies. For example, one limitation might be the limited number of subjects or an unreliable outcome measure.

3.2 Experimental Research

3.2.1 Purposes of Experimental Research

The researcher uses experimental methods to collect empirical data by manipulating independent variables and observing their effects, seeking maximum control of the data collection procedure and environmental conditions. An experimenter achieves *internal validity* when he or she is able to control extraneous variables that could affect the results (see Table 3–2). The degree of experimental rigor depends on these controls. Figure 3–1 shows the relationship between experimental research and clinical practice. Working together, their purposes are to

▶ compare the effectiveness of clinical treatment methods
▶ observe cause-effect relationships established in a laboratory

Table 3–2. Control of Extraneous Variables

Possible Confounding Extraneous Variables	Methods to Control Extraneous Variables
Demograpic variables (e.g., age, SES, gender, ethnicity, first language, handedness)	Establish screening criteria that includes range of ages, gender, ethnic groups, home language, or hand dominance
Cognitive variables (e.g., intelligence, academic achievement, processing abilities)	Administer a screening test to ensure equivalent groups
Test anxiety	Establish rapport, answer questions, and set the participant at ease prior to any data collection
Low motivation	Screen out individuals who show reluctance to participate in the study
Hawthorne effect	Establish a control group and ensure that each group within the study has equal attention
Test conditions	Ensure that environmental conditions (e.g., lighting, noise, temperature, presence of other people, distractions) do not interfer with data collection
Reliability and validity of the procedure	Use a double-blind control in which the data collector is not aware of the participant's group
Experimental bias	Ensure that all individuals collecting data have been trained and that interrater reliability is high
Data collection methods	Do a pilot study to examine the reliability and validity of the procedure, or use tests and procedures that have established high validity and reliability

▶ examine biopsychosocial factors underlying human responses

3.2.2 Comparison of Treatment Methods

Is treatment method "A" more effective than treatment method "B"? This question is a clinical problem affecting every individual treated by an occupational therapist in a hospital, home, or school setting. Nonetheless, the impact of clinical research remains limited. Many occupational therapists continue to cling to traditional methods of treatment without searching the literature to determine whether their effectiveness has been established experimentally. The classical research design employed in testing the relative effectiveness of clinical treatment methods is the paradigm:

PRETEST OF PATIENT	EXPERIMENTAL INTERVENTIONS	POSTTEST OF PATIENT
baseline function before treatment	→ treatment method versus control group	→ outcome dependent on treatment method

In this example, the experimental intervention represents the independent or manipulated variable, whereas the degree of improvement represents the dependent variable. A cause-effect relationship is observed directly by the experimenter.

Traditionally, the control group has been a nonintervention group or a comparative treatment group. In a nonintervention group, there is a possibility of a Hawthorne effect in which each group does not get

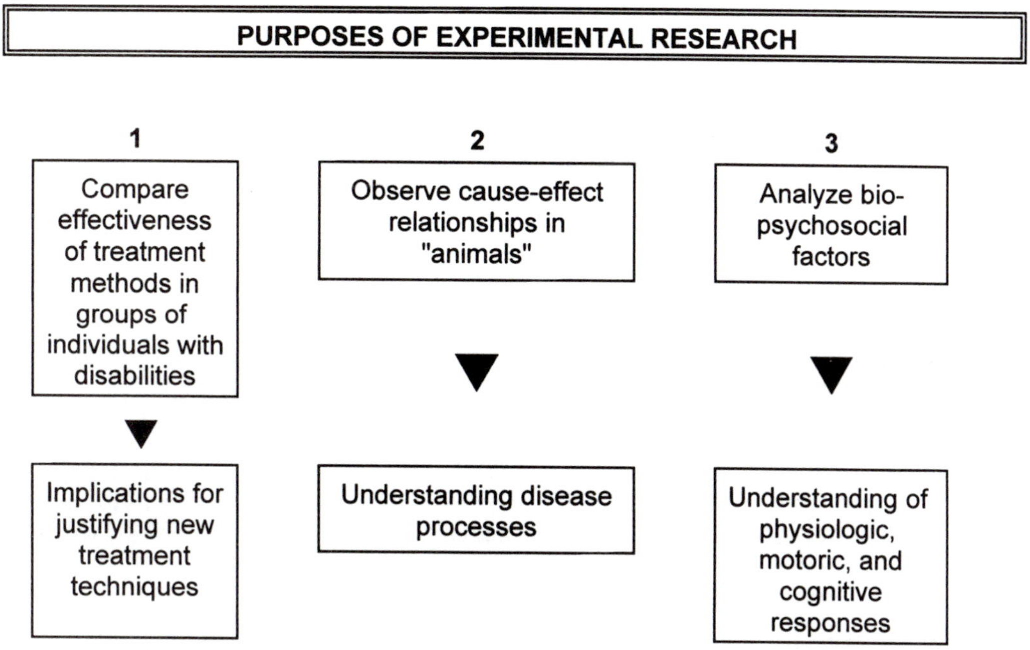

PURPOSES OF EXPERIMENTAL RESEARCH

1

Compare effectiveness of treatment methods in groups of individuals with disabilities

▼

Implications for justifying new treatment techniques

2

Observe cause-effect relationships in "animals"

▼

Understanding disease processes

3

Analyze bio-psychosocial factors

▼

Understanding of physiologic, motoric, and cognitive responses

Figure 3–1. Purposes of experimental research. Note that there are three purposes for research, all of which lead to implications for treatment or intervention.

equal attention, and the results may be attributable to the attention of the experimental group rather than to the treatment effect. Campbell and Stanley (1963), in their classical work on experimental design, used the term "quasi-experimental" to indicate experimental designs in which there is no comparative control group. For example, in a pilot study, a researcher may want to examine the effects of a stress management program on the reduction of depression by using an experimental group without a control group (Stein & Smith, 1989). This would be considered a quasi-experimental design.

An example of a clinical research design using a control group is a study by Callinan and Mathiowetz (1996). In this study, the researchers compared soft and hard resting hand splints on pain and hand function for 39 persons with rheumatoid arthritis. "A repeated measures research design was used to compare the two experimental conditions, wearing a soft splint versus a hard splint on the dominant hand

for 28 days at night only, and an unsplinted control period of 28 days" (p. 347).

Table 3–3 compares the features of two studies: Stein and Smith (1989) and Callinan and Mathiowetz (1996). Although the basic design is similar, the former study has no control group and uses a smaller sample.

3.2.3 Clinical Research

The clinician's major concern is the effectiveness of a specific treatment method for a specific client. The clinician evaluates the client, establishes treatment goals using RUMBA (i.e., relevant, understandable, measurable, behavioral, and achievable), applies appropriate treatment methods, re-evaluates the client's improvement made prior to discharge, and concludes that if the client improved, then the treatment intervention was effective. If the treatment method is effective, can the clinician assume that it could be applied to similar clients (*external validity*)? Before one can generalize

Table 3–3. Comparison of Quasiexperimental and Experimental Designs

	Quasiexperimental	*Experimental With Control*
Citation	Stein, F., & Smith, J. (1989). Short-term stress management programme with acutely depressed in-patients. *Canadian Journal of Occupational Therapy, 56,* 185–192.	Callinan, N. J., & Mathiowetz, V. (1996). Soft versus hard resting hand splints in rheumatoid arthritis: Pain relief, preference, and compliance. *American Journal of Occupational Therapy, 50,* 347–353.
Subjects	7 hospitalized patients with acute depression	39 clients with rheumatoid arthritis
Experimental group	7 hospitalized patients with acute depression	39 clients with rheumatoid arthritis using the soft and hard splints
Control group	None	Patients served as their own control when no splint was used
Design	Pre- and postdesign with no control group	Repeated measures design
Treatment program	Six sessions using various relaxation therapy techniques, including Benson relaxation response, progressive relaxation, visual imagery, back massage, biofeedback, behavioral rehearsal, deep breathing, and paradoxical intention	"Experimental treatment periods (28 nights each) included treatment with the soft splint, treatment with the hard splint, and unsplinted (control). The order of assignment to treatment periods was randomized" (p. 349).
Assessment of outcome	Stress Management Questionnaire, State-Trait Anxiety Invention, and self-evaluation	Arthritis Impact Measurement Scales, self-evaluation of pain localization, grip strength, diary, and a splint rating form
Results and conclusions	"Results showed that there was a significant reduction in anxiety…and patients indicated that the sessions had a positive effect in increasing their ability to relax and in learning to recognize individual stress reactions" (p. 185).	"The findings indicate that resting hand splints are effective for pain relief and that persons with rheumatoid arthritis are more likely to prefer and comply with soft splint use for this purpose" (p. 347).

the results, further data must be obtained to validate the results. Using evidence-based treatment is one way the clinician may validate treatment (Brown & Rodger, 1999). He or she may also postulate that the selected treatment method is better than other comparable methods. Again, this must be confirmed by comparing the effectiveness of various treatment methods. Another assumption is that the evaluation of treatment outcome is objective. The technique of measuring the effectiveness of a treatment method can make the difference between labeling it successful or ineffective. The test for an adequate outcome measure or evaluation of treatment effect-

iveness is its reproducibility by other clinicians. General application to other clients, relative effectiveness compared with other methods of treatment, and objective measurement of improvement are factors that clinicians must examine if their results are to be considered valid and generalizable.

Experimental research enables clinicians to compare the relative effectiveness of treatment methods. In clinical research, the occupational therapist carefully documents the effects of treatment over time. The therapist can carry out the research in a group experiment or single-subject design. (See Boxes 3–1 and 3–2, at the end of this section, for examples of research studies using experimental design with single subject or groups.) In a group experiment, the researcher compares treatment methods with groups of clients. Treatment groups are set up ahead of time, and clients are randomly assigned to each group. Analysis of results is by group statistics. In a single-subject design, the therapist may alternate different treatment methods with the same client (alternating treatments) who may act as his or her own control.

For example, in a group design, clients with arthritis are referred to occupational therapy for treatment. The clinician can employ physical agent modalities, exercise, purposeful activity, and hydrotherapy methods randomly. Functional skills, range of motion, and self-evaluation in the shoulder joint can be used as measures of improvement. Each treatment group is charted, and statistical analysis can be used to compare the relative effectiveness of each treat-

ment method. On the other hand, with a single-subject design, the effect of using an upper extremity inhibitive casting to reduce spasticity is used for a single child with cerebral palsy (Tona & Schneck, 1993). In this case, the investigators measured pre-post performance using the Modified Ashworth Scale, a clinical measure of spasticity. Results could not be generalized without further replication. Figure 3–2 illustrates how a clinical researcher could chart progress by using a graph.

Other variables that can potentially affect the results should be recorded for each client. In this way, systematic patterns can be noted. A data collection sheet containing information can be statistically analyzed later to compare the relative effectiveness of treatment methods and the systematic influence of extraneous variables. An example of a data collection sheet is illustrated in Figure 3–3.

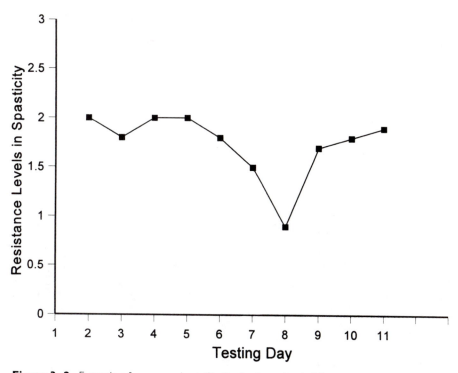

Figure 3–2. Example of progress chart. On the horizontal axis (X) are the testing days and on the vertical axis (Y) is the passive resistance to spasticity for each day. Adapted from Tona & Schneck, 1993.

DATA COLLECTION SHEET

Background Data

1 Patient code number (based on treatment group)

2 Gender   3 Date of Birth   4 Handedness

5 Diagnosis

6 Date of onset of illness

7 Occupation

8 Years of formal education

9 Marital status

10 Date of data collection

Test Data.

11   Pretest scores on dependent variable

12   Posttest scores   c 3 weeks _____
          a 1 week _____   d 4 weeks _____
          b 2 weeks _____   e 3 months _____

13 Treatment method

14 Other test data, including psychological tests, physiological measures and self-report

Figure 3–3. Example of a data collection sheet. The information contained on the sheet will change according to the needs of the researcher.

3.2.4 Designing Experimental Groups

The advantage of using clinical research is that the experimenter does not need large numbers of subjects to initiate research. The major disadvantage is the experimenter's lack of control in matching the groups on specific variables. For example, there will always be demographic and biopsychosocial differences between two treatment groups. Experimental research with matched groups increases the internal validity or rigor of the experiment.

In clinical research with groups, the investigator compares the effects of two or more independent variables in a patient population. If the clinical researcher wants to compare treatment method X_1 with treatment method X_2, he or she must create relatively equal groups and employ reliable and valid measures to test outcome. The design is illustrated below:

DEPENDENT VARIABLE MEASURE	GROUPS	DEPENDENT VARIABLE MEASURE
Pretest (Base State)	Treatment (Intervention)	Posttest (Outcome)
Y_1 before	—— X_1 ——	Y_1 after
Y_2 before	—— X_2 ——	Y_2 after

Experimental research with two or more groups can potentially eliminate the Hawthorne effect. Each group is given equal time and attention to control the effect. The procedure for guarding against the Hawthorne effect is described in Figure 3–4.

The foregoing sequential analysis illustrates the many controls necessary in isolating the experimental or treatment effect and in controlling for extraneous variables. In designing experimental research with a control group, it is important for the researcher to match the groups on variables that could potentially affect the results of the study, such as age, gender, socioeco-

nomic status, intelligence, and education. For instance, how can an investigator design an experiment applying biofeedback techniques in reducing hypertension in patients with postcardiac disease? The first step in this hypothetical design is to select a population of clients with cardiovasular disease by establishing a screening criteria for inclusion based on age, gender, diagnosis, length of hospitalization, and vital capacities. The number of subjects to be included in the study is determined by statistical and practical considerations. (See Chapter 7 for a discussion of these considerations.) Participants are then randomly assigned to an experimental group (e.g., biofeedback) and a control group (e.g., medication). The investigator should review the participants' backgrounds to determine if the groups are evenly matched on the relevant variables that are being considered. After two matched groups have been established, diastolic and systolic blood pressure is taken in various conditions (e.g., at rest and at several stages of exertion) to establish a baseline. Then the investigator checks to determine if both groups have approximately equal mean blood pressure scores. If not, the groups are re-formed until the researcher is satisfied that the two groups are comparable.

The two groups then undergo the experiment within a specified time period (e.g., two 2-hour sessions per week over a 3-month period). To avoid researcher bias, the test administrator would not know whether a subject was in the biofeedback group or medication group. Research assistants, who would not be told the purpose of the study, would be responsible for implementing the design. This method, called *double-blind control*, eliminates experimenter bias. Subject motivation, fatigue, anxiety, and distractibility or lack of cooperation are major factors that increase the error variance in experimental research and should be carefully monitored because these variables could affect the results. After the 3-month period, a posttest of blood pressures would be obtained from both groups.

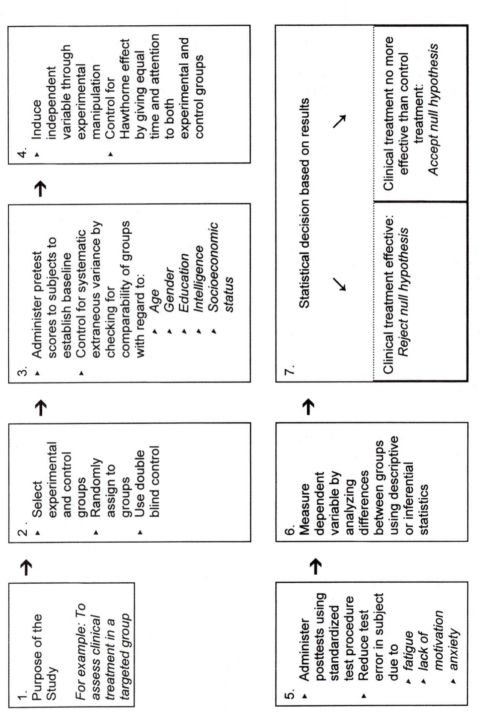

1.
- Purpose of the Study

  For example: To assess clinical treatment in a targeted group

2.
- Select experimental and control groups
- Randomly assign to groups
- Use double blind control

3.
- Administer pretest scores to subjects to establish baseline
- Control for systematic extraneous variance by checking for comparability of groups with regard to:
  - *Age*
  - *Gender*
  - *Education*
  - *Intelligence*
  - *Socioeconomic status*

4.
- Induce independent variable through experimental manipulation
- Control for Hawthorne effect by giving equal time and attention to both experimental and control groups

5.
- Administer posttests using standardized test procedure
- Reduce test error in subject due to
  - *fatigue*
  - *lack of motivation*
  - *anxiety*

6.
- Measure dependent variable by analyzing differences between groups using descriptive or inferential statistics

7.
Statistical decision based on results

| Clinical treatment effective: *Reject null hypothesis* | Clinical treatment no more effective than control treatment: *Accept null hypothesis* |

Figure 3–4. Sequential analysis of control factors in experimental research. Controlling for each of these factors helps prevent possible error due to the Hawthorne effect.

It would be expected that a training or Hawthorne effect would lower blood pressure in both groups; however, a null hypothesis would be proposed stating that there would be no statistically significant difference between the experimental and control groups. Statistical analysis would be performed to determine whether there is, in fact, a significant difference. A conclusion based on statistical analysis of the data could then be proposed by the researcher. Additionally, the researcher would examine the literature for similar studies to determine if the current results corroborate or contradict these findings. There are many variations of experimental research. One example of a factorial design is the interactional effect between medication and relaxation therapy in children with attention-deficit hyperactivity disorder (ADHD).

Before undertaking experimental research with human subjects, ethical and human rights factors must also be considered. Every subject should be informed of the experimental procedures and potential risks involved. (Further discussion regarding this topic is found in Chapter 7.)

3.2.5 Experimental Research Methods and the Effects of Clinical Treatment

Researchers and clinicians have various definitions of improvement. For researchers, improvement is operationally defined and measurable, and the variables that caused the improvement are clearly identified. Clinicians, who work with clients every day, use individual goals and, many times, subjective criteria for evaluating a patient's progress. In addition, clinicians present individual cases from their clinical practice to support or to negate a method of treatment. Table 3–4 summarizes the differences between researchers and clinicians in evaluating treatment outcome.

The problem of investigating the effectiveness of a treatment method is a complex issue. What criteria are used in evaluating

improvement? How can other variables in a patient's life space, such as family, friends, diet, activities, and work, be separated from the treatment procedure in the evaluation of improvement? How can the therapeutic relationship be separated from the treatment method in determining its effect on treatment outcome? The interactional effects between the therapist and client, treatment method and client, and external environment and client make it difficult for the experimenter to isolate the specific variables causing specific results. These interrelationships are schematically shown in Figure 3–5.

Before it is possible to determine if one treatment method is more effective than another, the clinical researcher must identify and control possible extraneous variables that could influence the results. Four areas of influence, as shown in Figure 3–5, include variables within the client, therapist, and environment, as well as within the treatment method. All of these factors potentially can affect outcome. Knowing this, the researcher must ask: What specific *treatment* method by what specific *therapist* for what specific *patient* in what specific *environment* is effective as measured by what specific *outcome instruments*? The interactional effects of these variables are shown in Figure 3–6.

3.2.6 Control of Factors Affecting Patient Improvement

When controlling for factors that may account for patient improvement, the researcher considers the following questions within each of the variables listed.

Therapist Variables

► Is the therapist's age or gender significant in affecting outcome?
► Is cognitive style (the characteristic way that the individual perceives the world) a factor?
► How does the therapist's personality affect change?

Table 3–4. Researcher-Clinician Comparison for Evaluating Treatment Outcome

Variable	Research Methods (Nomothetic Approach)	Clinician Methods (Idiographic Approach)
Treatment method	Experimental variable that is independent, mutually exclusive, and can be replicated in other studies	Clinical method that is modifiable, dependent on the observed needs of patient and the experiences of clinician
Other factors affecting treatment	Systematic extraneous variables that must be controlled (e.g., by matching, random assignment, or by narrowing the scope of the study)	Individual factors in the patient that account for some patients improving, while other patients remain the same or regress
Assessing improvement	Operational definition of measurement instruments for improvement and control for the Hawthorne effect	Clinical impression of patient's progress based on the clinician's initial evaluation and subsequent observed changes at discharge

▶ Is the therapist's level of education or expertise a factor in improvement?
▶ What part does the experience of the therapist play in client improvement?
▶ Are there cultural or ethnic factors in the therapist that facilitate or retard client progress?
▶ What other qualities of the therapist can potentially affect patient improvement?

Client Variables

▶ Do specific demographic factors (e.g., age, gender, or marital status) affect treatment outcome?
▶ What are the effects of diagnosis and severity of illness on treatment?
▶ How does the client's intelligence, education, occupation, and social class affect the treatment process?
▶ Does the congruence or conflict between the personality of the patient and therapist affect outcome?
▶ Is the patient's environment a factor?

Treatment Method Variables

▶ Does the therapist need special training to apply the treatment method?
▶ Is the treatment method reliable, that is, does it allow the therapist to apply a standard operational procedure or protocol to clients?
▶ Is there an underlying theoretical explanation for treatment effect on patient improvement?

Environmental Variables

▶ Does the setting where treatment takes place affect outcome? (Hospital, clinic, patient's home, classroom, special school, transitional housing, or supported employment are examples.)
▶ How does the timing (the length of individual treatment sessions and frequency of treatments during a week) affect outcome?
▶ Does group versus individual treatment affect outcome?
▶ What are the effects of interactions of cotherapists who are simultaneously treating the same patients?
▶ Do physical variables in the treatment setting (e.g., lighting, background, sound, color, temperature, atmospheric pressure, and visual distractions) affect treatment outcome?

In addition to these four variables (therapist, patient, treatment method, and environment), the researcher must pose the

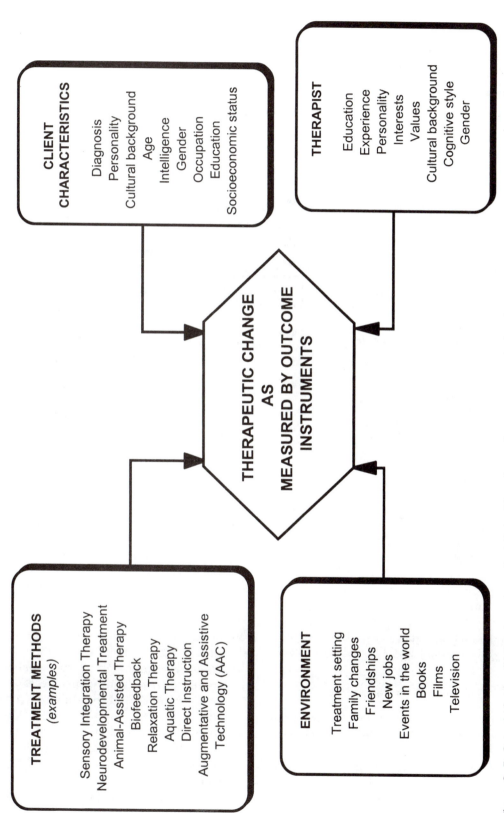

Figure 3–5. Potential factors affecting change in a patient. Each of these factors (i.e. treatment method, patient, treatment setting, and therapist) are multifaceted.

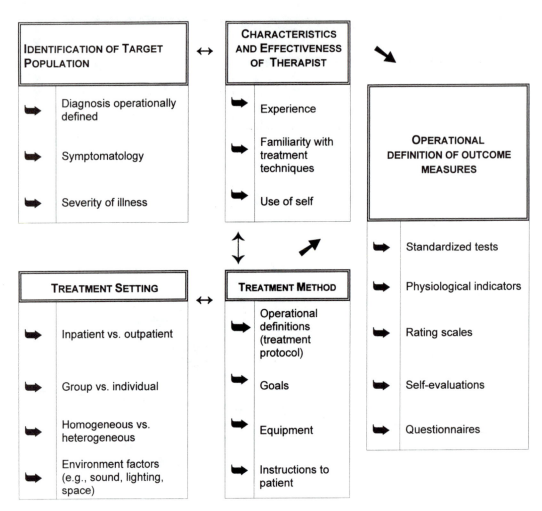

Figure 3–6. Interactional effects of treatment method, therapist, patient, and treatment setting. Although the operational definition remains the same, the results obtained on the outcome measures are dependent on the interactional effects of method, therapist, patient, and setting.

following questions regarding the measurement of outcome.

Measurement of Treatment

What criteria are used for measuring outcome? These criteria include the following:

▶ Change in physical capacity, such as grip stength, spasticity, fine motor dexterity, heart rate, upper extremity strength, gross motor abilities

▶ Increase in psychosocial functioning, such as the ability to work, improved self-esteem, improved interpersonal relationships (e.g., with family, peers, authority figures), and the ability to cope with stress

▶ Cognitive functioning, such as alertness, attention span, memory or information processing, problem solving, organization

▶ Improved behavioral performance with regard to insomnia, eating disorders,

smoking, substance abuse, or sexual dysfunction
▶ Increase in health-related knowledge, such as nutrition, stress management techniques, the use of activity or exercise, family relationships, and use of and compliance with pharmaceutical drugs

Interactional Effects on Treatment Outcome

The researcher must also account for interactional effects among variables. For example, a therapist with a penchant for order may be more effective using a behavioral modification treatment method than a therapist who has a personality characterized by a strong need for nurturing others. A treatment method that is effectively employed with one therapist may not be as effective with another therapist. The therapist's personality, values, and characteristics impact on their ability to work with specific clients and may affect the outcome. Therapists' preferences for working with specific patients are usually indicative of personality variables, although the self-selecting process of the therapists' preference for a

specific treatment method, in a specific treatment setting with a designated diagnostic group, may be limited by the therapist's education and experience. As therapists gain insight into their own skills and perceived effectiveness in working with patients, they develop specified preferences. For the researcher evaluating the effectiveness of a treatment procedure, a sensitivity to and awareness of the interactional effects of variables on treatment outcome is a necessity.

An example of a hypothetical research study examining the interaction between treatment methods in occupational therapy and therapists' characteristics is shown in Figure 3–7. In this example, four methods for treating ADHD in children are compared: behavior therapy, stress management, group psychodynamic, and psychoeducational. The therapists' characteristics in working with clients are typified as:

1. Laissez-faire: The therapist is permissive in approaching client
2. Authoritarian: The therapist is directive in working with the client
3. Democratic: The therapist allows the clients' input into treatment

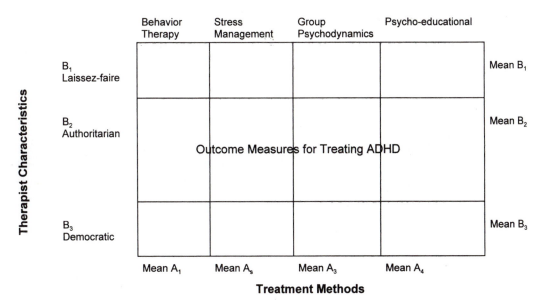

Figure 3–7. Interaction between treatment methods and therapist characteristics in treating clients with ADHD.

The hypothetical results may show that behavior therapy is most effective with therapists who are authoritarian and that a group psychodynamic approach may be most effective with a therapist who is laissez-faire. The stress managment or psychoeducational approaches may be most effective with therapists who use a democratic approach.

3.2.7 Analysis of Human Processes in Typical Subjects

Experimental research models have been used to investigate physiological, psychological, and sociological responses to various stimuli with typical ("normal") human subjects. In general, experimental research with typical subjects tends to be *nomothetic* in that the researcher seeks general laws of nature that govern kinesthetic, physiological, neurological, sociological, or psychological processes. The researcher might investigate the most effective means to encourage typical child development, for example. Such a study could involve selection of toys, specific teaching methods, nutrition, sensory motor stimulation, or physical activity. In all of these examples, the investigator can use experimental research to compare the different methods.

Potential relationships that can be studied with experimental research are the following:

▶ Exercise and mood in typical subjects
▶ Cooperative learning groups and achievement
▶ Cognitive style and choice of leisure activities
▶ Body alignment and mechanical stress on joints
▶ Dichotic listening and organization of auditory stimuli into meaningful patterns
▶ Movement patterns and sport skills
▶ Verbal reinforcement and learning
▶ Language stimulation and reading achievement
▶ Activity and normal aging

3.2.8 Operational Definitions of Normality

When defining normality and selecting typical subjects, the investigator should be guided by an a priori screening criteria setting forth attributes in the continuous range of typical functioning. Each screening criterion (e.g., intelligence, muscle strength, range of motion, blood pressure, heart rate, reading achievement) must be operationally defined and the range of scores determined to be typical or normal before the study begins. If this guideline is followed, the researcher can generalize the results from the data to all typical human subjects within the age ranges represented.

In some experiments, normality is defined as an ideal state of health without the presence of a disability or disease. In other cases, normality refers to a statistical average of a population where disease and disability are evenly distributed. The following example illustrates the fallacy of rigid criteria for defining normality: A physician evaluating an older individual's blood pressure would take into consideration the age of the individual in concluding that the blood pressure is normal. A pregnant woman would be expected to have a higher blood pressure than a nonpregnant woman. An obese individual would be expected to have a higher blood pressure than a nonobese individual, and so forth. The concept of normal blood pressure is dependent on age, gender, and weight as is indicated.

Relative normality needs to be considered when a researcher reports data for typical subjects. Many researchers assume that normality exists as an absolute and that the most healthy age is young adulthood. Concluding that young adults are usually healthy, the researcher many times is tempted to select young college students as representative samples of normally healthy individuals. The data derived from such a study would be representative only of a young adult population of college students, however. Whatever group is

Box 3–1. Example of an Experimental Case Study (Prospective Design)

1. **Bibliographical Notation**
   Stein, F., & Nikolic, S. (1989). Teaching stress management techniques to a schizophrenic patient. *The American Journal of Occupational Therapy, 43,* 162–169.

2. **Abstract**
   This paper describes a stress management training program used with a 26-year-old man with schizophrenia attending an outpatient day care program. In a seven-session program, the patient was taught to use various techniques in muscle relaxation and biofeedback to decrease anxiety and to cope with stress. The patients improvement on 7 of the 20 items of the State-Trait Anxiety Inventory demonstrated the effectiveness of even a short-term stress management program. (p. 162)

3. **Justification and Need for Study**
   The authors cited evidence for a biological basis for schizophrenia related to elevated dopamine levels. Increased anxiety leads to elevation in the levels of dopamine, resulting in an increase in schizophrenic episodes. Initial research has suggested that some individuals with schizophrenia can be taught ways to reduce anxiety and cope with psychosocial stressors. If, through occupational therapy, the anxiety in the client can be reduced, then the number of schizophrenic episodes might be reduced. The purpose of this study was to "teach stress management techniques to a schizophrenic man to help him reduce his anxiety level" (p. 163).

4. **Literature Review**
   Twenty-five references were cited in the study. Articles came from a wide variety of journals, such as *Journal of Consulting and Clinical Psychology, British Journal of Psychiatry, Perceptual and Motor Skills, Journal of Nervous and Mental Disease, Occupational Therapy in Mental Health,* and *Mental Health Special Interest Section Newsletter.* The majority of articles cited were published during the 1970s and 1980s.

5. **Research Hypothesis or Guiding Questions**
   The guiding question explicitly stated was "Can anxiety in schizophrenic patients be reduced through stress management training?" (p. 162)

6. **Methodology**
   The client was a 26-year-old single man who had been diagnosed with undifferentiated schizophrenia. His first hospitalization had been at age 19, and repeated hospitalization had occurred from that time. He was on neuroleptics and received occupational therapy for "poor grooming, inappropriate socializations, conflict with sexual identity, and impaired thought processes" (p. 163). "The patient agreed to stress management training because he had experienced intense levels of stress in the past and wanted to learn to deal with stress more effectively" (p. 163).

   Anxiety was measured through the S-scale on the State-Trait Anxiety Inventory (STAI; Spielberger, 1983). Qualitative measurements of coping behavior were measured through the Stress Management Questionnaire (SMQ; Stein, 1987). The program was carried out in six 1-hour weekly sessions using

continued

"practical stress management techniques that could be generalized to every-day living" (p. 165). The STAI was used as a pre- and posttest during all sessions except the first one. The patient was asked to complete the SMQ and use techniques learned during the sessions during the week. "A follow-up session to administer the SMQ and attain therapeutic closure was held 2 weeks after the sixth session" (p. 166).

A correlated *t* test was used to compare pre- and posttest scores on the STAI. The nonparametric sign test was used to examine changes in scores on the STAI over five sessions. The level of statistical significance for both statistical analyses was chosen at $p < .05$. Qualitative analysis of the SMQ was obtained regarding symptoms experienced, stressors, and activities to reduce stress.

7. Results

Significant changes in anxiety were noted over the sessions. The patient's mean posttest score on the STAI was statistically significantly lower than his pretest score. In addition, he "significantly reduced his anxiety on 9 of the 20 items [on the STAI] during the course of the study" (p. 166). Finally, changes in symptoms, stressors, and ways to reduce stressors changed over time.

> In summary, on the pretest [for the SMQ] during Session 1, the patient's primary symptom of stress was talking excessively, his primary stressor was being watched by others, and his primary activity to relieve stress was walking. In the follow-up Session 7, the patient's primary stress symptom was chest pains, his primary stressor was doing new things for the first time, and his stress-relieving activity was listening to music. (p. 167)

Two years after this study, the first author informally followed up on the patient's whereabouts and functioning. At that time, the patient had had no relapse and was maintaining successfully in the community.

8. Conclusions

Stein and Nicolic concluded the following:

1. A short-term stress management program using a combination of biofeedback and relaxation techniques can be used successfully with some individuals with schizophrenia.
2. The role of occupational therapists in a psychiatric setting can be enhanced by having them teach stress management techniques to individuals with schizophrenia.

9. Limitations of the Study

Since this was a case study, further research must be done if the findings are to be generalized to a larger population of individuals with schizophrenia.

10. Major References Cited in the Study

Acosta, F. X., Yamamoto, J., & Wilcox, S. (1978). Application of electromyographic biofeedback to the relaxation training of schizophrenic, neurotic, and tension headache patients. *Journal of Consulting and Clinical Psychology, 46,* 383–384.

Benson, H. (1975). *The relaxation response.* New York: William Morrow.

Hawkins, R., Doell, S., & Lindseth, P. (1980). Anxiety reduction in hospitalized schizophrenics through thermal biofeedback and relaxation training. *Perceptual and Motor Skills, 51,* 475–582.

Stein, F. (1987). *Stress management questionnaire.* Unpublished manuscript, University of Wisconsin-Milwaukee.

Box 3–2. Example of Experimental Research Group Study

1. Bibliographical Notation

Bulgren, J. A., Schumaker, J. B., & Deshler, D. D. (1994). The effects of a recall enhancement routine on the test performance of secondary students with and without learning disabilities. *Learning Disabilities Research and Practice, 9,* 2–11.

2. Abstract

The purpose of this study was to evaluate the effects of presenting mnemonic devices in conjunction with content information on the recall performance of students with and without learning disabilities" (p. 2). Forty-one students (18 students with learning disabilities, 23 students without learning disabilities) in grades 7 and 8 who were enrolled in two mainstreamed social studies classes were randomly placed in a control group and an experimental group. The two classes were team taught by a special educator and social studies teacher. After a class lecture in which important material had been verbally and visually cued (e.g., "This is important, write this down"), and a period of systematic review of some of the material, the students were given a multiple-choice test covering material from the class lecture. The systematic review differed for each group. The experimental group reviewed material through an enhanced memory routine designed to relate memory of information to specific mnemonic procedures. The control group was drilled repeatedly on the facts. Results of the data analysis indicated that students in the experimental group showed statistically significantly greater recall of information than the control group. In addition, more of the students in the experimental group received passing grades than did students in the control group. The researchers hypothesized that use of the memory enhancement system was beneficial in increasing recall of factual information for students with and without learning disabilities. (p. 2)

3. Justification and Need for Study

The investigator stated that the purpose of the study was to investigate ways in which students with learning disabilities could learn content material presented in lectures in the general classroom and the ways in which general educators could structure classroom lectures to facilitate and enhance learning for all students. The theoretical basis for the study was previous findings that when students with learning disabilities are taught mnemonic techniques, their ability to recall factual information increases. The study extended findings from previous research at the University of Kansas Center for Research on Learning (KU-CRL) regarding the needs of students with learning disabilities who are enrolled in general education classes.

4. Literature Review

Twenty-six references were cited in this article. Articles came from several different journals, including *American School Board Journal, Learning Disability Quarterly, Journal of Learning Disabilities,* and *Remedial and Special Education.* The

continued

authors cited in the references were well known in the field of learning disabilities, memory training, and strategy instruction.

5. **Research Hypothesis or Guiding Question**
   Implicit in the investigator's research design were the following nondirectional hypotheses: (a) There is no statistically significant difference between the experimental and the control group in the recall of reviewed facts; and (b) There is no statistically significant difference between the experimental and the control group in the recall of unreviewed facts. The latter hypothesis was raised to ensure that the two groups were similar.

6. **Methodology**
   Statistical analysis was carried out through a two-by-two analysis of variance (ANOVA) design comparing diagnosed and undiagnosed students in experimental and control groups. The experimental group reviewed factual material through an enhanced memory system, whereas the control group reviewed the same material through repeated questioning. Both groups were tested on nonreviewed material to determine similarities between the groups.

7. **Operational Definition of Variables**
   Independent variables
   a. control and experimental groups
   b. students with and without learning diabilities
   Dependent variables
   a. score obtained on reviewed facts
   b. score obtained on nonreviewed facts: used to determine similarity between groups

8. **Analysis of Results**
   The authors used an ANOVA to test their hypothesis. Results confirmed the first null hypothesis (there was no statistically significant difference between the two groups) and lead to rejection of the second null hypothesis (there was no statistically significant difference between the two groups in recall of reviewed material).

   A significant main effect for exceptionality was seen with nonreviewed and reviewed facts ($F = 12.197$, $p = .001$; $F = 10.173$, $p = .003$). This was expected, because there was a statistically significant difference between students with learning disability and students without learning disabilities. There was no statistical significance between group 1 and group 2 for nonreviewed facts, both of which contained students with and without learning disabilities; however, there was a statically significant difference between groups for reviewed facts ($F = 18.900$, $p = 000$).

9. **Stated Limitations of Study**
   a. "The practicality of incorporating the Recall Enhancement Routine into secondary lessons on an ongoing basis. . ." (p. 10) was not addressed.
   b. The ability of students to "generate their own mnemonic devices within mainstream setting" (p. 10) was not addressed. The students in this study were taught a mnemonic device and instructional modifications were made within the classroom setting.

c. "The levels at which LD students can perform in the mainstream secondary classroom" (p. 10) is a third limitation. Although more students with learning disabilities showed passing scores, approximately 25% of the students still failed, even when given extra accommodation and instruction.

10. **Major References in Study**

Bulgren, J., Deshler, D. D., & Schumaker, J. B. (1993). *Teacher use of a recall enhancement routine in secondary content classrooms.* Unpublished manuscript, University of Kansas, Center for Research on Learning, Lawrence.

King-Sears, M. E., Mercer, C. D., & Sindelar, P. T. (1992). Toward independence with keyword mnemonics: A strategy for science vocabulary instruction. *Remedial and Special Education, 13,* 22–33.

Mastropieri, M. A., Scruggs, T. E., McLoone, B., & Levin, J. R. (1985). Facilitating learning disabled students' acquisition of science classifications. *Learning Disability Quarterly, 8,* 299–309.

Scruggs, T. E., & Mastropieri, M. A. (1990). Mnemonic instruction for students with learning disabilities: What it is and what it does. *Learning Disability Quarterly, 13,* 271–280.

selected, the researcher must also demonstrate that the subjects had no physiological abnormalities that could influence results. In short, a research subject is considered typical only when compared to a priori screening criteria.

3.3 Methodological Research

3.3.1 Purposes of Methodological Research

The main purposes of methodological research in rehabilitation and special education are the design of assistive technology, the development of assessment instruments, the redesign of the physical environment for individuals with physical disability, the design of ergonomic interventions in the work place, and the development of curriculum and treatment protocols. Figure 3–8 outlines specific areas of applying methodological research to rehabilitation, occupational therapy, and habilitation.

As seen in Chapter 1, significant advances in medicine and rehabilitation oc-

curred because of technological advances via microscopes, X-Ray machines, electrocardiograms, augmentative communication, computer software, CT scans, and the numerous diagnostic scopes, all of which are results of methodological research. The introduction of psychophysiological measures and functional capacity evaluations are examples of the ongoing importance of methodological research and its relationship to clinical practice.

3.3.2 Strategies

In devising an assessment tool, treatment protocol, or assistive device, the researcher poses the question: What are the relevant factors that must be considered in devising a test instrument, treatment method, or self-care device? Factors to consider include developmental age, cognitive functioning, sensory-motor abilities, and educational level. The content and format of the instrument or test should be determined after a systematic review of related literature.

An example of a methodological research study involves developing a feasible

ASSISTIVE TECHNOLOGY

- Augmentative and alternative communication (AAC)
- Computer hardware and software
- Mobility (e.g., wheelchairs, environmental controls)
- Prosthetics/orthotics
- Self-help devices
- Sensory aids (visual, tactile)
- Switches and controls
- Vocational adaptations

ASSESSMENT INSTRUMENTS

- ADL scales
- Developmental inventories
- Functional capacity evaluations
- Interview schedules
- Outcome measures
- Perceptual-motor scales
- Questionnaires and attitude scales
- Rating scales

PHYSICAL EVALUATION

- Abnormal reflexes
- Biofeedback
- Grip strength
- Gross and fine motor
- Manual-muscle testing
- Pain sensitivity
- Range of motion
- Sensory (visual, auditory, tactile)

TREATMENT ENVIRONMENTS

- Adult day care programs
- Areas for animal-assisted therapy
- Community-based settings
- General and special education classrooms
- Halfway house
- Skilled nursing facilities
- Social milieus
- Supported employment
- Therapy clinic

CURRICULUM DEVELOPMENT

- Distance learning
- Field work (e.g., preceptor, mentoring, internships)
- Instructional aids (e.g., audiovisual tapes, CD ROMS, anatomical models)
- Module development
- Problem-based learning
- Software programs

TREATMENT PROTOCOLS

- Academic Instruction
- ADL/IADL programs
- Animal-assisted therapy
- Aquatic therapy
- Cognitive retraining
- Functional academics
- Neurodevelopmental therapy
- Relaxation therapy
- Sensory integration therapy
- Speech-language therapy

Figure 3–8. Methodological research: Purposes and content. This figure illustrates the application of methodological research to occupational therapy, rehabilitation, and habilitation.

method of independent feeding for a population of individuals with severe disabilities. The researcher needs to consider several aspects of feeding, including positioning, utensils, eye-hand coordination, motivational factors, instructional methods, and attention level of the clients. Another example is a researcher interested in devising therapeutic toys for children with cerebral palsy. In this case, factors relating to sensorimotor, cognition, psychosocial aspects, and language should be considered. The sequential analysis shown in Figure 3–9 describes the steps involved in

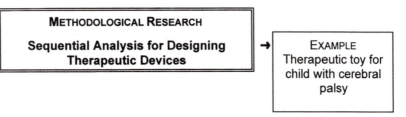

METHODOLOGICAL RESEARCH **Sequential Analysis for Designing Therapeutic Devices**	→	EXAMPLE Therapeutic toy for child with cerebral palsy

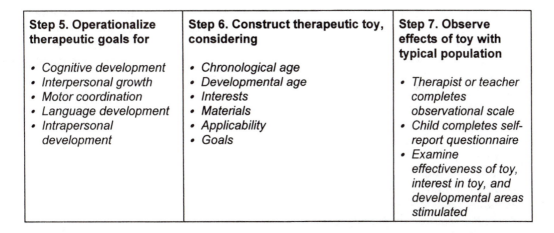

Step 1. Purpose *Devise toy to stimulate development in child with cerebral palsy*	**Step 2. Areas for literature review** • *Theory of play* • *Cerebral palsy* • *Child development* • *Toy construction*	**Step 3. Select subjects** *Screening criteria for cerebral palsy*	**Step 4. Analyze materials and construction** *Set up laboratory to design the toy*

Step 5. Operationalize therapeutic goals for • *Cognitive development* • *Interpersonal growth* • *Motor coordination* • *Language development* • *Intrapersonal development*	**Step 6. Construct therapeutic toy, considering** • *Chronological age* • *Developmental age* • *Interests* • *Materials* • *Applicability* • *Goals*	**Step 7. Observe effects of toy with typical population** • *Therapist or teacher completes observational scale* • *Child completes self-report questionnaire* • *Examine effectiveness of toy, interest in toy, and developmental areas stimulated*

Step 8. Redesign toy based on feedback from typical children	**Step 9. Use the toy with representative group of children with cerebral palsy**	**Step 10. Use feedback from consumers to modify toy**	**Step 11. Apply use of the toy in therapeutic treatment and evaluate its effectiveness**

Figure 3–9. Methodological research: Construction of a therapeutic toy. Note that the construction includes a literature review, operationalized goals, pilot testing on students with and without disabilities, and evaluation of effectiveness.

designing a therapeutic toy for children with cerebral palsy.

3.3.3 Designing Treatment Protocol

The treatment protocol is an operational definition of a treatment method. It includes all the details in the presciption, preparation, initiation, implementation, documentation, and evaluation. The number of treatments per day or week and the length of the sessions are also included. The treatment protocol should be modified or adjusted to meet the individual needs of the client.

What if an occupational therapist is interested in designing a new treatment protocol for cognitive retraining in adult patients who have had a traumatic brain injury (TBI)? How can the clinical researcher assist the occupational therapist in this investigation?

The overall design of the research is organized into five phases.

▶ *Phase I* is an examination of the need for developing a new cognitive retraining protocol that takes into consideration the incidence of TBI in the population as well as the family, social, and economic costs of TBI. The significance of the study is documented.

▶ *Phase II* includes a search of the literature reviewing the etiology, incidence and prevalence rates, and current treatment methods for cognitive retraining. As part of the literature review, the researcher would complete a descriptive meta analysis that evaluates and compares the research on cognitive retraining methods.

▶ *Phase III* considers the variables that enter into the design of a specific treatment protocol. The variables considered in devising the protocol are described in Table 3–5. In this phase, the clinical researcher's goal is to design the treatment method so that it can be used by trained occupational therapists to work with individuals with TBI.

▶ *Phase IV* includes the pilot testing of the treatment protocol. During this phase, the researcher is concerned with the refinement of the procedure and initial evaluation by occupational therapists working with TBI. A rating scale for assessing the clarity and relevancy of the treatment method is developed by the researcher and completed by clinicians. The actual testing of the effectiveness of the treatment protocol cannot be accomplished until the protocol has been operationally defined and then tested for its feasibility. The following issues must also be considered:

1. Are the instructions presented clearly to the client?
2. Are all theoretical assumptions considered when developing the method? For example, when developing a cognitive retraining protocol, the researcher must consider the encoding, storage, and retrieval aspects of information processing.
3. Should the treatment be shortened or lengthened in time?
4. Are there limitations to the treatment procedure? For example, clients with limited cognitive abilities may not benefit from a cognitive retraining protocol.

▶ *Phase V* includes the evaluation of the treatment protocol, its applicability to individuals with TBI, and the level of skill necessary to administer the treatment. The potential effectiveness of the treatment method compared with other procedures as identified in the literature review should also be considered.

3.3.4 Assessment Instruments

The design of assessment instruments is a traditional role for psychologists who are trained in measurement theory and test construction. Recently, clinicians of diverse disciplines in rehabilitation and special education have also become involved in developing new assessment measures that are directly related to clinical evaluation.

Table 3–5. Variables in Devising a Treatment Protocol

Patient	*Therapist*	*Method*
• Diagnosis	• Educational level	• Operationalized treatment goals
• Severity of illness	• Experience	• Time factors
• Gender	• Specific training	• Manual of directions
• Intelligence	• Cognitive style	• Individual versus group factors
• Education		
• Socioeconomic status		

For example, interest among occupational therapists in perceptual-motor functions and child development has led to the construction of new tests designed for specific treatment populations (Miller, 1988). Application and use of standardized tests is becoming an increasingly important task of the clinician who routinely evaluates the level of patient function. Even so, this area has generally not been incorporated into most undergraduate curriculums in the allied health professions. The construction of reliable and valid instruments for measuring human capacities is a relatively fertile area of methodological research in the allied health professions. A more in-depth discussion of testing and measurement is in Chapter 9. Figure 3–10 analyzes the steps involved in test construction.

3.3.5 Questionnaires and Interviews

The need to gather information regarding the characteristics and attitudes of populations has led to the wide abuse of interviews and questionnaires, especially in marketing research. Individuals are deluged by interviews and questionnaires asking whether they use a certain brand of toothpaste or deodorant, ad infinitum. Despite abuses, they can be useful tools in obtaining information about a target population. In constructing interviews or questionnaires, the researcher must resolve the following questions:

▶ Was there an overall theoretical framework or rationale for selecting the items?
▶ Do the items measure accurately what the researcher purports to measure? (Validity)
▶ Are the items clear, unambiguous, and consistent? (Reliability)
▶ Was a representative pilot sample selected for testing reliability?

For a further discussion of interviews and questionnaires see Chapter 9.

Rating Scales

Rating scales are a type of questionnaire that can be used to quantify information. Rating scales are employed most frequently in evaluating the performance of students, clients, and staff. Typically, the evaluator checks off the description most indicative of performance from a list of adjective phrases. Rating scales are usually of three types: numerical, dichotomous, and descriptive. In a numerical scale, often called a Likert scale, ratings are distributed along a continuum, such as in the following example:

> Rate each of the following items by circling the number that corresponds to your opinion. (Likert Scale)
> 1. Strongly agree
> 2. Agree
> 3. Neutral
> 4. Disagree
> 5. Strongly disagree

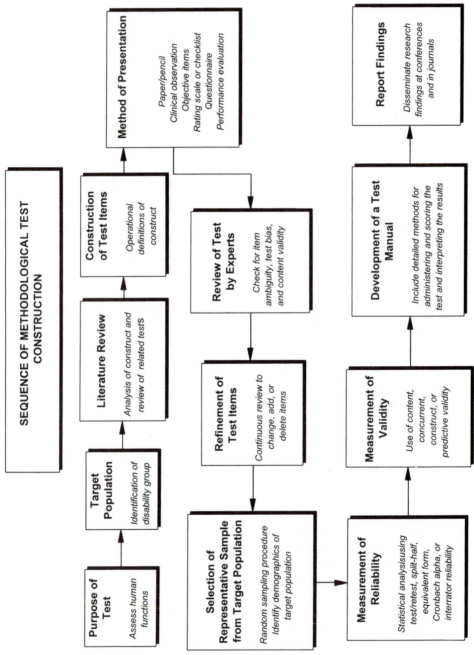

SEQUENCE OF METHODOLOGICAL TEST CONSTRUCTION

Purpose of Test

Assess human functions

Target Population

Identification of disability group

Literature Review

Analysis of construct and review of related tests

Construction of Test Items

Operational definitions of construct

Method of Presentation

*Paper/pencil
Clinical observation
Objective items
Rating scale or checklist
Questionnaire
Performance evaluation*

Review of Test by Experts

Check for item ambiguity, test bias, and content validity

Refinement of Test Items

Continuous review to change, add, or delete items

Selection of Representative Sample from Target Population

*Random sampling procedure
Identify demographics of target population*

Measurement of Reliability

Statistical analysis using test/retest, split-half, equivalent form, Cronbach alpha, or interrater reliability

Measurement of Validity

Use of content, concurrent, construct, or predictive validity

Development of a Test Manual

Include detailed methods for administering and scoring the test and interpreting the results

Report Findings

Disseminate research findings at conferences and in journals

Figure 3–10. Methodological research: Test construction, including rating scales and questionnaires. Note that there is a sequential order to the construction, with many validity checks while the task is being completed.

a. The United States   1 2 3 4 5
   should adopt a univer-
   sal health plan for all
   residents.
b. Medicare and Medicaid 1 2 3 4 5
   should be combined
   into one health care
   system

In a dichotomous scale, the extremes are identified, and the rater chooses the extreme that indicates the client's performance. For example:

The patient's ability to assemble small parts is adequate.
   1. Yes
   2. No

In a descriptive scale, the rater chooses a phrase from a presented list. For example:

Circle the descriptive phrase that is most accurate.

On a specific task (e.g., addressing envelopes) the worker in a supported employment needs supervision

▶ all of the time   ▶ rarely

▶ some of the time   ▶ none of the time

▶ once in a while

3.3.6 Treatment Facilities

How can a clinical researcher contribute to the design of an effective treatment environment for clients with disabilities? The tasks of designing sheltered workshops, adult day care, outpatient clinics, and halfway houses are a joint effort by architects, administrators, therapists, and other rehabilitation personnel. The researcher applying methodological research to the construction of a treatment environment should first pose the question: What factors must be considered in designing a therapeutic environment for clients? Using answers to this question, the researcher can generate a plan that considers several variables. A tentative outline for research follows.

3.3.7 Methodological Review: Treatment Facilities

1. Formulating the purposes for the treatment facility
   a. Disabilities serviced (e.g., individuals with mental illness, retardation, or physical impairments)
   b. Treatment goals (e.g., cognitive and physical development, functional skills, independent living)
   c. Demographic considerations for screening clients (e.g., age, gender, level of care)
   d. Location of treatment facility (e.g., urban, suburban, or rural area) and impact on neighborhood
2. Surveying need for treatment facility by documenting
   a. Number of potential clients to be serviced
   b. Number of other treatment facilities in service area
   c. Attitudes toward facility's location by potential clients, community residents, and health care providers
3. Reviewing literature describing similar programs
   a. Identifying model programs
   b. Architectural descriptions of physical layouts
   c. Analysis of staff functions and patient ratios
   d. Policies regarding patient admissions, discharges, and follow-up
   e. Evaluation research of treatment effectiveness
   f. Administrative considerations (e.g., budgeting, departmental responsibilities).
4. Stating guiding assumptions and rationale for
   a. Setting screening criteria for client admission and discharges
   b. Designing physical layout and geographical location
   c. Proposing staff positions
   d. Setting criteria for evaluating effectiveness
5. Surveying resources of community for
   a. Potential source of staff

   b. Transportation facilities
   c. Consultative services
   d. Community support
6. Survey cost-effectiveness factors
   a. Construction cost
   b. Cost of providing patient care and treatment
   c. Cost of providing supportive and maintenance services
   d. Sources of potential income
      (1) private pay
      (2) insurance and any third-party payments
      (3) government entitlements (Medicaid and Medicare)
      (4) state and federal grants
      (5) private foundations

3.3.8 Designing Education Curricula

The training of occupational therapists, dietitians, rehabilitation counselors, speech-language pathologists, audiologists, physical therapists, special educators, school psychologists, and other related professional groups involves interdisciplinary approaches. What knowledge in the areas of physiology, anatomy, psychology, and sociology are necessary? What interpersonal skills in working with clients with disabilities must be developed? What evaluation and treatment procedures should be taught? These questions regarding the content of educational curricula are continually reevaluated in light of the rapid growth of the occupational therapy profession. Parallel to the growth of the curricula content areas is the interest in designing methods for effectively communicating knowledge to occupational therapy students. How do students learn most effectively? What should be the role of problem-based learning, computer-assisted instruction, distance learning, technology, preceptor and intern supervision, and lecture in the educational curricula? These questions lend themselves to methodological research. The researcher objectively designs a curriculum after identifying the relevant factors from an extensive review of the literature.

3.3.9 Physical Evaluation Techniques and Treatment Hardware

Another area of methodological research that is appropriate to the allied health professions pertains to the use of machines and hardware for evaluating a patient's functional capacity. Electromyography (EMG), electrodiagnostic recording, perceptual-motor tests, visual, auditory and kinesthesis testing, and manual muscle testing are examples of the broad areas for potential research.

Occupational therapists may use physical agent modalities (PAMs), often in conjunction with physical therapists. PAMs include ultrasound, diathermy, infrared light, ultraviolet rays, hydrotherapy, electrical stimulation, hot packs, accupuncture, TENS, biofeedback, and paraffin. New methods of treatment, especially in muscle retraining, are now relying on electrophysiological methods involving oscilloscopes, telemetry, and computers. The growth in the area of prosthetics has been the result of the combined talents of researchers coming from backgrounds in engineering, neurophysiology, and occupational therapy. Orthotics, the development of splints and braces for individuals with physical disabilities, is another area for research development in occupational therapy.

Box 3–3 examines test-retest reliability of the Work Box®, which is used to "evaluate the manual dexterity and work skills of persons who have sustained injuries" (Speller, Trollinger, Maurer, Nelson, & Bauer, 1997, p. 517). This is an example of methodological research by occupational therapists.

3.4 Evaluation Research

3.4.1 Purposes of Evaluation Research

Evaluation research examines the effectiveness of programs that provide direct

---

Box 3–3. Example of Methodological Research

1. **Bibliographical Citation**
   Speller, L., Trollinger, J. A., Maurer, P. A., Nelson, C. E., Bauer, D. F. (1997). Comparison of the test–retest reliability of the Work Box® using three administrative methods. *The American Journal of Occupational Therapy, 51,* 516–522.

2. **Abstract**
   OBJECTIVE. The purpose of this study was to compare the test-retest reliability of three administrative methods of the Work Box®: (a) the original instructions, (b) a revised version of the original instructions, and (c) another revised version that was based on suggestions made by authors of the first two versions of the instructions.
   METHOD. Sixty subjects without disabilities were randomly grouped so that 20 subjects were tested per administrative method. The assessment was administered to each subject on two occasions, with a 7-day to 14-day period between tests. Scores were recorded as time in seconds, and intraclass correlation coefficients (ICCs) were used to calculate the reliability.
   RESULTS. The ICCs for assembly, disassembly, and total scores were .589, .604, and .654, respectively, for the original instructions; .424, .572, and .545 for the revised instructions; and .781, .579, .717 for the second revised instructions. Reliability was found to be higher for men than for women and for subjects who claimed to have more rather than less experience in similar manual dexterity tasks.
   CONCLUSIONS. On the basis of the reliability of each administrative method and comments made by subjects about their understanding of the instructions, the second revised version of the instructions is recommended as the standard method. The results also indicate that the assessment is most appropriate for a population of men with manual dexterity experience. With further standardization, the Work Box® could be a valuable assessment tool for therapists working in industrial rehabilitation settings. (Speller et al., 1997, p. 516)

3. **Justification and Need for Study**
   "Because of the discrepancies between the results of Feden and Black et al. and the need to further revise the administration methods, the present study attempted to clarify the administrative methods and to determine test–retest reliability with another subject group" (p. 518).

4. **Literature Review**
   The authors examined the literature on the standardization of tests-retest reliability for the Work Box®, general principals for standardization, work capacity evaluations, and the role of the occupational therapist as an evaluation. Thirty-three references were cited, selected from the following journals: *AJOT, Work: A Journal of Prevention and Rehabilitation, Journal of Hand Therapy, American Journal of Physical Medicine and Rehabilitation, Archives of Physical Medicine and Rehabilitation,* and *Hand Clinics.*

continued

5. **Research Hypothesis or Guiding Questions**
   "The specific research question, therefore, was What is the test–retest reliability for three administrative methods of the following scores on the Work Box®: assembly, disassembly, and total?" (p. 518).

6. **Methodology**
   Sixty subjects from a convenience sample were taken from (a) students at a university, (b) students at a community college, and (c) contract archaeologists. The subjects were between the ages of 14 and 69, had no interfering medical history, and had no experience with the Work Box®. Subjects were randomly assigned to one of three groups. Subjects assembled and disassembled the Work Box® and were retested 7 to 14 days later.

7. **Operational Definition of Variables**
   The Work Box® was described in detail [photograph included in the original article]. Data collection, testing procedures, and administrative method were also described.

8. **Flow Plan in Methodological Research** (Figure 3–11).

9. **Conclusions**
   This study of test-retest reliability of the Work Box® is one component of standardizing this assessment of manual dexterity. Of the three administration methods used, the revised instructions described in this study were found to be the most reliable, considering differences in scores and comments from subjects. . . . Development of the Work Box® depends on further research, including collect of normative data (to further standardize the assessment), studies determining validity, and examination of how experience relates to learning. (p. 521)

10. **Limitations of the Study**
    a. "The testing environment could have been better controlled by testing every subject at the same site" (p. 521)
    b. "Although pilot testing was performed to ensure that the two data collectors were using the same scoring and observation methods, minor individual differences between them may have affected the results" (p. 521).

11. **Major References in Study**
    Black, M. K. (1991). *Standardization of instructions and test–retest reliability of a manual dexterity* and work skills assessment tool. Unpublished master's thesis, Virginia Commonwealth University, Richmond.
    Black, M. K., Nelson, C. E., Maurer, P. A., & Bauer, D. F. (1993). Test–retest reliability of the Work Box®: A work sample with standard instructions. *Work: A Journal of prevention and Rehabilitation, 3*(4), 26–34.
    Feden, S. D. (1993). *Test-retest reliability of the Work Box® with nondisabled female subjects.* Unpublished research project, Virginia Commonwealth University, Richmond.

1	2	3
Establish need for a test for manual dexterity and work-skill	Search the literature for published tests in manual dexterity and work-skill	Develop a standardized test, including a manual and normative data

4	5	6
Obtain reliability and validity data with typical subjects (e.g., test-retest studies, concurrent validity)	Identify target population (i.e., assembly workers with disabilities) and compilation of data	Assess target population and compared with typical population

7
Obtain reliability and validity data with target population

Figure 3–11. Flow plan in methodological research. This example uses the plan from the development of the Work Box®.

health care, prepare health personnel, and administer services for private and governmental agencies. When engaged in evaluation research, the investigator considers a total corporate unit and the components that comprise it. Program effectiveness, quality of service, productivity, organizational communication, cost-effectiveness, stated objectives, and personnel practices are areas considered in evaluation research. Evaluation research is commonly applied in the following programs, services, and agencies:

▶ Certification of hospitals (e.g., Joint Commission on Accreditation of Hospital Organization [JCAHO])
▶ Accreditation of college or educational program (e.g., National College Accreditation of Teacher Education [NCATE] or Accreditation Commission of Occupational Therapy Education [ACOTE])

▶ Rehabilitation agency evaluation (e.g., The Rehabilitation Accreditation Commission [CARF])
▶ Analysis of cost-per-patient treatment (e.g., Medicare guidelines, Diagnostic Related Groups [DRGs])
▶ Outcome studies of patients or clients
▶ Needs assessment (e.g., community's health needs, available resources)
▶ Evaluation of program effectiveness using a priori criteria

A historical example of the impact of evaluation research on changing an institution was Abraham Flexner's (1910) report *Medical Education in the United States and Canada*, which was made to the Carnegie Foundation for the Advancement of Training. Flexner personally toured the 155 medical schools that existed at that time in the United States and Canada. Although he did not use a standardized questionnaire or test instrument for evaluation, he did apply specific criteria in evaluating the quality and effectiveness of medical schools in preparing physicians. These criteria were the following:

1. The entrance requirements for gaining admission to the medical school (e.g., minimal standards, high school graduation or equivalent, or college education)
2. The number of students in full-time or part-time attendance
3. The size of the faculty, including number of full-time professors and part-time instructors
4. The financial resources available to the college from endowments, student tuition, and clinical fees
5. The quality and adequacy of the physical plant, including laboratory classrooms, lecture halls, medical and laboratory equipment, refrigerator plants, amphitheater for observation of surgery and clinical interviews, and medical library
6. Professional supervision available to the students in the laboratories
7. The opportunities for student practice in clinics and availability of hospital patients.

On the basis of these criteria, Flexner found a wide discrepancy in standards of medical education in the schools he visited. He concluded, based on his observations, that many medical schools were doing a disservice to the public by preparing poorly educated physicians. He recommended that there be fewer medical schools.

Flexner's evaluations of the 155 medical schools led to dramatic changes in medical education that occurred between 1910 and 1925. He recommended that medical schools and hospitals enter into teaching relationships, that state boards reject applicants for medical degrees who graduate from medical schools that were inadequate, and that examinations for state licensure be rigorous. He hoped that "Perhaps the entire country may some day be covered by a health organization engaged in protecting the public health against the formidable combination

made by ignorance, incompetency, commercialism, and disease" (p. 173). All of these recommendations were eventually implemented and led to the founding of the American Medical Association (AMA). Evaluation research as used by Flexner was directed toward the improvement of an institution, specifically the medical profession.

When properly used, evaluation research can be useful (Weiss, 1972) in deciding whether to:

▶ continue or discontinue a program
▶ improve an agency's practices and procedures
▶ add or drop specific program strategies and techniques
▶ use a program as a model for new agencies
▶ utilize more fully the services of a program on a geographical basis,
▶ accept or reject theoretical approaches underlining an agency's program

These purposes are achieved only after the investigator has collected objective and valid data. The research steps include (a) the stated need for evaluation research; (b) a review of the literature, comprising a description of programs and criteria used; (c) an objective research design for collecting data through interviews, questionnaires, attitude scales, and clinical observation; (d) statistical analysis of records and examination of the physical plant; (e) comparisons of program with objective criteria; (f) separate sections on results and discussion of findings; and (g) the evaluation team's recommendation for reaccreditation, probation, or closing of the program. Figure 3–12 identifies examples of potential areas for evaluation research in occupational therapy, rehabilitation, and habilitation.

3.4.2 Strategies of Evaluation Research

The issue of researcher bias is of prime consideration in evaluation research. The underlying purpose of evaluation research is

TREATMENT PROGRAM LOCATED IN . . .	PREPARATORY AND ADVANCED EDUCATIONAL PROGRAMS FOR OCCUPATIONAL THERAPISTS
• General hospitals • Psychiatric facilities • Rehabilitation centers • Home-health services • Halfway houses • Residential treatment centers (RTC) • Independent living complexes • Special schools • Sheltered workshops • Clinics • Therapy departments	• Certified occupational therapy assistants • Basic professional (bachelors or master's degree) training program • Advanced professional degree program (masters or doctorate)

VOLUNTARY AND PRIMARY AGENCIES RELATED TO	GOVERNMENTAL AND NONGOVERNMENTAL AGENCIES
• AIDS • Alzheimer's disease • Arthritis • ADHD/ADD • Autism • Cancer • Cerebral palsy • Heart disease • Learning disabilities • Mental retardation • Multiple sclerosis • Muscular dystrophy • Psychosocial disorders • Spinal cord injury • Stroke • Traumatic brain injury	• Division of Vocational Rehabilitation • Department of Health and Human Services • Department of Corrections • Health maintenance organizations (HMOs) • Social Security Administration • National Institute of Mental Health • State Departments of Education • United States Department of Education • Veterans Administration

Figure 3–12. Potential areas for evaluation research in occupational therapy, rehabilitation, and habilitation.

to apply objective assessment to a facility, an agency, or a treatment program. How does a researcher objectively evaluate an organization? How are criteria established for measuring the effectiveness of a program? Are criteria established by the evaluation research team based on ideal theoretical considerations or by the treatment agency that is being evaluated? What expertise in research is needed in evaluating the competence and abilities of health professionals? What controls should be established in the research methodology to reduce investigator bias?

The following hypothetical example explores the process of evaluation research as applied to a residential school for adolescents who are disturbed:

1. Stated purposes of evaluation are set forth, such as:
   a. Continued school certification or accreditation
   b. Evaluation of treatment effectiveness
   c. Direct and indirect costs per student treatment
   d. Widening of services to include more diverse client groups
   e. Change in delivery of services to reduce residential population and to include more day care or community-based treatment
   f. The overall decision to cease operation
   Before evaluation research is undertaken, there must be a mutual understanding of the purpose between the evaluators and those being evaluated. If the purposes are unclear or if there is a hidden agenda, then the research objectivity could become undermined, and the evaluation could serve more as a political maneuver than as a means to collect objective data. For example, if the evaluators seek to close a program by collecting negative or damaging information and by omitting any positive attributes, then the evaluation is worthless as scientific research.

2. The formation of a research team of evaluators is dependent on the stated purposes of the evaluation and the specific areas considered. Expertise and experience in program administration, budgeting, treatment techniques, special education, vocational rehabilitation, research methodology, interviewing techniques, and familiarity with educational requirements and job descriptions of professional and nonprofessional staff members are necessary to provide appropriate expertise and knowledge levels for the members of an evaluation research team. Evaluation research demands a sophisticated level of expertise that is essential in the research process. The responsibility of judging the effectiveness of the program is delegated to the research team. As the level of effectiveness is a relative judgment, it is important that each member of the evaluation team understand and accept the criteria being used as the "measuring yardsticks." Experience of the members of the team in working in other treatment agencies and familiarity with the evaluation process, either as a supervisor in a clinic or in an educational environment, are necessary requisites for doing evaluation research. The size of the research team, responsibility based on the areas of expertise and experience represented, and the availability of consultants are considered in forming an effective evaluation research team.

3. The descriptive data will include:
   a. history of the organization, including why it was established and names and backgrounds of founders
   b. flow chart of administration, including lines of responsibility, and departmental components
   c. description of the physical plant, including a detailed layout of the facilities
   d. staff resumes, including education and experience of administrators, treatment staff, and supporting personnel
   e. job descriptions of work responsibilities
   f. rehabilitation and treatment services offered, including but not limited to medical, psychological, educational, child care, and prevocational
   g. formal and informal meetings, conferences, and patient staffings
   h. intake policies, orientation, and discharge procedures
   i. follow-up care and evaluation of discharges
   j. relationships with community and outside agencies

k. numerical data regarding maximum client capacity of facility, present number of clients, average length of residence, number of referrals, and discharges over time
4. Criteria of effectiveness are established by the research team. The criteria are based on a priori standards or objectives furnished by the administrator of the program. Areas for criteria include:
   a. *treatment effect:* percentage of clients who have made successful and unsuccessful adjustments after discharge (Definition of successful and unsuccessful outcome should be operationally defined.)
   b. *physical plant:* safety, health, and accessibility for those individuals with mobility impairment meeting the Americans with Disability Act (ADA, 1990) requirements; fire requirements
   c. *professional staff:* percentage of staff having professional educational backgrounds (resumes, number of years at facility, reasons for leaving previous position)
   d. *staff ratio:* number of clients per treatment staff
   e. *staff salaries:* average salaries as compared with national average or salaries in comparable agencies
   f. *continuing education:* opportunities for staff to attend conferences, workshops, or inservices
   g. *discharges:* number over time and reasons for client discharge
   Criteria can also be established by selecting characteristic patterns from programs considered to be successful models, although flexibility in employing these models is necessary when applying criteria. The severity of the disability in clients serviced and the financial resources available to an agency are factors that must be considered when analyzing outside criteria.
5. Interviews with staff and residents is necessary to transform the highly subjective process of "getting insights into a systematic method for the collection of social data" (Festinger & Katz, 1953, p. 327). The limitations of the interview process should be recognized by the researcher. The very nature of communicating feelings and attitudes is limited by the natural suspiciousness of the interviewee and his or her reliance on memory to provide information. It is not the authors' intent to discuss interviewing techniques in detail, but it shall be sufficient to note that researchers utilizing interview information must be certain that the interviewers have had training. Leading questions, long and complicated questions, and rambling and unrelated items, which untrained interviewers often use, provide data that subsequently bias the results. (See Festinger & Katz, 1953, for further information.)
6. The next process in evaluation research is the synthesis of objective descriptive data and objective interview material. The Results section of the report should be separated from the Discussion and Conclusions. Results are raw data that are objective findings. Results should not be "flavored" by subjective analysis or "undone" by interpretations. The results should remain separate from critical analysis. Table 3–6 lists hypothetical data that would be included in a Results section.
7. The interpretative summary consists of a qualitative discussion of the results apart from the quantitative results. Qualitative or naturalistic information could include, for example, staff opportunities to innovate new programs, the informality of the communication process, the accessibility of administrators, the feelings of hope and optimism generated by the staff, the willingness of the agency to change the consumer with disabilities' involvement in treatment planning, the use of community resources, the integration of new technology with present methods, and the facilitation of professional growth through supervision.
8. The conclusions and recommendations of evaluation research are a vital part of

Table 3–6. Hypothetical Results of a Residential Treatment Program

Variable	Number	Percentage
1. Capacity of program	55	100
2. Average daily attendance of residents during last 6 months	50	90
3. Average length of residence for each individual discharged in last 6 months	3 months	
4. Number of individuals in residence for over 1 year	15	30
5. Number of direct care workers (treatment personnel)	10	
6. Number of full-time professional staff, excluding administrators	6	
7. Number of part-time consultants	3	
8. Number of full-time teachers	5	

the report. How does the research team decide that a treatment program is effective and should have continued support by the community, or that a treatment program is ineffective, not responsive to the needs of a community, and should be terminated?

During the last 30 years, we have seen the decline and closing of large, isolated institutions that served individuals with physical and psychiatric disabilities who mainly came from poor backgrounds. These institutions were closed because they became custodial "warehouses" without providing for the needs of the individuals. Nevertheless, when the institutions were supported by governmental agencies in the United States in the 1920s up until the 1960s, there were few alternatives for community-based treatment. Did evaluation research play a role in the closing of institutions during the 1960s and 1970s?

The criteria identified in evaluative research must be consistent with the needs of the target population. These needs relate to values in human society, such as economic independence, social relationships, educational development, self-esteem, and whatever else the research team or agency sets forth as the goals and objectives. It should be clear that if an agency is not meeting "stated needs" of those individuals who are treated, educated, or serviced and alternative agencies or facilities are available, then the community should not continue to support an institution's existence.

The following research models are *ex post facto* in nature: heuristic, correlational, clinical observation, survey, and historical. Clinical observation is unique in that it can be either ex post facto (retrospective) or prospective. The data collection procedure in ex post facto research is retrospective because the presumed independent variable has already occurred. Kerlinger (1986) differentiated experimental research and ex post facto research on the basis of the lack of direct control by the researcher in ex post facto designs. For example, in experimental research, the investigator hypothesizes "if X then Y" and manipulates the X. In ex post facto research, the investigator observes Y (the dependent variable) and hypothesizes X (the independent variable). The researcher in ex post facto designs can only presume a past cause-effect relationship. In many ex post facto designs, the investigator seeks historically to reconstruct cause-effect relationships.

Suchman (1967) identified several areas of potential abuse as listed below.

▶ **"Eyewash"** is an attempt to justify an ineffective program by deliberately selecting only those aspects that appear successful and overlooking important parts of the program.

▶ **"Whitewash"** is an effort whereby the evaluators try to cover up program failure and inadequacies by avoiding these areas when evaluating the program. The evaluators may solicit "testimonials" to divert attention from the general failure of the program.

▶ **"Submarine"** or **"torpedo"** is a device to destroy a program regardless of its worth or usefulness in delivering health services. This often occurs in administrative power struggles when opponents and their programs are attacked.

▶ **"Posture"** is used by evaluators when they want to appear scientific and objective when, in fact, they carry out a superficial and incomplete evaluation.

▶ **"Postponement"** is a tactic of using evaluation research, for example, to answer public reaction to scandalous conditions in an institution. The real purpose of this ploy is to defuse public outrage by substituting research for action.

▶ **"Substitution"** is an attempt to hide an essential part of a program that is an obvious failure and to shift emphasis to areas that are controversial.

From the foregoing examples, it is evident that evaluation research can serve not only to provide objective data, but also as a tactic to keep an inadequate program operative or to discredit an effective program.

An example of evaluation research in occupational therapy is found in Box 3–4. The authors of this research study evaluated the effectiveness of an occupational therapy program with older adults who were living in independent housing.

3.5 Heuristic Research

3.5.1 Purposes of Heuristic Research

Kerlinger (1986) described a heuristic view of science as that which "emphasizes theory and interconnected conceptual schemata that are fruitful for further research" (p. 8). The main purpose of heuristic research is to discover relationships between variables as a means of generating further investigations. In heuristic research, the researcher "fishes" for correlational relationships as a means to build a theory and design further research.

The researcher engaged in heuristic research seeks to discover significant relationships by correlating variables with a specific disease or factors affecting treatment. Research in cardiovascular diseases, learning disorders, mental illness, arthritis, multiple sclerosis, cancer, and AIDS are appropriate areas for heuristic research, as well as investigations of space, time, and cost factors in the treatment environment.

3.5.2 Application of Pilot Studies in Heuristic Research

Pilot studies are innovative studies that examine a problem or question to determine if the research is viable. These studies often have a small number of participants. The investigator does not control all of the extraneous variables. Limitations of the research methodology are identified. While pilot studies are carried out in other research designs, pilot studies in heuristic research require both an exploration of a theoretical basis and recommendations for further research.

The following list gives examples of pilot studies from occupational therapy, medicine, and special education that are heuristic:

▶ Allen, S., & Donald, M. (1995). The effect of occupational therapy on the motor

Box 3–4. Example of Evaluation Research

1. **Bibliographical Citation**

   Clark F., Azen, S. P., Zemke R., Jackson, J., Carlson, M., Mandel, D., Hay, J., Josephson, K., Cherry, B., Hessel, C., Palmer, J., Lipson, L. (1997). Occupational therapy for independent-living older adults. A randomized controlled trial. *The Journal of American Medical Association, 278,* 1321–1326.

2. **Abstract**

   CONTEXT: Preventive health programs may mitigate against the health risks of older adulthood. OBJECTIVE: To evaluate the effectiveness of preventive occupational therapy (OT) services specifically tailored for multiethnic, independent-living older adults. DESIGN: A randomized controlled trial.

   SETTING: Two government subsidized apartment complexes for independent-living older adults. SUBJECTS: A total of 361 culturally diverse volunteers aged 60 years or older.

   INTERVENTION: An OT group, a social activity control group, and a non-treatment control group. The period of treatment was 9 months.

   MAIN OUTCOME MEASURES: A battery of self-administered questionnaires designed to measure physical and social function, self-rated health, life satisfaction, and depressive symptoms.

   RESULTS: Benefit attributable to OT treatment was found for the quality of interaction scale on the Functional Status Questionnaire (P=.03), Life Satisfaction Index-Z (P=.03), Medical Outcomes Study Health Perception Survey (P=.05), and for 7 of 8 scales on the RAND 36-Item Health Status Survey, Short Form: bodily pain (P=.03), physical functioning (P=.008), role limitations attributable to health problems (P=.02), vitality (P=.004), social functioning (P=.05), role limitations attributable to emotional problems (P=.05), and general mental health (P=.02).

   CONCLUSIONS: Significant benefits for the OT preventive treatment group were found across various health, function, and quality-of-life domains. Because the control groups tended to decline over the study interval, our results suggest that preventive health programs based on OT may mitigate against the health risks of older adulthood. (Clark et al., 1997, p. 1321)

3. **Justification and Need for Study**

   Findings from the literature suggest that effective activity-based intervention are capable of enhancing the lives of elderly individuals. "In response to this need, we conducted between 1994 and 1996 a randomized controlled trial, the Well Elderly Study, to evaluate the effectiveness of preventative OT specifically targeted for urban, multiethnic, independent-living older adults" (p. 1321).

4. **Literature Review**

   The authors examined the literature on normative aging, activity-theory and aging, quality-of-life issues in aging, and the role of occupational therapy with the elderly. Forty-three references were used, selected from the following journals: *Social Indicators Research, Social Science in Medicine, AJOT, International Journal of Aging and Human Development, Journal of Gerontology and Psychological*

Science, Journal of Gerontology, Journal of Clinical Psychology, Journal of the American Medical Association, and *Research in Nursing Health.*

5. **Research Hypothesis or Guiding Questions**
"We hypothesized that mere participation in a social activity program does not affect the physical health, daily functioning, or psychosocial well-being of well elderly individuals; and compared with participation in a social activity program or an absence of any treatment, preventative OT positively affects the physical health, daily function, and psychosocial well-being of well elderly individuals (1-sided alternative)" (p. 1322).

6. **Methodology**
Three hundred sixty-one elderly adults, ages 60 and above, were assigned randomly to three groups: an occupational therapy group, a social activity group, and a no treatment group. Participants came from government subsidized housing for independent living, private homes, and other facilities in the community. In the occupational therapy group, participants were exposed to didactic teaching of community living and use of adapted equipment, and performed activities emphasizing grooming, nutrition exercising, and shopping. Those in the social activities group were involved in "community outings, craft projects, films, played games, and attended dances" (p. 1322). Five questionnaires were used to measure outcome.

7. **Operational Definition of Variables**
Functional status, life-satisfaction, depression, perceptions of health, and physical and mental health status were evaluated through self-report.

8. **Conclusions**
The occupational therapy program in general was more effective than the other two groups. "The OT program enabled subjects to construct daily routines that were health promoting and meaningful given the context of their lives" (p. 1325).

9. **Limitations of the Study**
"The results may not generalize to older adults in different living situations (e.g., single-family dwellers, nursing home residents) or of different socioeconomic status" (p. 1326).

10. **Major References in Study**
Fisher, B. J. (1995). Successful aging, life satisfaction and generativity in later life. *International Journal of Aging and Human Development, 41,* 239–250.
Carlson, M., Fanchiang, S-P., Zemke, R., & Clark, F. (1996). A meta-analysis of the effectiveness of occupational therapy for older persons. *The American Journal of Occupational Therapy, 50,* 89–98.
Larson, K. O., Stevens-Ratchford, R. G., Pedretti, L. W., Crabtree, J. L. (1996). *ROTE: The role of occupational therapy with the elderly.* Bethesda, MD: American Occupational Therapy Association.
Levine, R. E., & Gitlan, L. N. (1992). A model to promote activity competence in elders. *The American Journal of Occupational Therapy, 47,* 147–153.

proficiency of children with motor/ learning difficulties: A pilot study. *British Journal of Occupational Therapy, 58,* 385–391.

▶ Cutler, S. K. (1992). *Executive functioning in middle school students who have learning disabilities.* Unpublished doctoral dissertation. University of New Mexico, Albuquerque.

▶ Dunn, W. (1990). A comparison of service provision models in school-based occupational therapy services: A pilot study. *Occupational Therapy Journal of Research, 10,* 300–320.

▶ Hoppes, S. (1997). Can play increase standing tolerance? A pilot-study. *Physical and Occupational Therapy in Geriatrics, 15,* 65–73.

▶ Lo, J., & Zemke, R. (1997). The relationship between affective experiences during daily occupations and subjective well-being measures: A pilot study. *Occupational Therapy in Mental Health, 13,* 1–21.

▶ Prince, F., Winter, D. A., Sjonnensen, G., Powell, C., Wheeldon, R. K. (1998). Mechanical efficiency during gait of adults with transtibial amputation: A pilot study comparing the SACH, Seattle, and Golden-Ankle. *Journal of Rehabilitation Research and Development, 35,* 177–185.

▶ Reid, D. T., & Jutai, J. (1997). A pilot study of perceived clinical usefulness of a new computer-based tool for assessment of visual perception in occupational therapy practice. *Occupational Therapy International, 4,* 81–98.

▶ Seidman, L. J., Biederman, J., Faraone, S. V., Weber, W., Mennin, D., & Jones, J. (1997). A pilot study of neuropsychological function in girls with ADHD. *Journal of the American Academic of Child and Adolescent Psychiatry, 36,* 366–373.

▶ Stefanyshyn, D. J., Engsberg, J. R., Tedford, K. G., & Harder, J. A. (1994). A pilot study to test the influence of specific prosthetic features in preventing transtibial amputees from walking like able-bodied subjects. *Prosthetics and Orthotics International, 18,* 180–190.

3.5.3 Assumptions Underlying Heuristic Research

In engaging in heuristic research, the investigator:

▶ seeks to discover statistically significant relationships between variables
▶ seeks data for theory building; the result of research provides the basis for theoretical formulations
▶ uses deductive methods to analyze a research problem
▶ analyzes a research problem retrospectively; that is, the researcher starts with the presumed effect (dependent variable) and works back to the presumed causative factors (independent variables)
▶ understands that results derived from heuristic research are not conclusive, implying that further investigation using prospective research is needed to substantiate cause-effect relationships

3.5.4 Method of Heuristic Research

The use of factor analytic studies with computer technology enables an investigator to correlate many variables and to systematically analyze interactional patterns. This method is especially appropriate in analyzing psychophysiological illnesses where there are a combination of presumed causative factors rather than a single etiological factor. Warren Weaver (1947) characterized research in the 17th, 18th, and 19th centuries as typifying the era of the two-variable problems in simplicity. In medicine during the early part of the 20th century, a single etiological factor was correlated with the effects of disease (two-variable research). Today, however, both modern medical research and social sciences research are engaged in investigating complex health problems that involve multiple causes. For example, drug addiction, mental retardation, arteriosclerosis, Alzheimer's disease, and dyslexia have multiple causes. An application of a two-variable model, where the investigator searches for the single cause of the disease, is inadequate in biopsychosocial research. On the other hand, heuristic research lends itself to the study of multiple factors that are interactive in nature. The Framingham studies of heart disease (Dawber, Meaders, & Moore, 1951) are an example of heuristic research. The strategy involved in these studies was to identify numerous risk factors that are significantly more frequent in patients with heart disease than in the normal population. The purposes of heuristic research are diagramed in Figure 3–13.

3.5.5 Identification of Correlating Factors

In heuristic research, the investigator seeks to derive the major factors that correlate

significantly to assess their relative importance. Descriptive and inferential statistics, as well as multiple regression, factor analysis, and path analysis are appropriate for analyzing the relative significance of factors that are important in generating further research.

A major problem in this research model is in the selection of a diagnostic group. It is critical that screening criteria be used in selecting a research sample. The researcher cannot assume that a patient's diagnosis is accurate. There is much controversy in the diagnosis of chronic illnesses such as asthma, schizophrenia, arthritis, fetal alcohol syndrome (FAS), and failure to thrive that requires the investigator to use rigorous methods for operationalizing diagnostic categories. After the investigator has developed

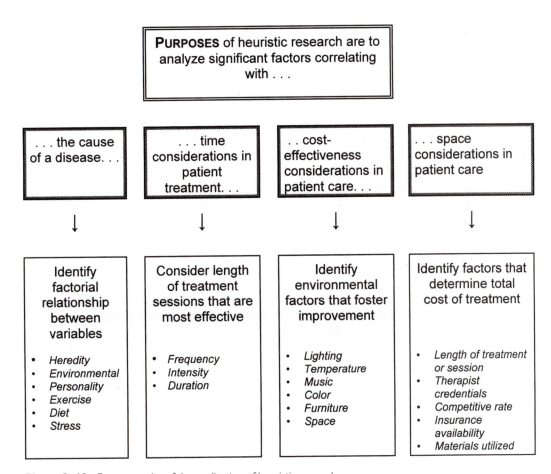

Figure 3–13. Four examples of the application of heuristic research.

and refined the screening criteria for subject selection, the next problem is to select a population of subjects that will be the source for a representative sample.

Parallel to the process of subject selection is the compiling of investigative variables. These variables are derived by analyzing the following areas:

▶ *Demographic:* age, gender, occupation, educational level, marital status, income
▶ *Psychosocial:* personality, intelligence, attitude, lifestyle
▶ *Biochemical:* physiological, somatotype, nutritional, genetic

3.5.6 Interactional Effects in Heuristic Research

Heuristic research requires the investigator to make an exhaustive search for variables that can potentially contribute to the onset of a disease. It is necessary for the investigator to take a holistic view of the problem of etiology so as to avoid the trap of two-variable research that lacks an analysis of interactional effects. As an example, let us suppose hypothetically that schizophrenia is a result of the interactional effects of genetics; child development; and lack of competence in educational, vocational, or social areas. In studying the exclusive relationship between genetics and schizophrenia, a researcher will have mixed results because other major factors have not been taken into

account. Results cannot be generalized to all patients with schizophrenia. Figure 3–14 illustrates hypothetically the interaction between the three independent variables (genetics, child development, and competence) and the dependent variable (diagnosis of schizophrenia).

The diagram shows that those individuals who have effective parenting and educational and vocational competence are the least likely to develop schizophrenia, even if they have a genetic vulnerability factor. Schizophrenia results only through the interaction of three variables: genetic, parental, and educational-vocational competence.

This hypothetical example shows the complexity of factorial designs that test the interactional effects of multiple causes. It is highly probable that many chronic illnesses result from this type of interactional pattern. Nonetheless, only through rigorous, painstaking research will it be possible to identify interactional effects. Heuristic research provides the framework to investigate multiple factors in the development of a disease process.

3.5.7 Analysis of Time Factors in Client Treatment

What are the determining factors in planning treatment time for patients? Why is 1 hour a week sufficient for some clients while 2 hours a week are prescribed for others? What proportion of treatment time

	Adequate Educational-Vocational Skills	**Inadequate Educational-Vocational Skills**
Effective Parenting	*Lowest Schizophrenic Risk*	
Ineffective Parenting		*Highest Schizophrenic Risk*

Figure 3–14. Interaction between independent and dependent variables in the risk of developing schizophrenia. An explanation of the development of schizophrenia must take into account all major variables, not just a single variable.

is a function of pragmatic issues, such as the availability of a therapist? What consideration for time is given to the physical and emotional needs of the client? How is treatment time planned for client groups? All of these questions are suitable for research analysis. In general, only a few studies have analyzed time factors in patient care (Clifton & Burcham, 1997; Lang, 1998). Yet time is one of the most basic factors in clinical treatment. An analysis of the factors considered in determining the length of time for treatments should consider both the ideal factors and pragmatic issues (Table 3–7).

3.5.8 Analysis of Cost Effectiveness Factors in Treatment

What are the real economic costs for treatment? What does it cost to treat a patient in a hospital compared with the treatment in an outpatient clinic? What are the costs for direct patient care by professionals as compared with nonprofessional health technicians trained for specific health purposes? What is the cost of a massive public health prevention program compared with existing costs for treating a specific disability group? What factors are considered in determining fees for health services? How are salaries for health workers determined? What is the economic worth of a health professional? These questions are typical of the pressing economic problems facing industrialized and developing countries where the demand for health care far outreaches the resources

that countries can allocate for prevention and treatment. If a society is to determine rationally how its economic resources can be used most effectively for implementation, then it must examine objectively the underlying factors affecting the costs of health care (Blumstein, 1997; Timpka, Leijon, Karlsson, Svensson, & Bjurulf, 1997).

3.5.9 Analysis of Space Factors in Patient Care

As with time and cost, space has received little attention from clinical researchers. Ethnologists and social anthropologists (e.g., Hall, 1966) analyzed the effect of space in animal behavior and health. There are a few studies that suggest a direct relationship between life space and psychological reactions (Crump, 1997; Hewitt, 1997).

In psychiatry it has been evident that space affects a client's emotions and behavioral patterns. Goffman (1961) described the syndrome of passivity and depersonalization as being the result of institutionalization. A contemporary definition of space is not limited to the traditional 19th century view that space represents *area*. Since Einstein's theory of relativity, space has taken on new meaning, implying in conceptual terms that space is the distance between two events. Space involves events, occurrences, or movement. An individual's space represents the potential area for movement. In this concept of space, factors related to increasing or diminishing space are appropriate. Hospitalization, imprisonment, and institutionalization are situations

Table 3–7. Analysis of Time Factors in Treatment

Ideal	*Pragmatic*
1. Time needed for application of treatment method: dependent on the client's treatment goals	1. Number of patients under care in proportion to the number of hours allocated for treatment (client load)
2. Time needed to meet short-term objectives or goals	2. Traditional practices (therapy schedules)
3. Time needed for preparation and progress notes	3. Third-party reimbursement for service (insurance)

in which the patient, prisoner, or inmate are deprived of space and consequently has fewer movements and events. In treating a patient, what considerations are given to space? Are wards or private rooms considered on any other basis than economic? Do groups occupying space limit the number of events or increase the movement of patients? Questions involving space are invariably linked to issues of group versus individual treatment. What is the relationship between the number of clients in a group, the area of movement, and the events taking place in a group? Issues related to the size of client groups in occupational therapy clinics involve space factors.

A researcher employing a heuristic research model seeks to discover underlying factors affecting space. For example, how would a researcher analyze the problem of determining the space needs of geriatric clients in a nursing home? Figure 3–15 illustrates this example. The first step is to define operationally the space of geriatric clients.

The next step is to discover the physical, psychological, and social needs of geriatric clients. A review of the literature and a survey of existing programs would provide the data. Maslow's (1954) theory of a hierarchy of needs and Havighurst's (1952) activity theory could be applied to an analysis of psychological and emotional needs. Theories of aging and health could provide the framework for setting physical and health goals.

The third step in the research process is to integrate the data derived from analyzing space factors in a nursing home with biopsychosocial needs. This is illustrated in Figure 3–16.

The goals of heuristic research in this example are to

▶ discover the factors comprising space in a nursing home
▶ analyze the effects of these factors in psychological adjustment, social relationships, and physical health maintenance
▶ identify in the literature the needs of the aged
▶ integrate space factors with need theory

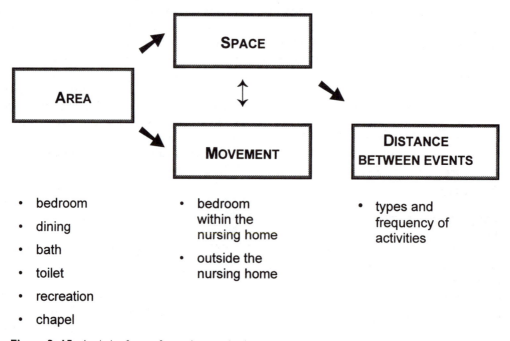

Figure 3–15. Analysis of space factors in a nursing home.

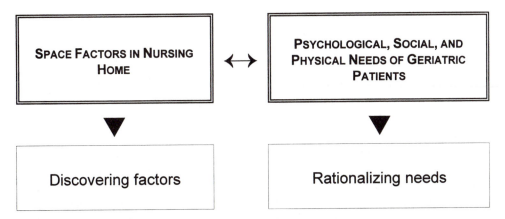

Figure 3–16. Integration of data with need theory. In this example, the data obtained from analyzing space factors in the nursing home with the needs of elderly patients (obtained through a literature review) is integrated.

The reader may be puzzled with the example in Figure 3–16. How, the reader may ask, does the heuristic researcher know that he or she has identified all the factors related to space and all the needs of geriatric patients? The answer is that researchers cannot conclude that the data collection is complete. Heuristic research is a method of discovery, and research in general is an ongoing process that functions as a feedback loop. As more information is gathered, analyzed, and integrated with previous data, the researcher comes closer to solving questions. Box 3–5 gives an example of heuristic research.

3.6 Correlational Research

3.6.1 Purposes of Correlational Research

Many studies published in occupational therapy are primarily correlational and retrospective. This research is analogous to experimental research in that the investigator tests a hypothesis. Unlike the experimental researcher, however, the investigator does not manipulate independent variables, nor does he or she simulate a cause-effect relationship. In correlational research, the investigator compares the relationships between variables by measuring differences. It is applied frequently to areas in the social sciences because the very nature of the problem limits the experimenter from inducing causal effects. If, for example, a researcher's purpose is to correlate characteristics in the individual who is alcoholic with causative factors, then he or she is limited to an ex post facto design where it is not possible to induce experimentally the onset of alcoholism. The researcher in this example is limited to a retrospective analysis of the assumed causes of alcoholism. Kerlinger (1986), in discussing the value of nonexperimental research, concluded that "social, scientific, and educational problems do not lend themselves to experimentation, although many of them do lend themselves to controlled inquiry of the nonexperimental kind" (p. 359).

A sequential analysis of correlational research is diagramed in Figure 3–17. These steps are reviewed in the section below.

3.6.2 Identification of Research Variables

As clinicians in the health fields, we are all concerned with the question of etiology. Why did this patient become schizophrenic? Why did this individual develop learning

BOX 3–5. EXAMPLE OF HEURISTIC RESEARCH

1. **Bibliographical Notation**
   Tona, J. L., & Schneck, C. M. (1993). The efficacy of upper extremity inhibitive casting: A single-subject pilot study. *American Journal of Occupational Therapy, 47,* 901–910,

2. **Abstract**
   This pilot study was designed to examine the effects of short-term (48-hr) upper extremity inhibitive casting, with an encased thermoplastic splint, on problems related to upper motor neuron damage. The subject was an 8½-year-old girl with left upper extremity spasticity. Three different measures were used: (a) rating of videotaped active movements of the child; (b) the Modified Ashworth Scale, a clinical measure of spasticity; and (c) The Biodex System, a measure of torque during passive elbow flexion and extension. After cast removal, subjective improvements were noted in the quality of active movement (through videotapes) and increased awareness and use of the casted hand by the child (through parents' reports). A trend toward decreased spasticity was demonstrated by the Modified Ashworth Scale and a statistically significant decrease in resistance to passive movement was shown by the Biodex recordings. However, this reduction in symptoms was temporary, lasting less than 3 days. The results of this study suggest that short-term inhibitory casting may prove efficacious in the treatment of the child with cerebral palsy, although further research is needed. (p. 901)

3. **Justification and Need for Study**
   The investigators stated, "Although several splints fabricated from thermoplastic materials have been identified in the literature as having tone-reducing effects on the upper extremity, the use of thermoplastic inhibitive splints encased within a plaster case has not been studied (p. 903).

4. **Literature Review**
   Fifty references were cited in the study. Articles came from a wide variety of journals, such as *American Journal of Occupational Therapy, Physical Therapy, Journal of Neurology, Neurosurgery and Psychiatry, Developmental Medicine and Child Neurology, Physical and Occupational Therapy in Pediatrics, Archives of Physical Medicine and Rehabilitation*, and *Canadian Journal of Occupational Therapy.* The majority of articles cited were published during the 1980s and 1990s.

5. **Research Hypothesis or Guiding Questions**
   The investigators hypothesized that "an upper extremity cast with an encased thermoplastic inhibitive splint when worn for a short period of time" (p. 903) would decrease spasticity in a child with cerebral palsy.

6. **Theoretical Assumptions**
   a. "Spasticity is defined as 'greater than normal resistance to externally imposed movements and this resistance increases with both movement amplitude and velocity' (Powers, Marder-Meyer, & Rymer, 1988, p. 115)" (p. 901).

    b. Inhibiting casting theoretically can decrease spasticity, but "The exact mechanism of spasticity reducing in casting is not known" (p. 902).

    c. "Serial casting procedures are based on the biomechanics of muscle length" (p. 902).

7. **Methodology**

An 8-year-old girl with cerebral palsy with spasticity in both lower extremities and in the left upper extremity paired with a control subject (8-year-old girl without pathology). The study was conducted over an 11-day period.

8. **Results**

"The study demonstrated that casting the upper extremity of a child with cerebral palsy for a short time did produce a statistically significant decrease in objectively measured positive symptoms of, as well as a decrease in subjectively rated positive symptoms of, UNM syndrome. Furthermore, it demonstrated that the reduction was temporary" (p. 907).

9. **Limitations of the Study**

"The main limitations of this study were a lack of interrater reliability in the videotape assessment, and insensitivity of the Biodex system to [measure] small changes in resistance" (p. 908).

10. **Recommendations for Further Research**

    a. Replication using "multiple subjects in a single-subject design" (p. 908)

    b. "Related efficacy studies using the Biodex system for spasticity measurement" (p. 908)

    c. Additional studies that "control for the amount of strength on the spastic muscle each testing day by setting consistent range of motion limits" (p. 908)

    d. "Effects of wearing a bivalved cast periodically throughout the day" (p. 908)

    e. "Effect of casting on abnormal motor patterns and whether periodic bivalved cast usage allows for greater relaxation of the limb and more efficacious learning the active motor movement" (p. 908)

    f. Study of changes in cast fabrication to "encase a long (forearm) cone splint or resting splint, to control for wrist extension and allow for easier cast application (p. 908).

11. **Major References Cited in the Study**

Bohannon, R. (1987). Inhibitive casting for cerebral-palsied children. *Developmental Medicine and Child Neurology, 29,* 122–123.

Feldman, P. A. (1990). Upper extremity casting and splinting. In M. D. Glenn & J. Whyte (Eds.), *The practical management of spasticity in children and adults.* Malvern, PA: Lea & Febiger.

Powers, R. K., Marder-Meyer, J., & Rymer, W. Z. (1988). Quantitative relations between hypertonia and stretch reflex threshold in spastic hemiparesis. *Annals of Neurology, 23,* 115–124.

Yasakawa, A. (1990). Case report—Upper extremity casting: Adjunct treatment for a child with cerebral palsy hemiplegia. *American Journal of Occupational Therapy, 44,* 840–846.

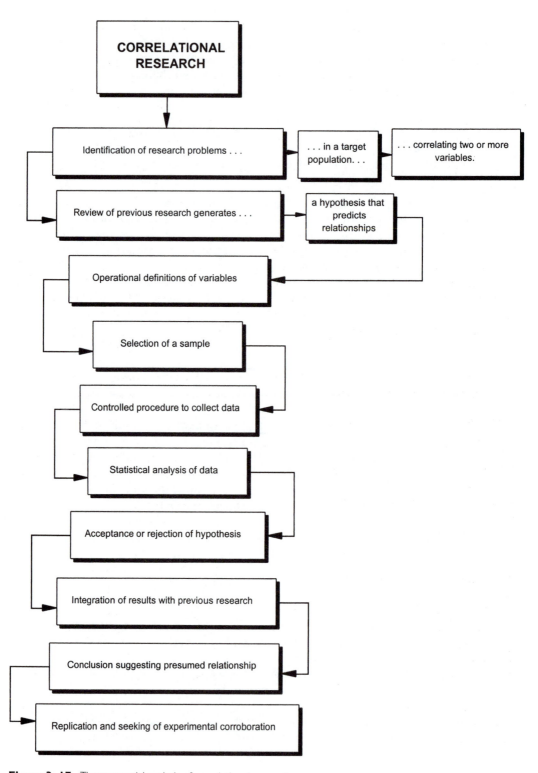

Figure 3–17. The sequential analysis of correlational research.

problems? What factors led to arthritis? What environmental factors contributed to juvenile delinquency? These questions regarding etiology and relationships between variables are feasible for correlational research.

The first step in correlational research is to identify the variables in a target population to be studied. These variables are presumed causative factors and may be genetic, neurophysiological, psychosocial, or cultural. The variables are identified from clinical observations, by examining previous studies or theoretical papers, or through deductive reasoning. The presumed independent variables and presumed dependent variables are identified. Because the researcher does not actively induce the independent variables, an associational or statistical relationship can only be assumed.

3.6.3 Formulating Hypotheses in Correlational Research

The researcher formulates an hypothesis after reviewing the related literature. The hypothesis can be directional, that is, predicting a significant positive or negative relationship between two variables. For example, the researcher predicts that there is an increase of abnormal reflexes in children with cerebral palsy compared with typical children. An hypothesis stated in a null form predicts no significant relationship. For example, the null hypothesis may be stated as, "There is no statistically significant difference between the presence of abnormal reflexes in children with cerebral palsy compared with typical children." The decision whether to formulate a directional hypothesis or null hypothesis is based on direct or implied evidence from previous research.

Other examples of directional hypotheses in correlational research are as follows:

▶ Individuals who are blind have a significantly greater kinesthetic ability than individuals with normal vision.

▶ Individuals with mental retardation educated in an inclusive setting will show higher self-concept than those educated in a self-contained program.

▶ Carpal tunnel syndrome occurs more frequently among individuals using a computer for 6 or more hours daily when compared with individuals using a computer for less than 4 hours daily.

▶ Children from dysfunctional, low-income families have better visual perceptual abilities than auditory processing abilities.

▶ There is a higher percentage of cancer among asbestos workers than in the population at large.

In all of the foregoing examples of directional hypotheses, the variables are associated with a target population. Analyzing the hypotheses one by one, we find the relationships shown in Table 3–8.

In the foregoing hypotheses, variables and populations are compared. Hypotheses can test the effects of multiple variables in one population or, conversely, the differences among multiple populations on one variable. A researcher cannot test multiple variables in multiple populations in one hypothesis. For example, it is fallacious to offer a hypothesis such as the following: High cholesterol level and hypertension are more prevalent among cardiac patients than among a normal population. Each variable, high cholesterol level and hypertension, should be stated in a separate hypothesis.

In stating a null hypothesis, the investigator states that there will be no statistically significant relationship between two variables. For example, a null hypothesis can be stated in the following way: There is no statistically significant relationship between smoking and heart disease. The decision whether to state a hypothesis in a directional form or as a null hypothesis should be an outcome of the literature review. If previous studies indicate directionality, then the researcher should state a directional hypothesis. On the other hand, if the researcher finds no evidence for a

Table 3–8. Associational Relationships Between Variables

Variables	Populations
Kinesthetic ability	Blind Normal vision
Self-concept	Children with mental retardation in inclusive settings Children with mental retardation in self-contained settings
Carpal tunnel syndrome	Computer operators using the computer 6 or more hours a day Clerical workers using the computer less than 4 hours a day
Visual-motor perception	Children from low-income, dysfunctional families
Auditory processing	
Cancer	Asbestos workers Typical individuals

directional hypothesis in a review of the literature, then a null hypothesis should be stated. The form in which the hypothesis is stated has implications when analyzing the data statistically. For those readers without statistical background, it will suffice to say that when a researcher is comparing statistically significant differences between two variables with a *t* test, a null hypothesis usually indicates a two-tail test of significance, and a directional hypothesis usually indicates a one-tail test of significance.

3.6.4 Operational Definitions of Variables

Before a hypothesis can be tested, the investigator must operationally define the variables stated in the hypothesis. The operational definition includes the specific test or procedure used in measuring a variable. For example, if an investigator is measuring self-concept, then a test such as *The Way I Feel About Myself: The Piers-Harris Self-Concept Scale* (Piers & Harris, 1984) might be indicated as the operational measure.

3.6.5 Selection of Sample

Screening criteria is necessary when selecting a sample. It is not sufficient simply to state that patients with diabetes or epilepsy will be compared with a typical population. The investigator must indicate how the patients have been diagnosed, the severity of the illness considered, and other demographics identifying the population such as age, gender, occupation, socioeconomic status, education, and geographical area. The screening criteria devised by the investigator serve as a reference point in generalizing the results to a population. Universality and external validity depend on the screening criteria devised for subject selection.

3.6.6 Data Collection Procedure

Can the test procedure be replicated? Has the investigator tried to reduce factors such as subject fatigue, anxiety, extraneous distractions, lack of cooperation, and any other factors that threaten the internal validity of the investigation? The test procedure should be described in detail by the investigator, including the time of day when the subjects are tested, the number in the group, the environmental conditions, the length of time for testing each subject, and the sequence in presenting the operational measures.

3.6.7 Interpretation of Results

In general, research has a cumulative effect. Usually, the results of one study are not sufficient to be conclusive. Many factors affect the results in correlational research that are not directly controlled by the investigator. These limitations affecting internal validity do not negate correlational research. The advantages of correlational research are that investigations can be easily replicated and subjects can be easily tested. Before an investigator proposes a conclusion based on the results of one study, he or she must integrate the results with previous research. If the results are contradictory, then perhaps further research is indicated. If the results are consistent with previous literature, then it may be valid to suggest that conclusive evidence has been found. There is a need in research to be conservative rather than premature.

An example of correlational research is found in Box 3–6.

3.7 Survey Research

3.7.1 Definition of Survey Research

Survey research, as defined in this text, is the descriptive study of populations. The main purpose of survey research is to obtain accurate objective descriptions about a specific universe of people or entities, such as a group of individuals with disabilities or the curriculum requirements in occupational therapy. The major task of the survey researcher is to obtain reliable and valid data from a representative sample of a population. In some cases, the researcher will be able to survey the total population or universe without relying on a representative sample.

3.7.2 Purposes of Survey Research

Health, social, and educational planners use descriptive survey research as the basis for needs assessment for developing health strategies, programs, and physical plants. The changing needs of populations as derived from surveys can contribute to the planning of health centers, inclusion practices for individuals with disabilities, allied health training programs, community mental health centers, and adult day care centers. Survey research should play an essential part in assessing the needs of a population where the planning of services is involved.

Along with community planning, survey research is an important tool for learning about the general attitudes of people. Many studies are sponsored by governmental agencies and legislators to solicit general opinion on topics such as national health insurance, malpractice in health, legalization of abortion, ethics in research, inclusion of individuals with disabilities in educational and community settings, and other controversial issues where majority opinion is used to formulate national policy and to guide the enactment of laws.

Survey research need not be limited to questioning individuals. Methodologies in survey research assessing the physical characteristics of groups are also applicable. Recently, governmental grants in health research have funded studies that screen a population for the presence of a disability. School populations are screened for deficits in hearing and vision acuity. Diabetes tests, chest X-Rays to detect tuberculosis and lung cancer, cardiovascular screening utilizing blood cholesterol counts, blood pressure measurements, and testing for HIV are some of the examples of survey research utilizing physical measurements to screen for health defects in large populations. Public health agencies use survey research as a means of identifying trends in the incidence of diseases and health problems. The information comprising the survey data is obtained from physicians, hospitals, clinics, and other health agencies that compile disease statistics. Table 3–9 from the *Morbidity and Mortality Weekly Report* is an example of epidemiological statistics, that

Box 3–6. Example of Correlational Research

1. **Bibliographical Notation**
   Keller, S., & Hayes, R. (1997). The relationship between the Allen Cognitive Level Test and the Life Skills Profile. *The American Journal of Occupational Therapy, 52,* 851–856.

2. **Abstract**
   OBJECTIVES. The purpose of this study was to further evaluate the validity of the Allen Cognitive Level Test (ACL-90) as a measure of the construct of "adaptive functioning" and to determine its effectiveness in discriminating between persons who live in the community and persons who are institutionalized.
   METHOD. Forty-one persons with schizophrenia living in the community and 17 persons with schizophrenia living in a long-term psychiatric hospital were assessed with the ACL-90 and the Life Skills Profile (LSP). Scores on the two measures were compared, as was the effectiveness of the two measures in discriminating between the participant groups.
   RESULTS. The ACL-90 scores correlated moderately with the LSP total, $r(56)=.54$, $p<.01$, and Self-Care Subscale, $r(56)=>53$, $p<.01$. Only the Nonturbulence subscale of the LSP discriminated between the community and institutionalized participant groups. The behavior of the participants living in the community was less turbulent than that of the participants who were institutionalized, $F(1,54)=15.24$, $p<.001$.
   CONCLUSION. Although the moderate correlations between the ACL-90 and the LSP measures support the ACL as a measure of adaptive functioning and reflect its theoretical perspective, additional information is needed to predict the community functioning and support needs of persons with schizophrenia. (p. 851)

3. **Justification and Need for Study**
   The investigators evaluated "aspects of the psychometric properties of the ACL to help clarify whether it reliably measures adaptive functioning" (p. 851).

4. **Literature Review**
   Thirty-one references were cited in the study. Articles came from a wide variety of journals, such as *Journal of Clinical Psychiatry, Perspectives in Psychiatric Care, Hospital and Community Psychiatry, Australian Occupational Therapy Journal, Australian and New Zealand Journal of Psychiatry, American Journal of Occupational Therapy, Occupational Therapy in Mental Health,* and *Schizophrenia Bulletin.* The majority of articles cited were published during the 1980s and 1990s.

5. **Research Hypothesis or Guiding Questions**
   The authors "hypothesized that persons with schizophrenia who obtain low scores on measures of adaptive functioning are more likely to be living in long-term institutional care than are persons with schizophrenia who obtain high scores on the same measures" (p. 852).

6. **Methodology**
   a. Seventeen adults from a long-term residential psychiatric hospital and forty-one adults from a community psychiatric rehabilitation unit participated in the study. Ages ranged from 20 to 57 years old. All participants

were receiving mediation; all were stable on the medication; and all had some form of schizophrenia.

    b. The ACL-90 and the Life Skills Profile (LSP) were administered in random order. The LSP rater was the primary caregiver for each participants.

7. Results

    a. The ACL correlated moderately with the LSP ($r = .54$).

    b. "Participants living in the community demonstrated considerably less turbulent behavior than did participants living in the hospital" (p. 854).

8. Conclusions

The authors concluded that "additional information is needed to predict the community functioning and support needs of persons with schizophrenia" (p. 851).

9. Limitations of the Study

    a. Unequal groups without randomization may have influenced the outcome.

    b. "Some of the difference is due to discrepancies in raters' scoring of the measures or to rater error, particularly for the LDP, which was rated by a different rater for each participant" (p. 854).

10. Sample of References Cited in the Study

Allen, C. K. (1992). Cognitive disabilities. In N. Katz (Ed.), *Cognitive rehabilitation: Models for intervention in occupational therapy* (pp. 1–21). Boston: Andover Medical.

Parker, G., & Hadzi-Pavlovic, D. (1995). The capacity of a measure of disability (the LSP) to predict hospital readmission in those with schizophrenia. *Psychological Medicine, 25,* 157–163.

Penny, N. H., Mueser, K. T., & North, C. T. (1995). The Allen Cognitive Level test and social competence in adult psychiatric patients. *American Journal of Occupational Therapy, 49,* 420–427.

Velligan, D. I., True, J. E., Lefton, R. S., Moore, T. C., & Flores, C. V. (1995). Validity of the Allen Cognitive Levels assessment: A tri-ethnic comparison. *Psychiatry Research, 56,* 101–109.

is, data showing cases of specified notifiable diseases in the United States.

3.7.3 Statement of Problem in Survey Research

The first step in survey research is to state the problem in question form. The problem should be researchable, requiring measurable data that can be collected and analyzed. In stating a problem in survey research, the investigator must operationally define the population to be surveyed in terms of geographical area and demographic characteristics, such as age, gender, socioeconomic level, education, and marital status. The identified population must be rigorously defined, otherwise there can be confusion in the *external validity* or in generalizing the results from the representative sample to the larger population. This, of course, is not a problem when the total population is surveyed. The following are hypothetical questions related to survey research:

▶ What is the present occupational status of clients who have been discharged

Table 3–9. Summary Cases of Specified Notifiable Diseases, United States, 1997

Disease	Cumulative Number
Acquired Immunodeficiency Syndrome	58,492
Botulism	132
Brucellosis	98
Chancroid	243
Chlamydia	526,671
Cholera	6
Cryptosporidiosis	2,566
Diphtheria	4
E. coli	2,555
Gonorrhea	324,907
Haemophilus influenzae (invasive disease)	1,162
Hansen disease (leprosy)	122
Hepatitis A	30,021
Hepatitis B	10,416
Hepatitis C	3,816
Legionellosis	1,163
Lyme disease	12,801
Malaria	2,001
Measles (rubeola)	138
Meningococcal disease	3,308
Mumps	683
Pertussis (whooping cough)	6,564
Plague	4
Poliomyelitis, paralytic	3
Psittacosis	33
Rabies, animal	8,105
Rabies, human	2
Rocky Mountain spotted fever	409
Rubella (German measles)	181
Rubella (congenital syndrome)	5
Salmonellosis	41,901
Shigellosis	23,117
Syphilis, total all stages	46,540
Syphilis, primary and secondary	8,550
Syphilis, congenital, age < 1 year	1,049
Tetanus	50
Toxic shock syndrome	157
Trichinosis	13
Tuberculosis	19,851
Typhoid fever	365
Varicella (chickenpox)	98,727

Note: Data from the *Morbidity and Mortality Weekly Report*, p. 20, by the Centers for Disease Control and Prevention, National Center for Health Statistics, 11/20/98. Data are cumulative through the week ending December 31, 1997 (52nd week). Available: http://www2.cdc.gov/mmwr/mmwr_wk.html or ftp://ftp.cdc.gov/pub/Publications/mmwr/wk/mm4654.pdf[1999, October 2].

from a supported employment program where they had been for a least 1 year?

▶ What are the minimal competencies required in different programs for teacher preparation in special education?

▶ What rehabilitation services do individuals with spinal cord injuries perceive as the most important?

▶ What are the socioeconomic characteristics of individuals using community mental health centers?

▶ What are the cholesterol levels of sedentary office workers?

▶ How are service dogs used by occupational therapists as adjunctive therapy?

▶ What are the specific treatment techniques that occupational therapists use in working with clients with AIDS?

▶ What methods are used for teaching reading in resource rooms?

3.7.4 Survey Research Methodology

After identifying a researchable problem, the target population, and the variables to be measured in the sample, the investigator formulates the procedure for collecting data and the measuring instruments. Sampling procedures (discussed in more detail in Chapter 7) should be objective and unbiased and provide a true description of the population. Random sampling, where the investigator selects a sample out of the total population, is the best method to achieve an unbiased, representative sample. The external validity of the results are, of course, increased as the percentage of the population sampled increases. For example, a random sample of 50% of the population will be more accurate than a random sample of 30% of the population. Use of stratified samples also increases the external validity. In a stratified sample, the sample is divided into strata, such as gender, age, diagnostic, or SES groups. Of course, the determination of how large a sample to include in a survey is many times based on practical considerations, such as the cost of the survey and the time allocated to the research project.

The principle methods for collecting data in survey research are the personal interview, mail (regular or E-mail), and telephone. Table 3–10 lists the relative merits of these three procedures.

3.7.5 Selection of Questionnaire

In selecting a measuring instrument for data collection, the survey researcher often is found in the position of devising a self-made questionnaire. Whether the questionnaire is custom-designed for a study or has already been published, the researcher must account for the reliability and validity of the instrument. Before the investigator devises the instrument, a thorough search of published questionnaires should be undertaken. The latest edition of *Buros' Mental Measurements Yearbook* (Conoley & Impara, 1995; http://www.unl.edu/buros/catalog.html#mmy), ERIC database for assessment and evaluation (http://ericae.net/aesearch.htm or http://ericae.net/scripts/ewiz/amain2.asp), other compendiums of tests and questionnaires, and abstracting journals are excellent sources for locating specific instruments for a study.

Surveys involving the measurement of physical variables in human research are also dependent on the reliability and validity of the instruments used. Procedures are employed for increasing the validity of a subject's response, such as taking three blood pressure readings or two different grip strength readings. Usually, the instruments used in collecting data are reliable and valid, such as the X-Ray, electrocardiogram, and blood typing, but sometimes, because of subject anxiety or variability caused by external circumstances, one test result can be inaccurate. Figure 3–18 describes the sequential steps in undertaking survey research.

3.7.6 Constructing a Questionnaire in Survey Research

The questionnaire is the most commonly used and most frequently self-devised

Table 3–10. Relative Merits of the Principal Survey Methods.

Personal Interview	Mail	Telephone
Advantages		
• Most flexible means of obtaining data because questions can be elaborated upon or revised during the interview • Open-ended questions are possible • Accountability of the respondent is increased • Nonverbal cues can be observed • Lack of response generally very low • Equalize the types of subjects (e.g., men vs. women) • Establishment of rapport may increase validity and reliability of the response	• Wider and more representative distribution of sample possible • No field staff • Cost per questionnaire relatively low • People may be more frank on certain issues (e.g., sex) • No interviewer bias; answers in respondent's own words • Respondent can answer at leisure; has time to "think things over" • Certain segments of population more easily approachable	• Cost per response relatively low • Control over interviewer bias easier; supervisor can be present at interview • Quick way of obtaining data • Flexibility possible by elaborating or revising questions • Current lists of telephone numbers easily obtained
Disadvantages		
• Likely to be most expensive of all methods • Training the interviewer is required • Dangers of interviewer bias that may result in skewed results (Halo or devil effect) • Scheduling • Time required for obtaining data	• Bias due to poor response rate (e.g., < 30%) • Control over who answers the questionnaire may be lost • Interpretation of omissions to questions may be difficult • Cost per return may be high if the response rate is poor • Open-ended questions may result in poorer response rate or difficulty interpreting • Only those interested in subject may reply • Certain segments of population are not available (e.g., those without E-mail) • Likely to be slowest response time of all	• Shortened interviews because of time • Questions must be short and to the point • Open-ended questions usually avoided because of possibility of misinterpretation • Certain types of questions cannot be used (e.g., visual material) • Certain segments of population are not available (e.g., those without telephones)

Source: Adapted from *Research Methods in Economics and Business* by R. Ferber and P. J. Verdoorn, 1962 (p. 210), New York: Macmillan. Copyright 1962 by The Macmillian Company.

measuring instrument. Simply defined, a questionnaire is a standardized list of objective questions or personal opinions. The purpose of a questionnaire is to obtain information directly from a sample. Ultimately, the goal may be to make generalizations to a larger population. The format of a questionnaire considers the following:

▶ Content, (e.g., demographic variables, personality characteristics, behavioral patterns, health history)

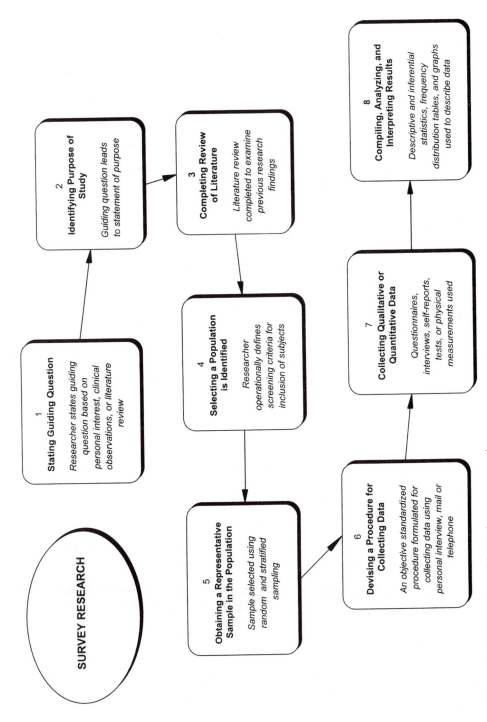

SURVEY RESEARCH

1
Stating Guiding Question

Researcher states guiding question based on personal interest, clinical observations, or literature review

2
Identifying Purpose of Study

Guiding question leads to statement of purpose

3
Completing Review of Literature

Literature review completed to examine previous research findings

4
Selecting a Population is Identified

Researcher operationally defines screening criteria for inclusion of subjects

5
Obtaining a Representative Sample in the Population

Sample selected using random and stratified sampling

6
Devising a Procedure for Collecting Data

An objective standardized procedure formulated for collecting data using personal interview, mail or telephone

7
Collecting Qualitative or Quantitative Data

Questionnaires, interviews, self-reports, tests, or physical measurements used

8
Compiling, Analyzing, and Interpreting Results

Descriptive and inferential statistics, frequency distribution tables, and graphs used to describe data

Figure 3–18. The sequential steps in survey research.

▶ Form of question, (e.g., forced-choice or open-ended)
▶ Level of data collected, (e.g., objective or attitudinal).

The steps in devising a questionnaire are listed in Table 3–11.

3.7.7 Item Construction

In constructing items, the researcher should be aware of the following:

▶ The choices available to the subjects should be exhaustive. On some items, a place for "other, please specify" should be provided.
▶ The choices should be mutually exclusive.
▶ The items presented should be unambiguous and precise. A pilot study testing the reliability of items is essential.

▶ Items should ask only one question. Avoid double-barreled questions.
▶ The respondent should have enough information to answer the item.
▶ The researcher should have a rationale for each item asked. The questionnaire should not be padded with irrelevant items.
▶ Negative questions should be avoided.
▶ Leading questions that force a response should be omitted. The respondents should not be in a position to give expected answers or opinions.

Examples of questionnaire items using various formats are described below:

▶ *Likert-type scales* rate subjects by their agreement or disagreement with a statement on a scale usually of 1–5 or 1–7. For

Table 3–11. An Example of the Steps in Creating a Mail Questionnaire

State research question	• What are the role functions of a public school occupational therapist?
Carry out literature review	• Locate studies on public school occupational therapists.
Identify key areas for items in the questionnaire	• Description of school environment, faculty, and staff • Description of occupational therapists • Occupational therapy facilities and space • Student demographics • Classification of students treated by occupational therapist • Treatment techniques employed by occupational therapists • Occupational therapy treatment goals for diagnostic groups • Treatment modalities used by occupational therapists • Outcome measures for diagnostic groups • Quality assurance through progress monitoring of individual students
Devise survey format	• Forced choice check off • Ranking priorities • Avoiding open-ended questions • Allowing opportunity for comment
Expert evaluation	• Send questionnaire to three public school occupational therapists asking them to evaluate each item using a specified form (see Table 3–12) and make suggestions for improvement • Send questionnaire to research design expert
Revise questionnaire	• Base revisions on expert recommendations • Limit time for completion to 10–15 minutes
Final draft	• Have local public school occupational therapist complete questionnaire before mailing to participants • Work out final "bugs" and consider aesthetics of format

example, if an investigator is interested in surveying the attitudes of the general public with respect to research on children, an item such as the following could be considered for inclusion in the study:

All experimental research with children is unethical.

1	2	3	4	5	6	7
Disagree Very Strongly	Disagree Strongly	Disagree	No Opinion	Agree	Agree Strongly	Agree Very Strongly

▶ *Multiple choice questions* can be used to elicit opinions or attitudes. Suppose a researcher is interested in surveying a group of patients with postmyocardial infarction on their attitudes toward the disability. The following multiple choice question is one example:

If I had a severe pain in my chest I would first do the following:
1. Call my private physician.
2. Call an ambulance.
3. Call the emergency rescue unit of the police.
4. Lie down and rest.
5. Other, please specify.

▶ *Rank order items* are used by researchers as a way of determining priorities. For example, a survey soliciting perceptions of treatment from former patients with psychiatric problems could include the following item:

From the list below of mental health workers, rank in order the most important persons who helped you improve in the hospital. Start numbering with 1 as the person who helped you most; 2, the second most helpful person, and so on:

Mental Health Worker	Rank
Attendant	_____
Nurse	_____
Occupational Therapist	_____
Psychiatrist	_____
Psychologist	_____
Social Worker	_____
Other: Please specify occupation:	_____

▶ *Incomplete sentences* are used in questionnaires to measure informational level, personality traits, and attitudes. For example:

Children with mental retardation are different from normal children in . . .

▶ *Multiple adjective checklists* can be used to elicit effective perception such as in the following example:

Circle the appropriate adjectives:

In general, older patients in nursing homes are:

independent	dependent
happy	sad
well nourished	poorly fed
active	passive
neglected	healthy
supervised	sick

▶ *Open-ended questions* are used in the interviews when the researcher wants the subject to discuss a particular issue in detail. Examples of such questions are:

What is your opinion of including students with disabilities in the general education program?

What do you think the purpose(s) of prisons are?

Do you think the United States should adopt a national health insurance program?

Depending on the ingenuity and creativeness of the researcher, other types of questionnaire items can be constructed, such as true-false questions, analogies, and rating scales. As with constructing any test instrument, it is critical that the investigator check the reliability and validity of the questionnaire before collecting data.

3.7.8 Evaluation of Survey

Once the survey has been developed, it will be important to have experts in the field evaluate it. This will improve reliability and validity and eliminate ambiguous questions. An example of an evaluation form is found in Figure 3–19. This form can be adapted as necessary.

Please read the survey.

1. For each question on the survey, indicate whether the question is stated clearly or if it should be restated or eliminated.
2. Add additional questions that you feel would improve the validity of the questionnaire.

Answer the following questions.

3. Do you feel the survey is too lengthy? _____ Yes _____ No
   If you feel the questionnaire is too long, please place a line through the questions that you would omit.
4. Do you find the questionnaire interesting? _____ Yes _____ No
   If you answered no, please tell us what you found uninteresting or irrelevant.

_____

_____

5. Were the questions arranged in a logical sequence? _____ Yes _____ No
   If you answered no, please indicate how you would rearrange the questions.

_____

_____

6. List further comments and include suggestions for decreasing research bias when administering questionnaire.

_____

_____

Thank you for your time. Any feedback you can give us will greatly enhance our study.

Figure 3–19   Evaluation form for survey questionnaires.

3.7.9 Application of Survey Research to Occupational Therapy

In the last 25 years, occupational therapists have expanded their role functions to include health planning and research. The future role of occupational therapists in planning community health services and health programs in schools is related to needs assessment research (Soderback & Paulsson, 1997). Figure 3–20 gives examples of the application of survey research and needs assessment.

Distribution of Health Care

One of the essential purposes of survey research is to guide the direction and planning of health services in a community. Health planners need hard data before they can recommend the construction of a health facility or hospital or the allocation of additional financial resources to a community health agency. Community health planning, therefore, is vitally linked to survey research. Legislators and developers who are persuaded by community pressures for new facilities need data to justify their positions. Survey research has taken on new importance in the current debate on whether the federal government should be responsible for the total health needs of the population. The data provided by survey research, such as the distribution of health personnel, the proportion of hospital beds for a designated population, and the number of various services provided in defined health catchment areas, can enable legislators to decide whether the present system of delivering health services is adequate for the country or whether a national system for health care would meet the needs of the population more equitably. Survey research can be combined with evaluation research in examining the effectiveness of a health delivery system.

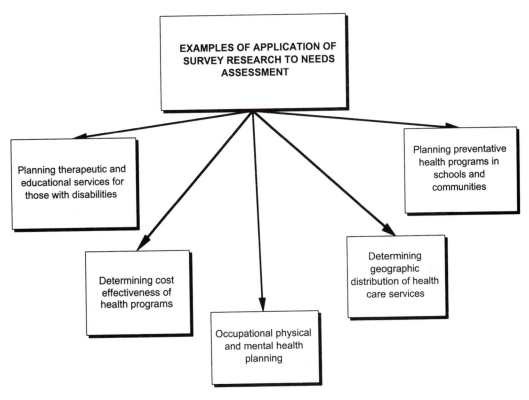

Figure 3–20. Application of survey research to allied health and education.

Planning Therapeutic Services

Community organization of health services is a good example of the applicability of survey research to the needs of a population. Questions such as "What are the health needs of a community?" and "What are the health resources available?" are areas that occupational therapy researchers can directly examine through survey research. Survey research in health is comparable to market research in advertising. In market research, the individuals in a business collect data regarding the need for a product in the community and the community's attitude toward the introduction of new merchandise. Health planners have sometimes failed miserably in surveying a community before introducing a halfway house, a clinic for treating individuals with addictions, or a child health center. The failure usually has been the result of unexpected resistance from the community to the apparent visibility of individuals with social or physical disabilities in a neighborhood. Survey research can be used to anticipate a community's negative attitudes or even to expose the unrealistic fears that are attached to individuals with disabilities.

Educational Planning

Educational planners and administrators often are asked by deans and presidents of colleges to determine if there is a need for a specific allied health training program (e.g., occupational therapy). Are there positions in schools, hospitals, or community agencies for occupational therapists when they graduate from a new program? Do vacancies in occupational therapy exist in hospitals and community clinics at present? Will there be an increased demand for occupational therapists in the future? In what geographic areas are the needs most pressing? These questions are directly accessible through survey research. Questions regarding level of training (i.e., associate, bachelors, graduate, postgraduate, and continuing education) can be answered through a survey methodology.

Other important concerns that health educators should consider in designing curriculums are course content, clinical reasoning, and skill knowledge. What theoretical content and level of training should the occupational therapy program provide? In designing curriculums, health educators must be aware of the expectations of administrators. Have graduates of an occupational therapy program been adequately prepared to provide services needed by individuals with disabilities? On what basis does the educator determine the content of a training program? The need for continual feedback and interaction between educators and health administrators is necessary to create meaningful development of the occupational therapy profession. The occupational therapy educator must decide whether the education provided is directly or indirectly related to the needs of the individual with disabilities. If the education of the occupational therapists is directed toward clinical practice and specialization, then occupational therapist educators must be responsive to the community's needs. Survey research can provide the data gathered from the community to answer many questions in educational planning in occupational therapy.

Occupational Health Planning

There is an increasing need to investigate the prevention of occupational injuries through ergonomics. Other areas include the relationship between mental health and job satisfaction, and the study of environmental conditions such as noise, ventilation, chemical contamination, and radiation. The distribution of accidents and the statistical relationship between occupation and disease are related to the application of survey research to occupational health. Occupational therapists in consultation with industrial researchers can provide information about workers' occupation patterns, nutritional needs, and protective equipment. Occupational health planning should not be done in a vacuum. There are obvious needs for descriptive data regarding frequency of diseases or accidents and the attitudes of workers toward using ergonomic methods before preventive programs can be implemented.

Research in occupational health must also consider psychosocial factors, such as the relationship between personality and accident-proneness; the effects of boredom, low morale, and poor motivation on job satisfaction and mental health; and the effects of job modification on productivity and injury prevention.

Preventive Programs in Schools and Communities

For the child from a low income or socially disadvantaged family, school represents the greatest potential escape from a life of deprivation and misery. The school is one of the few institutions that can help the child overcome parental neglect or other disadvantages. It was not by happenstance but through careful research that during the 1960s social reformers saw the need to incorporate Head Start programs, work-study curriculums, nutritional programs, and vocational education into schools located in inner-city slums and poor rural regions. Survey research has been used in the past as a means to justify the existence of new programs in the schools, but there has been a backlash to the abuse of survey research in areas where data have been gathered and the needs of a community identified without any program implementation. Community leaders are now suspicious of researchers who come into a neighborhood or community for the purpose of determining the need for services and promise to start new programs, only to leave without any follow-up.

Occupational therapists, in conjunction with allied health professionals and educators, have much to contribute in the areas of nutrition, health education, career planning, recreation, and developmental screening in schools and community centers. Survey research can provide the data for planning these services. Nonetheless, community support and follow-up are necessary if survey research is to have any impact on planning preventive programs. Box 3-7 gives an example of survey research.

Box 3–7. Example of Survey Research

1. **Bibliographic Notation**
   Stonefelt, L. L., & Stein, F. (1998). Sensory integrative techniques applied to children with learning disabilities: An outcome study. *Occupational Therapy International, 5,* 252–272.

2. **Abstract**
Learning disabilities are the most frequently reported causes of functional limitation among school-age children (McNeil, 1995). Many children with learning disabilities have an underlying sensory integrative dysfunction (Hoehn & Baumeister, 1994), therefore, sensory integration therapy has been widely used in treating those children. Research on the effectiveness of sensory integration therapy in treating children with learning disabilities has shown conflicting results; many studies supported the use of sensory integration therapy, while others did not. Most of the literature indicates a need for further study in this area. The current study focused on the effectiveness of sensory integration therapy in treating children with learning disabilities as perceived by their parents, teachers, and occupational therapists. Thirty surveys were sent to participants in the Midwest: 10 each to parents, teachers, and occupational therapists. Twenty three surveys were returned for a response rate of 77%. Most of the respondents identified that sensory integration therapy was extremely or somewhat effective in helping the children improve function in 12 skill areas. All parents reported doing activities in the home to help their child and all teachers reported making adaptations in the classroom to better accommodate the child. The sensory integrative techniques most frequently used by the therapists were linear activities, tactile stimulation, games, and jumping/bouncing. Seven of the therapists reported using another treatment method in addition to sensory integration. These seven noted that a combination of treatments, a multi-modal approach, was more effective than sensory integration alone. This study was consistent with previous research that showed that sensory integration is an effective treatment method for children with learning disabilities. However, further research is needed using prospective designs involving single subject or group studies where extraneous variables are rigorously controlled. (p. 252)

3. **Justification and Need for Study**
   Many children with learning disabilities have problems in sensory integration, to which some of all of their learning difficulties can be attributed. Although

continued

sensory integration therapy has been used in treating many people with various disabilities, it has been applied primarily to children with learning disabilities. Whether or not sensory integration therapy is an effective treatment for this population, however, is a controversial issue. (p. 253)

4. **Literature Review**

Recent articles and papers from 1972 to 1996 primarily from the special education, pediatrics, and occupational therapy are cited by the investigators. Examples of journals include *American Journal of Occupational Therapy, Journal of Learning Disabilities, Occupational Therapy Journal of Research, Journal of the American Medical Association (JAMA), Physical and Occupational Therapy Pediatrics,* and *The Journal of Pediatrics and Child Health.*

5. **Research Hypotheses for Guiding Questions**

The guiding question was as follows: How effective is sensory integration therapy for children with learning disabilities as reported by parents, teachers, and occupational therapists?

6. **Methodology**

The following questionnaire was sent to parents, teachers, and occupational therapists (10 each). The occupational therapists used sensory integrative techniques in their therapy. Five of the occupational therapists had used these techniques for 3 to 4 years.

Survey/Data Collection Form
(Questions 1–21 were included on surveys completed by all participants.)

Think of an actual child with a learning disability that you have provided sensory integration therapy to (if you are an occupational therapist), a child in your classroom who has received sensory integration therapy for a learning disability (if you are a teacher), or your own child diagnosed with a learning disability (if you are a parent). Please answer the following questions based on your observations of that child.

1. What is your relationship to the child?
   a. parent
   b. teacher
   c. occupational therapist

2. What specific types of learning disabilities does the child have?
   a. developmental speech and/or language disorder
   b. developmental reading disorder
   c. developmental writing disorder
   d. developmental arithmetic disorder
   e. attention deficit disorder
   f. attention deficit hyperactivity disorder
   g. motor skills disorder
   h. coordination disorder
   i. other, please list _____

3. How old was the child when the learning disability was diagnosed?
   a. <5 years

    b. 5–6 years
    c. 7–8 years
    d. 9–10 years
    e. 11–12 years
    f. other _____

4. How long has the child been receiving occupational therapy services?
    a. less than 1 year
    b. 1–2 years
    c. 2–3 years
    d. 3–4 years
    e. other _____

5. How often does the child receive therapy?
    a. once a week
    b. twice a week
    c. three times a week
    d. other, please specify _____

6. How long do the therapy sessions last?
    a. less than 15 minutes
    b. 15–30 minutes
    c. 30–45 minutes
    d. 45–60 minutes
    e. more than 1 hour

7. Does the child have any other disabilities?
    a. yes Which ones? _____
    b. no

8. Which, if any, other special services does the child receive?
    a. physical therapy
    b. speech therapy
    c. counseling
    d. other, please specify _____
    e. none

9. Which of the following best describes the child?
    a. is excited about therapy and participates willingly
    b. goes to therapy willingly
    c. is reluctant to go to therapy, but participates
    d. dislikes going to therapy and refuses to participate

Please answer questions 10–21, according to the following scale:
1 - extremely effective
2 - somewhat effective
3 - not very effective
4 - not effective at all
5 - irrelevant

continued

How effective do you think sensory integration therapy was in helping the child improve function in each of the following skill areas?

10. Mathematics	1	2	3	4	5
11. Language	1	2	3	4	5
12. Reading	1	2	3	4	5
13. Gross Motor Skills (e.g., kicking a ball, riding a bike)	1	2	3	4	5
14. Fine Motor Skills (e.g., buttoning a shirt, writing)	1	2	3	4	5
15. Balance	1	2	3	4	5
16. Coordination	1	2	3	4	5
17. Self-Esteem	1	2	3	4	5
18. Behavior	1	2	3	4	5
19. Social Skills	1	2	3	4	5
20. Attention	1	2	3	4	5
21. Overall	1	2	3	4	5

(The following two questions were included only on the surveys completed by the parents of children with learning disabilities who are receiving sensory integration therapy.)

22. How noticeable are the effects of sensory integration therapy at home?
    a. very noticeable
    b. somewhat noticeable
    c. not noticeable

23. What activities are you doing in the home to help your child?
    a. hiring a tutor for your child
    b. doing activities suggested by your child's teacher
    c. doing activities suggested by your child's occupational therapist
    d. other, please specify _____
    e. other, please specify _____
    f. other, please specify _____

(The following four questions were included only on the surveys completed by the teachers who have the child with a learning disability in their classroom.)

22. Are the effects of sensory integration therapy readily noticeable in the classroom?
    a. yes
    b. no

23. What is the attitude among the other children toward the child with a learning disability?
    a. friendly
    b. supportive
    c. indifferent
    d. unfriendly
    e. other _____

24. Have you made any adaptations in the classroom to facilitate learning for the child with a learning disability?
    a. yes
    b. no

25. If you answered yes to the previous question, what types of adaptations have you made?
    a. changing the seating arrangement
    b. allowing the child more time to complete assignments
    c. providing alternative methods of instruction for the child
    d. other _____
    e. other _____
    f. other _____

(The following seven questions were included only on the surveys completed by the occupational therapists providing sensory integration treatment to the child.)

22. How long have you been practicing in the school system?
    a. <1 year
    b. 1–2 years
    c. 3–4 years
    d. 5–6 years
    e. 7–8 years
    f. 9–10 years
    g. 10+ years

23. How long have you been practicing sensory integration therapy?
    a. <1 year
    b. 1–2 years
    c. 3–4 years
    d. 5–6 years
    e. 7–8 years
    f. 9–10 years
    g. 10+ years

24. What specific types of sensory integration therapy have been used with the child? (Choose all that apply.)
    a. rotary activities
    b. linear activities
    c. tactile stimulation
    d. games
    e. jumping/bouncing
    f. therapy balls
    g. equilibrium discs
    h. activities involving food
    i. massage
    j. deep pressure
    k. other, please list _____

continued

25. Based on your opinion, rank order beginning with 1 (from most effective to least effective) the specific treatments that have been used in treating the child. (Put a 0 next to the treatments that have not been used).
    ____ rotary activities
    ____ linear activities
    ____ tactile stimulation
    ____ cognitive games
    ____ other games
    ____ jumping/bouncing
    ____ therapy balls
    ____ equilibrium discs
    ____ activities involving food
    ____ massage
    ____ deep pressure
    ____ other, please specify _____
    ____ other, please specify _____
    ____ other, please specify _____

26. Is another treatment (e.g., NDT, perceptual-motor) combined with sensory integration?
    a. yes
    b. no

27. If you answered yes to question 26, which other treatments are used?
    _____

    Does the combination seem to be more effective than sensory integration therapy alone?
    a. yes
    b. no

28. What is your rationale for using sensory integration therapy with children with learning disabilities? _____
    _____
    _____

7. **Analysis of Results**

The parents, teachers, and occupational therapists included in this study perceived sensory integration therapy to be an effective method in treating children with learning disabilities. Their perceptions concur with findings from studies conducted by Wilson and Kaplan (1994) and Fanchaing (1996). However, the study by Wilson and Kaplan showed that significant gains were only sustained in the area of gross motor skills. In this study, coordination and behavior were the functional areas in which sensory integrative techniques were perceived to be the most effective. Other areas in which sensory integrative techniques had a significant effect were fine motor, gross motor, balance, and coordination. (p. 266)

8. **Conclusion of Study**

   "This study, along with other studies, has shown sensory integrative techniques to be effective in treating children with learning disabilities, however, there is still a pressing need for further research in this area" (p. 267).

9. **Stated Limitations of the Study**
   a. The validity and reliability of the survey can be questioned because it was not standardized.
   b. The survey was conducted in two Midwestern states and may not be representative of students in other areas of the country.
   c. Seven of the occupational therapists used a multi-modal approach. One might question whether improvement is a result of the sensory integration technique, another technique, or a combination of a multi-modal approach.
   d. Additional activities and adaptations were made by the parents and teachers that may have confounded results.
   e. Discrepancies in diagnostic information was noted between parents, teachers, and occupational therapists.

10. **Major References in the Study**

    Ayres, A. J. (1972). Improving academic scores through sensory integration. *Journal of Learning Disabilities, 5,* 24–28.

    Fanchaing, S. P. C., (1996). The other side of the coin: Growing up with a learning disability. *The American Journal of Occupational Therapy, 50,* 277–285.

    Hoehn, T. P., & Baumeister, A. A. (1994). A critique of the application of sensory integration therapy to children with learning disabilities. *Journal of Learning Disabilities, 27,* 338–350.

    McNeil, J. M. (1995). Disabilities among children aged <17 years–United States, 1991–1992. *Journal of the American Medical Association, 274,* 1112–1114.

    Polatajko, H. J., Kaplan, B. J., & Wilson, B. N. (1992). Sensory integration treatment for children with learning disabilities: Its status 20 years later. *The Occupational Therapy Journal of Research, 12,* 323–341.

    Wilson, B. N., & Kaplan, B. J. (1994). Follow-up assessment of children receiving sensory integration treatment. *The Occupational Therapy Journal of Research, 14,* 244–266.

3.8 Summary

Quantitative research offers occupational therapy clinicians the means to demonstrate the effectiveness of their treatment protocols. The importance of evidence-based practice is established primarily through the results of quantitative research. The various quantitative research models described in this chapter can assist clinicians in developing new ways to evaluate outcome, design treatment methods, and implement a needs assessment. Action research provides the occupational therapist with data to solve clinical problems at the local level. Qualitative research, as described in the next chapter, can be integrated with quantitative research to investigate research problems more thoroughly.

CHAPTER

Qualitative Research Models

Gwynnyth Llewellyn, Ph.D., Susan K. Cutler, Ph.D., NCSP,
and Franklin Stein, Ph.D., OTR/L

---

*It is undesirable to believe a proposition when there is no
ground whatever for supposing it is true.*
—Bertrand Russell, *Sceptical Essays* (p. 1)

All great truths begin as blasphemies.
—George Bernard Shaw, *Annajanska* (p. 262)

Operational Learning Objectives

By the end of this chapter, the learner will

1. Identify the characteristics of qualitative research
2. Explain the qualitative research process
3. Recognize the difference between quantitative and qualitative research designs
4. Identify qualitative data collection methods
5. Identify the principles of qualitative data analysis
6. Critically analyze examples of qualitative research from the allied health literature

4.1 Defining Qualitative Research

Qualitative research is defined as the study of people and events in their natural setting.

Qualitative research is multi-method in focus, involving an interpretive naturalistic approach to its subject matter. This means that qualitative researchers study things in their natural settings, attempting to make sense of or interpret phenomena in terms of the meanings people bring to them. Qualitative research involves the studied use and collection of a variety of empirical materials—case study, personal experience, introspective, life story, interview, observational, historical, interactive, and visual texts—that describe routine and problematic moments and meaning in individuals' lives. (Denzin & Lincoln, 1994b, p. 2)

In this method, researchers use multiple and interconnected methods, seeking to explore perceptions and experiences to understand phenomena in terms of the meanings that people bring to them. These phenomena are examined in context and from the individual's point of view. In rehabilitation settings, the phenomena investigated include the experience of disability or of a chronic medical condition. The people involved may be clients, their family members, or medical and allied health personnel.

Among health and rehabilitation personnel, there is a rapidly growing interest in exploring the views of clients and their families (Ferguson, Ferguson, & Taylor, 1992; Llewellyn, 1995; Morse, 1994). This interest is being shaped by two forces. The first is the disability movement. Consumers of health and related services are actively campaigning for a less medical approach to disability and a more positive acceptance of people with disabilities' place in society (French, 1994). The second is the coming together of researchers in medical and social science disciplines. This has led to the demise of the traditional illness-based view of disability. In its place, disability is regarded as a social construction. This view takes into account the ways in which particular societies regard impairments and the influence of situational factors such as poor socioeconomic conditions on the incidence of disability (Oliver, 1991).

Exploring the viewpoint of individuals requires different research designs from those usually employed in the medical and health sciences. Allied health researchers are turning to sociology (the study of groups) and to anthropology (the study of cultures) for more appropriate research models. Investigators in these disciplines have been "unraveling" the complex interactions between individuals since the turn of the century (Parsons, 1964).

Qualitative research models differ from those in the positivist quantitative tradition in three fundamental ways. First, qualitative researchers are interested in "participatory and holistic knowing" (Reason, 1988, p. 12). This contrasts with the distance and objectivity found particularly in experimental research designs. Second, there is a focus on critical subjectivity in qualitative research. This involves researchers acknowledging their primary subjective experience.

The researcher becomes his or her own "research instrument." This is in direct contrast to the notion of the objective researcher in experimental research designs. Third, researchers working in the qualitative tradition hold the view "that knowledge is formed in and for action" (Reason, p. 12). Action, as it naturally occurs, is viewed as the appropriate context for the development of knowledge.

4.2 Characteristics of Qualitative Research

There are four fundamental characteristics of qualitative research:

▶ Phenomena are investigated and interpreted in their natural settings, taking into account the socio-cultural-historical context
▶ Multiple methods are used to understand and offer interpretations of the meanings held by participants about these phenomena
▶ The researcher occupies a central place in the qualitative research process
▶ An inductive process is used to develop general principles from the study of specific instances

Phenomena are investigated and interpreted in their natural settings, taking into account the socio-cultural-historical context. Qualitative research takes place in the field. Qualitative researchers get involved in the natural setting to understand the meanings held by participants about the phenomena under investigation. From this involvement and understanding, qualitative researchers develop knowledge. This knowledge may be in the form of patterns or themes or a fully developed theory about the phenomena studied. Whatever the case, the resulting knowledge is grounded in direct field research experience rather than imposed a priori through hypotheses or deductive propositions (Glaser & Strauss, 1967).

Multiple methods are used to understand and offer interpretations of the meanings held by participants about the phenomena under investigation. Qualitative researchers use an array of methods to collect information about, describe, and interpret events and meanings in individuals' lives. The basic methods used for gathering data are interviewing, observation, and documentary analysis. The strategies most commonly used to analyze data include content or theme analysis, grounded theory procedures, and story analysis. These strategies are employed in the search for regularities in the meanings that participants hold about the phenomena under investigation. For some researchers, these regularities are viewed as a form of conceptual order; for others, their interest lies in the repetition of patterns across the data.

The researcher occupies a central place in the qualitative research process. In qualitative research, the researcher is acknowledged as an individual located within a historical context and within a research tradition or traditions. Researchers bring to the research process particular sets of beliefs about the world that guide their actions. In contrast to experimentally based research designs, however, qualitative researchers do not impose preexisting expectations on the phenomena or setting under study. Rather, the researchers' set of beliefs functions as an interpretive framework (Guba, 1990). This interpretive framework guides the research purpose and also shapes the research questions and the methods employed to address these questions. In addition to an interpretive framework, qualitative researchers become familiar with the literature and develop a guiding question to focus the purpose of the research.

An inductive process is used to develop general principles from the study of specific instances. In qualitative research, the analysis begins with specific instances of data and builds toward general principles. This contrasts with the deductive process employed in the quantitative tradition in which hypotheses are constructed prior to data

collection and then tested. In qualitative research, preparing the research text is the final stage of the inductive analysis process. The research text is a construction that integrates and interprets data and researcher understanding of the area of study. The completed product is the public text, which may be delivered either as a research report, journal article, book, or seminar paper.

4.3 Types of Qualitative Research

Qualitative research is a term widely used to indicate methods that subscribe to the characteristics described above. Tesch (1990), for example, listed 46 different research approaches under the rubric of qualitative research. Some research methods more closely fit the characteristics described; others are less closely associated. Several qualitative methods have become standard in the medical literature and in the related health professional literature (Morse, 1994). These include case study, field study, focus group research, ethnography, and oral history (Table 4–1). Other methods, such as ethnoscience, discourse analysis, transformative research, and hermeneutics are not as familiar.

Discourse analysis and ethnoscience are concerned with the study of the characteristics of language as a communication tool and as culture, respectively. Transformative research involves the research subjects as active participants in developing and implementing the research project to overcome the usually passive nature of the research process by turning this into a "transforming" activity. Researchers employing hermeneutics take as their central theme, the understanding of events in relation to the context of which these are part, with special reference to the historical context.

Tesch proposed that working with words is a basic requirement of qualitative research. She developed a continuum of qualitative research types based on the degree of focus on language. At one end of

Table 4–1. Five Approaches to Qualitative Research

	Case Study (Retrospective or Prospective)	Grounded Theory or Heuristic Study	Phenomenological	Ethnography or Field Study	Biographical
Defined	• Exploration of an individual, organization, program, or event through an in-depth data collection using multiple sources of information (Creswell, 1998)	• General method for generating or discovering theory during the data collection (Strauss & Corbin, 1994)	• "From the individual descriptions, general or universal meanings are derived, in other words, the essences of structures of the experience" (Moustakas, 1994, p. 13)	• Examination of a cultural or social group through extended participant observations to determine the meanings of behavior, language, and interactions of the group (Creswell, 1998; Vidich & Lyman, 1994)	• Study of an individual; this study may be through "portrayals, portraits, profiles, memoirs, life stories, life histories, case studies, autobiographies, journals, diaries, and on and on—each suggesting a slightly different perspective under consideration" (Smith, 1994, p. 278)
Example of Study	Emerson, H., Cook, J., Polatajko, H., & Segal, R. (1998). Enjoyment experiences as described by persons with schizophrenia: A qualitative study. *Canadian Journal of Occupational Therapy, 65,* 183–192.	Creighton, C., Dijkers, M., Bennett, N., & Brown, K. (1995). Reasoning and the art of therapy for spinal cord injury. *American Journal of Occupational Therapy, 49,* 311–317.	Hasselkus, B. R., & Dickie, V. A. (1993). Doing occupational therapy: Dimensions of satisfaction and dissatisfaction. *American Journal of Occupational Therapy, 48,* 145–154.	Frank, G., et al. (1997). Jewish spirituality through actions in time: Daily occupations of young orthodox Jewish couples in Los Angeles. *American Journal of Occupational Therapy, 51,* 199–206	Frank, G. (1996). Life histories in occupational therapy clinical practice. *American Journal of Occupational Therapy, 50,* 251–264.
Methods of Data Collection	• Interviewing • Naturalistic observational techniques		• Mute evidence • Personal experience		

this continuum is research primarily concerned with the characteristics of language. At the other end is research with an interest solely in reflection. In between, some types of research focus on the discovery of regularities in text; others focus on the comprehension of the meaning of text or action. Those approaches that focus on language are more structured and employ more codified methods of data collection and analysis. In contrast, the approaches that rely mainly on reflection employ more holistic procedures that "build on intuition and on insight that are achieved through deep immersion in and dwelling with the data" (Tesch, 1990, p. 60).

Another way of classifying the different approaches used in qualitative research is by the research purpose. Some approaches are ideal for identifying regularities, patterns, or themes. Others are better suited to generating and refining tentative theoretical propositions. Still others are more useful for intense, intimate study of a particular phenomenon using personal reflection. There is ongoing debate in the qualitative research literature about this diversity of approaches and associated methodological issues (Denzin & Lincoln, 1994a; Higgs, 1997). Each approach has adherents in the core disciplines of psychology, psychiatry, sociology, and anthropology.

It is not by chance that many of the important contributions in the social sciences have emerged from clinical observation methods (Dukes, 1965). Sigmund Freud in his search for an understanding of the psychodynamics of mental illness, Arnold Gesell's (1928) rigorous observation of child development, Jean Piaget's (1926) conceptualization of cognitive development through detailed analysis of clinical responses, and Jules Henry's (1971) naturalistic observation of families of children with emotional disturbance have all made a significant impact through qualitative research. Clinical observation as a research method has the potential to contribute greatly to the fields of occupational therapy and special education. Table 4–2 lists some of the major studies in the social sciences based on clinical observation research methods.

Clinical observation research employs four methods: individual case study, child development studies, field observation (ethnography), and operations research. The definition, purposes, procedure, and application to occupational therapy and special education are listed in Table 4–3.

4.3.1 Case Study

There is much criticism by experimentalists of the case study approach as a model for research, primarily directed toward the subjectivity of the researcher and the inability to generalize to a population on the basis of one subject. The most important purpose of the case study is in the intensive investigation of one individual. Through a thorough study the researcher can examine factors that ordinarily would be difficult either in an experimental study involving a group of subjects or in a correlational study. To illustrate, let us suppose an investigator is interested in learning why patients who are older and living in a nursing home develop feelings of hopelessness and disengage from the mainstream of society. The researcher poses the question: What factors in an older person's life contribute to feelings of hopelessness and disengagement? In this study, the investigator is limited to an ex post facto research model. It would be possible to answer this question by comparing a group of older individuals who display feelings of hopelessness with another group of older individuals who are actively engaged in independent activities. In this hypothetical study, the researcher could test whether individuals who have personalities characterized by an external locus of control feel more hopeless than a similar geriatric sample who characteristically have more internal locus of control and feel less hopeless. The reader will recognize this research model as correlational. In a correlational model, the researcher is restricted by the test instruments used in measuring the variables of locus of control

Table 4–2. Major Contributions From Clinical Observation Methodologies in the Social Sciences

Social Scientist	Major Works	Methods	Publication Dates	Fields of Investigation
Sigmund Freud and Josef Breuer	*Studies in Hysteria*	Case study	1895	Psychiatry
Margaret Mead	*Coming of Age in Samoa*	Field observation	1928	Cultural anthropology
Arnold Gesell	*Infancy and Human Growth*	Developmental observation	1929	Child development
Jean Piaget	*The Psychology of Intelligence*	Developmental observation	1947	Cognitive development
Stanton and Schwartz	*The Mental Hospital*	Operations research	1950	Psychiatry
Robert White	*Lives in Progress*	Case study	1952	Personality
Jules Henry	*Pathways to Madness*	Field observation	1965	Family casework
Rene A. Spitz	*The First Year of Life: A Psychoanalytic Study of Normal and Deviant Development of Object Relations*	Developmental observation	1965	Child psychiatry
Joseph Church	*Three Babies: Biographies of Cognitive Development*	Case study	1966	Cognition
Oscar Lewis	*La Vida*	Field observation	1966	Cultural anthropology
Bruno Bettelheim	*The Empty Fortress*	Case study	1967	Child psychiatry
Robert Coles	*Children of Crisis*	Field observation	1967	Social psychiatry
Eric Berman	*Scapegoat*	Field observation	1973	Family casework
Mary Ainsworth et al.	*Patterns of Attachment*	Clinical observation	1978	Social psychology
Jack Fadely and Virginia Hosier	*Case Studies in Left and Right Hemispheric Functioning*	Case study	1983	Perception
Stephen Marks	*Three Corners: Exploring Marriage and the Self*	Case study	1986	Family relationships
Sylvia Kenig (Ed.)	*Who Plays? Who Pays? Who Cares? A Case Study in Applied Sociology, Political Economy and the Community Mental Health Centers Movement*	Case Study	1992	Community mental health
Kelley Johnson	*Deinstitutionalizing Women: An Ethnographic Study of Institutional Closure*	Case Study	1998	Deinstitutionalization

Table 4–3. Application of Clinical Observation Methods

Methods	Purposes	Procedures for Collecting Data	Application to Fields
Individual case study	Understanding of underlying dynamics of illness	• interviewing • testing • examination of personal documents • case research	Investigation of • health problems • chronic diseases • individual factors
Child development studies	Description of the sequential, hierarchical processes in human development	• objective observation in a controlled setting • mechanical audiovisual recordings	Examination of normal and abnormal patterns in development
Field observations (ethnography)	Examination of the interaction between members of a social group, educational group, or family	• naturalistic observation • process recordings of interactions • unobtrusive measurement	Description of group interaction in: • dysfunctional families • halfway houses • residential treatment programs • education classrooms • socioeconomic units
Operations research	Analysis of administrative problems in organization systems	• flow charts of organizational structure • job descriptions • communication patterns • decision-making process	Examination of interrelationships among systems • political • economic • health care • educational

and hopelessness and by the limitations in controlling for the individual differences among participants. On the other hand, a case study approach would allow the investigator the freedom to search for individual factors that could easily be overlooked in a correlational study, but on closer investigation prove to be a critical variable in generating dependency and hopelessness. The flexibility of a case study and the creativity afforded to the researcher compensate for the apparent lack of external validity or the ability to generalize to a representative population.

The general outline of case study research is similar to all aspects of research in that the researcher justifies the need for investigation, reviews previous literature, states guiding questions for data collection,

and obtains data through observation. In contrast to experimental and correlational research, in the case study the researcher does not initially state a statistical hypothesis or collect group data from a representative sample of a population. Rather, inferences are drawn from an analysis and review of data collected from and about the individual during the study. The general format of a case study follows.

Need for the Study

The need for the study comes from a broad societal context, such as aggression and hopelessness in youth, obesity, or underachievement in gifted students. In this section of the study, the investigator explores the multiple effects of a problem on family, educational and health institutions, and society in general. The investigator examines the prevalence of the problem and its relationship to occupational therapy or special education. The investigator should also discuss the appropriateness of using a qualitative case study model in contrast to an experimental or correlational design. If a case study is used as a pilot study or preliminary study, such as to collect data about a problem before undertaking a larger study, then it should also be stated. A case study should not be used in place of an experimental or correlational study. For example, a case study is more appropriate than experimental or correlational methods in an in-depth study of a complex chronic disability. The investigator should also consider the indirect effects of a problem, such as economic loss to society due to the inability of the individual with disabilities to work and the emotional and family turmoil that accompany chronic disability. The number and percentage of a population affected by a problem should be documented. What statistics are available regarding mortality rates, hospitalization admissions, physician visits, special education, and related services? What evaluation tests and treatment methods are provided by allied health or educational professionals at present, and what is the potential of generating therapeutic techniques? These questions are pertinent in demonstrating the need for a study. The investigator should also discuss in this section what the possible implications of the results from a case study could provide. Investigations into the dynamic factors affecting the onset of arthritis, schizophrenia, delinquency, stuttering, dementia, reading or math disability, and attention deficit-hyperactivity disorder are particularly appropriate for case study research.

Review of Literature

The investigator should do an extensive review of the literature on the question and critically examine the variables in the case study. Research related to etiology and treatment is particularly important in a case study. The literature review should provide the investigator with a general overview of the current state of knowledge. Research journals, textbooks, and conference proceedings, electronic databases, and other sources of information should be reviewed. An outline should guide the investigator in deciding what aspects of the research problem to include, the extensiveness of the review, and the sources used to obtain information. (For a more detailed discussion on reviewing literature, see Chapter 6.)

The literature review also should include an examination of case study methods for collecting data, such as interviewing, reliability of case records, medical history recording and psychological testing. These areas are especially important to the investigator who is unfamiliar with the case study methods.

Research Methodology

In this section, critical variables are operationally defined, a screening criteria for subject selection is delineated, a procedure for interviewing and testing the subject is stated, test instruments are identified, and reliability and validity data are reported. A screening criteria should be based on a rationale considering representative statistical data for a target population. For example, if an investigator is interested in doing a case study of a youth who is delinquent, he or she would consider gender, age when most delinquency occurs, socioeconomic group factors, school status, cognitive level, family, and delinquent acts committed. The variables identified should be obtained from a review of the literature, statistical abstracts, and clinical observations. From these sources the researcher operationalizes the screening criteria as outlined in Table 4–4.

The investigator should also consider exclusional criteria, that is, factors that should not be present in the subject. These could include brain damage, mental illness, language difficulty, or language difference. After the researcher has determined in-

Table 4–4. Example of Screening Criteria (Delinquent Youth)

Age:	16 years old
Gender:	Male
Socioeconomic factor:	Working-class family
Intelligence:	Average nonverbal I.Q.
Family:	Dysfunctional, nonintact due to divorce, separation, or parent desertion
School status:	Special education setting
Geographic area:	Urban
Behavior:	Delinquent, with vandalism, truancy, and deviant behavior that results in adjudication, probation, or referral to residential treatment setting

clusional and exclusional criteria, the next task is to plan a procedure for selecting a subject or subjects if the project involves several case studies (Llewellyn, Sullivan, & Minichiello, 1999). This entails contacting a juvenile facility, a court, or an agency working with delinquent youth. The cooperation of the agency is crucial to the research. The participant and the parent or guardian must be told of the purposes of the study through informed consent. The plan for collecting data is another important part of the research methodology. This includes the following questions:

▶ At what setting will the study take place?
▶ What psychological tests, evaluation instruments, questionnaires, and interview schedules will be employed?
▶ During what period of time will the study take place (e.g., hours of day, school time or evening, time of year)?

Results

The data gathered for a case study include the subject's history, informal and formal assessments, collateral information from case records, interviews with the individual and family members, and clinical reports. Difficulties can arise in a case study

that threatens the researcher's objectivity. Robert White (1952), in his classic study *Lives in Progress* felt, "It is impossible to study another person without making evaluations, and it is hard to keep the evaluations from being seriously distorted by one's personal reactions to the subject" (p. 99). The investigator must acknowledge this limitation of a case study. One way to do this is to have more than one interviewer obtain an independent history on the same individual. In this way, the investigator bias and personal views can be isolated. Another method is to make the investigators aware of their own rigidities, assumptions, and prejudices "through increased familiarity with their own personalities" (p. 100). Most important, however, is the need to acknowledge that there will always be investigator influence in the conduct and reporting of any study, particularly in intensive works such as a case study. The preferred way to demonstrate that the reported results accurately reflect the case study individual or individuals, and the investigors's perceptions, is to ensure that the investigator states (a) his or her perspective up front and (b) the interpretative framework used to examine the case material. Most investigators, in reporting a case study, use a chronological outline starting from the subject's early childhood and continuing through his or her current age. A topical biography is another way to organize data. For example, in a case study of a subject with arthritis, the investigator may want to report data under subject headings, such as possible etiological factors (joint injuries, allergies, emotional disturbances, endocrine disorders) or treatment intervention (occupational therapy, physical therapy, chemotherapy, and psychologic counseling). An interpretive summary and a recommendation for further research follow the reporting of results.

In short, case study research is a viable method for obtaining credible data pertaining to the life of an individual with disabilities. It is an idiographic approach to research that considers individual differences in etiology of disease and specific adaptations in coping with a disability. Box 4–1 gives an example of a qualitative case study.

4.3.2 Operations Research

Ackoff and Rivett (1963) described the three essential characteristics of operations research: "(1) systems orientation, (2) the use of interdisciplinary teams, and (3) the adaptation of scientific method" (p. 10). Operations research was developed in Great Britain during World War II mainly for the purpose of using radar effectively to combat German air attacks (Crowther & Whiddington, 1948). Subsequently, during the 1950s, large corporations employed operations research teams to analyze production methods as a way of increasing efficiency. Norbert Wiener's (1948) contribution in cybernetics and the application of the feedback principle expanded systems theory to biological, sociological, and psychological dimensions. Using the technology of cybernetics, the methodology of operations research, and systems theory, researchers have examined the physiology of respiration (Pribram, 1958), equipment design, and human engineering (United States Department of Defense, Joint Services Steering Committee, 1963), political

life (Easton, 1961), and the city as a system (Blumberg, 1972), clinical rotation (Reid, Seavor, & Taylor, 1991), higher education (Cheng, 1993), family planning (Huezo, 1997), and obstetric care (Sibley & Armbruster, 1997).

Efficiency in industrial production has been one of the areas in which operations research has been widely applied. Feigin, An, Connors, and Crawford (1996) applied operations research to restructure IBM's manufacturing strategy. The goal of the efficiency expert in a factory is to minimize expenditures and maximize production. By analyzing the industrial system of production, the operations researcher can determine where costs can be reduced and production increased. Factors such as competitive costs of raw materials and plant machinery, redeployment of labor, employee morale, and distribution of goods are all considered in operations research. Essentially, operations research analyzes a system by identifying all those factors that affect input or raw materials and output or finished product. The feedback in this system represents the critical analysis of input and output and the resultant changes in the total system of production.

The concept of operations research and systems theory can also be applied to research problems in health care. For example, hospital management provides an excellent area for operations research. For hospital administrators, the problems of expanding costs and depersonalized care for health consumers have become increasingly more aggravated during the last two decades. Although society seeks improved

---

SIMPLE FEEDBACK MODEL

input → process → output
▼ ▼ ▼
expenditure → feedback → product
loop

Box 4–1. Example of Qualitative Case Study

1. Bibliographical Notation
Richardson, G. M., Kline, F. M., & Huber, T. (1996). Development of self-management in an individual with mental retardation: A qualitative case study. *Journal of Special Education, 30,* 278–304.

2. Abstract
Ethnographic methodology was used to explore the development of self-management skills in an 18-year-old woman with Down Syndrome. Triangulation of data types and the constant comparative method of data analysis were employed. Outcomes suggested the individual's family culture had a large impact on development of self-monitoring and that early and continuing intervention and "expectation of normalcy" were critical. (p. 278)

3. Justification and Need for Study
The authors stated that their purpose was "the development of self-monitoring in an individual who is mentally retarded" (p. 282) and that a case study was appropriate because the study involved a single participant.

4. Literature Review
Thirty-five references were cited in the study. Articles came from a wide variety of sources, including books on mental retardation, *Education and Training in Mental Retardation, International Journal of Disability, Development and Education, American Journal of Mental Retardation,* and *Remedial and Special Education.*

5. Research Hypothesis or Guiding Questions
The guiding question explicitly stated was the authors' "curiosity about how Sandy had developed self-management abilities" (p. 278).

6. Methodology
"The issue studied was the development of self-monitoring in an individual who is mentally retarded. This study was accomplished by exploring her recollections and interpretations over her 18 years of life, conducting extensive interviews with other key informants, and reviewing the records of her development, preserved by school and family" (p. 282).

Analysis of data was completed through "a 'broad strokes' analysis" (p. 294), and finally through a detailed analysis of those items initially coded as cognitive.

7. Results
The results indicated five major outcomes, including
- the ability to self-monitor personal behaviors
- influence of the nuclear family in the development and use of self-monitoring behaviors
- part played by the extended family in the development of self-monitoring and other cognitive abilities
- parental child rearing beliefs were supported by the family, school, and community contexts
- evidence for the developmental stages of self-monitoring

continued

8. Conclusions

The authors concluded that the development in self-regulation was due, in part, to the "practical expectation of normalcy. . . Expectations from Sandy's family were normal, but practical in light of Sandy's functional limitation" (p. 302). The findings have implications for the development of self-regulation in other individuals with mental retardation.

9. Limitations of the Study

Because this was a case study, further research must be done if the findings are to be generalized to a larger population of individuals with mental retardation.

10. Major References Cited in the Study

Cole, C. L., & Gardner, W. I. (1983). Teaching self-management skills to the mentally retarded: A critical review. In O. C. Karan & W. I. Gardner (Eds.), *Habilitation practices with the developmentally disabled who present behavioral and emotional disorders* (Research Report No. 179–202). Madison: University of Wisconsin, Research and Training Center in Mental Retardation. (ERIC Document Reproduction Service No. ED 270–957)

Hughes, C. A., Korinek, I., & Gorman, J. (1991). Self-management for students with mental retardation in public school settings: A research review. *Education and Training in Mental Retardation, 26,* 271–291.

Whitman, T. L. (1990). Development of self-regulation in persons with mental retardation. *American Journal of Mental Retardation, 94,* 247–362.

---

expanded health care for larger portions of the population, hospitals have to find more efficient methods to service more clients and to provide them with sophisticated diagnostic methods for detecting and treating illnesses with the most advanced technology. Specifically, these problems include (a) architectural design, (b) medical equipment, (c) hospital staffing including availability of consultants, (d) cost sharing for using expensive machinery, and (e) issues such as managed care. Operations research as applied to the fields of allied health and rehabilitation uses observational data and systems analysis to identify critical issues and solve problems. Health problems appropriate for operations research include the following:

▶ the lack of health care workers in rural areas (Rosenblatt, 1991)
▶ depersonalization of clients in long-term care (Kliebsch, Sturmer, Siebert, & Brenner, 1998).

▶ inadequate funding for long-term care (Xakellis, Frantz, Lewis, & Harvey, 1998)
▶ recurrence of chronic disease among vulnerable populations (Woods, et al., 1997)
▶ lack of rehabilitation services in forensic psychiatry (Lloyd, 1995)
▶ inefficient emergency care in urban hospitals (Ernst, Houry, & Weiss, 1997)
▶ day care for elderly or adults with severe disabilities (Macdonald, Epstein, & Vastano, 1986).

In all the foregoing problems, the underlying assumption is that a system, a unified interconnected whole, exists. The systems researcher analyzes the specific components of the system and their interrelationships. In these examples, the systems are identified as rural health, long-term care, legislation process, general hospitals, chronic illness, emergency care, and adult day care. Box 4–2 provides an example of an operational research study.

Box 4–2. Example of Operations Research

1. Bibliographical Notation
Hester, P. H. (1994, November). *A contextual analysis of classroom interaction at the university level: An operations research approach.* Paper presented at the Annual Meeting of the Mid-South Educational Research Association, Nashville, TN. (ERIC Document Reproduction Service No. ED 382-139)

2. Abstract
This study sought to demonstrate how an interactive model can be used as a "semiotic" tool to reconcile contrasting views of the role of the college professor. The study used concepts of group dynamics to study classroom leadership, climate, and expectations and a social-psychological perspective was used to analyze group interaction patterns as they were phenomonologically described. The study used a case study approach employing descriptive statistics. Subjects were 22 graduate students enrolled in an Introduction to Education Administration course. In Phase 1, they were trained as participant observers, given a course syllabus with objectives, a list of students, forms for recording their classroom responses, and a time sheet to record how many hours they studied each week. In Phase 2, data from tools distributed to the subjects were collected and tabulated weekly for 10 weeks. In Phase 3, the data were analyzed. Findings showed that a research and teaching strategy could be used to reconcile the polarity which exists when professors at higher education institutions see a conflict between the dual roles they are expected to perform—as teachers and researchers.

3. Justification and Need for Study
After stating that "all is not well in the classroom" (p. 3), the author noted that this research is important as it would show "how professors can improve their teaching process by modeling themselves as constructive motivators, subject-matter organizers, and relevant conveyors of instruction in the classroom" (p. 3). The author further stated that "the intent of the study was to provide the university professor with an exportable teaching and research tool for strengthening class instruction via students' interaction (p. 21).

4. Literature Review
Twenty-five references were cited in the study. Articles came from a wide variety of literature, including books and journals. Journals included *Teacher College Record, Review of Education Research,* and *American Educator Research Journal.* The majority of studies cited were from the 1980s and 1990s.

5. Research Hypothesis or Guiding Questions
The guiding questions explicitly stated were:
- What is the relationship between study time and student class participation?
- What is the relationship between extrovert/introvert personality types and the amount of study time devoted to the subject matter?
- Is increased study time congruent with absolute relevant student responses as contrasted to irrelevant responses? (p. 4)

continued

6. Methodology

A case study approach using techniques of small group research (Hare, Borgatta, & Bales, 1965) was used with students in a college class. Participants recorded the number and relevance of declarative sentences used by their classmates. Data were also collected on the time spent studying each week. Introvert/extrovert data was determined by an interaction matrix in which the amount of time spent talking was transformed into a measure of introversion or extroversion. Analysis of the data was completed through Spearman's rank order correlation and a Chi-square test.

7. Results

According to the author, results showed

- moderate correlation between study time and class participation
- a high correlation between personality types and study time
  a high correlation between increased study time and absolutely relevant response rates
- no significant difference in interaction patterns between male and female students.

In addition, "The findings from this study show that a research and teaching strategy can be used to reconcile the polarity which exists between professors at higher education institutions who see a disparity between the dual roles that are expected to perform as teachers and researchers" (p. 19).

8. Conclusions

Hester concluded that this type of research provides tools to "enable the professor to 'harvest' an easy source of valuable data that can increase research productivity. In addition it can have a positive impact on the quality of instruction and students' performance" (p. 20).

9. Limitations of the Study

Constraints include time and resources. Limitations included the small number of participants.

10. Major References Cited in the Study

Carroll, J. B. (1963). A model of school learning. *Teacher College Record, 64,* 723–733.

Hare, P. A., Borgatta, E., & Bales , R. (Eds.). (1965). *Small groups: Studies in social interaction.* New York: Alfred A. Knopf.

Katz, J., & Mildred, H. (1988). *Turning professors into teachers.* New York: American Council on Education. Macmillan.

Magoon, J. (1977). Constructivist approaches in education research. *Review of Educational Research, 47,* 651–693.

Simpson, R. (1993). Balancing teaching and research. *Innovative Higher Education, 17,* 227–229.

4.3.3 Developmental Observations

"Experimental observation, with conditions so clearly defined that they can be duplicated and so delimited that only a single variable remains for study is scientifically a goal to work toward" (Gesell, 1928, p. 23). This description stated almost three-quarters of a century ago remains the benchmark for research on child development. Developmental observation research is concerned with the rigorous investigations into the process, stages, and hierarchical steps in human development. How does speech develop? What are the sequential stages in the areas of language, ambulation, psychosocial development, cognition? These and other questions are examples of research problems that lend themselves best to developmental observation methods. The investigator seeks to identify the processes involved in development, the approximate ages when landmarks are reached, and the biopsychosocial factors that shape development.

A key assumption in developmental research is that human behavior unfolds at critical stages. In Table 4–5, some examples of approximate ages are given for achieving a developmental landmark. The typical child is expected to pass a test item related to chronological age. The child's rate of development is relative to the norm response for specific chronological age groups. The basic assumption in the DDST-II (Frankenburg, Dodds, Archer, Shapiro, & Bresnick, 1990) test is that human development progresses in a linear direction originating from genetic forces. In this model, the child is ready at specific ages to learn to walk, play games cooperatively with other children, write, speak, or perform any number of other developmental tasks. Environmental experiences provide the opportunities for development to occur.

Stating the Guiding Question

The first task of the researcher is to state a research question that generates data. Piaget (1926), in the first sentence of his book *The Language and Thought of the Child* stated: "The question which we shall attempt to answer in this book may be stated as follows: What are the needs which a child tends to satisfy when he talks?" (p. 1). Gesell

Table 4–5. Denver Developmental Screening Test—Revised

Developmental Skills	Hierarchical Sequential Activities from Birth to 6 Years
Gross motor	*Lifts head at 2 months* to *walks backward (heel to toe) at 6 years*
Fine motor	*Visually tracks objects to midline at 2 months* to *draws a man with six distinct parts at 6 years*
Language	*Responds to bell at 2 months* to *defines six words at 6 years*
Personal-social	*Regards face at 2 months* to *dresses without supervision at 5 years*

Note. From normative data, age levels were established as to when children develop individual skills. Normal limits (upper and lower) were validated for each hierarchical activity. Adapted from *The Denver Developmental Screening Test–II* (DDST–II) by W. R. Frankenburg, J. B. Dodds, P. Archer, H. Shapiro, & B. Bresnick, 1990, Denver, CO: Denver Developmental Materials. Copyright 1990 by Denver Developmental Materials.

and Thompson (1923), in their research on infant behavior, also began with a guiding question: "When does this orthogenetic patterning of the human individual begin?" (p. 9).

The potential areas for research using developmental observation are considerable. An outline of the broad areas of development and specific research questions, listed in Table 4–6, demonstrates the wide perspective in doing developmental research.

The questions listed in Table 4–6 represent only a fraction of the potential research appropriate for developmental observation. The area of development selected by a researcher and the research questions generated provide the engine for the study. The justification and need for the study are based on practical and clinical issues.

Need for Study in Developmental Observation

For the occupational therapist and special educator, developmental research provides the data for evaluating clients or students. Is this individual functioning within normal limits? To answer this question, data

regarding normal development are needed. Developmental studies therefore provide benchmarks for (a) interpreting the developmental level and (b) constructing sequential treatment programs. In children with developmental disabilities, such as cerebral palsy, mental retardation, autism, or severe social deprivation, data from developmental observations are used by therapists to monitor the progress within the treatment or intervention. The rationale behind this approach is that development progresses sequentially and hierarchally in the typical child, but is delayed, incomplete, or impaired in the child with a developmental disability. The developmental therapist reconstructs the sequential stages in an area of development and treats the child by facilitating progress through each stage. Steps along a linear developmental progression are programmed for the individual child starting at his or her base level of performance.

The results of developmental observation research have a direct effect on evaluating and treating children with developmental disabilities. After delineating the need for the study, the researcher designs an observational method for collecting data.

Table 4–6. Suggested Areas for Research Questions

Areas of Development	Examples of Research Questions
Social	What are the sequential stages that lead to cooperative play in children?
Emotional	What are the origins of anxiety?
Cognitive	What types of logic are used by 3-year-old children?
Language	What is the most favorable age for learning a second language?
Academic	What cognitive processes are related to reading?
Moral	What factors facilitate moral learning in 8-year-old children?
Motor	What are the sequential stages of development in eye-hand coordination?
Feeding	What is the relationship between obesity in infancy and obesity in adolescence?

Observational Methods for Collecting Data

> The technique of observation of infant behavior is not a subject that lends itself to free and easy generalization. Nor does the question, what is the best technique, permit a simple answer. Observation methods must vary considerably with the age of the infant and, of course with the objectives in view. (Gesell, 1928, p. 23)

The observational method that the developmental researcher selects should provide objective descriptive data that are representative of the child's repertoire of behavior. This is accomplished by providing the child with a stimulus that will elicit the desired behavior, schematically represented in Figure 4–1.

The researcher selects the stimulus after operationally defining the area of development in terms of the behavioral response. Tests for assessing a child's level of development such as the Bayley Scales of Infant Development–2 (BSID–2; Bayley, 1993) and the Miller Assessment for Preschoolers (MAP; Miller, 1988) are examples of this method. In the BSID–2, cognitive abilities are operationally defined by the following tasks:

DEVELOPMENTAL FACTORS	OPERATIONAL DEFINITION
Object Permanence	An object is wrapped in a sheet of paper while the child is watching. The child is asked to find the object.
Manual Dexterity	Child puts pegs into a peg board in a timed or untimed condition. The time taken to complete the task is age specific.

Questions arise in this context. How does the researcher know that all aspects of a developmental factor are being considered

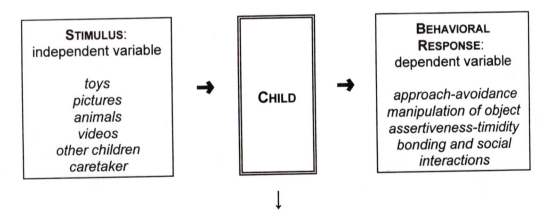

Figure 4–1. Schematic representation of observational research. Notice that the subject is provided with stimuli so as to elicit a response. The data collected are the behaviors elicited by the stimuli.

and that the operational definition of a developmental factor is valid? These questions are pertinent in developmental research, and they demand a rationale from the investigator.

In reporting developmental data, the researcher should describe factors in the child that affect the results. These factors include age, gender, intelligence, education, socioeconomic status, family structure, and experiences. The selection and control of these factors by inclusion in the research eliminates ambiguity in interpreting the results.

As well as operationally defining the developmental factors and identifying variables within the child, the researcher must construct an objective environment for collecting valid data. Examples of experimental environment in developmental research are shown in Figures 4–2 and 4–3. Arrangements for observation are part of a standard procedure. Adaptations in this method include the use of a photographic dome as developed by Gesell (1928) or the use of experimental rooms with one-way mirrors, where the observer is not seen by the subject. Box 4–3 gives an example of a study using developmental research.

4.3.4 Longitudinal Research (Prospective Designs)

Are there developmental factors over a period of time that cause changes in a person's anatomical and physiological processes, predisposing him or her to illness? Does prolonged exposure to smog cause lung cancer? Do obese adults develop heart disease when they are middle-aged at a higher rate than nonobese adults? Do children who have high IQs become leaders in the society when they are adults? What is the prognosis for high-risk children who come from socially disadvantaged environments? What is the relationship between occupational hazards and the later onset of disease? These problems are all affected by time factors.

Longitudinal research is a method used in observing the effects of independent variables on dependent variables over a determined period of time. The investigator uses longitudinal research to predict an outcome based on the presence of causative factors. For example, a team of researchers may study groups of individuals over a period of 20 years from young adult to middle age and observe whether certain groups are more vulnerable to heart attacks than other groups. In occupational therapy, a researcher may examine the long-term effects of sensory integration on academic achievement in children with learning disabilities. Box 4–4 provides an example of longitudinal research relating cholesterol to coronary heart disease.

4.3.5 Field Observation (Ethnography)

About the same time that Gesell was experimenting with his photographic dome, cultural anthropologists developed scientific methods for collecting data describing the

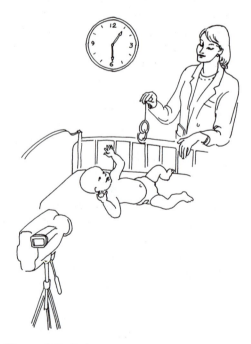

Figure 4–2. Position of the camera and baby when taking observational data.

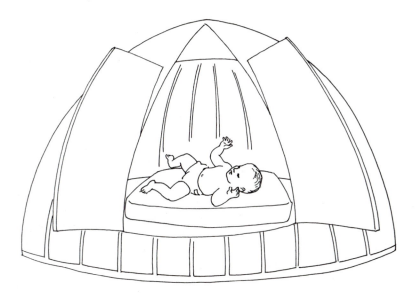

Figure 4–3. Illustration of a photographic dome used by Gesell (1928) in observational research.

everyday lives of aboriginal people. Franz Boas, the noted anthropologist, wrote in the foreword to Margaret Mead's classic study *Coming of Age in Samoa* (1928) the following, which summarized field research:

> Through a comparative study of these data and through information that tells us of their growth and development, we endeavor to reconstruct, as well as may be, the history of each particular culture. Some anthropologists even hope that the comparative study will reveal some tendencies of development that recur so often that significant generalizations regarding the processes of cultural growth will be discovered. (p. xiii)

Mead attempted to answer the question "Are the disturbances which vex our adolescents due to the nature of adolescence itself or to the civilization?" (pp. 6–7). She lived in Samoa for 6 months, and there she analyzed the life and development of 68 girls between the ages of 8 and 20. She was particularly concerned with three villages on the island of Tau.

In her field study, Mead painted a vivid and complete picture of the island life of adolescent girls. She felt that certain characteristics, basically Samoan, enable adolescent girls to pass through puberty without the storms and crises that are part of living in Western society. Chiefly, a Samoan girl may leave her immediate household and go to live with another family at any time, especially if she feels put upon. Other characteristics concern life roles, absence of double standards, familiarity with disasters such as death, casual family relationships as opposed to intense ones, and a specific place in society for each member. Further, the author pointed to a tolerance for sexually diverse behavior and concomitant lack of guilt feelings about such behavior, absence of extreme poverty, and a less stressful environment as reasons for a more serene adolescence than that found elsewhere in the world.

Mead's pioneering research led to the field of ethnography: to reconstruct accurately a particular culture and to search for patterns that can be generalized to a specific population. The observations occur in a natural setting, such as in a primitive village, urban neighborhood, family home, playground, street corner, Israeli kibbutz,

---

BOX 4–3. EXAMPLE OF DEVELOPMENTAL OBSERVATION

1. **Bibliographical Notation**

   McConnell, D. B. (1994). Clinical observations and developmental coordination disorder: Is there a relationship? *Occupational Therapy International, 1,* 278–291.

2. **Abstract**

   This exploratory investigation examined the validity of using Wilson's format of clinical observations to assess children with developmental coordination disorder (DCD). Wilson's Clinical Observations format closely follows the original format by Johnson and is based on the work of A. J. Ayres. Forty-five children 6–9 years of age, including 15 children with DCD, 15 children below average and 15 children average or better in their motor skill performance were assessed using clinical observations. Differences among these three groups of children were significant or approached significance on 19 out of 36 observations. The implications of the findings for using clinical observations to assess children with DCD are discussed. (p. 278)

3. **Justification and Need for Study**

   To date, however, the relationship between items in any format of clinical observations and the motor skill performance of children with DCD has not been investigated. Whether it is valid to use any format of clinical observations to assess children with DCD is, therefore, not known. The aim of this investigation was to examine the relationship between items in the format of clinical observations most commonly used in Australia, namely, the formats developed by Wilson (1984), and the motor skill performance of children with DCD. (p. 279)

4. **Literature Review**

   Thirty-seven references were cited in the study. Articles came from a wide variety of journals, such as *American Journal of Occupational Therapy, Occupational Therapy Journal of Research, Journal of Child Psychology and Psychiatry, British Medical Journal, Developmental Medicine and Child Neurology, Australian Occupational Therapy Journal,* and *Child: Care, Health and Development.* The majority of articles cited were published during the 1980s and 1990s.

5. **Research Hypothesis or Guiding Questions**

   The guiding question implicitly stated was What is the "usefulness of Wilson's (1984) Clinical Observations format for assessing children with DCD?" (p. 287).

6. **Methodology**

   Two measures, the Bruininks Oseretsky Test of Motor Proficiency (BOTMP), Short Form (Bruininks, 1978) and the Wilson's (1984) Clinical Observations

---

or mental hospital. Examples of field studies are Stanton and Schwartz's (1954) analysis of the interactional communication patterns among staff members in a mental

hospital, Bruno Bettelheim's (1969) investigation of the child-rearing patterns among families living in an Israeli kibbutz, and Oscar Lewis' (1965) study of a Puerto Rican format, were administered to 45 children, ages 6–9, over a period of 16 weeks. The assessments were videotaped and reassessed for interrater reliability. Clinical observations included motor and postural difficulties. Group 1 was composed of children from waiting list for occupational therapy services. Group 2 were children who were perceived as having poor motor coordination and who were referred by teachers from a participating school. Group 3 were typical children with age-appropriate motor skills.

7. **Results**
An analysis of variance (ANOVA) revealed differences between the three groups. "Findings of this investigation suggest ten [of the 24] observations in Wilson's (1984) Clinical Observation format are related to DCD, with another nine observations potentially related." (p. 289).

8. **Conclusions**
Further research is needed with a larger population to confirm the findings and to examine the causal relationship between developmental coordination disorder and motor skills.

9. **Limitations of the Study**
Limitations include (a) the size of the sample, (b) the associational relationship between variables rather than the causal relationship between variables, and (c) possible bias in teacher judgement.

10. **Major References Cited in the Study**
Ayres, A. J. (1972). *Sensory integration and learning disorders*. Los Angeles: Western Psychological Services.
Ayres, A. J. (1976). *Interpreting the Southern California Sensory Integration Tests*. Los Angeles: Western Psychological Services.
Laszlo, J. I. (1990). Child perceptuo-motor development: Normal and abnormal development of skilled behaviour. In C. A. Hauert, (Ed.), *Developmental psychology: Cognitive, perceptuo-motor and neuropsychological perspectives* (pp. 278–308). Amsterdam: Elsevier Science.
Smyth, T. R. (1991). Abnormal clumsiness in children: A defect of motor programming? *Child: Care, Health and Development, 17*, 283–293.
Wilson, E. B. (1984). *Occupational therapy for children with minimal handicaps*. Unpublished manual.
Wilson, B., Pollock, N., Kaplan, B. J., Low, M., & Faris, P. (1992). Reliability and construct validity of the Clinical Observations of Motor and Postural Skills. *American Journal of Occupational Therapy, 46*, 775–783.

family coping with slum life in New York City. (See also Hall, 1966; Jessor, Colby, & Shweder, 1996.)

Jules Henry's (1971) in-depth study of five families in which a child with psychosis was present is a bleak and brilliant example of field observation. He proposes that the main difference between "them and us" is "that they [families with a child with psychosis] seem to go to extremes and do too many things that are upsetting"(p. xx). Henry detailed communication

BOX 4–4. EXAMPLE OF LONGITUDINAL RESEARCH

1. Bibliographical Notation

Kinosian, B., Glick, H., & Garland, G. (1994). Cholesterol and coronary heart disease: Predicting risks by levels and ratios. *Annals of Internal Medicine, 121,* 641–647

2. Abstract

Objective: Comparison of four measures of cholesterol for predicting men and women who will develop coronary heart disease within 8 to 10 years.

Design: Cohort study.

Patients: 1898 men who received placebo (the placebo group of the Lipid Research Clinics (LRC) Coronary Primary Prevention Trial (CPPT), 1025 men and 1442 women who participated in the 1970–1971 Framingham Heart Study biennial examination, and 1911 men and 1767 women without coronary heart disease who were from the LRC Population Prevalence Study.

Measurements: Total cholesterol, low-density lipoprotein (LDL) cholesterol, ratio of total cholesterol to high-density lipoprotein (HDL) cholesterol, and the ratio of LDL to HDL. Outcomes were coronary heart disease in the CPPT and Framingham studies and death from coronary heart disease in the Prevalence Study.

Results: Independent information in the total cholesterol/HDL ratio added risk-discriminating ability to total cholesterol and LDL cholesterol measures ($P < 0.02$), but the reverse was not true. Among women, a high-risk threshold of 5.6 for the total cholesterol/HDL ratio identified a 0% to 15% larger group at 25% to 45% greater risk in the Prevalence and Framingham studies, respectively, than did current guidelines. Among men in the same studies, a risk threshold of 6.4 for the total cholesterol/HDL ratio identified a 69% to 95% larger group at 2% to 14% greater risk than did LDL cholesterol levels alone. Eight-year likelihood ratios for coronary heart disease ranged from 0.32 to 3.11 in men and from 0.59 to 2.98 in women for total cholesterol/HDL ratios (grouped from < 3 to ≥ 9).

Conclusions: The total cholesterol/HDL ratio is a superior measure of risk for coronary heart disease compared with either total cholesterol or LDL cholesterol levels. Current practice guidelines could be more efficient if risk stratification was based on this ratio rather than primarily on the LDL cholesterol level. (p. 641)

3. Justification and Need for Study

The authors conducted this study to gain a better understanding of the relationship between the total cholesterol/HDL ratio when used as a measure of risk for coronary heart disease.

4. Literature Review

Twenty-seven references were cited in the study. Articles came from a wide variety of journals, such as *Journal of American Medical Association (JAMA),*

Circulation, American Heart Journal, Archives of Internal Medicine, Journal of Chronic Diseases, and *The American Journal of Epidemiology.* The majority of journals came from the 1990s.

5. **Research Hypothesis or Guiding Questions**
The guiding question implicitly stated was, What is the relationship between cholesterol level and heart disease over a 8- to 10-year period?

6. **Methodology**
This was a longitudinal study using participants from two general populations. The researchers examined whether the total cholesterol/HDL ratio could predict different risks for coronary heart disease. The at-risk population was a randomized, double-blind, placebo-controlled intervention trial that included 3806 men with primary hypercholesterolemia (type IIA). The comparison group included men and women from the Framingham Heart Study, a longitudinal observational study with biennial follow-up of 5209 men and women, between the years of 28 to 62 at study inception.

7. **Results**
When using the total cholesterol and LDL as the primary measures, statistically significantly high and low-risk groups were identified by measures of total cholesterol/HDL and LDL/HDL ratios.

8. **Conclusions**
The total cholesterol/HDL ratio was superior in predicting subsequent coronary heart disease to either the total cholesterol level or the LDL cholesterol level.

9. **Limitations of the Study**
The limitation of the study is that it is a correlational design that looks at the relationship between cholesterol and heart disease, rather than an experimental study in which the independent variable is manipulated.

10. **Major References Cited in the Study**
Glick, H,. Kinosian, B., Garland, G. (1993). Effectiveness and efficiency of lipid modification directly estimated from the Coronary Primary Prevention Trial (CPPT). *Medical Decision Making, 13,* 386.

Jacobs, D. R., Mebane, I. L., Bandiwala, S. I., Criqui, M. H., & Tyroler, H.A. (1990). High density lipoprotein cholesterol as a predictor of cardiovascular disease mortality in men and women: The follow-up study of the Lipid Research Clinics' Prevalence Study. *American Journal of Epidemiology, 131,* 32–47.

Levy, D., Wilson, P. W., Anderson, K. M., & Castelli, W. P. (1990). Stratifying the patient at risk from coronary disease: New insights from the Framingham Heart Study. *American Heart Journal, 119,* 712–771.

National Institutes of Health Consensus Development Panel on Triglyceride, High-Density Lipoprotein and Coronary Heart Disease. (1993). *Journal of the American Medical Association, 269,* 505–510.

patterns, physical interaction, and positions of power in each of the five families. He faithfully recorded the emotional content of the parents' communication patterns and their effects on their children. To record accurately, he lived with four of the five families for a short time and relied on a trained observer to supply similar observations about the fifth family. The five studies involved field visits to each family once a week. Rapport was established when the investigator informed each family that this kind of observation would perhaps aid other children with psychosis. He maintained confidentiality in the study by altering some of the details of family life and all of the names of the families.

A study entitled *Clinical Observation of Ghetto Four-Year-Olds: Organizational, Involvement, Interpersonal Responsiveness and Psychosexual Content of Play* by Borowitz, Costello and Hirsch (1971) is a good example of field observation methodology. In this study, children were observed while playing in semistructured settings. The play sessions were filmed on 16-mm silent movie film and tape-recorded simultaneously. The data were analyzed later by independent raters using play behavior scales developed by the authors.

The Application of Field Observation (Ethnography) to Occupational Therapy

What research problems are appropriate to field observations? Some possibilities are as follows:

▶ Research involving the culture of individuals with disabilities living in specialized environments such as halfway houses, forensic units, adult day care, psychiatric hospitals, communities for individuals with physical disabilities, and residential institutions for the individuals with profound mental retardation (Gleason, 1990; McColl & Peterson, 1997)
▶ Client advocacy (Sachs & Linn, 1997)

▶ Occupational therapy practice (Fitzgerald, Mullavey-O'Byrne, & Clemson, 1997)
▶ Meaning of play (Gleason, 1990)
▶ Mental health day programs (Townsend, 1996)
▶ Inclusionary settings for individuals with special needs (Falk-Ross, 1996; Miller, 1990)
▶ Daily occupations of Orthodox Jewish couples (Frank et al., 1997)
▶ Cultural diversity (Adger, 1994; Luera, 1994; Malave & Duquette, 1991; Whiteford, 1995)

Advantages of Field Observation

The main purpose of field observation or ethnography is to describe accurately the social structure and social processes engaged in by a group of people. The investigator observes the interactions between members of a group, records their responses, describes their formal codes for communications and the unwritten rules that guide their behaviors (Frederick, 1928; Mead, 1928). In the field study, the investigator structures observations while being as unobtrusive as possible in the environment to minimize the influence of one's presence on those being observed. One major advantage of the field observation is that data obtained from this method are not affected by artificial laboratory conditions. Another advantage is that the investigator observes behavior directly rather than eliciting verbal responses, such as through group personality tests. A third advantage is that the observer, who is not a part of the culture, will recognize patterns and behaviors differently from the way that these are acknowledged by those within the culture. Indeed, the "outsider" assists in bringing to the forefront patterns that, being embedded in "insider" behavior, are not readily described or easily recognized by members of the group.

Which research method would be appropriate for examining the interactions in a residential school for individuals with profound retardation? It is not possible to construct experimental conditions or control for all of the possible variables that could affect the dependent variable, which is, in this example, the rate of development in the child who is profoundly retarded. The most appropriate method would be qualitative research, where the investigator observes, like an ethnographer in a natural setting, the structures and processes of the institution and the transactions and interactions between all the participants in the institutional setting.

Methods of Field Observation

The investigator using field observation research is initially guided by research questions that focus on the important issues in social structures and social processes, such as education, vocational preparation, health care, child-rearing practices, sexual expression, ethical standards, peer relationships, leisure patterns, and recreation (Box 4–5). Broad areas selected for field observation are decided before the investigator collects data. The preparation for field observation is detailed in the Research Design section. Here the investigator decides:

▶ The total time period for field observation
▶ The methods used in establishing rapport with the group
▶ The broad areas in a social structure to be investigated
▶ The observational recording devices to be used (e.g., camcorders, audio tapes)
▶ Methods for preserving the confidentiality of group and obtaining informed consent
▶ Test instructions for collecting data (e.g., rating scales, questionnaires, and attitude surveys)

4.3.6 Historical Research

Definition

Historical research is a systematic method for reconstructing events that happened in the past to describe and understand them. As applied to occupational therapy, historical research pertains to (a) the chronology of events in occupational therapy, (b) the interrelationship between these events, and (c) the critical factors influencing them. For example, one might want to describe the events and identify the individuals that led to the formation of the discipline of occupational therapy in 1917. In studying historical data in occupational therapy, the investigator examines the individuals who were significant in shaping events and creating change and the institutions or organizations that were part of the historical process. The scientific approach to collecting historical data is similar to all methods of research in that the investigator proposes a research problem, states guiding questions, collects data, interprets the results, and arrives at conclusions and implications. The main differences between historical research and other types of research models are in the format of guiding questions and in the use of related literature. In historical research the guiding questions serve as the generating rationale for collecting data and the literature review provides the data, while the literature review generates guiding questions in other qualitative methods.

Purposes

Fraenkel and Wallen (1990) suggested five purposes for historical research:

1. "To make people aware of what has happened in the past so they may learn from past failures and sucesses" (p. 411): For example, cone stacking has been used rather than craft activities to increase fine motor coordination. The craft activity is client centered and increases motivation, whereas the cone stacking is a nonmeaningful repetitive activity.
2. "To learn how things were done in the past to see if they might be applicable to the present day problems and concerns" (p. 411): The model used in adult day centers from the 1950s and 1960s was

Box 4–5. Example of Ethnographic Research

1. Bibliographical Notation
Yau, M. K-S. (1997). The impact of refugee resettlement on southeast Asian adolescents and young adults: Implications for occupational therapist. *Occupational Therapy International, 4,* 1–16.

2. Abstract
After the change of governments in Vietnam and Cambodia and amidst turmoil in the mid 1970s, many Southeast Asians, fearing reprisals, emigrated from these countries. Among them were children, many of whom were separated from their families prior to, or during, their escape. Many of them have been resettled in the Western countries from the refugee camps, and now are adolescents or are entering into young adulthood. With memories of the war and the stress of separation from family and adaptation to different cultures, psychosocial problems are common in this population. Occupational therapy can help these clients by providing opportunities to: (1) practice appropriate human occupations and establish more satisfying relationships; (2) facilitate release and sublimation of emotional drives; (3) enhance smooth transition and adaptation to the new environment; and (4) assist in the adoption of appropriate occupational roles. General principles are proposed for developing occupational therapy services that are appropriate and culturally relevant to the needs of this client group. Occupational therapists can play an important role in assisting the clients in resettlement, pursuing better quality of life and being a contributing member of the society. (p. 1)

3. Justification and Need for Study
The author justified the study by showing the need for occupational therapists to help refugees cope with lifestyle changes.

4. Literature Review
Forty-eight references were cited in the study. Articles came from a wide variety of journals, such as *Australian Journal of Occupational Therapy, American Journal of Occupational Therapy (AJOT), Social Science and Medicine, Hospital and Community Psychiatry, American Journal of Psychiatry, Journal of the American Academic of Child and Adolescent Psychiatry,* and *Archives of General Psychiatry.* The majority of journal citations are from the 1980s and 1990s.

5. Research Hypothesis or Guiding Questions
The guiding question stated was, What is the "impact of the refugee resettlement process on the Southeast Asian adolescents and young adults' mental health, and to highlight the implications for occupational therapy practice?" (p. 2)

6. Methodology
From the author experiences and a review of the literature, the author's identified four factors as critical in the adjustment of Southeast Asian adolescents

and their mental health. Implications for therapy were addressed: "The nature of occupational therapy practice with its diverse skills, holistic view of clients and focus on human's occupational role, occupational performance and the associated performance components within one's physical social and cultural environments affords the profession a vital role in all aspects of adaption and resettlement" (p. 9).

7. Results

"Based on the author's clinical experience and the available occupational therapy literature in this area of practice... 10 general principles are proposed to guide planning cluturally relevant therapeutic interventions for Southeast Asian refugee clients, particularly adolescents and young adults" (p. 10).

8. Conclusions

The author concluded that although

there is a lack of literature to highlight the role of occupational therapists in working with Southeast Asian adolescents and your adult client groups, the extensive nature of the literature review provides an overview of the unusually traumatic experiences endured by the Southeast Asian refugee population and, in particular, highlights the unique needs of the adolescent, within the community in Western host countries. It is hoped that highlighting areas of need for further research and general consideration may also prove useful to the health care professionals' research endeavors. (pp. 13–14)

9. Limitations of the Study

The author stated that "These suggestions may seem idealistic given the unclear perceived role of occupational therapists within a multidisciplinary team to work with the client group, in a limited treatment time" (p. 13).

10. Major References Cited in the Study

Axelson, J. A. (1993). *Counseling and development in a multicultural society.* Pacific Grove, CA: Brooks/Cole.

Bemak, F., & Greenberg, B. (1994). Southeast Asian refugee adolescents: Implications for counseling. *Journal of Multicultural Counseling and Development, 22,* 115–122.

Dillard, M., Andonian, L., Flores, O., Lai, L., MacRae, A., & Shakir, M. (1992). Culturally competent occupational therapy in a diversely populated mental health setting. *American Journal of Occupational Therapy, 46,* 721–725.

Kinebanian, A., Stomph, M. (1992). Cross-cultural occupational therapy: A critical reflection. *American Journal of Occupational Therapy, 46,* 751–757.

Yau, M. K. (1995). Occupational therapy in community mental health: Do we have a unique role in the interdisciplinary environment? *Australian Occupational Therapy Journal, 42,* 129–132 successful in treating individuals with psychosocial illnesses. Adult day care centers now use this model in caring for individuals with Alzheimer's disease.

3. "To assist in prediction" (p. 412): Special education has alternated between placing students with special needs into self-contained classrooms and into the general education program. Examination of mainstreaming in the 1980s demonstrated that these students will not succeed in the general education program without support from special educators, occupational therapists, and other allied health personnel.

4. "To test hypotheses concerning relationships or trends" (p. 412): Over the last 80 years, an examination of trends of employment settings has shown a change for occupational therapists from primarily hospital-based settings to schools and home health care.

5. "To understand present educational practices and policies more fully" (p. 412): To understand Medicare reimbursement, occupational therapists study previous legislation and litigation leading to the present policies.

Hypothetical Questions Examined in Occupational Therapy

▶ How did occupational therapists treat individuals with polio during the 1950s?
▶ What treatment techniques were used by occupational therapists in large mental hospitals during the 1930s?
▶ What are some of the experiences and education of noted individuals in occupational therapy?
▶ How is occupational therapy treated in the literature by individuals who write about their disability experiences?
▶ How have different philosophical viewpoints in occupational therapy influenced treatment in the schools?
▶ What is the history of the use of arts and crafts in occupational therapy?
▶ What are the major theories that impact on clinical treatment?

Format of Historical Research

The outline of historical research is as follows:

Part I: The statement of problem and significance of the study (e.g., how the study impacts on occupational therapy)

Part II: Guiding questions and methods for collecting data

Part III: The results, including the collection of data from primary and secondary sources

Part IV: A discussion of the results based on previous data from other studies

Part V: Conclusions, implications of results, and recommendations for further study

Part I: The Statement of Problem and Significance of the Study. What are potential areas for historical research in occupational therapy? How does one determine its significance? These are issues of concern for the historical researcher or historiographer planning a study. Jacques Barzun (1974), in a discussion of psychohistory, stated that the primary purpose of the new history is explanation, and the ulterior motive is action. He stated, "The type of explanation sought is the scientific; that is, showing a connection ('durable link') between the facts and a definable cause. Classification, then analysis, then prediction is the sequence that leads naturally to action" (p. 60). Barzun suggested that the historiographer's main motive is to obtain evidence in support of a cause. In effect, the historical researcher is a tool for change. This approach to medicine and health care can lead to research supporting causes that advocate change in the delivery of health care, public health education, the training and preparation of health professionals, and the training of special educators. The vulnerability of this approach is that the researcher could subjectively determine what evidence to cite. The historiographer should start with a relevant problem and objectively collect data. Table 4–7 outlines the relationship between the researcher's motive and the problem being investing using the historical research model.

Part II: Guiding Questions and Methodology. After narrowing the area of investigation to a researchable question, the researcher states any assumptions underlying the study. These assumptions are the researcher's preliminary opinions, attitudes, and knowledge in the area. For example, if a researcher is interested in what factors led to the development of the rehabilitation movement in the 20th century, tentative assumptions could be proposed. These are:

▶ The rehabilitation movement developed in response to the health needs of the individual who is chronically disabled.
▶ The rehabilitation movement was facilitated by governmental legislation related to social security.
▶ The industrialized countries were first to educate specialized rehabilitation workers.
▶ World War I and World War II generated the need for developing a technology for restoring function in soldiers who were severely wounded.
▶ The first leaders in the rehabilitation movement were social reformers.

Continuing with the above examples, the researcher generates the following questions:

▶ What was the historical chronology of the rehabilitation movement?
▶ How did social welfare programs influence rehabilitation legislation?
▶ How did advances in medical treatment influence rehabilitation of individuals who were chronically disabled?
▶ When did the allied health professions emerge and affect the rehabilitation movement?
▶ What scientific technology facilitated advances in rehabilitation medicine?
▶ Who are the leaders and supporters of the rehabilitation movement?

These guiding questions provide the content areas for the literature search and collection of data. The plan for collecting the data should be carefully formulated. The research plan is the outline of primary and secondary sources to be used in the data collection procedure. These sources include the following:

Table 4–7. Relationships Between Researcher's Motive and Investigated Problem

Motive of Researcher	Statement of Problem
• Establishing the occupational therapist as an independent practitioner	• How did the independent health practitioner evolve historically?
• Including the individual with mental retardation in the community	• What factors led to the institutionalization of individuals with mental retardation from 1900 to 1950?
• Incorporating wellness in health education of public schools	• What is the history of health education in public schools?
• Assuring the right of access to primary health for every individual	• Historically, what are the determining factors regarding access to health care?
• Gaining parity in health insurance coverage for psychosocial disabilities	• Why have insurance companies typically restricted reimbursement for psychosocial disabilities?

- Published books, periodicals, newspapers, and pamphlets
- Unpublished conference proceedings and minutes of meetings
- Official records and vital statistics
- Governmental documents, archives, and publications
- Personal letters, diaries, and memoirs
- Collateral interviews of eyewitnesses
- Tape recordings and films

Part III: Data Collection. The essential task of the historical researcher is to collect reliable and valid data. By obtaining various sources of information, one is able to cross-check the data, thereby substantiating one's conclusions. This procedure is called *triangulation*. Primary sources that represent "first hand" data, such as eyewitnesses and contemporary documents, are the best evidence for the historical researcher. In comparison, secondary sources are the interpretations and critiques of historical evidence based on primary data. Primary sources are the raw data for historical research, while secondary sources serve as supportive evidence. In researching a problem the investigator should seek evidence that is direct, objective, and verifiable. It should be clear that one unit of datum is not conclusive. The "personal equation," which is the observer's effect on what is being observed and measured, must be controlled by the investigator's substantiating evidence from more than one primary source as eyewitness account.

Secondary sources such as encyclopedias, textbooks, and critical essays are useful in initially obtaining an overview of an historical problem. These sources represent the generally accepted versions of historical events that have been "retold" in a reductive manner. The critical historiographer need not accept any evidence until primary data can substantiate the facts.

Part IV: Discussion of Results, and Part V: Conclusions and Recommendations. The raw data of an historical study must be critically analyzed by the investigator for its validity before any conclusions or generalizations can be made. The historical researcher must examine every document and piece of evidence with a skeptical eye, seeking substantiating proof for the authorship and the accuracy of its contents. *External criticism* of a document is a testimony of its authenticity. The Hippocratic writings are an example of unknown authorship and unknown copyright date. It is important for the historical researcher to substantiate the author of every document, the date it was written, and the place of origination or presentation, as evidence for external validity. Indirect means for collecting evidence are frequently used by historians. These methods include archeology and paleography (e.g., study of ancient manuscripts and examination of art objects). Ancient medical instruments used in surgery were discovered through archeological evidence. Questions that might be asked when examining external validity are (Fraenkel & Wallen, 1990):

- Did the purported author actually write the document or report the event?
- Do we know the exact the date that the document was written?
- Do we know where the document was written or where the observation took place?
- Are we sure that the writing of the document or observation data were not influenced by external events or individuals?
- Are we sure the document is genuine?

The next step of the historical researcher is to establish the validity or truth contained in a document. This process is called *internal criticism*. The purpose of this process is to establish as near as possible the actuality of an event. Fraenkel and Wallen (1990) suggested the following types of questions:

- Was the author an eyewitness to the event?
- Did the author participate in the event?

▶ What expertise did the author have to discuss or report the event?

▶ Was the author biased or subjective in the observation, or did the author have a vested interest in the event?

Historical surveys of medical progress are frequently filled with interpretative statements that go beyond the evidence and selective omissions that fail to give a true perspective of events or individuals who had an impact on treatment. It is left to the historical researcher in occupational therapy to carefully evaluate the biases of the authors when interpreting evidence. Generalizations and synthesizing statements should be carefully documented. In examining the causes of events, the historiographer takes a multidimensional point of view looking at the influences of contemporary practices of treatment, discoveries, patterns of dysfunction, governmental and community intervention, war, and natural disasters. One variable rarely changes the course of history.

A good example of historical research is a scholarly manuscript by Saul Benison (1972), "The History of Polio Research in the United States: Appraisal and Lessons." In this article, Benison documented the chronological events that led to a safe and effective vaccine for preventing polio. He analyzed the problem from three perspectives: (a) time of events, (b) settings where research took place, and (c) individuals and scientists who had an impact on the problem and facilitated progress in the development of a vaccine. These three factors are detailed in Table 4–8.

In documenting the chronology of events and the individuals who made important contributions to the development of a successful polio vaccine, Benison used the following primary sources:

▶ contemporary accounts of the early polio epidemics from 1894 to 1910
▶ autobiographical notes
▶ history of the Rockefeller Institute

Table 4–8. History of Polio Research in the United States

Time	Event	Setting	Contributors
1884	Polio epidemics identified in U.S.		
1907	Initial research in polio	Rockefeller Institute	Flexner
1910–1913	Poliovirus implicated	Rockefeller Institute	Flexner and associates
1920–1930	Transmission of polio	Rockefeller Institute	Olitsky et al.
1938	Warm Springs Foundation	Georgia	Roosevelt et al.
1938	Electron microscope	Germany	Borries
1946	Immunization of monkeys	Johns Hopkins	Morgan
1948–1951	Identification of poliovirus	U. California Johns Hopkins U. of Pittsburgh	Kessel Bodian Salk
1949	Cultivation of poliovirus	Harvard	Enders et al.
1952	Salk vaccine (dead intramuscular [i.m.] vaccine)	U. Pittsburgh	Salk
1954	Mass vaccinations	U. Michigan	Francis
1958	Sabin Vaccine (oral live vaccine)	U. Cincinnati	Sabin

Note: Adapted from "The History of Polio Research in the United States: Appraisal and Lessons" by S. Benison. In *The Twentieth-Century Sciences: Studies in the Biography of Ideas*, pp. 308–343, by G. Holton, New York: W. Norton. Copyright 1972 by W. Norton.

▶ foreign journals
▶ scholarly articles by Flexner (1910) and associates
▶ conference proceedings
▶ research articles
▶ Bulletin of the History of Medicine
▶ National Foundation Archives
▶ history of Warm Springs
▶ private communication
▶ minutes of committees
▶ files from the National Foundation
▶ biographical essays
▶ final reports of research grants
▶ congressional hearings

In total, Benison used 117 citations to document his article. He concluded that the development of a successful polio vaccine was a cooperative effort by researchers in major universities funded by two private organizations—The Rockefeller Foundation and the National Foundation—with external support from the United States Public Health Service. Benison's lesson in the article was that modern medical progress is a cooperative effort where researchers from diverse settings are supported by the federal government, private foundations, and voluntary heath agencies.

The historical research article by Benison is an example of rigorous documentation providing strong external validity. Benison's article should serve as a model for research in occupational therapy. (See Box 4–6 for another example of historical research.)

Potential areas for historical research in occupational therapy include:

▶ biographies of founders of the discipline of occupational therapy
▶ development of innovative assistive technology
▶ development of social attitude toward psychosocial illness
▶ chronological analysis of the treatment of a disability
▶ history of the occupational therapy discipline
▶ history of a hospital, health facility, organization, or institution

▶ history of reimbursement practices
▶ history of movements in occupational therapy (e.g., rehabilitation and normalization)

4.4 Collecting Qualitative Data

There are many ways to collect qualitative data. Table 4–9 gives some examples. These are more fully explained in the following paragraphs.

4.4.1 Interviewing

The most common data collection method in qualitative research is interviewing. Using interviews as a research method rests on the assumption that "the perspective of others is meaningful, knowable, and able to be made explicit" (Patton, 1990, p. 270). In short, researchers conduct interviews to find out about things that cannot be directly observed. Everyday familiarity with conversational or therapeutic interviews can lead novice researchers to regard interviewing for research purposes as quite straightforward; but to effectively use interviewing as a research method requires knowledge of, and practice with, available techniques.

Research interviews take several forms. Interviews can be done face-to-face, over the telephone, or in a group. The format may be structured, semistructured, or open-ended. Interviewing may be used to collect personal experiences, to understand particular phenomena, or to identify the perspective of a particular group of people. Interviews may be brief or lengthy, they may be "one-off," or part of a series.

Oftentimes investigators will employ a combination of interviewing approaches if this suits the purpose of the research and the research questions. For example, an interview may begin with a standardized, structured format, followed by sections made up of semistructured questions. Alternatively, the interview may begin with an unstructured, open-ended format and conclude with a set of standardized questions.

Box 4–6. Example of Historical Research

1. **Bibliographical Notation**
   Sachs, D., & Sussman, N. (1995). Historical research: The first decade of occupational therapy in Israel: 1946–1956. *Occupational Therapy International, 2,* 241–256.

2. **Abstract**
   The present study examined the first decade of the development of occupational therapy in Israel: 1946–1956. The structural-functional approach to the study of professions, which provided the theoretical framework for this study, identifies three formal organizations in the professions: the practice, the educational system, and the association. The purpose of this article was to follow the development of occupational therapy and to examine the interrelations of the profession's three formal organizations in the reviewed period. The methodology of the study was based on qualitative historical methods. Data collection included oral histories, and published and unpublished written material. Data organization and analysis were within the framework of the structural-functional approach. Data analysis indicated that "expansion" was a major theme affecting the development of occupational therapy, the reason for which lies within the historical background of the period under investigation. In addition, data indicated that the practice was the strongest and most active organization in occupational therapy and that expansion in practice was beyond the capacity of both the educational system and the professional association. The interrelations of the three formal organizations, and the rapid expansion of occupational therapy practice, had a lasting effect on the development of occupational therapy in Israel. (p. 241)

3. **Justification and Need for Study**
   Because "historical research sheds light on present behaviors and practices," this study was completed to "understand current theories and practices more accurately, and to plan intelligently for the future" (p. 242).

4. **Literature Review**
   Forty-two references were cited in the study. Articles came from a wide variety of sources, including files at the Occupational Therapy School at the Hebrew University from 1947 to 1954; archives of Hadassah 1941–1949; *Israeli Journal of Occupational Therapy; Health services in Israel: A ten year survey 1948 –1958;* and *Trade Unions in Israel.*

5. **Research Hypothesis or Guiding Questions**
   The guiding questions explicitly stated were (a) "How did the practice [in occupational therapy] develop and how did it adapt itself to the growing needs of the healthcare services?" (b) "How did the educational system cope with practice needs?" and (c) "How did the association [Israeli Occupational Therapy Association] meet the needs of the profession?"

continued

6. Methodology

Interviews were held with nine female occupational therapists who had been practicing between 1946 and 1956 and who were considered prominent leaders in the development of occupational therapy in Israel. Primary documents including memoirs and archived materials were accessed by the investigators. These materials were analyzed using the structural-functional approach (Parsons, 1939) The credibility of the data was obtained by validating oral testimonies with contemporary documents.

7. Results

The historical development was organized into three periods, each covering the practice, the education system, and the professional association: (a) Preliminary Period, 1941–1945; (b) The Formative Years, 1946–1948; and (c) Expansion: 1949–1956.

8. Conclusions

"Analysis of the data indicates that the practice was the strongest and most active organization [as compared with education and professional association] in the function of occupational therapy. Expansion in the practice was beyond the capacity of the education and the association. . . . By employing historical research methods and a conceptual framework to the study of professions, this study exposed the origin of some of the problems faced by occupational therapy in Israel" (pp. 254–255).

9. Limitations of the Study

The study only interviewed nine individuals when collecting the bulk of the data. Also, some contemporary documents were not available and presumed to have been lost due to war conditions.

10. Major References Cited in the Study

Archives of Hadassah (1941–1949). *Occupational therapy correspondence services* (RQ, 1 HMO, Box 51), New York: Hadassah

Files at the occupational therapy school, 1st class. (1947–1949). Jerusalem: Hebrew University.

Files at the occupational therapy school, 2nd class. (1949–1951). Jerusalem: Hebrew University.

Files at the occupational therapy school, 3rd class. (1952–1954). Jerusalem: Hebrew University.

Goldschmidt, R. (1968, May). 20 years of the occupational therapy school (Hebrew). *Israeli Journal of Occupational Therapy,* 19–28.

Grushka, T. (1959). *Health services in Israel: A ten year survey 1948–1958.* Jerusalem: Ministry of Health.

Grushka, T. (1968). *Health services in Israel.* Jerusalem: Ministry of Health.

Sussman, N. (1989). *The history of occupational therapy in Israel: The first decade—1946–1956.* Unpublished masters thesis: New York University: New York.

Table 4–9. Methods of Collecting Data in Qualitative Research

Type	Definition	Research Example
Interviewing	Data collection method for obtaining information through face-to-face verbal exchange or mailed or through telephone surveys. Interviews can occur in a single session or over multiple sessions. Interviews can be group or individually obtained and can be structured, semistructured, or unstructured. Structured interviews have specific questions that are answered by the interviewee, whereas unstructured interviews have no specific questions but may have general areas of discussion. Semistructured interviews are a combination of both (Fontana & Frey, 1994).	Focus groups: Semistructured group interview. • Lau, A., Chi, I, & McKenna, K. (1998). Self-perceived quality of life of Chinese elderly people in Hong Kong. *Occupational Therapy International, 5,* 118–139.
Naturalistic observational techniques	• "the act of noting a phenomenon, often with instruments, and recording it for scientific or other purposes" (Morris, 1973, p. 906). Qualitative observation occurs in the natural setting among the targeted population without intervention by the observer. The focus of naturalistic observation is to examine "trends, patterns, and styles of behavior" (Adler & Adler, 1994, p. 378). • Naturalistic observation occurs through videotaping, audio taping, photography, or through participant observation.	Observational case study • Henry, J. (1971). *Pathways to madness.* New York: Random House.
Mute evidence	Primary sources, such as field notes, diaries, memos, letters, and official records (e.g., marriage licenses, banking statements, driving records), but not audio tapes or videotapes that can be heard or viewed.	Historiography • Benison, S. (1972). The history of polio research in the United States: Appraisal and lessons. *The twentieth-century sciences: Studies in the biography of ideas* (pp. 308–343). New York: W. Norton. • Jonsson, H. (1998). Ernst Westerlund—A Swedish doctor of occupation. *Occupational Therapy International 5,* 155–171.
Personal experience	Understanding of someone's life story through questioning who we are through the narrator, through our relationship to the text, and the way we interpret the text (Clandinin & Connelly, 1994). The life stories told by an individual become a means of educating self and others. Autobiography, case histories, and life stories are all part of personal experience.	Personal journals • Jung, B., & Tryssenaar, J. (1998). Supervising students: Exploring the experience through reflective journals. *Occupational Therapy International, 5,* 35–48.

The type of interview that will best suit the research purpose needs particular care and thought.

Structured Interviewing

In this type of interview, the interviewer uses a preestablished set of questions in a uniform manner. Although the questions may be open ended, the interviewer cannot alter the predetermined format. The aim of this structured approach is to achieve as close as possible a standard format across interviewers and respondents. One disadvantage of this approach is that the interviewer is not able to pursue topics of interest that arise during the interview.

Semistructured Interviewing

This type of interviewing utilizes a general interview guide. The issues to be covered in the interview are predetermined; however, question format and exact content are not prespecified. Rather, the interviewer uses a guide that can be adapted, as necessary, during the interview. Semistructured interviewing is an effective use of time while still allowing the interviewer to build up rapport and conduct the interview in a flexible way. This approach is particularly appropriate for group interviews where it can be used to encourage all participants to contribute to the topic under discussion.

Unstructured Interviewing

Unstructured interviews are sometimes referred to as informal conversational interviews or in-depth interviews. The purpose of this approach is to interview respondents without imposing any a priori categories on the content or format of the interview. The emphasis is on listening and on understanding each interviewee's individual point of view, not on explaining interviewees' perspectives within a predetermined interpretive framework (Holstein & Gubrium, 1995).

Unstructured interviews often occur as part of observation in field research. They may also be used with a specific purpose in mind, such as exploring one or more issues in depth. In unstructured interviewing, most of the questions flow from the immediate interview context. Specific questioning techniques are used to elicit, as clearly as possible, the way that each interviewee constructs meaning. For example, Spradley (1979) suggested three types of questions: descriptive, contrast, and structural. Patton (1990) also listed a number of alternative questioning formats. Whichever techniques are used, the researcher's primary task is to understand as fully as possible the interviewee's point of view.

Unstructured interviews are particularly useful for interviewing individuals over a period of time. Later interviews can be used to elaborate information gathered in earlier interviews to help build a comprehensive picture of the topic being investigated. One disadvantage of unstructured interviewing is the time involved. Another is the resources needed to analyze the quantity and variety of information gained.

Group Interviews

Interviewing people in groups is gaining popularity in allied health research. Group interviews are commonly called focus groups. Focus groups may be structured, semistructured, or unstructured. Group interviews are a cost-effective and efficient way to gather information. Interviewers need to be experienced in managing group processes, however. For example, aspects of group interaction, such as the tendency of one or more members to dominate the group or the group members sliding into "group think," may impede the interview process (Frey & Fontana, 1995).

Attentive Listening

The role of self is critical in interviewing. Interviewing requires a commitment to, and an interest in, understanding another's point of view. Developing skills as an attentive listener are as important, if not more so, than becoming a skilled questioner. To resist the temptation to fit individuals into predetermined response categories requires careful listening and skillful questioning. Questions need to be as unambiguous, focused, and value-free as is humanly possible. Compiling such questions and learning how to create a context in which interviewees are willing to answer openly and honestly require effort and practice. The rewards are well worth the time spent.

Using a Tape Recorder

Using a tape recorder is an efficient and accurate method to record an interview, although this needs to be done unobtrusively so as not to inhibit interviewees' responses. Researchers can easily become dependent on using a tape recorder, and disaster strikes if for any reason a taped account is not possible. Not using a tape recorder requires a methodical approach and self-discipline to make sure that the researcher's notes are adequate. This is essential if the researcher is to gather the richest possible information in as many situations as possible.

There are instances in which tape recording is not a suitable means of documenting information. Using a tape recorder may invade the privacy of the participant by drawing attention to the interviewee. Circumstances may mitigate against adequate sound recording, particularly in open and crowded public places such as a shopping center. Tape recording may be inappropriate when the aim is to keep interviews as informal as possible.

Experience suggests that interviewees frequently share valuable information when tape recording is not possible, for example, on the sidewalk or just after the machine is turned off. No matter how relaxed interviewees become with a tape recorder, occasions still occur when information is withheld for privacy reasons or because of personal embarrassment. It is, therefore, most unwise to rely on taped interviews. Alternative procedures are described in the section on field notes (Section 4.4.3) discussed later in the chapter.

4.4.2 Observation

Observation is essential to understanding human and natural phenomena. As Adler and Adler (1994) noted, "as long as people have been interested in studying the social and natural world around them, observation has served as the bedrock source of human knowledge" (p. 377). Observation in qualitative inquiry goes by several terms: participant observation, direct observation, field research, or qualitative observation. Whatever the term employed, the essence of observation "lies in the prolonged and unobtrusive presence of a *sensitive* and *trained* observer among the people being studied" (Edgerton & Langness, 1978, p. 339, italics added). All observational methods require disciplined training and rigorous preparation.

The primary purpose of observation in qualitative research is to describe. Description includes the setting, the activities taking place, the participants, and the meaning of the setting and its activities from the perspective of the participants. Observing activities as they take place provides the researcher with direct first-hand experience. This is essential to a full understanding of the phenomena under investigation. There are a number of sources of data in fieldwork settings. These include the physical setting, social interactions and activities (both planned and informal), the language used, nonverbal communication, unobtrusive indicators, program documents and "notable nonoccurrences" (Patton, 1990). In any setting, however, there is far more happening than can be accurately observed and documented. Therefore, qualitative researchers usually employ a framework to guide their fieldwork observations.

Several dimensions to observing need careful consideration in the research design phase. These are the role of the observer, portrayal of role and purpose, and duration and focus of observation.

Role of the Observer

The first dimension relates to the extent to which the observer not only observes but participates in the setting. There are several typologies of observer involvement in research settings. For example, Gold (1958) outlined four modes: the complete participant, the participant-as-observer, the observer-as-participant, and the complete observer. The latter is rarely used now owing to the ethical concerns about covert observation.

Adler and Adler (1994) suggested three roles for researchers as observers: the complete-member-researcher, the active-member-researcher, and the peripheral-member-researcher. These roles fall along a continuum. The role chosen will depend on the purpose and nature of the research study. The peripheral-member-researcher is part of a setting while remaining removed from the core activities. The active-member-researcher participates in the core activities of the setting. The complete-member-researcher is one who already has full membership in the setting or converts to genuine membership during the study.

Portrayal of Role and Purpose

Researchers may explicitly explain their observer role and purpose, may choose not to disclose any information about their observational role, or may portray their role somewhere in between these two extremes. The nature of the research questions and the access the researcher has to the setting and their position within that setting will influence how much others are told about the researcher role. For example, in primarily evaluative research, there will usually be full and complete explanation of the observational component. As Patton succinctly noted, "People are seldom deceived or reassured by false or partial explanations— at least not for long" (p. 212). By contrast,

in research of a more public nature, there may be little need to describe exactly what will be observed, or when, how, and why it will be observed.

Duration and Focus of Observation

Observation may occur once only, happen for a limited period, or be of varying duration carried out multiple times over an extended period. The duration of the observational period relies heavily on the purpose of the research. For example, research investigating complex processes that change over time, such as adaptation to acquired disability, require prolonged observation. In contrast, the timeliness and resources available for evaluation research often determine how much—or how little— observation occurs.

Not everything in a single research project warrants observation. The focus and scope of the observation need to be considered when framing the research question. Decisions will need to be made, for example, about whether to observe a small number of occasions in great depth or many occasions in less depth.

4.4.3 Field Notes

Field notes are the basic tool of the qualitative researcher. As Patton noted, "There are many options in the mechanics of taking field notes. . . . *What is not optional is the taking of field notes*" (Patton, 1990, p. 239, italics in original). Taking field notes can be used to substitute for tape-recording interviews. Note taking can also be used to expand the taped account, for example, with enriching descriptions of visual "pictures" of participants' facial expressions, gestures, and other nonverbal behaviors. Taking notes also expands the opportunities to collect data. For example, taking notes can provide a documented account of participants' reactions and interactions.

As noted above, researchers need to learn to observe methodically. Similarly, learning to systematically document observations requires the researcher to develop disciplined methods. The first step in this process is to decide on a format. Field notes can be in one notebook or can be contained in a file system. The second step is to organize the different types of field notes according to their content, which will vary according to their purpose. The purposes of field notes include maintaining a transcript file, a personal log, or an analytical log (Minichiello, Aroni, Timewell, & Alexander, 1995).

The transcript file contains descriptive data about the observation or interview setting. This includes where the observation took place, who was present, and what social interactions and activities took place. This file may also contain a diagram of the setting. The transcript file also contains either a transcription of the interview or a written account of the observation. The secret of making good field notes for the transcript file is to be descriptive, concrete, and detailed. The researcher needs to avoid interpretation or judgment, loosely defined comparisons, and abbreviations that, although making sense at the time of documenting, may mean nothing at all when reviewing the file. This file should also contain direct quotations of what the research participants say. The quotations may be documented in the actual transcript of a recorded interview. If not, it is critical that the researcher record relevant information in the participants' own words. Participants' words can be differentiated from the researcher's descriptions by using quotation marks.

The personal log is the repository for the researcher's thoughts on the field research. This log includes personal feelings, reactions to the fieldwork experience, and personal and methodological reflections during the study. Writing this log needs to be done as soon as possible after each encounter in the field. It is not possible at the end of a study to go back and capture the feelings, reactions, and reflections that occurred during fieldwork. Keeping the personal log in the form of a journal may be helpful. Using headings and subheadings will help to organize the material and make it easier to review the contents in the analysis stage. The headings will vary according to research focus. For example, headings can be used to organize the material according to the sequence of events.

The analytical log contains the researcher's insights and reflections on data collection and analysis in the context of the theoretical framework of the study. Minichiello et al. (1995) suggested that this is where the researcher asks and answers questions such as: What is it that I know so far? What do I not know? What do I need to know? How do I collect this information? This log also provides a record or audit trail of the analysis and theoretical propositions as these develop throughout the study.

4.4.4 Political and Ethical Context for Research

The political context sets the background for any research project. This context ranges from the micropolitical of personal relationships to the macropolitical of government sponsorship of research. Feminist research and research about race and ethnicity have highlighted the potential nature of research as a political activity. Grappling with the political context may seem overwhelmingly daunting to the beginning researcher. This is more so because little is written about how experienced researchers understand and deal with the political dimensions of the contexts in which they are working (Shaffir & Stebbins, 1991). Consideration of the political context is crucial in the research design phase.

Much has been written about the stages of fieldwork, particularly strategies for entering and leaving the field (see, for example, Schatzman & Strauss, 1973, and Shaffir & Stebbins, 1991). Personal factors such as age, race, and gender of both the researcher and the research participants affect fieldwork. Other influences on fieldwork include the nature and status of the researcher's institution and the institution where the research occurs, for example, a prestigious teaching hospital compared to a community health center. Gatekeeping—the term used to describe institutional power holders blocking access to people served by their institution—does occur in the health and welfare fields. For example, family workers may be unwilling to inform client families about a proposed research project or may tell only some families and not others. This may be done on the grounds that some families are more likely to be willing to participate, are more articulate, or are more able to withstand yet another intrusion into their lives. Frequently, however, those families not informed are less well educated, from minority ethnic groups, or are disadvantaged parents. Professional gatekeeping of these families may result in nonrepresentative samples for the research.

Professional associations, academic institutions, funding bodies, and medical facilities have ethical standards and convene human ethics committees. These have a mandate to permit or disallow proposed research according to federal and state regulations. Traditionally, the ethical precepts of biomedical research have been applied to social science research, although this research is more likely to be of a qualitative nature. These regulations, although providing a useful framework, may offer little guidance for the proper and ethical conduct of research in the field. Of primary interest to field researchers are issues of consent, privacy, confidentiality, trust, and betrayal (Bulmer, 1982).

Gaining the informed consent of research participants is essential to the ethical conduct of any research. Informed consent, however, is not as straightforward as it first appears. What happens, for example, to individuals' behaviors if they are informed a priori that they will be observed? What constitutes "informed" consent under circumstances such as mental illness, cognitive limitations, extreme youth, and extreme age? Research in the medical, rehabilita-

tion, and allied health fields is often carried out with individuals identified as vulnerable subjects on ethics clearance forms. Obtaining informed consent from research participants in these groups may require special procedures (Booth & Booth, 1994; Llewellyn, 1995).

A major aim for ethical researchers is to protect the privacy and confidentiality of research participants. Typical ways that this is done include keeping data in locked storage, destroying identifying material, and using pseudonyms in research reports. Safeguards also need to be in place against less obvious intrusions on participant privacy and confidentiality. For example, the researcher's institutional affiliation, the description of the research context, or the bibliography of the research report may give away the research location and the likely participants.

Finishing a field research study presents a further ethical concern. At the beginning of a research study, intense effort, possibly over weeks, months, or even years will have gone into building trust with the research participants. At the end of the study, the researcher leaves while the participants remain. After a period of engagement, the participants may feel betrayed or, at the very least, let down. There are no simple rules to deal with this possibility. Each researcher must find a way to leave the field in an acceptably ethical manner. Fontana and Frey (1994) suggested a three-point guide to exercising moral responsibility toward research participants: "to our subjects first, to the study next and to ourselves last" (Fontana & Frey, 1994, p. 373).

4.5 Analyzing Qualitative Data

There is a diverse variety of methods for analyzing qualitative data (for example, see Bryman & Burgess, 1994; Miles & Huberman, 1994; Strauss & Corbin, 1998; Van Manen, 1990). Qualitative data analysis methods are based on the following general principles.

4.5.1 Principles

The first principle is that the analysis is conducted concurrently with data collection. This means that as analysis occurs, the researcher develops further questions that guide ongoing data collection. The researcher analyzes the data, proposes new questions or tentative propositions, and then "checks these out" by returning to the data. This proposing and verifying process illustrates the movement between inductive and deductive procedures typical of qualitative analysis procedures.

The second principle is that the analysis process is systematic. Methods vary according to schools of thought and the researcher's interpretive framework. All methods make use of systems that involve reflection, are open to examination, and can be applied to more than one researcher. Miles and Huberman (1994) described their system as follows: "Margin notes are made on the field notes, more reflective passages are reviewed carefully, and some kind of summary sheet is drafted. At the next level are coding and memo writing" (p. 432). These memos are analytic in nature and result from reflection on the data. Memos help the process of generating an increasingly more abstract conceptualization from the concrete field data (Miles & Huberman, 1994).

The third principle is that, during the analytic process, the data are "divided" into segments. These segments of data, however, remain part of the whole. Dividing the data into segments is carried out by using content analysis procedures. The researcher reviews the data from transcribed interviews or questionnaire responses or field notes and gives a name or code to each unit of meaning. This process is called *open coding* (Strauss & Corbin, 1998). The names or codes given to these units of meaning are developed directly from the text data or are generated from previous studies, from the relevant literature, or from a combination of all these sources.

The fourth principle is that comparison is the main intellectual tool employed by the researcher in doing the analysis. Comparison is used to "discern conceptual similarities, to refine the discriminative power of categories, and to discover patterns" (Tesch, 1990, p. 96). Glaser and Strauss (1967) developed the term *constant comparative analysis* to describe the process whereby the researcher compares and contrasts elements of data in a search for recurring regularities. These regularities are further compared and contrasted to develop concepts. These concepts are then compared and contrasted to form internally consistent and mutually exclusive categories.

The fifth principle is that the researcher refines the category organizing system as familiarity with the data develops. Using the comparative process, the researcher clusters together categories that are alike. The organizing system remains flexible, becoming more conceptually sound and parsimonious as the researcher develops a deeper understanding of the phenomena under study. This occurs as the categories are expanded and elaborated, which occurs by building on existing information, making links between items of information, and proposing and verifying new information. Category organization is continually refined until "theoretical saturation" is reached (Glaser & Strauss, 1967). Theoretical saturation is said to occur when new data lead to redundancy and the categories appear to be conceptually sound.

The sixth and final principle is that the goal of qualitative analysis is synthesis of the data into a higher level of conceptualization. In this process, a qualitative researcher has dual roles. The first is to describe phenomena as they exist—the what, how, when, and where. The second is to interpret and explain these phenomena as concepts. Patton (1990) suggested that this involves "discovering" and "uncovering."

Discovering involves elaborating concepts that are obvious to participant and researcher alike. *Uncovering* requires clarifying or elaborating already existing sociological concepts or building new concepts from the research setting. In summary, the aim in qualitative research designs is not casual determination, prediction, or generalization as in quantitative research. Rather, qualitative researchers aim to elucidate relationships, investigate and interpret connections and, by so doing, develop an understanding about particular phenomena and their place within existing theoretical knowledge about the social world.

4.5.2 Practice

Qualitative data is, most frequently, text derived from interview transcripts, questionnaire responses, field notes, and documents such as case records. The researcher may also use photographs and video (Harper, 1989). The volume of text data gathered can create a data management challenge. Miles and Huberman (1994) provided a useful summary of storage and retrieval requirements (Table 4–10).

Qualitative researchers need to develop a data management system that suits their own style or that of the research team and the purpose of the research. Traditional methods for organizing data using notebooks, file folders, card systems, filing cabinets, and the like. Newer methods include word-processing programs, databases, spreadsheets, and other computer-based programs. Storage and retrieval of data can be done quickly and efficiently using computer software.

Recent developments in computer software mean that researchers can also get help with data analysis. Several computer-based text analysis programs are available. The researcher needs to be aware of the assumptions underlying the design of the software and to decide whether such assumptions are congruent with the research purpose and design. For example, a common assumption is that concepts are of a

hierarchical nature (such that *A* is an instance of a higher order concept *B*, and so on). Three widely known programs are NUD.IST 4 (Richards & Richards, 1997), NVIVO (Richards & Richards, 1999), Ethnograph (Seidel, 1989), and ATLAS/ti (Muhr, 1991). Comprehensive reviews of available programs, their functions, advantages, and shortcomings are available (Miles & Huberman, 1994; Weitzmann & Miles, 1995).

4.6 Credibility in Qualitative Research

In qualitative research designs, the aim is to make sense of the meanings that people bring to phenomena in the social world. Qualitative researchers therefore want to make sure that their research findings are credible in the everyday sense of being plausible, believable, and trustworthy (Morse, 1994). Researchers using experimental designs and quantitative methods for collecting and analyzing data use constructs of reliability and validity. Many investigators have written on ways to address credibility in qualitative research. These range from applying of the experimental concepts of reliability and validity to suggesting alternative concepts better suited to qualitative designs (see, for example, Kirk & Miller, 1986, and Lincoln & Guba, 1985). Among these writers, there is general agreement that three elements of the inquiry process must be addressed. These are the research techniques used, the researcher's credibility, and the assumptions underpinning the study.

Credibility of the research techniques can be checked by testing rival explanations, by searching for negative cases, and by triangulation. The first, testing rival explanations, requires the researcher to consider and "test out" alternative explanations to that proposed and then to report the results. Searching for negative cases is a related process. In this instance, the researcher searches for cases that do not fit the pro-

Table 4–10. What to Store, Retrieve From, and Retain

- Raw material: field notes, tapes, site documents
- Partially processed data: write-ups, transcriptions. Initial version and subsequent corrected, "cleaned," "commented-on" versions
- Coded data: write-ups with specific codes attached
- The coding scheme or thesaurus, in its successive iterations
- Memos or other analytic material: the researcher's reflections on the conceptual meaning of the data
- Search and retrieval records: information showing which coded chunks or data segments the researcher looked for during analysis, and the retrieved material; records of links made among segments
- Data displays: matrices or networks used to display retrieved information, along with the associated analytic text; revised versions of these
- Analysis episodes: documenting of what was done, step by step, to assemble the displays and write the analytic text
- Report text: successive drafts of what is written on the design, methods, and findings of the study
- General chronological log or documentation of data collection and analytic work
- Index of all the above material

Note: Adapted from *Qualitative Data Analysis. An Expanded Sourcebook,* (2nd ed.), by M. B. Miles and A. M. Huberman, 1994, p. 48. Thousand Oaks, CA: Sage. Copyright 1994 by Sage.

posed patterns or themes identified from the data. Identifying negative or outlier cases increases understanding of the commonly occurring cases and, therefore, the totality of the phenomenon under investigation. The last way to check credibility is by a process called triangulation.

Triangulation has come to mean the use of multiple methods, sources, analysts, or theoretical perspectives to verify the information gained in different arenas. The aim of triangulation is "to guard against the accusation that a study's findings are simply an artifact of a single method, a single source, or a single investigator's bias" (Patton, 1990, p. 470). Triangulation of methods may involve collecting both quantitative and qualitative data for comparison and potential reconciliation. This helps to expand and elaborate the quality of information gained by one method alone.

Triangulation of sources involves comparing the consistency of information derived from varying sources, for example, comparing the data gathered from interviews and observations, from public and private documents, or from informants making the same claim independently. Triangulation across analysts is becoming more common. This can take the form of agreement between the field notes of one observer and the observations made by another, for example. Lastly, some investigators have suggested triangulation of theoretical perspectives. This means applying more than one theoretical perspective to the research findings to reveal any differences and similarities (Patton, 1990).

As mentioned at the beginning of this chapter, the researcher is an integral part of the qualitative research process. Concern for researcher credibility is therefore an inherent part of the verification process. Researcher credibility is dependent on training, experience, and acknowledgment of the researcher role in the research process. Most of all, credibility requires a clear and concise explanation of the researcher role and contribution to the study findings. It is the researcher's responsibility to explain the extent of possible researcher effect on the study and whether changes in perceptions or responses occurred during the study or whether any predispositions or biases influenced the study findings. Describing the researcher's interpretive framework allows the reader to understand exactly how the researcher framed the research question and collected and analyzed the data.

The final element is the need for concise clarification by the researcher of the philosophical orientation underpinning the study. For example, there is continuing debate about the place of objectivity in scientific inquiry. This often takes the form of competition between the two paradigms of quantitative and qualitative research (Guba, 1990). Clear explanation by the researcher of the philosophical orientation of the study helps to place the study findings within a particular interpretive framework and allows readers to judge the authenticity of the study results for themselves. Frank and open explanation in reporting research enhances credibility (Miles & Huberman, 1994).

Readers of qualitative research need a method to evaluate study credibility and the contribution to knowledge of the study findings. Some tests deal specifically with evaluating qualitative studies, (e.g., Higgs, 1998). The following questions proposed by Schwandt and Halpern (1988) and cited in Miles and Huberman (1994, p. 439) provide useful criteria for readers in the medical and rehabilitation research literature:

▶ Are findings grounded in the data? (Is sampling appropriate? Are data weighted correctly?)
▶ Are inferences logical? (Are analytic strategies applied correctly? Are alternative explanations accounted for?)
▶ Is the category structure appropriate?

▶ Can inquiry decisions and methodological shifts be justified? (Were sampling decisions linked to working hypotheses?)
▶ What is the degree of researcher bias (premature disclosure, unexplored data in field notes, lack of search for negative cases, feelings of empathy)?
▶ What strategies were used for increasing credibility (second readers, feedback to informants, peer review, adequate time in the field)?

In summary, qualitative research offers a diversity of methods well suited to the interests of researchers in the medical and rehabilitation fields. The increasing popularity of these methods in these fields is evident in the growing number of qualitative studies reported in the allied health literature and the appearance of journals devoted specifically to qualitative research studies.

Until recently, however, the positivist experimental tradition (quantitative research) was predominant in the medical profession and in rehabilitation and related health professions. Several authors (e.g., Ottenbacher, 1992) have noted that the pendulum appears to be in danger of swinging to an exclusive focus on using qualitative research designs in occupational therapy. As this book makes clear, both quantitative and qualitative research approaches contribute to the development of scientific inquiry in clinical research. The challenge for researchers in occupational therapy is to incorporate qualitative and quantitative approaches into their research studies. A recent example of integrating both qualitative and quantitative research was carried out by McKinney and Leary (1999) in a study of multifetal pregnancy reduction.

CHAPTER

The Research Problem

> The great working hypotheses in the past have often originated in the minds of the pioneers as a result of mental processes which can best be described by such words as 'inspired guess', 'intuitive hunch', or 'brilliant flash of imagination'.
> —J. B. Conant, *Science and Common Sense* (p. 48)

Operational Learning Objectives

By the end of this chapter, the learner will

1. Identity a feasible research topic in an area of clinical practice, administration, or education
2. Write a paragraph justifying the need for a research study
3. Identity a feasible research problem
4. Formulate relevant questions pertaining to a research problem
5. Identify possible psychological blocks in the investigator and flaws in research designs that could potentially deter the research
6. Outline a general plan for data collection

5.1 The Need for Problem-Oriented Research in the Health Professions

During the last 55 years, health research in the United States has multiplied beyond the volume that could have been predicted a century earlier. One hundred years ago, a medical scientist could easily have read most of the published research in a wide range of health specialties. A scholar in the sciences in the 19th century would also be familiar with the literary and artistic worlds. Today it is impossible. C. P. Snow (1964) in his discussion of the two worlds of science and humanities was one of the first to rec-

ognize the isolating effect of specialization in the 20th century. Scientists and humanists now live in two cultures, deprived of the sharing and communication that existed in the 18th and 19th centuries. Specialization and the narrowing of interest in scientific topics have led to a multiplicity of professional associations and published journals.

Currently, there are thousands of scientific journals published monthly, semimonthly, and quarterly. There is also a growing trend toward electronic publication where scholars can read articles directly from the Internet. A gap exists between the methods used in social science research and research in the biological and physical sciences. Quantitative research is more prevalent in the biological and physical sciences, while the social sciences apply more qualitative research methods for collecting data. Research in the social sciences is most vulnerable to criticism because of the subjective nature of qualitative research. On the other hand, there is a pressing need for social progress (e.g., the reduction of alcoholism, drug addiction, juvenile crime, and mental illness). The gap between research in the social sciences and its impact on social problems has led to criticism of applied research. Yet one need only examine the history of medical progress to realize the tremendous gains science has made through applied research, such as in the reduction of heart disease and surgery for cataracts. There is also a strong need for basic research in areas that may not seem relevant at the moment, as with cellular research and microbiology, where theory and basic research carried out 50 years ago have led to practical results in understanding the immune system and how it impacts on AIDS. There is a need for basic research into life processes, such as in DNA, muscle metabolism, and neurological and cognitive areas of human development. The need exists for problem-oriented research that can be applied in the areas from health, medicine, occupational therapy, and special education. A research study begins with establishing the need, significance, and implications of the results.

5.2 Selecting a Significant Research Problem

How does a researcher select a significant area for investigation? What factors in an individual's personal life, education, or clinical experience generate a research interest? William Harvey in the introduction of his book *On the Motion of the Heart and Blood in Animals,* written in 1628, described his purpose in investigating the problem of circulation of blood in the following quotation.

Since, therefore, from the foregoing considerations and many others to the same effect, it is plain that what has ... been said concerning the motion and function of the heart and arteries must appear obscure, inconsistent, or even impossible to him who carefully considers the entire subject, it would be proper to look more narrowly into the matter to contemplate the motion of the heart and arteries, not only in man, but in all animals that have hearts; and also by frequent appeals to vivisection, and much ocular inspection, to investigate and discuss the truth. (p. 73)

Harvey selected the problem of investigating the circulatory system after he evaluated the previous studies as contradictory and inconclusive. His motivation to study the problem was based on his desire to bring clarity to an area of medicine that is vital to human survival. This desire to clarify is an important motivating force in the researcher. There are numerous examples in the history of scientific research of individuals seeking to understand the basic anatomical and physiological processes of man.

Other motivating forces can also generate research. Individuals can pursue a research area because they seek insight into a disease or disability that has touched their own life or the life of a family member or close friend. In 1847, Ignaz Semmelweis, a relentless investigator, pursued the causes of puerperal fever (i.e., blood poisoning associated with childbirth) after the death of a friend. Louis Braille, blinded at the age of four, became a teacher of the blind and in 1824 devised a reading method for the blind. Some situations that may motivate an individual to pursue an area of research include:

▶ A clinician becomes a researcher after becoming aware of the need for more effective treatment methods or diagnostic instruments. There are many instances in the history of medicine where practitioners became part-time researchers and made notable contributions through their efforts. For instance, A. R. Luria, a Russian neuroscientist, became interested in the way the brain worked after evaluating neurological injuries occurring in soldiers. He used case study research to explore neurological disorders and from this developed a concept of how an undamaged brain works.

▶ A dramatic increase in the incidence of a disease produces national priorities for research. In the United States during the last 50 years, there has been a significant amount of research effort directed at cancer, cardiovascular disease, and AIDS. These areas have received added attention from researchers partially because of the dramatic increases in the incidence of these illnesses and partially because of the availability of federal grant support. It is no secret that a research investigator's career can become determined by national politics and priorities. On the other hand, the abuse of federal grant support in the opportunism of research can also become an overriding problem in neglecting research areas that are significant, yet receive little interest from the granting foundations and governmental agencies.

▶ An interest in a content area is generated by an inspiring teacher. There is no doubt that universities are an ideal place for research because they can play an active yet neutral role in facilitating research efforts. Universities need not be caught in political decisions.

▶ A student develops an interest in a research area through intellectual curiosity spurred by intense reading and study. As the student gains more understanding in a specific area, more questions are raised, which motivate research.

From these motivating forces and others, the researcher selects an area of investigation. From this point, how does one maintain momentum and nurture research interests sometimes in the face of insignificant results and tedious, laborious work? The story of Fleming's discovery of penicillin in 1929 is an example of persistence. The impetus for Fleming's investigation was the catastrophic rate of death that occurred during World War I from infected wounds. Fleming sought a chemical substance that would destroy the pathogenic germs entering the body from an open flesh wound. After 10 years of painstaking laboratory work that involved growing bacterial colonies and observing the reactions of chemicals, he was successful in discovering a powerful therapeutic agent that would eventually change the course of medical practice. There were two landmark events in his work. The first occurred in 1922 when he noticed that a foreign chemical substance prevented a bacterial colony from growing. At this point in his work, he was unable to isolate or identify the chemical substance. In 1928, he noticed that a bacterial culture of staphylococci had accidentally become contaminated by mold. He found that the mold produced a substance that retarded the growth of the bacteria. The chemical substance was later identified by an American mycologist, Thom, as *Penicillium notatum*. After the substance was identified, Fleming was able to produce penicillin in the laboratory and experiment with its effect on bacteria and on normal human tissues. It was not until 1943, about 20 years after Fleming's original investigations, that penicillin was mass produced in Great Britain and the United States. In analyzing Fleming's discovery, a combination of persistence and responsiveness to accidental discovery was the key factor. Fleming first asked a researchable question: Is there a chemical substance that can stop the growth of harmful bacteria in the bloodstream without destroying normal human tissue? He persisted in his efforts to solve the problem over a period of 25 years until his successful discovery of penicillin.

Compared to medicine, research originating from occupational therapy fields is in the beginning stages of development. Potential directions for research abound in the areas of evaluation and treatment and in the areas of professional education and administration. These areas can be described as two triangles as depicted in Figure 5–1.

In diagram 1 of the figures, research originates out of the relationship between the evaluation and treatment of a specific disability. By analyzing a disability, the clinical researcher tries to determine where the major gaps in knowledge exist. For instance, in evaluating and treating the client with arthritis, are there effective evaluative instruments? What treatment methods have been demonstrated to be effective? What factors in the client's life affect the course of the illness? From this analysis, the researcher can identify a research problem. This same process of generating research also is evident in analyzing the educational and administrative aspects of occupational therapy in addressing such questions as the admission of students into a program, effective supervision and evaluation of staff, maintenance of morale in job satisfaction, design of the curriculum. The need for research is justified when a researcher can establish the significance of the results. For example, the researcher should ask, "If I collect this data, what impact will the results have on treatment, education, or administration?" A researcher should clearly state the implications of the study, relating it to the evaluation or treatment of a specified disability or the educational or administrative practices that could be affected by the results. Before data are collected, the researcher should be able to think through the impact of the results. An *if* (results positive or negative) . . . *then* (recommendations and options taken) contingency is the initial strategy proposed by the researcher.

5.3 Identifying Problems Resulting From a Disability

In selecting a disability area for research, investigators can be guided by their own clinical experience in an area of specialization. For example, the significance of a problem can be gauged by the leading causes of death and the leading causes of hospitalization. The 15 leading causes of death in the United States in 1993 and 1997 are shown in Table 5–1.

For the researcher, these disabilities and diseases represent significant health problems. Evaluation and diagnosis are ongoing concerns for the therapist. Methodological research such as in diagnostic hardware, clinical observational methods, screening procedures, and objective tests can become the focal point of an investigation. The development of specific treatment techniques or protocols that can be generalized to

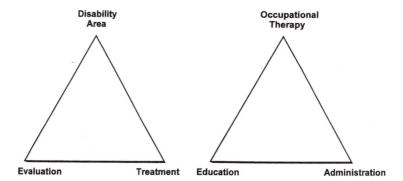

Figure 5–1. Potential directions for research in occupational therapy. Note that the relationship between evaluation and treatment leads to research in disabilities, whereas the relationship between education and administration leads to research in occupational therapy.

Table 5–1. Fifteen Leading Causes of Death for 1993 and 1997

Cause	1993		1997	
	Number	Rank	Number	Rank
All causes	2,268,553	—	2,314,245	—
Heart disease	722,736	1	726,672	1
Malignant neoplasms	528,501	2	539,219	2
Cerebrovascular disease	149,064	3	159,682	3
Chronic obstructive pulmonary disease	101,634	4	171,254	4
Injuries, including motor vehicles	90,342	5	94,884	5
Pneumonia and influenza	83,556	6	85,627	6
Diabetes mellitus	54,204	7	62,484	7
Suicide	31,619	9	30,085	8
Nephritis, nephrotic syndrome, and nephrosis	24,980	10	25,456	9
Chronic liver disease and cirrhosis	24,660	12	25,456	10
Alzheimer's disease	16,754	15	23,142	11
Septicemia	20,250	13	23,142	12
Homicide and legal intervention	24,844	11	2,082	13
HIV infection	37,267	8	1,619	14
Atherosclerosis	17,020	14	1,619	15

Note. The table shows the number and rank for the top causes of death in the United States in 1993. The data include all races and are based on the National Vital Statistics Report published by the Centers for Disease Control and Prevention. Taken from the *Monthly Vital Statistics Report*, Vol. 42, No. 12, May 13, 1994, *Monthly Vital Statistics Report*, 44(7-Supplement), February 29, 1996; and the *National Vital Statistics Reports*, Vol. 47, No. 19, June 30, 1999.

a population with disabilities represents another fertile direction for researchers. Treatment techniques such as sensory-integration therapy (SI), neurodevelopmental therapy (NDT), aquatic therapy, hippo therapy, stress management, and biofeedback are a few examples of research areas generated from examining the needs of people with disabilities.

5.4 Identifying Significant Issues in Professional Education

Who should become occupational therapists? Are there specific abilities, personalities, intellectual potentials, or academic achievements necessary before entering a professional preparatory program? What is the rationale for each characteristic? How are admission requirements for entrance to an occupational therapy program determined? Who among the faculty and staff in the occupational therapy departments determines policy for admission? These questions examine the assumptions underlying the education of occupational therapists. The recruitment, screening, and selection of students pose realistic problems to the occupational therapy educator that should provide significant areas for investigation.

Along with the admission process, the curriculum is a potential area for research. The educational curriculum includes the classroom teaching methods, curricular content, audiovisual aids, clinical education, problem-based learning, and student evaluation. Examples of these potential areas of research in educating occupational therapy students are listed in Table 5–2.

Administration of clinical programs, personnel policies, budgetary planning, physical plant layouts, and job satisfaction are often neglected areas of research, although the effect of administrative policies sometimes has more impact on the course of a client's disability than the direct effects of treatment. Public health policies to mass vaccinate a population, the access to health care, and the staff morale are all critical areas of concern that have important implications in the total health needs. These are all potential areas for research.

5.5 Justifying the Research Problem

Once a research area is identified by the investigator, statistical data should be cited (see Table 5–3 as an example of statistical data) that indicate the extent of the problem. A problem involving one of the 10 leading causes of death or hospitalization is obviously significant. Nonethless, how does one justify investigating a rare disease, such as amyotrophic lateral sclerosis (ALS), that affects proportionately few people? On the other hand, should the freedom of an investigator be restricted by governmental agencies deciding which areas to fund research? The question of research significance does touch on societal values. Priorities are established by nations in areas of health that realistically affect research efforts. It is assumed that the individual scientist should have the freedom to pursue any area of investigation as long as it does not endanger the lives of the subjects. Yet, research should not be isolated from the pressing needs of a society. If, for example, osteoarthritis becomes a problem of epidemic proportions in the United States in the early 21st century, then society should justly allocate a large percentage of its health resources to those researchers seek-

Table 5–2. Methodology and Content of Professional Programs in Occupational Therapy

Classroom Teaching Methods	Curricula Content	Presentation Methods	Clinical Education	Student Evaluation
• Case studies • Laboratory experiences (e.g., testing or treatment) • Lecture • Problem-based learning • Role playing • Seminar • Student-oriented group projects	• Basic sciences • Dynamics of interactions • Evaluation and treatment techniques • Practice areas (e.g., geriatrics, mental health, pediatrics, physical disabilities) • Research design • Supervision and administration	• Audiovisual methods • Computer-assisted instruction • Distance learning • Internet • Presentation software (e.g., PowerPoint) • Videos	Level 1: Short-term experiences with or without supervision • Observations (single day) • Clerkships (weekly) Level 2: Two 3-month affiliations with supervision • Internships or Affiliations • Optional affiliations in a specialty area	• Grades: number and letter grades • Grades: pass/fail • Individual counseling • Observation of students in clinical settings • Competency-based evaluation

Table 5–3. Number of Selected Reported Chronic Conditions per 1,000 Persons

Impairment	All Ages
Visual impairments	892
Color blindness	156
Cataracts	574
Glaucoma	341
Hearing impairment	1,638
Tinnitus	618
Speech impairment	589
Absence of extremities (excludes tips of fingers or toes only)	126
Paralysis of extremities, complete or partial	213
Deformity or orthopedic impairment	3,455
Back	1,433
Upper extremities	377
Lower extremities	1,552

Note: The information contained in this table is based on data from the *Vital and Health Statistics, Prevalence of Selected Chronic Coniditons: United States, 1990– 1992*, Series 10, No. 194, Table 26, by J. G. Collins, 1997, Centers for Disease Control and Prevention, National Centers for Health Statistics, p. 42. This publication is available through http://www.cdc.gov/nchs/products/pubs/pubd/series/ sr10/199-190/se10_194.htm

ing means to reduce the incidence of osteo-arthritis. Establishing research priorities in a democratic society involves the participation of a broad spectrum of groups who represent the policy makers, clinicians, consumers, and researchers. Governmental agencies, universities, pharmaceutical companies, and private foundations are the primary sources for the financial support of research, and thus, the policy makers for research. The recipients of research grants are those clinical practitioners, students, educators, and administrators who have convinced policy makers of the significance and validity of their research proposals.

In summary, the researcher justifies an investigation by establishing the need for a study based on an analysis of a health problem and the implications of the results. The need for an investigation is documented by the following statistical data:

▶ The *incidence* (initial occurrences) and *prevalence* (existing cases in the population) of a disability, derived from primary statistical data

▶ The leading causes of death as reported by national and international centers for health statistics (e.g., World Health Organization)

▶ The number of first admissions and readmissions to a hospital caused by a disability, obtained from national and state public health agencies

▶ The number of physicians and outpatient visits reported as the result of a disability

▶ The days lost at work because of specific health problems, compiled from Department of Labor Statistics and Workers Compensation

▶ The incidence of social disabilities (i.e., alcoholism, drug addiction, adult crime, juvenile delinquency, and child abuse), available through the national and state public health agencies and the state attorney general's office

▶ The number of occupational therapists employed in the United States as provided by professional organizations, the *Occupational Outlook Handbook* (published by the United States Department of Labor), and state employment agencies

▶ Statistics on the number of hospitals, outpatient clinics, state institutions for individuals with mental retardation and mental illness, rehabilitation centers, and other patient care facilities, usually available from public health agencies or through directories published by municipal and state organizations and private social service agencies.

5.6 Narrowing the Investigation

Problem-oriented research is a process of asking questions and gathering data. The investigator generates a question and intellectually ponders the possible outcomes. This ability to formulate research questions and to predict outcomes is an essential part of the research process. The Socratic method of teaching is based on this principle of questions and answers that invariably lead to other questions and answers until a topic is exhausted. This method is also used in problem-based learning where students examine a case study by asking relevant questions and developing hypotheses.

Brainstorming a problem is another method for generating questions by creative free association. The researcher must be able to freely generate questions that on initial examination may seem unrelated or unfeasible. Many great discoveries, when they were first reported publicly, seemed like "hair-brained" ideas that would never work. Roentgen, a physicist, accidentally discovered X-Rays when examining the results of passing electricity through a vacuum tube. He then proceeded to ask himself

questions regarding its applicability to medical diagnosis. On hearing of Roentgen's discovery in 1895, people in the streets were incredulous. Many felt that X-Rays would be used like a camera to spy on people or to expose them. Later medical scientists raised questions regarding the potential of X-Ray in diagnosis and in the treatment of cancerous growths.

This process of asking questions and observing the outcome is the essential part of research. At first, the question may be general, ill-conceived, unclear, and incongruous. As the researcher explores and defines what is actually being asked, the research question becomes sharper until, as Graham Wallas (1926) stated:

> Our mind is not likely to give us a clear answer to any particular problem unless we set it a clear question, and we are more likely to notice the significance of any new piece of evidence, or new association of ideas, if we have formed a definite conception of a case to be proved or disproved. (p. 84)

The persistent effort on the part of the researcher to brainstorm a problem, to think it through, to ponder silently, or to discuss it with a colleague brings the researcher closer to a solution. For some investigators, the problem incubates, while for others the problem stirs. Whatever the style is, the researcher must be able to stay with a problem while trying to overcome the apparent pitfalls and cul de sacs that are created. Many a researcher is stymied by the assumption of others that the problem is too complex or impossible to solve or by the knowledge that others have failed. The investigator must persist in working through the problem. For example, low back pain is a significant health problem that affects a large number of sedentary and manual workers. It directly affects industrial production, psychological well-being, and participation in sports and leisure activities. Although it is widespread in the population and it has significant implications, practitioners have been only partially successful in treating this disability. Experienced occupational therapists observe that low back pain is an elusive syndrome that is difficult to diagnose and sometimes difficult to separate from malingering or psychosomatic effects. Other clinicians are hesitant to investigate the problem because of the subjective nature of measuring pain. Others state that the neurophysiology is too complex to investigate. These reactions to low back pain should not deter research. Investigators entering into an area of research can become overwhelmed by the immensity of a problem, but they need not try to solve all aspects of the problem, including objective diagnosis and successful treatment. Researchers should instead attempt to "slice off" a portion of a research problem that is feasible within the limitations of time and resources available. The process of formulating a research problem by a clinician is summarized in Figure 5–2.

Let us examine hypothetical examples of research questions derived from significant health problems (Table 5–4). These research questions are derived directly from an analysis of a health problem. The specificity of the question depends on the uniqueness of the investigator's interests. After researchers identify an area of investigation and document the significance of the study, they are faced with the task of narrowing the area of investigation into a feasible chunk within a designated time span. Some researchers devote their entire professional life to a specific area of research; others drastically change their research areas as they broaden their interests.

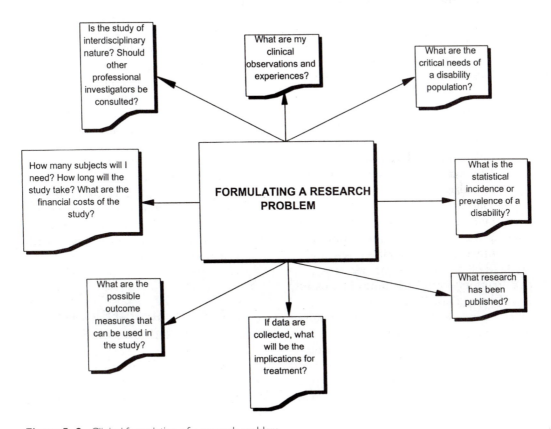

Figure 5–2. Clinical formulation of a research problem.

Table 5–4. Hypothetical Research Questions Related to Disability

Disability	Research Question
AIDS:	How can prescriptive exercise help in reducing symptoms?
Cerebral palsy:	Is development sequential and hierarchical in children with motor lesions in the cerebral cortex?
Depression:	What is the role of exercise in increasing serotonin?
Hypertension:	Can blood pressure rates be self-regulated through biofeedback techniques?
Learning disability:	What are significant factors in facilitating handwriting?
Mental retardation:	How does the environment facilitate or restrict learning?
Multiple sclerosis:	What are the effects of stress on "triggering" episodes?
Schizophrenia:	Can relaxation therapy help the individual to manage stress?
Social deprivation:	How is language acquisition affected by the parent talking with the child?
Stroke:	How does client motivation significantly affect recovery of function?
Traumatic brain injury:	What issues need to be addressed if school re-entry is to be successful?

5.6.1 Determining Feasibility

In the process of narrowing the investigation to a feasible study, the investigator should, as a preliminary procedure, carefully examine the following questions:

1. How long will data collection take?
   a. Laboratory experiments—the length of time required for preparing and collecting data for each participant
   b. Travel time—the length of time required to get to and from the data collection site
   c. Interview time—time for each subject multiplied by total number of subjects equal total interview time
   d. Mail survey—researcher must account for response time and possibly a second mailing
   e. Correlational study—individual or group testing time periods
   f. Methodological—consideration of time for constructing instrument and obtaining reliability and validity data
2. What measuring instruments are available for testing constructs and variables?
   a. Cost—expenses incurred to obtain test instruments
   b. Expertise—level of competency or experience needed to administer and interpret test results
3. Are participants readily available? Where can participants be obtained?
   a. Screening criteria—used to determine participant inclusion
   b. Incentives for the participants—will payment or some other incentive be given to the participants?
4. What expertise is needed to carry out the treatment procedure?
   a. What are the total financial costs of the research, and who will finance them?
   b. How long will it take for approval by the institutional review board (IRB) of ethical standards?

5.7 Psychological Blocks in Selection of a Research Problem

Many times, graduate students confronted with the task of completing a thesis, dissertation, or study that involves collecting primary data are stymied in selecting a researchable topic. Students often belabor the the process and frequently change their research area. In the process of selecting a feasible research problem, the student can become frustrated and blocked. In overcoming these psychological blocks, the student should examine the consequences of a research study and its potential significance. The following examples are typical of the psychological blocks that interfere with selecting a research problem.

▶ A research topic is dropped prematurely because the investigator fails to locate enough published studies related to the topic.
▶ The investigator is overwhelmed by the multiplicity of studies published in an area and concludes that further research is not necessary because the area has already been researched sufficiently. The investigator drops the topic without rigorously evaluating the validity and conclusiveness of results.
▶ The research topic selected is too broad, considering the time constraints of an investigator. Instead of narrowing the research topic to a feasible study the investigation is terminated.
▶ A preliminary investigation of a research area reveals difficulty in measuring an outcome variable. The investigator drops the study without seeking to construct an instrument that could reliably and validly measure the outcome.
▶ An investigator is motivated to explore a research area with the goal of making an important and original contribution to the body of knowledge. The investigator refuses to delimit a study after realizing the amount of time necessary to complete the study and subsequently terminates the investigation.

Selecting a researchable problem should be an ongoing process where the investigator explores the relevance, feasibility, applicability, and significance of a study. The worksheet guide in Box 5–1 lists the areas that a researcher should be aware of in the process of selecting and narrowing a researchable problem.

5.8 Worksheet Guide for Selecting a Research Problem

Box 5–1. Worksheet Guide for Selecting a Research Problem

1. **What is the target population?**
   a. group with disabilities
   b. allied health profession
      1. student
      2. clinician

2. **What are the perceived needs of the population?**
   a. investigating causes of disability
   b. evaluation and diagnostic methods
   c. student performance
   d. evaluation of therapists' effectiveness
   e. investigation of treatment techniques
   f. evaluation of personnel factors

3. **What are the primary and secondary sources relevant to responses 1 and 2?**
   a. journal articles
   b. annual reviews

continued

    c. textbooks
    d. statistical compendiums

4. **Are independent and dependent variables identifiable?**
    a. independent variables: (presumed causes)
    b. dependent variables: (presumed effects)

5. **How can the research impact on**
    a. treatment
    b. education
    c. administration

6. **Can research variables be operationally defined?**

7. **What explanation or theory accounts for the presumed relationship between variables?**

8. **What research models are relevant to the study? State research question relative to research model.**
    a. quantitative
        1. experimental (pretest/posttest)
        2. methodological (construction of instrument)
        3. evaluation (evaluation of health care system)
        4. correlation (relationship between variables)
    b. qualitative
        1. survey (description of population)
        2. historical (reconstruction of events)
        3. clinical or naturalistic observation (dynamic analysis of subject)
        4. heuristic (discovery of relationships)

9. a. State the research problem.
   b. State the hypothesis in null or directional form.
   c. State the guiding question.

10. **To which groups are the research findings directed?**
    a. clinicians
    b. individuals with disabilities
    c. students
    d. academicians
    e. program administrators

11. **Feasibility check**
    a. Where can participants be obtained?
    b. How many participants are necessary?
    c. What tests, instruments, or apparatuses will be necessary to measure outcome?
    d. What are financial costs?
        1. travel
        2. mailings
        3. tests
        4. protocols
        5. clinical time

6. apparatus
7. computer analysis
8. books and duplicating
9. clerical and typing
10. laboratory analysis of findings

12. **Analysis of Time (List the projected time sequence or dates for completion of research phases)**

Initiation of study	Review of literature	Preparation for data collection	Approval from IRB	Collection of results	Writing discussion chapter	Completion of study

5.9 Why Research Proposals Are Disapproved

The following list of major reasons for the disapproval of research proposals is based on the authors' experiences as raters on governmental and university committees. The list is summarized in Table 5–5.

▶ *The research problem is insignificant, and the results will have little impact on clinical practice currently or in the future.* An example of an insignificant problem is an investigation of the relationship of low birth weight with the incidence of cerebral palsy. A literature search in this area already confirms that low birth weight is one among many risk factors for cerebral palsy. Nonetheless, not all infants with cerebral palsy are born prematurely nor are all infants with low birth weight destined to have cerebral palsy. This study will have little impact on our understanding of the causes of cerebral palsy and will not provide insight into the prevention and treatment. The projected results from this type of study would have a splintering effect where one variable is linked to a disability that has already been found to have multiple causes. A better study in a related area

would be to examine the effects of low birth weight on one area of development, such as motor function. In this way, the investigator can narrow the research and control for extraneous variables that could have a potential effect on the results.

▶ *The hypothesis presented is not supported by scientific evidence and seems speculative.* As a hypothetical example, a researcher proposes that a computer software program in cognitive rehabilitation is effective in treating individuals with brain injuries. The investigator equates improvement with the client's ability to learn a computer game. The investigator does not demonstrate through a literature review that there is a carryover of this computer skill to the learning of functional skills in independent living. A better study is to investigate the types of skills that are facilitated while learning with a computer.

▶ *The research problem is more complex than the investigator presents, and it needs to be narrowed down.* For example, a researcher proposes to examine the effects of sensory integration therapy on children with Attention Deficit Hyperactivity Disorder (ADHD). Both variables are complex and must be operationally

Table 5–5. Reasons Why Research Proposals Are Denied

---

1. The research problem is insignificant, and the results will have little impact on clinical practice currently or in the future

2. The hypothesis presented is not supported by scientific evidence and seems speculative

3. The research problem is more complex than the investigator presents, and it needs to be narrowed down

4. The anticipated results from the study will be of only local significance and lacks external validity or generalizability

5. The research proposed has too many uncontrolled elements

6. The research methodology seems overly complex and difficult to replicate

7. The proposed outcome measures are either inappropriate, unstandardized, unreliable, or invalid

8. Extraneous variables are left uncontrolled and may have an influence on the results

9. Overall design of the study seems incomplete and not well conceived

10. The statistical tests suggested for analyzing the data are not appropriate

11. Selection of subjects for the study is not representative of a target population

12. The treatment procedure under investigation has not been adequately defined in enough detail to replicate

13. The literature review seems outdated and lacks landmark studies in the area of investigation

14. The equipment identified in the study is outmoded or unsuitable

15. The investigator has not proposed adequate time for completion of the study

16. Resources are inadequate to complete the study

17. The setting and environment for the study are unsuitable

18. The investigator has not considered the ethical nature of the study, such as stating the potential physical and psychological risks to participants in an informed consent form

---

defined. Sensory integration therapy includes a number of components in treatment, whereas ADHD is a complex disorder with multiple causes. A better study is to identify one aspect of sensory integration therapy, such as vestibular stimulation, and evaluate its effectiveness with a measurable variable, such as motor proficiency, as assessed by the *Miller Assessment for Preschoolers* (MAP; Miller, 1988).

▶ *The anticipated results from the study will be of only local significance and lacks external validity or generalizability.* An example of a flawed proposal is when a researcher designs a survey of job satisfaction for occupational therapists in a local school district without considering the generalizability to a larger sample or population. The data collected from this study would have only local interest and

could not be generalized to teachers in other schools. In a better study of job satisfaction among occupational therapists, the researcher would determine first the demographics of an average occupational therapists, considering age, gender, and educational level. These variables could be used to determine if the occupational therapists are representative of a larger population. The survey would be designed with the intention of applying it to a more general sample. Questions would be generated that examine the broad issues of job satisfaction among occupational therapists in general, rather than looking at local issues that affect job satisfaction in that particular school district.

▶ *The research proposed has too many uncontrolled elements.* For example, a researcher wants to study the effects of in utero exposure to alcohol on children born with Fetal Alcohol Syndrome (FAS). The amount of alcohol exposure is unknown and is dependent on the mother's self-report, which is often unreliable. In addition, the home environment and genetic makeup are variables that may play a part in the child's behavior. These variables are difficult to measure and are often neglected by the researcher. A better approach is a retrospective case study analysis of an infant with FAS and the child's mother, exploring the dynamics of the case.

▶ *The research methodology seems overly complex and difficult to replicate.* For example, a researcher wants to examine the relationship between the onset of a depressive episode and an individual who is vulnerable. The interaction between family relationships, work situations, and personal attitudes are complex and make it difficult to identify the interactive factors that result in depression. Because of the individuality of each episode, replication of the study using a group method or survey would be difficult and might distort results. A better study would include a qualitative research method using an in-depth case study approach to identify within each individual the interactive effects that trigger depression.

▶ *The proposed outcome measures are either inappropriate, unstandardized, unreliable, or invalid.* A researcher investigating the effects of exercise on depression creates a scale for depression without testing for its reliability or validity. A better approach to measurement is to use more than one instrument to measure outcome (triangulation). For example, the investigator can use a physiological measure, a standardized test, and a client self-report. These three measures will increase the internal validity of the study in assessing outcome.

▶ *Extraneous variables are left uncontrolled and may have an influence on the results.* For example, a researcher wants to examine the effect of a specific treatment method on improving motor skills. Al-

though the researcher is careful to administer pre- and posttests, extraneous variables, such as practice at home, additional interventions, or sessions per week, are not included in the analysis. These variables will most certainly affect the results. A better study would be to take frequent measures of performance, perhaps at the beginning and end of each therapy session, to determine changes in skill level. Another possibility is to have the client and researcher keep a log describing motor performance.

▶ *Overall design of the study seems incomplete and not well conceived.* In this example, elements of the research proposal are missing, such as controlling for extraneous variables that could possibly influence the results, or a large section of the literature review is omitted. It is important for the researcher to work with an outline that lists the essential components of a research proposal.

▶ *The statistical tests suggested for analyzing the data are not appropriate.* An investigator has collected ordinal data, such as ranking of students on an achievement test. Rather than using a nonparametric test, such as the Spearman Rank Order Correlation used for ordinal type data, the researcher inappropriately applies a parametric test, such as the Pearson Correlational Coefficient statistical test used for interval scale data. The statistical test applied should be based on the measurement scale of data. The assumptions of parametric statistics, such as normality of data distribution, should be followed. The appropriate statistics are based on the assumptions underlying the statistical tests.

▶ *Selection of subjects for the study is not representative of a target population.* If it is known that the incidence of traumatic brain injuries (TBI) is higher for males than females by more than 2 to 1 and that more than 50% of clients with TBI are between the ages of 15 and 24, then the investigator should try to select participants who reflect these statistics. This is especially true for studies where the investigator intends to generalize results to a representative sample. Nonetheless, there are studies in which the investigator is interested in examining a nonrepresentative sample that is a portion of the target population, such as females or children with TBI. Then the investigator must delineate clearly the target population in the title of the study.

▶ *The treatment procedure under investigation has not been adequately defined in enough detail to replicate.* An investigator identifies the independent variable as counseling; however, not enough detail is given regarding the type, frequency, and duration of counseling. Therefore, this study cannot be replicated.

▶ *The literature review seems outdated and lacks landmark studies in the area of investigation.* In reviewing the literature, it is wise to first examine current secondary texts or to survey articles in the area to identify the major landmark studies that are cited frequently. An up-to-date literature review also can be found by scanning the current journals in a subject area and by looking at the journal's yearly index.

▶ *The equipment identified in the study is outmoded or unsuitable.* For example, a test that has been standardized on adults is used for children. This is inappropriate and unsuitable for the study.

▶ *The investigator has not proposed adequate time for completion of the study.* In outlining the proposal for a study, the researcher should set up a time line graph that breaks down the components of the study into time periods. (See Box 5–1: Worksheet Guide in Section 5.8.)

▶ *Resources are inadequate to complete the study.* For example, a research plan includes a request for funds to pay assistants to collect data. The funds requested for support are insufficient to complete the study.

▶ *The setting and environment for the study are unsuitable.* In this instance, the investigator attempts to complete a complex study without securing an appropriate environment for the study, such as a fully equipped laboratory or testing area that is free from distracting noise.

▶ *The investigator has not considered the ethical nature of the study, such as stating the potential physical and psychological risks to subjects in an informed consent form or has not received approval from an Institutional Review Board (IRB) regarding human subjects.* For example, a researcher begins to collect data for a study on apraxia and its relationship to students with learning disabilities before the IRB has approved the research design. This is unethical, and data collected cannot be used in the final analysis.

CHAPTER

Review of the Literature

> That "the library" as yet unspecified—is the repository of by far the largest part of our recorded knowledge needs no demonstration. The author of an active article on West Africa who reports that the annual rainfall in Fernando, PA, is 100 inches found this information in the library—in a book. It is most unlikely that he measured the rain himself.
> —Jacques Barzun and Henry Graff, 1970,
> *The Modern Researcher* (p. 63)

Operational Learning Objectives

By the end of this chapter, the learner will

1. identify the main purpose of a literature review
2. initiate a computer-based library search, such as OT BibSys, MEDLINE, CINAHL, ERIC, or HealthStar
3. compare and contrast referral and primary sources
4. initiate a search of the literature identifying relevant research articles
5. critically evaluate the validity of research studies
6. outline a comprehensive search of the related literature

6.1 The Need for a Literature Review

Good research is part of a cumulative process in which information expands in many directions. Breakthroughs in knowledge do not occur suddenly. The scientist exploring solutions to problems first masters the previous literature to determine (a) what has been accomplished, (b) where the cul de sacs are, and (c) what research is in the forefront of knowledge. A search of the literature involving the location of relevant studies is a critical part of the research process. It is impossible to conceive of a researcher devising a research plan without first examining previous findings. The literature search is not only a method of uncovering; it is also a way for the researcher to attain an historical perspective and overview of a problem.

Scientific research is a force that advances knowledge. For many scientists, discovery of new information or technology is a process of juxtaposing research from diverse fields in relation to an identifiable problem.

Norbert Wiener (1948) in his work on cybernetics, which eventually led to the invention of the computers, attained success by brainstorming with engineers, psychiatrists, educators, and physicists. These specialists were able to share their ideas, and their collaboration stimulated the examination of a problem from many perspectives. Wiener, from this experience, developed a theory of thinking based on the integration of physical science theory with behavioral observations. The lesson from Wiener's careful research is that investigators exploring the literature should not only examine studies directly related to a problem, but also try to find studies from other fields that have an indirect or implied relationship to their question.

If, for example, a researcher is interested in examining the relationship between staff morale and treatment effectiveness, he or she would need to search the literature in management psychology if a preliminary search reveals a lack of studies in occupational therapy. The diversity of findings adds strength to a study, especially if corroboration of data appears from different professions. The Hawthorne effect, which was first noted in factory workers, is now widely accepted as a factor in clinical treatment. Spinoffs from research in the space programs, such as the advances in nutrition, computer programming, temperature control, and monitoring of vital bodily functions, are examples of applying data generated from a seemingly unrelated field.

The main goals of the investigator in searching the literature are to

▶ make an exhaustive search for related studies
▶ identify the landmark studies that have an important impact in the area investigated
▶ evaluate the validity of the research findings
▶ integrate and synthesize the results into subject areas
▶ summarize the findings from previous studies, highlighting areas where results are either inconclusive or controversial

These goals are part of the overall preliminary process of research that precedes data collection.

6.2 Conceptual View of a Literature Search

The steps involved in a conceptual view of the literature search is shown in Figure 6–1. Each of these steps is described below.

1. The first step in initiating a literature search is to identify the key words in the study. The key words may be identified through (a) reading a secondary source, (b) experience with a particular population, (c) reviewing a journal article, or (d) examining a thesaurus of terms such as MEDLARS or ERIC. These key words can be linked to the independent variable (e.g., treatment technique), dependent variable (e.g., desired outcome), outcome measure (e.g., ACL), target population (e.g., individuals with spinal cord injury), contextual setting (e.g., assisted living center), age range (e.g., elderly), or frame of reference (e.g., occupational behavior). Key words are important for researchers when initiating a computer search because they help to differentiate between similar materials. For example, if a researcher wants to examine the literature on sensory integration, use of the key words "sensory integration" will eliminate studies that examine NDT.

2. The next step in a literature search is to locate a textbook or review article in which the researcher can obtain an overall summary of the major research in the specific area. For example, a researcher may be interested in the effectiveness of occupational therapy on the achievement of students with learning disabilities. The researcher would examine a recent textbook on pediatric occupational therapy to gain an overall view of treatment and to identify recent refer-

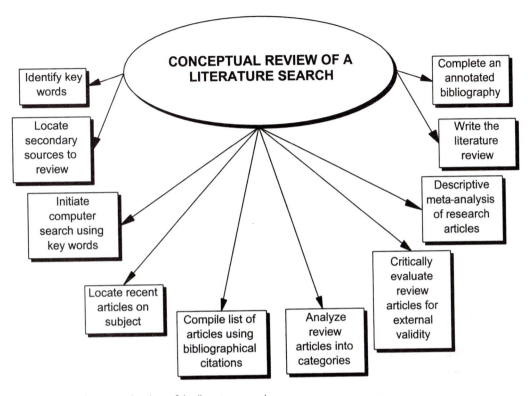

Figure 6–1. Conceptual review of the literature search.

ences. The textbook may help in the identification of key words and in narrowing the focus of the study.

3. Next, the researcher is ready to do a computer search of recent articles in the field. MEDLINE, CINAHL, or ERIC are examples of databases that can be used. Another way to examine recent articles is to look at the article in current issues or the cumulative yearly index in the journals. The *American Journal of Occupational Therapy* (AJOT) and *Occupational Therapy International* (OTI) are two examples of referral sources. Examining the bibliography in relevant articles may also help to locate other articles. After the researcher has identified relevant articles, it is important to file the bibliographic citations and abstract for later use. (See discussion of bibliographic citations later in this chapter.)

4. The next step is the categorization of the articles into types of publications, such as review, research, or theoretical papers (see Table 6–1). Articles can also be categorized into subject areas for easier review.

5. The researcher must critically evaluate each article for external (i.e., generalization of results) and internal validity (i.e., rigor of the methodology). The researcher examines how the variables were controlled, the subject selection, the randomness of the selection, reliability and validity of the outcome measures, and the operational definition of the independent variable.

6. A descriptive meta-analysis of research studies identified by the literature review is the next step. The researcher designs a table that includes the title of the study, the date of publication, the authors or researchers, number of subjects, treatment methodology, outcome measures, statistical results, and conclusions (Table 6–2).

Table 6–1. Categorization of Publications

Types of Publications	Examples of Publications
Primary data research	Journal articles Dissertations Theses Conference proceedings Government documents Statistical surveys
Review articles	Journal articles Monographs
Evaluation findings	Joint Commission on Accreditation Results Special commissions
Conceptual or theoretical papers	Journal articles Monographs Conference proceedings
Position papers	Journal articles Associational and organizational statements Monographs Editorials
Secondary and tertiary information	Popular magazines *Scientific American* Encyclopedias College texts
Other publications	Test manuals Reference books for test instruments Book reviews Software programs and reviews Manuals for self-help devices
Bibliographic references	*Books in Print* Information retrieval system Directories of reference

7. The researcher is now ready to write the literature review from an outline. The review should include an integrated summary of the various articles.

8. Finally, the researcher should develop an annotated bibliography. Articles should be organized by subject heading, with research articles listed separately from theoretical articles. The annotated bibliography includes the published abstract. The annotated bibliography serves as a primary data source for the research study. It also helps the reader gain an overview of the research study.

6.3 Locating Sources of Related Literature

More than 4,000 periodicals are currently published every year in medical and health related areas. The task of searching the literature would be enormous if the investigator had to review each and every periodical individually. How can the investigator quickly obtain a list of studies that are relevant so as to narrow the search and reduce the number of hours examining the on-line catalog and library stacks? For the compulsive investigator seeking to identify *every*

Table 6–2. Effect of Exercise on Depression: Example of Descriptive Meta-Analysis

Study	Subjects	Treatment Technique	Outcome Measures	Results
Blue, R. F. (1979). Aerobic running as a treatment of moderate depression.	2 adult patients with chronic depression	Aerobic running program 3 times per week, for 9 weeks	Zung Self-Rating Depression Scale (Zung, 1965)	Significant reduction of depression.
Bosscher (1993). Running and mixed physical exercises with depressed psychiatric patients.	24 men and women diagnosed with depression and hospitalized in psychiatric hospital	E₂: short-term running therapy, 3 times a week for 8 weeks C: Mixed physical and relaxation exercises, 3 times a week for 8 weeks	Zung Self-Rating Depression Scale (SDS; Zung, 1965)	Significant improvement for running group; no significant improvement for mixed physical and exercise group.
Brollier et al. (1994). Aerobic exercises: A potential occupational therapy modality for adolescents with depression.	4 adolescent boys from a private psychiatric hospital with diagnosis of depression	Brisk walking and running 3 times a week for 1 hour over 65-day period	Beck Depression Inventory (BDI; Beck et al., 1961)	Results showed a general decrease in depression scores of all subjects.
Doyne, E. J. et al. (1983). Aerobic exercise as a treatment of depression in women.	4 women with major depressive disorder (MDD)	Aerobic exercise for 6 weeks	Beck Depression Inventory (BDI; Beck et al., 1961) Depression Adjective Check-Lists (DACL; Lubin, 1981)	Significant reduction in depression scores compared with pre-exercise screening phase.
Doyne, E. J. et al. (1987). Running versus weight lifting in the treatment of depression.	40 women diagnosed with depression	E₁: walked/ran on indoor track in 7-minute intervals for 8 weeks E₂: used weight-lifting machine for 8 weeks C: no treatment	Beck Depression Inventory (BDI; Beck et al., 1961); Hamilton Rating Scale for Depression (HRDS; Hamilton, 1960); Depression Adjective Check-Lists (DACL; Lubin, 1981)	Both aerobic and weight-lifting groups showed significant improvement in depression; no change in control group.
Greist et al. (1979). Running as a treatment for depression.	13 men, 15 women, aged 18 to 30	E: 10 patients ran 3–4 times/week C: 18 in psychotherapy	Response Symptom Checklist (Greist et al., 1979)	Running as treatment for moderate depression was as effective as psychotherapy.

(continued)

Table 6–2. *Continued*

Study	Subjects	Treatment Technique	Outcome Measures	Results
Kaplan et al. (1983). The effect of a jogging program on psychiatric inpatients with symptoms of depression.	12 women, 6 men, aged 15 to 38, patients in acute care psychiatric ward	Warm-up and cool-down exercises; 20 minutes of graded walking/jogging on indoor track; short discussion of exercise and health-related topics	*Self-report questionnaire* (5-point Likert scale); observation by coleaders	Decreased sleep disturbances and increased self-esteem.
Martinsen et al. (1985). Effects of aerobic exercise on depression: A controlled study.	43 subjects, ages 17–60 with MDD	E_1: 9 patients receiving tricyclic antidepressants (TCAs) and aerobic exercise for 1 hour 3 times week for 9 weeks E_2: 15 patients receiving aerobic exercise but no TCAs C_1: 14 patients receiving TCAs and OT 3 times a week for 9 weeks C_2: 5 patients receiving OT but not TCAs	*Psychopathological Rating Scale* (CPRS; Åsberg et al., 1978); *Beck Depression Inventory* (BDI; Beck et al., 1961)	Significantly lower depression scores for those participating in aerobic exercises than others; maximum oxygen uptake noted in aerobic training groups resulted in greater antidepressive effects.
Martinsen et al. (1989). Comparing aerobic with nonaerobic forms of exercise in the treatment of clinical depression: A randomized trial.	90 inpatients of a psychiatric hospital with diagnosis of depression	E: 43 patients, brisk walks and jogging 3 times a week for 8 weeks C: 47 patients; muscular strength, flexibility and relaxation, exercises 3 times week for 8 weeks	*Beck Depression Inventory* (BDI; Beck et al., 1961); *Montgomery and Åsberg Depression Rating Scale* (MADRS; Montgomery and Åsberg 1979)	Depressed scores in both groups were reduced significantly, but no significant difference between groups
Rape, R. N. (1987). Running and depression.	21 Caucasian males running 15 or more miles per week 21 Caucasian males, nonexercisers	Matched two-group design comparing runners with nonexercisers	*Beck Depression Inventory* (BDI; Beck et al., 1961)	Runners were significantly less depressed than were non-exercisers

Note: E refers to the experimental group. C refers to the control group.

study conceivable, the task could be endless. Realistically, the investigator accepts the limitation that some published and unpublished studies will not be located. For example, studies published in foreign journals that have not been translated, recent unpublished papers presented at conferences and institutes, ongoing research where the investigator has not published the findings, and research studies by students presented in unpublished theses, dissertations, or special studies may not be found. These are realistic limitations to every study. Nonetheless, with the availability of computer systems for information retrieval, the present-day investigator is able to locate a vast portion of the literature.

The literature search is divided into two areas: referral sources and primary sources of data. These two areas are outlined in Table 6–3.

The first step in searching the literature is to locate where the relevant studies are reported, that is, in which journal, source book, or dissertation. The referral source supplies bibliographical information locating a specific study. The use of key words allows the student or researcher to identify more easily those studies that cover a particular topic. Frequently, the key words for a specific article are listed immediately before or after the abstract. This is illustrated in Figure 6–2, in which the key words (adolescence, learning disabilities, school-based,

Table 6–3. The Literature Search in Occupational Therapy

Referral Sources	*Primary Sources of Data*
• Information retrieval systems	• Journals
• Abstracting periodicals and bibliographic indexes	• Theses
• Directory of references	• Conference proceedings
• Annual reviews	• Government documents
	• Statistical compendiums
	• Unpublished studies

Ethical Dilemmas in
School-Based Therapy:
Implications for Occupational
Therapy

Josephine Mae Smith

Key Words: adolescence•learning disabilities•school-based•
ethics•occupational therapy•decision making

Abstract: An analysis . . .

Figure 6–2. An example of key words listed before the abstract and journal article. The use of these key words will lead the reader to other related articles.

ethics, occupational therapy, decision making) have been listed before the abstract. A student or researcher looking for related articles would use one or more of these key words in the computer search.

Each database has its own thesaurus that contains key words or concepts by using a controlled vocabulary. The controlled vocabulary provides a structure for classifying articles into given topics. Subjects or key words used by each database can be found in a thesaurus that is available in hard copy or on the CD-ROM used in the search process. The researcher or student will want to refer to the appropriate thesaurus to obtain the correct term for the database used. For more specialized words, such as names of tests, specific intervention theories (e.g., sensory integration, cognitive-behavioral, or NDT), the exact term will suffice to locate the articles. One database, MEDLINE, uses MeSH subject headings.

MeSH is the National Library of Medicine's controlled vocabulary thesaurus. Thesauri are carefully constructed sets of terms often connected by "broader-than," "narrower-than," and "related" links. These links show the relationship between related terms and provide a hierarchical structure that permits searching at various levels of specificity from narrower to broader. Thesauri are also known as "classification structures," "controlled vocabularies," and "ordering systems."

MeSH consists of a set of terms or subject headings that are arranged in both an alphabetic and a hierarchical structure. At the most general level of the hierarchical structure are very broad headings such as "Anatomy," "Mental Disorders," and "Enzymes, Coenzymes, and Enzyme Inhibitors." At more narrow levels are found more specific headings such as "Ankle," "Conduct Disorder," and "Calcineurin." There are nearly 19,000 main headings in MeSH and nearly 800 specialized descriptors called Qualifiers. In addition to these headings, there are 103,500 headings called Supplementary Concept Records (formerly Supplementary Chemical Records) within a separate chemical thesaurus. There are

also thousands of cross-references that assist in finding the most appropriate MeSH Heading, for example, Vitamin C see Ascorbic Acid.

MeSH Applications

▶ The quality of an information retrieval system is determined by the effective selection and assignment of thesaurus terms in order that items of interest may be readily found. MeSH, one of the world's preeminent controlled vocabularies, is a vital component of NLM's [National Library of Medicine] computer-based information retrieval system.

▶ The MeSH thesaurus is used by NLM for indexing articles from more than 4,200 of the world's leading biomedical journals for the MEDLINE® database and for other NLM-produced databases that include cataloging of books, documents, and audiovisuals acquired by the Library. Each bibliographic reference is associated with a set of MeSH terms that describe the content of the item. Similarly, a retrieval query is formed using MeSH terms to find items on a desired topic.

▶ MeSH is the source of the headings used as index terms in NLM's Index Medicus® and is fundamental to the organization of this monthly guide to articles from nearly 3,300 international journals. (National Library of Medicine, 1999c, p. 1)

An outline of the MEDLARS structure of categories is listed in Table 6–4. These categories are divided into subcategories and Medical Subject Headings (MeSH), allowing for a very specific search of terms.

Most information retrieval systems use *Boolean logic* as the strategy to build search statements. Boolean logic uses the logical operators *and*, *or*, and *not* to represent relationships between topics in a symbolic manner (see Figure 6–3). Some systems also use the search operators of *with* and *in*. The use of the term *with* identifies those articles in which the connected terms are

Table 6–4. MEDLARS Category Headings

A. Anatomy

B. Organisms

C. Diseases

D. Chemicals and Drugs

E. Analytical, Diagnostic, and Therapeutic Techniques and Equipment

F. Psychiatry and Psychology

G. Biological Science

H. Physical Sciences

I. Anthropology, Education, Sociology, and Social Anthropology

J. Technology, Commerce, and Industry

K. Humanities

L. Information Sciences

M. Named Groups

N. Health Care

Z. Geographical

used in the same field (e.g., traumatic brain injury with cognitive-behavior therapy), whereas the use of the term *in* specifies the particular field (traumatic brain injury in title). By combing search terms with these logical operators, the researcher can limit or enlarge the search. For example, if a researcher is looking for articles regarding the treatment of traumatic brain injury using cognitive-behavior therapy in occupational therapy settings, the search term would be written as

traumatic brain injury and cognitive-behavior therapy and occupational therapy

Use of these terms as well as the delimiter *and* would limit the search to only those articles in which both traumatic brain injury and cognitive-behavior therapy have been discussed. Articles that contain only etiology or only treatment will not be obtained. If, on the other hand, the researcher is

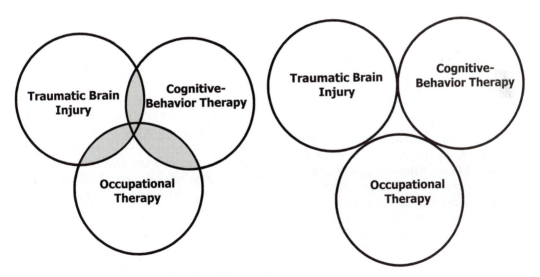

Figure 6–3. An example of Boolean thinking. In this example, the researcher is interested in information about traumatic brain injury **AND** cognitive-behavior therapy **AND** occupational therapy. The articles retrieved from the search will be found in the intersection that contains all three terms. In the second example, articles about traumatic brain injury, cognitive-behavior therapy, **OR** occupational therapy will be found. The first example is a more specific search that yields a smaller number of articles.

interested in articles that describe either traumatic brain injury or cognitive-behavior therapy, the search statement is written as

(Traumatic brain injury and occupational therapy) or (cognitive-behavior therapy and occupational therapy)

Articles that examine traumatic brain injury or cognitive-behavior therapy and occupational therapy, or both traumatic brain injury and cognitive-behavior therapy will be obtained. Thus, this search statement produces a larger list of citations, including the citations from the first search statement. Because each system uses a slightly different search technique, it will be necessary to obtain specific information about search strategies for the system used (e.g., OT BibSys, MEDLINE, or ERIC).

6.3.1 Information Retrieval Systems

Automated systems for storing and retrieving information have revolutionized libraries. Through computer technology, research librarians now are able to provide printouts of studies and their sources. The studies, sources, and key words are stored on CD-ROMS or hard drives, allowing for direct random access and interactive searching. In using a computer-based retrieval system the research proceeds as shown in the following box.

Information retrieval systems using CD-ROMs are limited by the information stored on the CD-ROM. Although these CD-ROMs are updated frequently, there can be a lag of up to 6 months from the time of publication of a journal article to the time of its inclusion in the computer memory bank. The production of the CD-ROM also is delayed, resulting in a possible lag of up to a year in the information stored on the database. The journals included in the system, the number of citations, and the years reviewed are important considerations in using these systems for research. A more

INPUT	COMPUTER PROCESS	OUTPUT
Researcher provides descriptors from a list of terms obtained from a thesaurus, a controlled vocabulary list, previous articles, or specialized terms	Titles of journal articles stored on disk or CD-ROM are scanned, and relevant titles are retrieved	Printout of studies (containing author, title, source, abstract, and sometimes the entire article) are obtained, either directly or through E-mail

up-to-date list of articles can be obtained through on-line databases; however, these may be costly, and many students do not have access to them if they are not available in the university or college library.

In spite of these limitations, computer-based retrieval systems should be one of the first referral sources used to locate relevant literature. There are two major advantages in using them: (a) the amount of time saved from laboriously reviewing individual journals or printed lists of journal articles (e.g., *Psych Abstracts, Medicus Indicus*), and (b) the ability to limit the articles by combining a number of key terms (e.g., Fetal Alcohol Syndrome, children, and Native Americans). On the other hand, computer-based retrieval systems are not inclusive as indicated in the foregoing, and they should not be the sole method of locating bibliographical references. The major information retrieval systems relevant to research in medicine, rehabilitation, health care, and education are described below.

MEDLARS®

The Medical Literature Analysis and Retrieval System (MEDLARS®) is a database system using computer subsystems (ELHILL® and TOXNET®), which contains more than 18 million citations in more than 40 databases derived from over 3,900 journals indexed for *Cumulative Index Medicus,* as well as about 700 selected journals indexed in the *Index to Dental Literature* or the *International Nursing Index.* Citations are available as far back as 1964. Articles are indexed using a list of more than 19,000 medical subject headings (MeSH) and 800 specialized descriptors or qualifiers. Use of one or more of these MeSH headings combined with the qualifiers allows an individual to search for articles and obtain citations of articles on a particular topic. Table 6–5 has an example of a printout for a complete MEDLINE unit record. Although any or all of these data elements can be printed within the computer printout of the search, usually the researcher requests only the author, title, source (location of the article), MeSH headings, and abstract.

The MEDLARS system consists of a number of different on-line databases. MEDLINE® (acronym for MEDlars onLINE) is the most widely used medical database. MEDLINE® and its companion databases (OLDMEDLINE and PREMEDLINE) contain citations in all languages for all areas of biomedicine. SDILINE® is a monthly update and contains citations of newly indexed articles to be published in the monthly *Index Medicus.*

Table 6–5. Sample MEDLINE Unit Record[a]

Unique Identifier
99109678

Authors
LaBan MM. Martin T. Pechur J. Sarnacki S.

Institution
Department of Physical Medicine and Rehabilitation, William Beaumont Hospital, Royal Oak, Michigan, USA.

Title
Physical and occupational therapy in the treatment of patients with multiple sclerosis. [Review] [31 refs]

Source
Physical Medicine & Rehabilitation Clinics of North America. 9(3):603-14, vii, 1998 Aug.

NLM Journal Code
cx9

Country of Publication
United States

MeSH Subject Headings
Bladder Diseases / pc [Prevention & Control]
Contracture / pc [Prevention & Control]
Decubitus Ulcer / pc [Prevention & Control]
Disease Progression
Fatigue / pc [Prevention & Control]
Fractures, Stress / pc [Prevention & Control]
Human
Intestinal Diseases / pc [Prevention & Control]
*Multiple Sclerosis / rh [Rehabilitation]

Multiple Sclerosis / th [Therapy]
Muscle Spasticity / pc [Prevention & Control]
Muscle Weakness / pc [Prevention & Control]
*Occupational Therapy
Osteoporosis / pc [Prevention & Control]
Patient Care Team
*Physical Therapy
Venous Thrombosis / pc [Prevention & Control]

Abstract
The interdisciplinary approach to the management of MS patients includes the services of both physical and occupational therapy. These professions complement one another in their concerted effort to mobilize the patient, thereby minimizing the symptoms of progressive weakness, fatigue, and spasticity. The ambulant patient is far less likely to develop complications of inactivity such as contractures, decubitus ulcers, venous thrombosis, or osteoporosis (with its associated fatigue fractures), as well as bowel or bladder complications. [References: 31]

ISSN
1047-9651

Publication Type
Journal Article. Review. Review, Tutorial.

Language
English

Entry Month
199904. Entry Week: 1999041.

[a]From MEDLINE database, Unique Identifier #99109678. Bolded terms are called field names. A researcher can ask for any or all of these field names when searching for citations. Only the field names pertinent to the citation are included in the record.

Internet Grateful Med was released to the public on April 16, 1996, and the current V2.6 was released September 2, 1998. It offers free searching in MEDLINE on NLM's PubMed system and in 14 other databases on the MEDLARS® computer system. To use Internet Grateful Med, point a compatible WWW browser such as Netscape Navigator or Microsoft Internet Explorer at the IGM URL: http://igm.nlm.nih.gov. (National Library of Medicine, 1999a, p. 2)

There are 31 specialized on-line databases included in MEDLARS. These databases include such subjects as acquired immunodeficiency syndrome (AIDS) and related subjects (AIDSLINE), drugs used in clinical trials for AIDS (AIDSDRUGS), biotechnological journals not covered in MEDLINE® (CATLINE®), major cancer topics (CANCERLIT), nursing and allied health literature (CINAHL), and bibliographic citations regarding toxicological, pharmacological, biochemical, and physiological effects of drugs and other chemicals (TOXNET® and TOXLINE® systems).

MEDLINE® refers to MEDLARS onLINE and is the database most commonly used by medical and allied health researchers throughout the world.

What is MEDLINE? MEDLINE is the NLMs on-line database that contains almost 10 million references to journal articles in the health sciences. Some facts:

Time covered. 1966 to the present
Source. 3,900 journals in 40 languages; 52% published in the U.S.; 88% of the current references are to articles in English. 76% of the references have English abstracts.
Weekly update. 7,300 references are added weekly (almost 400,000 yearly)
Broad coverage. Basic research and the clinical sciences (including nursing, dentistry, pharmacy, and allied health)
(National Library of Medicine, 1999c, p.1)

The computer base for MEDLARS is located in the National Library of Medicine in Bethesda, Maryland. More than 400 medical schools and hospital libraries in the United States have access to the MEDLARS system. A back-up system of eight regional medical libraries in the United States provides MEDLARS searches for health scientists in hospitals that do not have computer terminals. These federally designated regional medical libraries also provide consultative services and interlibrary loan privileges to other medical libraries within their region. The regional medical libraries are listed below:

▶ Toll-free phone number for all regional medical libraries: (800) 338–7657
▶ For general information contact **National Network of Libraries of Medicine,**
National Network Office,
National Library of Medicine,
8600 Rockville Pike,
Bldg. 38, Room B1-E03,
Bethesda, Maryland 20894
Phone: (301) 496-4777
Fax: (301) 480-1467
URL: http://www.nnlm.nlm.nih.gov
▶ **Middle Atlantic Region**
The New York Academy of Medicine
1216 Fifth Avenue
New York, NY 10029
Phone: (212) 822-7396
Fax: (212) 534-7042
URL: http://www.nnlm.nlm.nih.gov/mar
States served: DE, NJ, NY, PA
▶ **Southeastern/Atlantic Region**
University of Maryland
Health Services Library
601 West Lombard Street
Baltimore, Maryland 21201-1583
Phone: (410) 706-2855
Fax: (410) 706-0099
URL: http://www.nnlm.nlm.nih.gov/sea
States served: AL, FL, GA, MD, MS, NC, SC, TN, VA, WV, the District of Columbia, Puerto Rico, and the U.S. Virgin Islands
▶ **Greater Midwest Region**
University of Illinois at Chicago
Library of the Health Sciences
1750 W. Polk St.

Chicago, IL 60612-7223
Phone: (312) 996-2464
Fax: (312) 996-2226
URL: http://www.nnlm.nlm.nih.gov/gmr
States served: IA, IL, IN, KY, MI, MN, ND, OH, SD, WI

▶ **Midcontinental Region**
McGoogan Library of Medicine
University of Nebraska Medical Center
Regional Medical Library
986706 Nebraska Medical Center
Omaha, Nebraska 68198-6706
Phone: (402) 559-4326
Fax: (402) 559-5482
URL: http://www.nnlm.nlm.nih.gov/mr
States served: CO, KS, MO, NE, UT, WY

▶ **South Central Region**
Houston Academy of Medicine
Texas Medical Center Library
1133 M. D. Anderson Boulevard
Houston, Texas 77030-2809
Phone: (713) 799-7880
Fax: (713) 790-7030
Internet: nnlmscr@library.tmc.edu
URL: http://www.nnlm.nlm.nih.gov/scr
States served: AR, LA, NM, OK, TX

▶ **New England Region**
University of Connecticut Health Center
Lyman Maynard Stowe Library
263 Farmington Ave.
Farmington, CT 06030-5370
Phone: (860) 679-4500
Fax: (860) 679-1305
URL: http://www.nnlm.nlm.nih.gov/ner
States served: CT, MA, ME, NH, RI, VT

▶ **Pacific Northwest Region**
Health Sciences Libraries and Information Center
Box 357155
University of Washington
Seattle, Washington 98195-7155
Phone: (206) 543-8262
Fax: (206) 543-2469
Internet: nnlm@u.washington.edu
URL: http://www.nnlm.nlm.nih.gov/pnr
States served: AK, ID, MT, OR, WA

▶ **Pacific Southwest Region**
University of California, Los Angeles (UCLA)

Louise Darling Biomedical Library
12-077 Center for the Health Sciences
Box 951798
Los Angeles, California 90095-1798
Phone: (310) 825-1200
Fax: (310) 825-5389
URL: http://www.nnlm.nlm.nih.gov/psr
States served: AZ, CA, HI, NV, and U.S. Territories in the Pacific Basin

The locations of medical libraries providing MEDLARS services are available from the National Library of Medicine. Because the use of automated information retrieval systems has been expanding at an extremely rapid rate, the researcher must keep abreast of the innovations and changes occurring in this field. The costs and services connected to the MEDLARS system vary throughout the country.

In addition to the MEDLARS system, the National Library of Medicine houses a National Information Center on Health Services Research and Health Care Technology (NICHSR; see Box 6–1). For more information on NICHSR, contact:

▶ National Information Center on Health Services Research and Health Care Technology (NICHSR)
National Library of Medicine
8600 Rockville Pike
Building 38A, Mail Stop 20
Bethesda, MD 20894
Voice: (301)496-0176; Fax: (301)402-3193
E-mail: nichsr@nlm.nih.gov; Internet: http://www.nlm.nih.gov/nichsr/nichsr.html

OT BibSys (http://www.aota.org/search/logon.asp)

OT BibSys is a bibliographic database that requires payment of a yearly fee. It was developed and is owned by the American Occupational Therapy Association. Many occupational therapy programs pay the site fee so that their students and faculty can have access to the database. The database covers literature in the disciplines of occupational therapy and related subject areas, such as rehabilitation, education, psychiatry or psychology, and health care delivery or administration. On the Web site, information that identifies the material and the abstract necessary for obtaining the full text of the indexed resources is available. The depository for the official documents for AOTA is located in the Wilma L. West Library.

Cardiopulmonary Technology

Physical Therapy

Emergency Service

Physician Assistant

Health Education

Radiologic Technology

Medical/Laboratory

Technology Therapy

Medical Assistant

Social Service/ Health Care

Medical Records

Surgical Technology

Occupational Therapy

The Wilma L. West Library (WLWL) owns a copy of all the material indexed in OT BibSys. While searchers will find material from related or supporting disciplines in this database, the primary purpose is to bring together the literature of occupational therapy in one database. To this end, we are gradually expanding coverage of non-OT journals in OT BibSys on a selective basis; that is, only articles written by occupational therapists or of definite interest to occupational therapists will be included. There may be times, therefore, when OT BibSys is not appropriate for retrieving information on a particular subject, such as a rare syndrome or a more sociological issue. Consult a librarian at your institution for guidance in selecting the database that covers the literature you are seeking. You may also visit our listing of useful WWW links or rehabilitation-related databases for further information. . . . Nominal charges apply to obtaining photocopies of journal articles from the Library. (American Occupational Therapy Association, 1999, p. 1)

CINAHL (Cumulative Index to Nursing & Allied Health; http://www.cinahl.com)

This database, updated monthly, covers English-language journals and literature from 1983 to the present in the disciplines of nursing and allied health, including emergency services, health education, and social services in health care. Publications from the following allied health fields are indexed:

Selected journals are also indexed in the areas of consumer health, biomedicine, and health sciences librarianship. In total, more than 500 journals are regularly indexed; online abstracts are available for more than 150 of these titles. The database also provides access to healthcare books, nursing dissertations, selected conference proceedings, standards of professional practice, educational software, and audiovisual materials in nursing. Although not a part of MEDLARS, the format of citations and search strategies are based on the MEDLARS MeSH subject headings. "More than 6,400 CINAHL subject headings provide specific access to NAHL citations. Approximately 70 percent of CINAHL headings also appear in MEDLINE®. CINAHL supplements these headings with 2,000+ terms designed specifically for nursing and allied health" (Cinahl Information Systems, 1997, p. 1). This database is also available on CD-ROM and is updated regularly. More information about CINAHL can be found at http://www.biomedsearch.lib.umn.edu/ ovidweb/fldguide/nursing.htm

ERIC (http://www.accesseric.org/searchdb/ searchdb.html)

ERIC is an acronym for Educational Resources Information Center, a component of the National Library of Education (http:// www.ed.gov/NLE/). The database is available on CD-ROM (Silver Platter) in most university libraries and contains citations for more than 70,000 publications in educational journals and technical reports, documents of program descriptions, curricular materials, and papers presented at national conferences. An on-line edition is updated monthly and is available for those with access to the Web. Unpublished articles cited in ERIC are available as ERIC documents on microfiche in many university libraries. As with MEDLINE, the records for each citation include a number of fields (e.g., author, title, citation, language, year of publication, search descriptors, and target audience). A thesaurus of descriptors is available in hard copy and as part of the CD-ROM for those unsure of the proper search term.

PsychINFO (http://milton.mse.jhu.edu/dbases/psychlit.html)

PsychInfo is an online database that covers the disciplines of psychology and related fields, including psychiatry, sociology, anthropology, education, pharmacology, physiology, linguistics, and psychopharmacology. Journal articles, technical reports, and dissertations published since 1967 are included in the database. It is also available on CD-ROM. As with ERIC, a thesaurus of descriptors is available in hard copy and as part of the on-line database or CD-ROM. The CD-ROM, available in most libraries, is updated regularly. PsychLit summarizes English language chapters and books in psychology and related disciplines worldwide published from 1987. The database is updated monthly.

REHABDATA (http://www.naric.com/search)

This database, sponsored by the National Rehabilitation Information Center (http://www.naric.com/), lists citations of research reports, monographs, and other material that focus on rehabilitation of individuals with physical or mental disabilities. The database, funded by the National Institute on Disability and Rehabilitation Research (NIDRR), is committed "to serve anyone, professional or lay person, who is interested in disability and rehabilitation, including

consumers, family members, health professionals, educators, rehabilitation counselors, students, librarians, administrators, and researchers" (National Rehabilitation Information Center, n.d., p. 1).

ABLEDATA (http://www.abledata.com/index.htm)

ABLEDATA, also funded by NIDRR, provides information in the area of assistive technology.

> The ABLEDATA database contains information on more than 25,000 assistive technology products (17,000 of which are currently available), from white canes to voice output programs. The database contains detailed descriptions of each product including price and company information. The database also contains information on non-commercial prototypes, customized and one-of-a-kind products, and do-it-yourself designs. (National Institute on Disability and Rehabilitation Data, n.d., p. 1)

CHID (http://chid.nih.gov)

This database, which stands for Combined Health Information Database,

> provides titles, abstracts, and availability information for health information and health education resources.
> CHID lists a wealth of health promotion and education materials and program descriptions that are not indexed elsewhere. New records are added quarterly and current listings are checked regularly to help ensure that all entries are up to date and still available from their original sources. Some older records are retained for archival purposes.
> CHID is updated four times a year. The updated database is available at the end of these months: January, April, July, and October.
> CHID is a cooperative effort among several Federal agencies. Recognizing the need for a single source of health information, the participating agencies combined their information files into one database—

thus creating the Combined Health Information Database or CHID. CHID has been available to the public since 1985. Since then, new topics have been added and will be added in the future. Each topic is updated on a quarterly basis.

At present, CHID covers 18 topics. You can search either individual topics or the entire database. The topics are:

► AIDS Education (AD)
► Alzheimer's Disease (AZ)
► Arthritis and Musculoskeletal and Skin Diseases (AR)
► Cancer Patient Education (CA)
► Cancer Prevention and Control (CP)
► Complementary and Alternative Medicine (AM)
► Deafness and Communication Disorders (DC)
► Diabetes (DM)
► Digestive Diseases (DD)
► Disease Prevention/Health Promotion (NH)
► Epilepsy Education and Prevention (EP)
► Health Promotion and Education (HE)
► Kidney and Urologic Diseases (KU)
► Maternal and Child Health (MC)
► Medical Genetics and Rare Disorders (MG)
► Oral Health (OH)
► Prenatal Smoking Cessation (PS)
► Weight Control (WC)

(CHID Technical Director, n.d., p. 1)

Other Databases

► **Rhoda Weiss**'s home page lists several additional links and databases useful for occupational therapists:
http://www.readap.umontreal.ca/InternOT/home.html
► **OTDBase** is provided for a modest fee and contains abstracts from about 18 international occupational therapy journals. The system is user friendly and cross-indexes articles.
http://www.otdbase.com/
► **OVID** accesses several databases (e.g., MEDLINE and CINAHL). AGELine (http://www.usc.edu/isd/elecresources/gateways/ageline.html) is a database specializing in social gerontology (i.e., study of aging in psychological, health-related, social, and economic contexts). Because additional databases are being developed, the reader may want to explore library sources and on-line services for additional information.

6.3.2 Bibliographic Indexes and Abstracting Periodicals

There is a growing trend in the medical, educational, and allied health fields to group together published articles under specific headings or separate publications. Consequently, indexes to the literature on arthritis, cardiovascular disease, stroke, gastroenteritis, cancer, and dyslexia, special teaching methods, and others are being published with the aid of computer technology. Because of the change in technology and the use of CD-ROMs and on-line services, these sources are being discontinued quickly. Until they disappear, however, these sources can provide an additional means of obtaining information.

When using a bibliographic index, the researcher should be aware of the specified journals cited and the frequency of publication. Although more tedious to use, these indexes supplement the CD-ROMs because of their more frequent updates. Articles referenced after the production of the CD-ROM will be listed in the monthly updates.

Bibliographic indexes and abstracting periodicals are hard-copy sources for lists of recent studies from a multitude of journals grouped under a specific subject heading. Usually, they include concise summaries (abstracts) of articles or investigations. The purpose of the abstract is to provide the reader with a quick overview of the problem under investigation, the methods used in data collection, the results reported, and the conclusions. The abstract is an intermediary step between the bibliographical citation and the complete journal article. Because the abstract is a self-contained summary, it can provide the researcher with all the information desired in a specific research area. More frequently, researchers use abstracting periodicals to select pertinent articles for further examination. Bibliographic indexes and abstracting journals most frequently used by allied health and special education providers are listed below.

▶ *Index Medicus* is published monthly as a bibliographic listing of references to current articles from more than 3,300 worldwide biomedical science and clinical medicine journals. There is a separate bibliography of medical reviews. This index is the major index for journals in basic biomedical sciences and clinical medicine. Since 1976, the index has also published selected conference publications and multi-authored monographs. The index is the hard copy of MEDLARS. Citations use both author and subject headings. Journal articles are cited under the same major MeSH terms as found in MEDLARS (Table 6–4), with an additional list of about 9,000 technical terms arranged in subheadings. These subheads are arranged alphabetically, with cross references in categorized lists. A search for articles in a specific topic is more arduous with this index than with MEDLARS because the researcher must examine all the articles under a given subject rather than narrowing the search through the use of delimiting terms such as *and, and not,* or *or.* Nonetheless, use of this index allows the searcher to find the most recent articles not yet included on the CD-ROM.

▶ *Cumulated Index Medicus* is published, since 1960, by the National Library of Medicine in conjunction with the U.S. Department of Health, Education, and Welfare (DHEW), Public Health Service, and National Institutes of Health. It includes the culmination of the 12 monthly issues of *Index Medicus.*

▶ *Cumulative Index to Nursing and Allied Health Literature (CINAHL)* is available through CINAHL, 1509 Wilson Terrace, Glendale, CA 91206. This is the hard-copy edition of the CINAHL database. The index includes references to all the major nursing periodicals published in the English language. Journals, book reviews, pamphlets, illustrated material, films, filmstrips, and recordings are cited. More than 250 periodicals are indexed and nonnursing databases (e.g., PsychLIT, ERIC) are scanned for articles of specific interest to nurses and allied health professionals.

▶ *Excerpta Medica Abstract Journals* (http://hilly.com/spd/embase/emaj1.html) is by far the most complete medical abstracting service in the world. Forty-one abstract journals are published monthly under separate covers. The world medical literature consisting of almost 3,500 current journals are reviewed. Of particular interest to occupational therapists are the abstracts in *Arthritis and Rheumatism, Cancer, Cardiovascular Disease, Chest Diseases, Drug Dependency, Epilepsy, Gerontology and Geriatrics, Neurology, Occupational Health, Psychiatry, Public Health,* and *Rehabilitation and Physical Medicine.*

▶ *ErgoWeb* (http://www.ergoweb.com/Pub/Company/comhome.shtml), established in 1992 at the University of Utah's Department of Mechanical Engineering, is a resource for researchers investigating topics in ergnomics.

▶ *Mental Health* (http://www.mentalhealth.com/p.html) is a free Web database that provides information on the 50 most common mental disorders.

▶ *Health Education Research* contains abstracts of theses and dissertations from colleges offering graduate programs in health education. Studies are listed by areas that include community and public health, curriculum development, education, health careers, health institutions, environmental health, nutrition, weight control, and others.

▶ *Hospital and Health Administration Index* (previously *Hospital Literature Index*), first published in 1945, cites studies on administration, planning, and financing of hospitals and related health care institutions, and the administrative aspects of the medical, paramedical, and repayment fields. It is published quarterly.

▶ *Psychological Abstracts,* the hard-copy format of the *PsychLIT* database, provides international coverage of journals, books, government research reports, and dissertations in all disciplines of psychology. The information is arranged by subject with author and subject indexes provided. *Psychological Abstracts* contains nonevaluative summaries of the world's literature from more than 850 journals, technical reports, monographs, and other scientific documents. Each monthly issue contains abstracts listed under numerous major classifications including the following: general psychology, psychometrics and statistics, perception and motor performance, cognitive processes and motivation, neurology and physiology, developmental psychology, cultural influences and social issues, social behavior and interpersonal processes, communication, language, personality, professional, personnel, physical and psychological disorders, treatment and prevention, educational psychology, and applied psychology.

▶ *Sociological Abstracts* (http://www.csa.com/) is the hard-copy edition of the on-line service. More than 150 journals from sociology are represented in *Sociological Abstracts,* published five times a year. Articles of particular interest to allied health are included under subheadings such as sociology of health and medicine, demography and human biology, and social problems and social welfare.

▶ *Social Work Research and Abstracts* (http://www.lib.umn.edu/index/about/a-swabs.html) was previously entitled *Abstracts for Social Workers.* It contains abstracts from journals related to the field of social work. Both print and CD-ROM are available. These abstracts are grouped under major headings, such as fields of service, social policy and action, service methods, the social work profession, history of social work, and related fields in the social sciences. Subhead-

ings of particular interest to allied health professionals and special educators include aging, health and medical care, mental retardation, mental health, interprofessional relations, and psychiatry and medicine.

▶ *Dissertation Abstracts* (http://www.lib.umn.edu/index/about/a-dsa.html) contains doctoral dissertations abstracts from more than 550 colleges and universities in the United States, Canada, and Europe. Masters theses are available from selected colleges. Dissertations are available through three sources, (microfilm, photocopy, and computer output). Citations for doctoral dissertations are available from 1861. Information is updated at least quarterly.

▶ *Biological Abstracts* and *Biology Digest* report the world's bioscience research. These periodicals are published semimonthly with the cooperation of individual biologists, biological industries, and biological journals. Approximately 9,300 journals from 100 different countries are indexed in areas related to life science, genetics, anatomy, physiology, environmental pollutants, nutrition, psychiatry, and public health. The articles are arranged by topic, with author, biosystem, and subject indexes.

▶ *Science Citation Index* (*SCI*; http://www.lib.umn.edu/index/about/a-scie.html) is an international, interdisciplinary index to the literature of science, medicine, agriculture, technology, and the behavioral sciences. "Bibliographic citations, plus author abstracts 'for approximately 70% of the articles in the database.' Each citation also includes a list of references cited in the source article. In addition, it is possible to retrieve a list of works that have cited a specific author or a specific earlier work" (University of Minnesota Libraries, 1998, p. 1).

▶ *Current Contents*® (http://www.lib.umn.edu/index/about/a-ccon.html) is published weekly by the Institute of Scientific Information, Inc. It offers access to the table of contents in seven different subject areas, including social and behavioral sciences and provides complete bibliographic information, title, word, and author index, and author and publisher addresses. Separate editions cover life sciences, social and behavioral sciences, clinical medicine, engineering technology and applied sciences, and the arts and humanities. A computer disk is available, as well as a hard copy.

▶ *NIH Office of Extramural Research* (http://www.nih.gov/grants/award/award.htm) is an on-line data base that contains information about health research currently supported by various agencies of the National Institutes of Health, thereby allowing scientists and administrators of science programs to identify current research activities in areas relating to their own endeavors.

▶ *Annual Reviews Inc* (http://www.AnnualReviews.org/) is published yearly and contains integrated summaries of topical issues by recognized authorities. They publish the following Annual Reviews of interest to the researcher in occupational therapy.

Annual Review of Neuroscience

Annual Review of Biomedical Engineering

Annual Review of Genetics

Annual Review of Medicine

Annual Review of Gerontology and Geriatrics

Annual Review of Psychology

Annual Review of Public Health

Annual Review of Sociology

Annual Review of Rehabilitation

Annual Review of Nutrition

6.3.3 Sources for Health Statistics

Statistical information is an essential part of the literature search. The incidence of dis-

eases, hospitalization rates, occupational accidents, infant mortality rates, and the leading causes of death are examples of data compiled by government agencies and published in periodicals available to researchers. A common source of primary statistical information, located at http://www.cdc.gov/nchswww/default.htm, is the National Center for Health Statistics. FEDSTATS, available at http://www.fedstats.gov, gives additional information. Statistical reports are issued periodically. The National Center for Health Statistics complies several series of statistics. The series listed below may be useful to health care researchers.

▶ *Series 1: Programs and collection procedures:* Reports that describe the general programs of the National Center for Health Statistics and its offices and divisions, data collection methods used, definitions, and other material necessary for understanding the data.

▶ *Series 2: Data evaluation and methods of research:* Studies of new statistical methodology including experimental tests of new survey methods, studies of vital statistics collection methods, new analytical techniques, objective evaluations of reliability of collected data, and contributions to statistical theory.

▶ *Series 3: Analytical and epidemiological studies:* Reports presenting analytical or interpretive studies based on vital and health statistics, carrying the analysis further than the expository types of reports in the other series.

▶ *Series 4: Documents and committee reports:* Final reports of major committees concerned with vital and health statistics and documents, such as recommended model vital registration laws and revised birth and death certificates.

▶ *Series 5: International vital and health statistics reports:* Analytical and descriptive reports comparing U.S. vital and health statistics with those of other countries.

▶ *Series 6: Cognition and survey measurement:* Measurement using methods of cognitive science to design, evaluate, and test survey instruments.

▶ *Series 10: Data from the National Health Interview Survey:* Statistics on illness, accidental injury, disability, use of hospital, medical, dental, and other services, and other health-related topics, based on data collected in a continuing national household interview survey.

▶ *Series 11: Data from the National Health Examination Survey, the National Health and Nutrition Examination Surveys, and the Hispanic Health and Nutrition Examination Survey:* Data from direct examination, testing, and measurement of national samples of the population provide the basis for two types of reports: (a) estimates of the medically defined prevalence of specific diseases in the United States and the distributions of the noninstitutionalized population with respect to physical, physiological, and psychological characteristics; and (b) analysis of relationships among the various measurements without reference to an explicit finite universe of persons.

▶ *Series 12: Data from the institutional population surveys:* Statistics relating to the health characteristics of persons in institutions and on medical, nursing, and personal care received, based on national samples of establishments providing these services and samples of the residents or patients. This series was discontinued after 1969. Information in this series appears in Series 13.

▶ *Series 13: Data from the National Health Care Survey:* Statistics on the utilization of health manpower and facilities providing long-term care, ambulatory care, and family planning services.

▶ *Series 14: Data on health resources: manpower and facilities:* Statistics on the numbers, geographic distribution, and characteristics of health sources including physicians, dentists, nurses, other health manpower occupations, hospitals, nursing homes, outpatient and other inpatient facilities.

▶ *Series 20: Data on mortality:* Various statistics on mortality other than as included in regular annual or monthly reports. Special analyses by cause of death, age, and other demographic variables; geographic and time series analy-

ses; and statistics on characteristics of death not available from the vital records based on sample surveys of those records.

For a complete list of series reports, access http://www.cdc.gov/nchswww/products/pubs/pubd/series/ser.htm

The World Health Organization of the United Nations has compiled the following statistical compendiums.

▶ *World Health Statistics Report* is published quarterly by the World Health Organization, Geneva, Switzerland. It reports articles both in English and French and contains two parts: statistics on diseases and specific topics of current interest, such as certain causes of death and morbidity.

▶ *World Health Statistics Annual* is a result of a joint effort by national health and statistical administrations of various countries, the statistical offices of the United Nations, and the World Health Organization. It consists of three parts: (a) Volume I, vital statistics and causes of death; (b) Volume II, infectious diseases, causes, death, and vaccination; and (c) Volume III, health personnel and hospital establishments. It is printed simultaneously in English and French.

Other statistical compendiums include the following:

▶ *Demographic Yearbook,* published by the statistical office of the United Nations, Department of Economic and Social Affairs, New York. Statistics compiled from 250 countries of the world are included. Topics include population rates, mortality rates by disease, life expectancy tables, and marriage, divorce, and migration statistics.

▶ *American Statistics Index: A Comprehensive Guide and Index to the Statistical Publications of the United States Government,* published by Congressional Information Service, Inc. This index contains all data collected by the federal government in various subjects.

► U.S. Bureau of the Census
► U.S. Bureau of Labor Statistics
► U.S. Department of Agriculture

6.3.4 Directories of References

Directories of references are books that provide a comprehensive source for locating studies in specified fields. They provide lists and short reviews of available textbooks, journals, bibliographies, dictionaries, atlases, databases, and government documents. The following directories are a sample of the many reference resources available to the clinical researcher. The main limitation of directories is the rapidity with which new sources of information are created, which makes it almost impossible for a directory to be up to date. When using a directory the researcher should be aware of the copyright date.

► Armstrong, C. J. (Ed.). (1993). *World Databases in Medicine.* London: Bowker-Saur. The author states in the preface:

> *World Databases in Medicine* is the first in a series of directories whose overall aim is to map the databases in twenty-three clearly defined subject disciplines—twenty-three disciplines which encompass all of mankind's knowledge. As its name implies, this directory like the others to follow, is attempting worldwide coverage and includes databases from Australasia, CIS, Europe, Scandinavia and the Far East as well as from UK and North America. (p. v)

The book provides comprehensive information about each database, including commentaries and reviews about the database and links to similar databases. Journals and periodicals connected to databases are also identified, making it easy for the reader to find hard-copy material.

► Blake, J. B., & Roos, C. (Eds.). (1967). *Medical Reference Works 1679–1966: A Se-*

lected Bibliography. Chicago: Medical Library Assoc.

Listed in the publication are indexes and abstracts, bibliographies, proceedings of Congress, dictionaries, periodicals, and directories related to such areas as medicine, anatomy, medical education, hospitals, neurology, psychiatry, nursing, nutrition, pediatrics, physical medicine and rehabilitation, psychology, public health research in progress, and sociology. The purpose of the publication, as stated by the editors, is "To survey the world's bioscientific, medical, and allied health literature and select and organize from it an annotated list of the major works useful in gaining access to publications or frequently needed data" (p. iii).

► Bowker Company (1999). *Medical and Health Care Books and Serials in Print: An Index to Literature in the Health Sciences.* New York: R. R. Bowker Co. (http://www.bowker.com/catalog/home/entries/p10_c2.html)

The index covers a wide range of books and serials related to the major health sciences disciplines (e.g., medicine, dentistry, human health, nursing, nutrition, veterinary medicine, psychiatry, psychology, behavioral sciences, and other associated health sciences that are currently available from publishers. This book is a companion to *Books in Print* and *Serials in Print.*

► **NELINET** (http://mailboss.nelinet.net/cdrates/pchome.htm) is a valuable list of data bases organized by name and vendor. Although Web sites for individual databases are not provided, the vendor name is helpful for locating the databases online.

► **RESNA:** http://www.resna.org/
The Rehabilitation Engineering and Assistive Technology Society of North America (RESNA), founded in 1979, is

> an interdisciplinary association of people with a common interest in technology and disability. Our purpose is to improve the potential of people

with disabilities to achieve their goals through the use of technology. We serve that purpose by promoting research, development, education, advocacy, and the provision of technology and by supporting the people engaged in these activities. (Rehabilitation Engineering and Assistive Technology Society of North America, [RESNA], n.d., p. 1)

▶ Reish, W. T. (Ed.). (1998). *Encyclopedia of Bioethics.* New York: Macmillan Library Reference, Simon and Schuster. This five-volume encyclopedia explains terms and concepts related to bioethics. The encyclopedia includes a bibliography and an index.

▶ Roper, F. W., & Boorkman, J. A. (1994). *Introduction to Reference Sources in the Health Sciences* (3rd ed.). Methven, NJ: Scarecrow.
The book contains bibliographic and informational sources of monographs, periodicals, abstracting services, databases, U.S. government documents and technical reports, conferences, medical and health statistics, and audiovisual reference sources.

▶ Walters, L. (Ed.). (1998). *Bibliography of Bioethics* (Vol. 24). Washington, DC: Georgetown University, Kennedy Institute.
This bibliography of bioethical topics is published annually and provides a comprehensive cross-disciplinary listing of journals, newspaper articles, monographs, essays, court decisions, and audiovisual materials. The bibliography is designed for anyone concerned with bioethics, including scientists, health professionals, and legal scholars.

6.3.5 Current Research

Current research not included in computer retrieval systems or annual reviews can be found in the most recently published periodicals. Most university and medical libraries have reading rooms where current scientific journals are placed on open shelves.

A perusal of newly published articles may be helpful in gaining an overview of a topic and establishing an up-to-date bibliography of related literature. Key words often will be listed under the abstract. Use of these key words to identify additional literature through databases and indexes may result in additional material. Current journals will also be helpful in locating individuals engaged in ongoing research, allowing researchers to request current reprints of articles, unpublished research, and conference papers. In general, most scholars will be flattered to receive requests from individuals genuinely interested in their work, and they will respond readily. The standard format in requesting reprints is to list the bibliographical citation (i.e., journal, volume, date, and title) as in the example in Figure 6–4.

6.3.6 Journals

A list of occupational therapy journals published around the world is supplied in Table 6–6. A Web site link to 150 biomedical journals, including *JAMA, International Journal of Medicine, American Heart Association, New England Journal of Medicine* is http://www.medstudents.com.br/link/journal.htm.

6.4 Recording Information From Research Articles

The beginning researcher should develop a system for recording, organizing, and storing information related to a content area. It is important to develop this system early in the process by recording bibliographic information from all sources at the time it is obtained, even if the use of the material is questionable (Englehart, 1972). The reconstruction of bibliographic sources at a later time can be time consuming and difficult. An effective method of organizing data is to use a letter-size folder for each subject heading or variable in a study. Some inves-

```
                                    19524 E. Lewis Avenue
                                    Marketplace, AK 99872
                                    July 15, 1999


Dear Dr. Clark:

Please send me a reprint of your article: Occupational Therapy
for Independent-Living Older Adults: A Randomized Controlled
Trial published IN JAMA (1997)Volume 278, pp. 1321-1326


                                    Sincerely,



                                    John Walker
```

Figure 6–4. An example of a request for an article. Notice that the request includes the author, title of article, date of article, journal, and page numbers. If the article is unpublished, the request should state that.

tigators photocopy studies from periodicals or newspapers that relate to a specific area. Using information obtained from each of these articles, researchers are able to compile an up-to-date annotated bibliography.

In recording notes from a study, 3×5 index cards are helpful when compiling a bibliography, while 5×8 index cards may be useful for more extensive information, such as long quotes or abstracts. An example of a card is shown in Figure 6–5. The card should contain the following information from each study:

1. A bibliographical notation that includes all information used in a citation (see Chapter 9 for examples of citations)
2. Library call number or ERIC number can be helpful also, as this allows the researcher to find the publication quickly
3. Abstract of study including number of subjects, data collection methodology, test instruments, results, and conclusions
4. Important quotations (including page numbers) that can be cited in literature review

5. Any reactions to the article, such as evaluation of the validity of results or generalizations offered

By recording this information accurately, the researcher saves the time and effort it would require to return to the library and look up a bibliographical notation or other missing information.

Researchers should obtain information from many different types of publications. Although primary sources are used the most, valuable information can be obtained from secondary and tertiary sources.

6.5 Evaluating Validity of Research Findings

The finding and citing of research are not the final processes in reviewing literature. A critical analysis is a vital task of the investigator. One of the more difficult tasks in a literature review is the ability to review the articles in an integrated fashion. One cannot

Table 6–6. Compendium of Journals in Occupational Therapy

- **American Journal of Occupational Therapy (AJOT)**
  http://www.aota.org/nonmembers/area7/links/link3.html
  4720 Montgomery Lane,
  P.O. 31220
  Bethesda, MD 20824-1220

- **Australian Occupational Therapy Journal (AOTJ)**
  http://www.blacksci.co.uk/products/journals/xajot.htm
  Blackwell Science Pty Ltd.,
  54 University Street,
  Carlton, Victoria 3053, Australia
  E-mail: 100036.2660@compuserve.com
  home page: http://www.blackwell-science.com/australi

- **British Journal of Occupational Therapy (BJOT)**
  http://www.iop.bpmf.ac.uk/home/trust/ot/otcot.htm
  6-8 Marshalsea Road,
  London, SE1 1HL, England

- **Canadian Journal of Occupational Therapy (CJOT)**
  http://www.caot.ca/pages/publications%26products/periodicals.html
  Carleton Technology and Training Centre
  Suite 3400-1125 Colonel By Drive
  Ottawa, Ontario, Canada, K1S 5R1

- **Chinese Journal of Occupational Therapy**

- **Dutch Journal of Occupational Therapy**

- **Ergotherapie & Rehabilitation [Germany]**
  http://www.ergotherapie-reha.de/Ergo/Ergotheraphie.html

- **Hong Kong Journal of Occupational Therapy**
  http://www.polyu.edu.hk/hkota/journal.htm

- **Indian Journal of Occupational Therapy**

- **Irish Journal of Occupational Therapy (IrJOT)**
  Editorial Committee
  c/o AOTI, Unit 4, Argus House
  Greenmount Office Park
  Harold's Cross
  Dublin 6, Ireland

- **The Israeli Journal of Occupational Therapy (IJOT)**
  Gefen Publishing House
  7 Ariel Street
  P.O. Box 6056
  Jerusalem, 91060, Israel 91060
  Alternative Address:
  P.O. Box 101
  Woodmere, NY 11598

- **Journal D'Ergotherapie [France]**
  http://www.bois-larris.com/centrdoc.html

- **Journal of Occupational Science [Australia]**
  Editorial Office
  School of Occupational Therapy
  University of South Australia
  North Terrace
  Adelaide, South Australia, 5000, Australia

- **Journal of Occupational Therapy Students**
  http://www.aota.org/nonmembers/area7/links/link4.html

evaluate and critique each article separately; rather, the integration of the information must be done by synthesizing the information (Finley, 1989). One outcome of this type of evaluation is that the reader begins to build a conceptual framework, thereby allowing for a more mature evaluation of other literature in the field.

The quality of the research and the validity of the conclusions need to be evaluated before the research can be integrated with other results. When contradictory results arising from different studies occur, the in-vestigator should seek to offer an explanation based on the research methodologies. Occasionally, investigators reviewing literature cite the results and conclusions of previous research without determining the size of sample, data collection procedures, and measuring instruments used. It should be obvious to the reader that results of studies involving small samples and using tests that have low reliability are not as valid as large-scale studies in which rigorous methodology and reliable measuring instruments are used. In reporting previ-

Table 6–6. *Continued*

- *Journal of Japanese Association of Occupational Therapists (JJAOT)*
- *Journal of the Otago Polytechnic Occupational Therapy Department (JOPOT)*
  Occupational Therapy Department
  Otago Polytechnic
  Private Bag 1910
  Dunedin, New Zealand
  E-mail: irenem@tekotago.ac.nz
- *La Revue Qubecoise d'ergotherapie (LRQD)*
  Title/Abstracts Translated from French
- *New Zealand Journal of Occupational Therapy (NZJOT)*
  http://www.asianmediaaccess.com.au/lmm/
  mediadata1/123363.html
  PO Box 36-223
  Aukland, 1330, New Zealand
- *Occupational Therapy in Health Care (OTHC)*
- *Occupational Therapy in Mental Health (OTMH)*
- *Physical and Occupational Therapy in Pediatrics (POTP)*
- *Physical and Occupational Therapy in Geriatrics (POTG)*
  The four journals above are from
  http://web.spectra.net/haworth/
  Haworth Document Delivery Center,
  10 Alice Street, Binghamton, NY 13904
- *Occupational Therapy International (OTI)*
  http://www.allenpress.com/catalogue/index/occ_

therapy_international/index.html
Whurr Publishers Ltd.,
19b Compton Terrace,
London N1 2UN, ENGLAND

- *Occupational Therapy Journal of Research (OTJR)*
  http://www.slackinc.com/otpt/otjr/otjrhome.htm
  Slack, Inc.
  6900 Grove Road
  Thorofare, NJ 08086-9447
- *Occupational Therapy Practice (OTP)*
  http://www.aota.org/nonmembers/area7/links/
  link1.html
  American Occupational Therapy Association
  4720 Montgomery Lane
  Bethesda, MD 20814-3425
- *Praxis Ergotherapie (PE)*
  [Title/Abstracts Translated from German]
- *Scandinavian Journal of Occupational Therapy (SJOT)*
  http://www.scup.no/journals/journals.html
  Dept. of Physical Medicine and Rehabilitation
  Umeå University SE-901 87
  Umeå, Sweden
- *South African Journal of Occupational Therapy*
  Editor Daleen Casteleijn
  E-mail: sajot@cis.co.za
- *World Federation of Occupational Therapists Bulletin (WFOT)*
  http://fohweb.macarthur.uws.edu.au/ot/wfot.htm

---

ous literature, the investigator should consider the following factors in evaluating the validity of the research findings:

▶ The size of the sample, sampling procedure, and representativeness
▶ Control of extraneous variables that can potentially affect results
▶ Evidence of research bias in conclusions that are not consistent with results
▶ Selection of reliable and valid measuring instruments
▶ Data collection procedures
▶ Statistical techniques employed

In addition to these factors, the reader should ask a number of questions about the article. These questions are summarized in Table 6–7.

6.6 Outlining the Literature Review Section

Whether the researcher is reporting results in a journal article or preparing a thesis, he or she must decide how much of the background literature should be cited. The *Publication Manual of the American Psychological*

Braverman, S. E., Spector, J., Warden, D. L., Wilson, B. C., Ellis, T. E., & Bamdad, M. J. (1999). Multidisciplinary TBI inpatient rehabilitation programme for active duty service members as part of a randomized, clinical trial. <u>Brain Injury</u>,13(6), 405-415.

OBJECTIVE: To evaluate the effectiveness of a multidisciplinary rehabilitation program for military service members with moderate brain injury

DESIGN: Randomized control trial

SETTING: Impatient rehabilitation program in a U.S. military tertiary care hospital

PATIENTS: 67 active-duty individuals with moderate to severe TBI

INTERVENTION: "Eight week rehabilitation program combining group and individual therapies with an inpatient milieu-oriented neuropsychological focus. Group therapies included. fitness, planning and organization, cognitive skills, work skills, medication, and milieu groups, and community re- entry outings. Individual therapy included neuropsychology, work therapy, occupational therapy, and speech and language pathology" (p. 405)

                                                                    Continued

DESIRED OUTCOME: Successful return to work and return to duty.

RESULTS: At 1-year follow-up, 64 individuals returned to work (96%), and 66% (44/67) returned to duty.

CONCLUSION: The multidisiplinary rehabilitation program demonstrated an effective approach to rehabilitate military service members with TBI.

REACTION:
-   may not be generalizable to nonmilitary personnel
-   doesn't operationationally define outcome measures
-   can the research design be replicated?

Figure 6–5. An example of an index card used in collecting information from articles.

Table 6–7. Critically Reviewing a Research Article

Introduction
- Does the introduction state the hypothesis directly or implicity?
- Does the literature review support the hypothesis?
- Are the choices of outcome measures relevant to the study?
- Is the study feasible and further knowledge in the field?

Methodology
- Based on the information presented in the study, can the study be replicated?
- How were the participants chosen for the study?
- Are the demographics of the participants adequately described?
- Were unusual circumstances or extraneous variables (e.g., use of medication, time of testing) described?
- What were the reliability and validity of the outcome measures?
- Were appropriate tests used for the population studied?
- Were the measures free from external bias?
- Were appropriate statistics used?

Results and Discussion
- Were the results reported in an understandable and clear manner?
- Are the figures and tables clear and consistent with the text?
- Was the discussion related to the findings?
- Was there discussion regarding the acceptance or rejection of the null hypothesis?
- Did the investigator discuss limitations of the study and the need for future research?

Note: Adapted from material "A Reader's, Writer's, and Reviewer's Guide to Assessing Research Reports in Clinical Psychology," by Brendan A. Maher, 1978, *Journal of Clinical and Consulting Psychology, 46*, 835–838. Copyright 1978 by American Psychological Association.

Association (1994) recommends that a writer of a journal article should:

> Discuss the literature but do not include an exhaustive historical review. Assume that the reader has knowledge in the field for which you are writing. . . . A scholarly review of earlier work provides an appropriate history and recognizes the priority of the work of others. Citation of a specific credit to relevant earlier works is part of the author's scientific and scholarly responsibility. . . . Cite and reference only works pertinent to the specific issue and not works of only tangential or general significance. If you summarize earlier works, avoid nonessential details; instead, emphasize pertinent findings, relevant methodological issues, and major conclusions. Refer the reader to general surveys or reviews of the topic if they are available. (p. 11)

In contrast to the journal article, the writer of a master's thesis or doctoral dissertation should include extensive background literature, which demonstrates to the reader that the researcher is cognizant of the important findings with which the present study rests. The continuity of findings should be documented by the researcher. The literature review in a master's thesis or doctoral dissertation serves as a vehicle for presenting chronologically the progression of knowledge in a specific area. Thus, the literature review should reflect the development of a problem by first presenting general background findings and then gradually narrowing to the significant variables identified in the title of the study.

A search of the literature will result in identifying literature that is directly related to the topic at hand, literature less directly related but that should be read, and literature that is unrelated. Although it will be important to peruse all of these, only the articles directly related to the topic will be used in a literature review. Locke, Spirduso, and Silverman (1987) suggested that the literature review "is made to serve the reader's query by supporting, explicating, and illuminating the logic now implicit in the proposed investigation" (p. 59). A well-written literature review allows the reader to (a) understand the significance of the research question, (b) validate the connection between previously conducted research directly related to the present research question, and (c) grasp the reasons for the proposed methodology.

The plan for presenting previous literature should include a logical development that incorporates both a chronological sequence and a topical order. By using an outline, the researcher begins to organize the data found in reviewing the literature. The outline is a working tool. It should change to accommodate new ideas and evidence.

One way to develop an outline is by organizing the index cards into groups by topic, which makes the writing easier for a number of reasons. First, by examining and reviewing the cards, important themes and topics may emerge. Second, because the cards have been organized by subject, the writer does not waste time looking through the articles and other references for related material. Third, by placing the cards into groups, they can be further organized into a logical outline or sequence.

Although actually writing the literature review can be challenging, the completed product gives the researcher a sense of accomplishment. The literature review section of a study should represent an extensive process that is the basis for implementing the research design. The worksheet in Box 6–1 describes this process.

BOX 6–1. NATIONAL INFORMATION CENTER ON HEALTH SERVICES RESEARCH AND HEALTH CARE TECHNOLOGY (NICHSR)

The 1993 NIH Revitalization Act created a National Information Center on Health Services Research and Health Care Technology (NICHSR) at the National Library of Medicine to improve "... the collection, storage, analysis, retrieval, and dissemination of information on health services research, clinical practice guidelines, and on health care technology, including the assessment of such technology."

The Center works closely with the Agency for Health Care Policy and Research (AHCPR) to improve the dissemination of the results of health services research, with special emphasis on the growing body of clinical practice guidelines.

The overall goals of the NICHSR are: to make the results of health services research, including practice guidelines and technology assessments, readily available to health practitioners, health care administrators, health policy makers, payers, and the information professionals who serve these groups; to improve access to data and information needed by the creators of health services research; and to contribute to the information infrastructure needed to foster patient record systems that can produce useful health services research data as a by-product of providing health care.

Products and Services

NICHSR coordinates the development of information products and services related to health services research. HealthSTAR is the online bibliographic database that provides access to the published literature of Health Services Technology, Administration, and Research. HealthSTAR became available in 1996 through the merging of two former NLM databases, the HEALTH (Health Planning and Administration) database, initiated in 1978 with the cooperation of the American Hospital Association, and the HSTAR (Health Services/Technology Assessment Research) database, initiated in 1994 by NLM's NICHSR.

HealthSTAR contains approximately 3 million citations (with abstracts if available) to journal articles, monographs, technical reports, meeting abstracts and papers, book chapters, and government documents from 1975 to the present, including selected records from NLM s MEDLINE® database as well as unique records specially indexed for it.

HSRProj, a database of citations to research-in-progress funded by federal and foundation grants and contracts, became available in 1995. HSRProj builds upon a database developed in prototype by staff of the Association for Health Services Research and the Cecil Sheps Center at the University of North Carolina with funding from the Pew Charitable Trust. It includes over 5,000 citations to ongoing or recently completed research funded since 1995.

HSTAT (Health Services/Technology Assessment Text), a full-text resource for clinical practice guidelines, became available in 1994. The system, developed by NLM's Lister Hill Center, allows those interested in clinical practice guidelines to search for and read them on computers in their offices via the Internet or modem. It includes Agency for Health Care Policy and Research evidence reports, guideline documents, and technology assessments, NIH Consensus Development Conference Statements and Technology Assessment Workshop Reports, NIH Clinical Center active research protocols, the U.S. Task Force on Preventive Services' Guide to Clinical Preventive Services, HIV/AIDS Treatment Information Service (ATIS) approved guidelines, and Substance Abuse and Mental Health Services Administration (SAMHSA) treatment improvement protocols. It also provides a link to the Centers for Disease Control and Prevention (CDC) Prevention Guidelines Database.

DIRLINE®, NLM's Directory of Information Resources onLINE, has a special subfile covering health services research organizations including those involved in technology assessment and development of practice guidelines.

In addition to its online databases, NICHSR and other NLM staff develop guides, fact sheets, bibliographies, and other products targeted to health services researchers. Like other NLM publications, HSR publications are available from the NLM home page, and via file transfer protocol (ftp) from NLM's publications server. (National Library of Medicine, 1999d, p.1)

(This material was obtained from the NICHSR fact sheet, available at http://www.nlm.nih.gov/pubs/factsheets/nichsr_fs.html)

6.7 Worksheet for Literature Review

Box 6–2. Worksheet for Literature Review

1. State the research problem in question form

2. Identify variables in the study
   - Independent variables
   - Dependent variables

continued

- Target populations
- Specific setting for study (e.g., hospital, clinic)

3. **Checklist for locating references (list titles)**
   - Information retrieval systems
   - Directories of references
   - Bibliographical indexes
   - Annual reviews
   - Abstracting periodicals
   - Textbooks
   - Personal communication from experts

4. **Primary Sources Utilized (list)**
   - Journals
   - Statistical compendium
   - Conference proceedings
   - Theses and dissertations

CHAPTER

Research Design and Methodology

> *The quality of research depends not only upon the adequacy of the research design but also upon the fruitfulness of the data-collection techniques which are employed. The purpose of the various data-collection techniques is simply to produce precise and reliable evidence which is relevant to the research questions being asked. Fulfillment of this purpose, however is rarely simple.*
>
> —M. Johoda, M. Deutsch, and S. W. Cook, 1951,
> *Research Methods in Social Relations* (p. 92)

Operational Learning Objectives

By the end of this chapter, the learner will

1. State a research hypothesis or guiding question
2. Operationally define a research variable
3. Identify any assumptions underlying a proposed research study
4. Diagram a research study
5. Identify the possible methodological limitations in a research study
6. State the theoretical rationale underlying a proposed research study
7. Design a procedure for selecting participants for a study
8. Design screening criteria for participant inclusion
9. Define and contrast the terms *random sampling, random assignment, conven-*ience sampling, representative sampling, and *target population*
10. Define test reliability and test validity
11. Evaluate the feasibility, reliability, and validity of a published test or measuring instrument
12. Compare and contrast the four scales of measurement
13. Understand the concept of internal validity
14. Design a data collection procedure for a proposed research study
15. Understand ethical principles underlying human research
16. Outline a research proposal including an informed consent protocol
17. Understand the concept of external validity
18. Describe the major research designs and methodological limitations of a study

7.1 Proposing a Feasible Research Question

The initial step in research is asking the right questions. Science progresses along the continuum of knowledge by researchers seeking solutions to key problems. Historically, researchers gain advanced knowledge by posing feasible questions. For example:

▶ What are the basic anatomical structures and physiological functions of human beings?
▶ How are diseases transmitted?
▶ What chemical substances destroy specific microorganisms that cause diseases?
▶ How can we detect the presence of trace chemicals in food and blood?
▶ What are the causes of specific diseases?
▶ What effect does a child with disabilities have on the family?
▶ What is the effect of including a child with disabilities in a general education classroom?
▶ What are the most effective methods for rehabilitating individuals with traumatic brain injury?

Scientists have raised numerous questions that have guided research and led to solutions. In the research design section, the investigator raises specific testable or feasible questions that guide the data collection.

In proposing research, the investigator reviews the following six areas:

1. Statements of hypotheses or guiding questions
2. Operational definitions of variables
3. Underlying assumptions of the study
4. Diagrammatical relationship between variables
5. Methodological limitations of the study
6. Overall theoretical rationale guiding the study

7.2 Statement of Hypothesis

A *hypothesis* is a statement predicting the relationship between variables. In logic, it is stated as an *if-then* contingency. For example, consider the hypothesis: There is a positive, statistically significant relationship between obesity and heart disease in sedentary workers. In this hypothesis, there is a predicted relationship between obesity and heart disease among sedentary workers expressed as "*if* obesity (in sedentary workers), *then* heart disease." The hypothesis contains the question and predicts a directional relationship. (A direction can be either positive or inverse.)

How does the investigator arrive at a hypothesis or guiding question? The review of literature as discussed in Chapter 6 serves as the generating force in guiding the proposed hypothesis or guiding question. The relationship between a research question, a guiding question, and a hypothesis is described in Table 7–1. The hypothesis is a specific statement that can be derived from a research question or guiding question. Table 7–2 shows the relationship between a research model and a statement of hypothesis or guiding question.

In quantitative research, the investigator needs to state a guiding question or hypothesis that leads to data collection. In qualitative research, the guiding question or hypothesis can arise during data collection. For example, a researcher who is initially interested in the problems associated with obtaining employment for individuals with schizophrenia may change his or her focus to an examination of the relationship between stress and employment. The qualitative researcher has more flexibility in stating guiding questions or hypotheses than the quantitative researcher who must state the question prior to collecting data. Once the guiding question or hypothesis is stated, the researcher needs to operationally define the variables.

7.3 Operationally Defining a Variable

Variables are operationally defined by stating or describing (a) the treatment procedure (presumed independent variable),

Table 7–1. The Relationship Between a Research Question, a Guiding Question, and a Hypothesis

	Definition	*Purpose*	*Example*
Research question	A broad inquiry into a general area of investigation	Leads researcher into an extensive literature review	What is the relationship between repetitive motion and hand injuries?
Guiding question	A statement of inquiry that leads to data collection	Identifies factors that relate to a specific research question	What factors in repetitive motion injury are related to carpal tunnel syndrome?
Hypothesis	A detailed statement that can be tested through inferential statistics	Evaluates effectiveness or significant relationship between variables	There is no statistically significant difference in the use of biofeedback versus splinting in remediating the symptoms of carpal tunnel syndrome.

(b) the outcome measure (dependent variable), and (c) screening criteria for participant selection. Operational definitions make it possible for researchers to replicate a research study. Many differences arising from the inconsistent results of several investigators often can be traced to different operational definitions of the same stated conceptual variables. For example, the following variables could become ambiguous unless one describes in detail how they are measured or procedurally defined:

▶ Cognitive rehabilitation (treatment procedure)
▶ Intelligence (screening criterion for participant inclusion)
▶ Language disorder (dependent variable or screening criterion for participant inclusion)
▶ Muscle strength (dependent variable or screening criterion for participant inclusion)
▶ Spasticity (dependent variable or screening criterion for participant inclusion)
▶ Sensory-integration therapy (treatment procedure)
▶ Visual motor ability (dependent variable or screening criterion for participant inclusion)
▶ Work hardening (treatment intervention)
▶ Individuals with low back pain (screening criterion for participant inclusion)

Research became rigorous when researchers described experimental procedures in detail so that other investigators could duplicate the exact experiment or study. The rigor in operationally defining a variable is associated with *internal validity*. Results cannot be accepted unless it is known how the investigator defined the variables. Conflicts over the effectiveness of treatment techniques, descriptions of target populations, and measurements of outcome are caused by comparing seemingly similar variables, which are, in fact, different because of the way they are measured. How many definitions are there for self-perception, cognitive disability, language therapy, manual dexterity, work capacity, and low back pain? The conceptualization of variables described by investigators may be entirely different if they are not operationally defined. Ineffectual research is typified by the omission of operational definitions. The problem is compounded when investigators synthesize findings in an area by "lumping" studies. For example, if visual perception is defined operationally through group tests, individual tests, clinical observations, and functional performance, then conflicts will arise when examining the relationship between visual perception and a variable such as ADL. A researcher's often fallacious interpretation of the literature and subsequent invalid conclusions are a result

Table 7–2. The Relationship Between the Research Model and the Hypothesis

	Statements	Examples of Research Questions
Quantitative Research Models		
Experimental (prospective research design)	Hypothesis: directional or null	How effective is exercise in reducing symptoms of depression?
Methodological	Guiding question	What factors must be considered in designing a (specific) instrument or test for measuring pain?
Evaluation	Guiding question	How effective is the occupational therapy department in preventing rehospitalizations?
Heuristic (retrospective research design)	Guiding question	What risk factors are related to the etiology of multiple sclerosis?
Correlational	Hypothesis: directional or null	Is there a statistically significant positive relationship between perceptual motor abilities and reading?
Survey	Guiding question	What are the personality characteristics of the leaders in the field of occupational therapy?
Qualitative Research Methods		
Individual case study	Guiding question	What are the dynamic factors and processes underlying the cause of schizophrenia in a specific individual?
Operations research	Guiding question	What is the impact of the prospective payment system on the quality of home health care?
Child development studies	Guiding question	What are the sequential steps in a child's development of the palmer grasp?
Longituditional research (prospective designs)	Guiding question	What are the long-term effects on children exposed to cocaine in utero?
Field observation (ethnography)	Guiding question	How do parents' attitudes toward a child with Down syndrome affect the child's development?
Historical	Guiding question	What are the historical roots of the concept of humanism in occupational therapy?

of equating variables even though the operational definitions are different.

In operationally defining a variable, the investigator should consider the following questions:

▶ What is the theoretical rationale underlying the definition?
▶ What is the accepted definition of a variable as stated in a dictionary or occupational therapy textbook?
▶ How can the variable be measured?

▶ Does the investigator need to establish the screening criteria in defining a target population?
▶ Is the variable defined by a standardized procedure (e.g., employing a treatment technique)?
▶ Can a mathematical formula be employed in the definition (e.g., in ergonomics when defining work output)?

Traditionally, government agencies have operationally defined specific criteria (National Center for Health Studies, 1974). The following information was obtained from *Your Guide to Choosing a Nursing Home*, published by the United States Department of Health and Human Services, Health Care Financing Administration (n.d.).

▶ **Home and Community Care:** A person who is ill or disabled may be able to get help from a variety of home services that might make moving into a nursing home unnecessary. Home services include Meals on Wheels programs, friendly visiting and shopper services, and adult day care. These programs are found in most communities . . . Some nursing homes may provide respite care and admit a person in need of care for a short period of time to give the home care givers a break. Depending on the case, Medicare, private insurance, and Medicaid may pay some home care costs that are related to medical care.

▶ **Subsidized Senior Housing (Non-Medical):** There are Federal and State programs that help pay for housing for older people with low to moderate incomes. Some of these subsidized facilities offer assistance to residents who need help with certain tasks, such as shopping and laundry. Residents generally live independently in an apartment within the senior housing complex.

▶ **Assisted Living (Non-Medical Senior Housing):** [Individuals who] only need help with a small number of tasks, such as cooking and laundry, or reminders to take medications, assisted living facilities may be an option worth considering. "Assisted living" is a general term for living arrangements in which some services are available to residents who still live independently within the assisted living complex. In most cases, assisted living residents pay a regular monthly rent, and then pay additional fees for the services that they require.

▶ **Board and Care Homes:** Board and Care homes are group living arrangements designed to meet the needs of people who cannot live independently, but do not require nursing home ser-

vices. These homes offer a wider range of services than independent living options. Most provide help with some of the activities of daily living, including eating, walking, bathing, and toileting. In some cases, private long-term care insurance and medical assistance programs will help pay for this type of living arrangement. . . . [M]any of these homes do not get payment from Medicare or Medicaid and are not strictly monitored.

▶ **Continuing Care Retirement Communities (CCRCs):** CCRCs are housing communities that provide different levels of care based on the residents' needs from independent living apartments to skilled nursing care in an affiliated nursing home. Residents move from one setting to another based on their needs, but continue to remain a part of their CCRC community. . . . Many CCRCs require a large payment prior to admission and also charge monthly fees. For this reason, many CCRCs may be too expensive for older people with modest incomes. (pp. 2–4)

▶ **Nursing Home:** A nursing home is a residence that provides a room, meals, skilled nursing and rehabilitative care, medical services, and protective supervision to residents. It also provides residents with help with daily living and recreational activities. Many nursing home residents have physical, emotional or mental impairments which keep them from living independently. Nursing homes are certified by State and Federal government agencies to provide levels of care which range from custodial care to skilled nursing care that can only be delivered by trained professionals. (p. 1)

Hospital services are defined by the Joint Commission on Accreditation of Healthcare Organizations (JCAHO; 1998) as follows:

▶ **Home Health Services:** Services provided by health care professionals in an individual's place of residence on a per-visit or per-hour basis to patients who have or are at risk of an injury, an illness, or a disabling condition or who are terminally ill and require short-term or long-term intervention by health care professionals. These services may include dental, medical, nursing, occupational therapy, pediatric, physical therapy, speech-language pathology, audiology, social work, and nutrition counseling services and may be provided directly or through contract with another organization or individual.

▶ **Hospice:** An organized program that consists of services provided and coordinated by an interdisciplinary team at a frequency appropriate to meet the needs of patients who are diagnosed with terminal illnesses and have limited life spans. The hospice specializes in palliative management of pain and other physical symptoms, meeting the psychosocial and spiritual needs of the patient and the patient's family or other primary care person(s). The program also includes a continuum of interdisciplinary team services across all settings where hospice care is provided, the availability of 24-hour access to care, utilization of volunteers, and bereavement care to the survivors, as needed, for an appropriate period of time.

▶ **Hospital:** A health care organization that has a governing body, an organized medical staff and professional staff, and inpatient facilities and provides medical, nursing, and related services for ill and injured patients 24 hours per day, seven days per week. For licensing purposes, each state has its own definition of a hospital. (p. 1)

7.4 Stating Assumptions

A researcher undertaking an investigation may make certain assumptions that are usually unstated. These assumptions can be on a general level, such as:

▶ All diseases have a cause.
▶ Intelligence is the result of the interaction between genetic structure and environmental opportunities.

▶ Obesity is the result of overeating and inactivity.
▶ Language development is maturational.
▶ Disengagement from social activity is a learned behavior rather than a biological determinant.
▶ Learning is a complex variable that is not entirely based on external reinforcement.

Other assumptions can be more subtle, such as:

▶ Rehabilitation of individuals with severe disabilities should have a high priority in a society.
▶ People with alcohol dependency should be treated as persons with medical problems rather than as criminals.
▶ Individuals with mental retardation should be integrated into community schools rather than isolated in large institutions.
▶ Home health care is more cost-effective than hospitalization.

In designing a research study, the investigator should be aware of all the assumptions underlying the study. Whether the assumptions are made explicit in reporting the results is at the discretion of the researcher. Nonetheless, in preparing a research proposal, the researcher must state all assumptions.

When distinguishing an assumption from established evidence, it should be clear from the previous examples that assumptions are controversial or inconclusive theory that can also reflect the investigator's values or biases. Many assumptions are tacitly implied by an investigator who assumes that all people accept certain beliefs or hold certain opinions. A researcher should try to identify all assumptions being made in the study as an indication of his or her own subjective biases and beliefs. Whenever possible, a reference should be used when stating assumptions. The reference could be either theoretical or supported by research.

7.5 Diagrammatical Relationships Between Variables

In clarifying the research design, it is helpful for the investigator to diagram the study, especially in a proposal, showing the relationship among variables, populations sampled, and operational definitions.

▶ *Experimental model:* For example a researcher is interested in testing two therapeutic interventions for students with moderate mental retardation who have difficulty in self-care activities. The experimental model is used in this study. The diagrammatical relationship between variables is depicted in Figure 7–1.
  - In this hypothetical example, the guiding question is, "Is the cognitive approach more effective than the behavioral approach in increasing self-care abilities among individuals with moderate mental retardation."
  - An operational definition of moderate mental retardation is required (IQ score obtained on an individual test between 40 and 55; subaverage adaptive behavior skills in two or more areas [e.g., leisure, communication, social skills] and occurrence in the developmental years). Age, gender, ethnicity, and socioeconomic status should be considered.

▶ *Correlational model:* A correlational model would be diagramed in a hypothetical study involving coma. The variables are now considered to have an associational or statistical relationship, not a cause-effect relationship. The hypothetical relationship between variables is diagramed in Figure 7–2. In this model, the independent variable is not experimentally induced; therefore, it is considered to be presumed.
  - In this model, the guiding question for the hypothetical example is, "Is there a statistically significant relationship between the number of days in a coma and the severity of cognitive deficits?"

  - An operational definition of the population and the severity of cognition deficits are required. In the hypothetical example, the population is defined as those individuals who (a) have sustained a traumatic brain injury from a motor vehicle accident (MVA), (b) are participating in a rehabilitation program, and (c) have gained consciousness after being in a coma for at least 1 hour. Age, gender, socioeconomic status, and handedness must also be considered. Measurement tools include the Glascow Coma Scale and the Halsted-Reitan Neuropsychological Battery.

▶ *Methodological model:* Using methodological research, such as in developing a test, the researcher outlines the study by using the diagram found in Figure 7–3. In this model, there is no hypothesis; rather, the researcher proposes a guiding question.
  - In the hypothetical question, the researcher wants to design a reliable and valid instrument for assessing the ability to cope with stress. The construct of stress needs to be defined based on theoretical concepts from a literature review. Individuals who deal well with stress and individuals with mental illness who have difficulty dealing with stress participate in obtaining normal values for the instrument. Stratification of age, gender, and socioeconomic status would occur by examining the differences that may occur because of these variables.

▶ *Evaluation model:* In evaluation research, the investigator determines the effectiveness of a health system in meeting the defined objects. This model is diagramed in Figure 7–4. As in methodological research, a guiding question is used by the researcher to propose the research. The researcher must determine the a priori objectives of the system. In the hypothetical example, the investigator would determine the mission statement

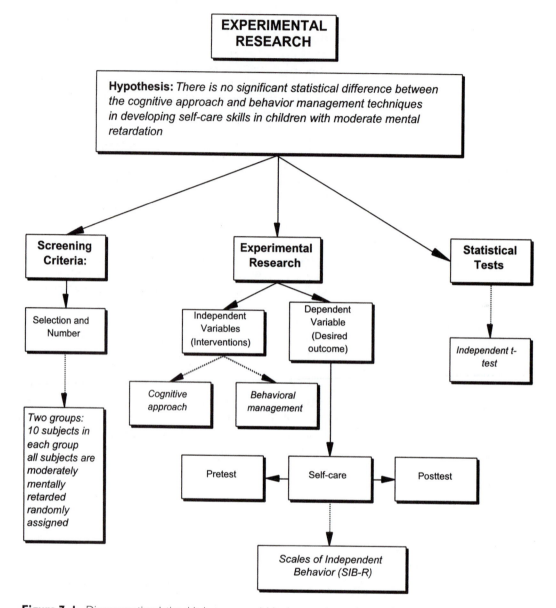

Figure 7–1. Diagrammatic relationship between variables in experimental research.

and the objectives of the Iowa health care system, then would use these criteria to determine the effectiveness of the system. General criteria for comparison purposes also would be used. In the example, statistical information would be used to compare Iowa's health care system with those of other states.

▶ *Heuristic model:* A researcher using a heuristic model seeks to understand and discover the relationship between heuristic factors. In a hypothetical study, such as discovering risk factors for a disease, the researcher seeks to identify the factors that are significantly related to the disability. The hypothetical example, using heart disease, is depicted in Figure 7–5. In this example, the risk factors for heart disease are identified through literature review. The population studied

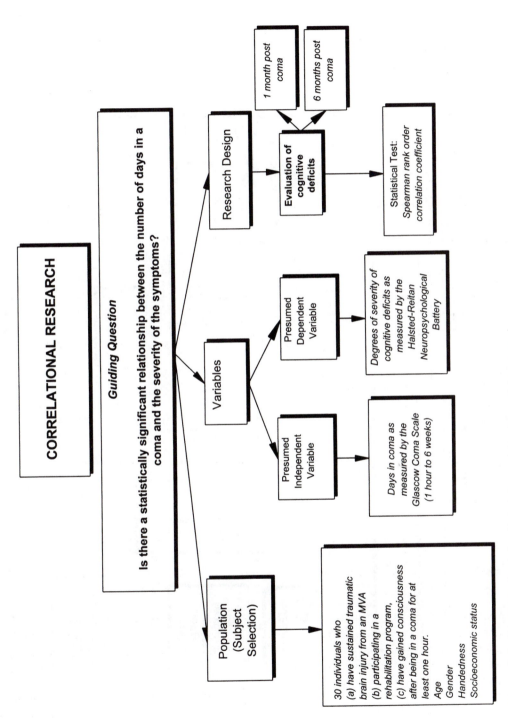

Figure 7–2. Diagrammatic relationship between variables in correlation research.

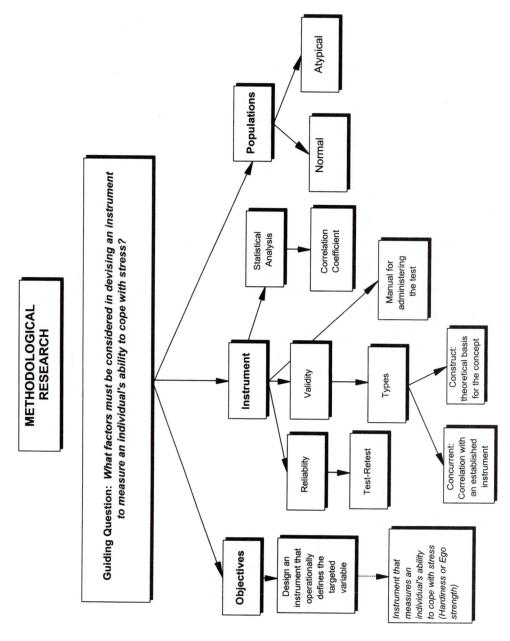

Figure 7–3. Diagrammatic relationship between variables in methodological research.

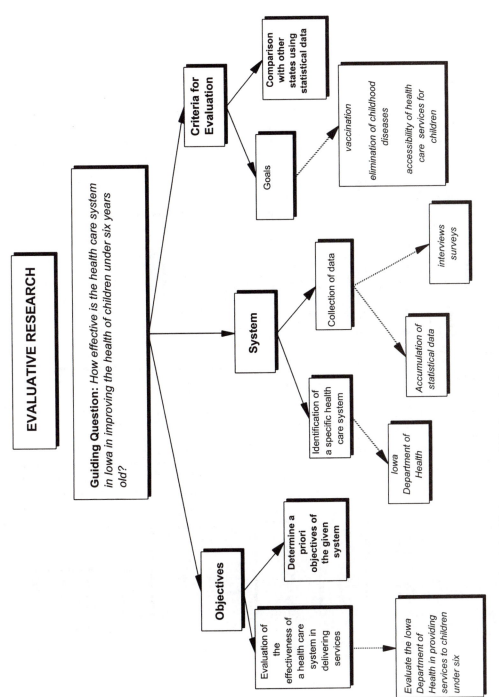

Figure 7–4. Diagrammatic relationship between variables in evaluation research.

233

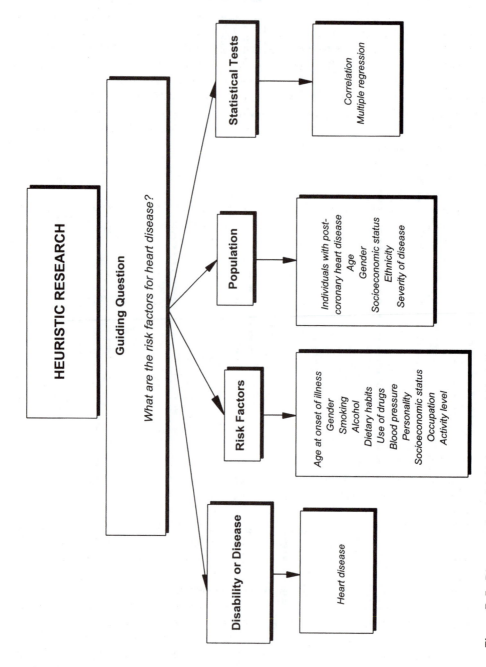

Figure 7-5. Diagrammatic relationship between variables in heurestic research.

include individuals with postcoronary heart disease. Control factors include age, gender, socioeconomic status, ethnicity, and severity of disease.

▶ *Survey model:* In this model, the researcher is interested in identifying characteristics of a homogeneous population. For example, in a hypothetical study, the researcher is interested in examining the level of job satisfaction among occupational therapists in the United States (see Figure 7–6). After the survey is completed, the results can be compared with a similar study focusing on another professional group, such as nursing.

  • The population is identified, but only a sample of the population receives the survey. Of those receiving the survey, it is expected that 50% will respond. Thus, in a population of 60,000 occupational therapists in the United States, only 6,000 will receive the survey, and only 3,000 are expected to respond.

  • The survey is sent to a striated sample of the population giving a representative sample of the distribution of occupational therapists in the United States. Although the striation is based only on geographical location, the statistical analysis from the results of the survey separates job description (e.g., pediatrics, physical dysfunction, psychosocial) and demographics (e.g., age, gender, socioeconomic status, ethnicity).

  • In the methodology, the researcher must design a valid and reliable questionnaire. Statistical analysis consists of descriptive statistics, including a frequency distribution table, a statistical pie, and histograms.

▶ *Qualitative models:* Qualitative research models include

  • Individual case study
  • Operations research
  • Child development studies
  • Longitudinal research (prospective designs)

  • Field observation (ethnography)
  • Historical research

Figure 7–7 depicts a hypothetical study of a family in which a child has a bipolar disorder. In selecting a family, the researcher would consider the child's diagnosis, severity of illness, family constellation, and cooperativeness of the family to participate in a study. Additional considerations include the research methods used for data collection and for analyzing the results.

7.6 Theoretical Rationale

Theory generates research, and research generates theory. Research should be a planned activity based on a theoretical rationale. Why are variables correlated? Why do we think this treatment will work? Why do we project these results? What factors justify the conclusions proposed? The researcher is not only interested in the questions *Does it work?* or *Is it curative?* but also *Why is the treatment effective? Why is there a relationship between causative factors and the onset of illness?* Theories in science are in a continual state of change. As knowledge progresses in an area, theory changes to accommodate the new information. Researchers do not assume that theories and knowledge are static. What currently is accepted as truth may be revised later when new research data are obtained.

  The investigator needs to state the underlying theory generating the research design, even if it is meager and incomplete. Research is not justified if we collect meaningless bits of information for future analysis. For example, if a researcher working on techniques to improve motor skills in children with severe mental retardation finds a statistically significant difference between behavior modification and a comparable method in motivating the children to use motor skills but does not explain why behavior modification is effective, the research is

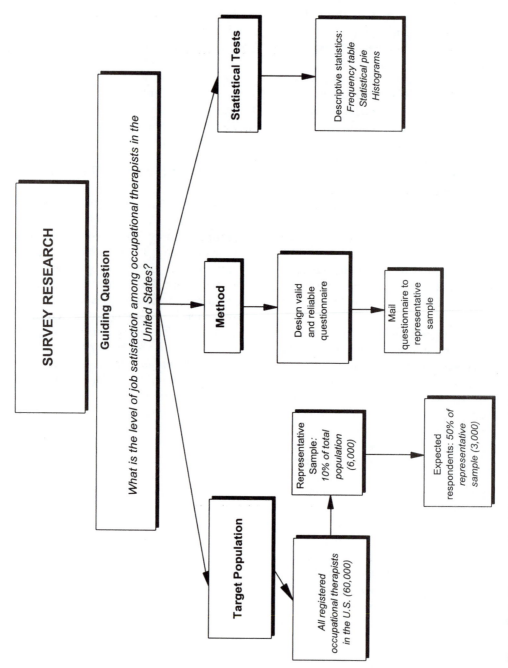

Figure 7–6. Diagrammatic relationship between variables in survey research.

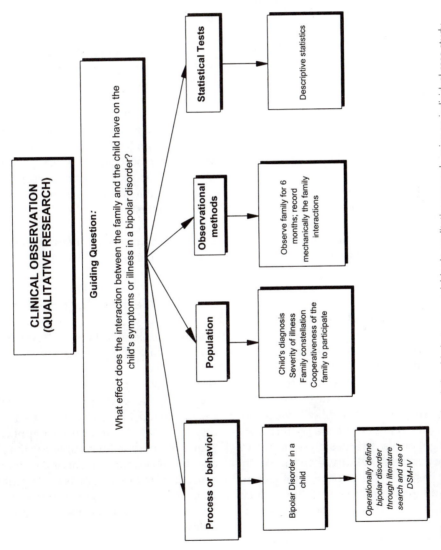

Figure 7–7. Diagrammatic relationship between variables in qualitative research, using an individual case study.

The following text appears within the figure:

CLINICAL OBSERVATION (QUALITATIVE RESEARCH)

Guiding Question:

What effect does the interaction between the family and the child have on the child's symptoms or illness in a bipolar disorder?

Process or behavior

Bipolar Disorder in a child

Operationally define bipolar disorder through literature search and use of DSM-IV

Population

Child's diagnosis
Severity of illness
Family constellation
Cooperativeness of the family to participate

Observational methods

Observe family for 6 months; record mechanically the family interactions

Statistical Tests

Descriptive statistics

incomplete. If, in this example, the group that received behavior modification realized significantly improved motor skills more than the control group did, the reader is left to speculate the causes for the differences. Was the Hawthorne effect controlled? Are there other explanations? The absence of a theoretical explanation leaves a gap in the research and leaves it open to the reader to speculate why motor development was enhanced. Speculations are raised, such as:

▶ Interpersonal relationships influenced motor learning
▶ Treatment stimulated motor development
▶ Reinforcement used in behavior modification was more effective than that used in the comparable methods
▶ Tests selected were unreliable and inappropriate

The reader can make many speculations in the absence of a theoretical rationale. Research should be guided by theory and explanation rather than merely presenting data that describe the relationships between variables.

7.7 Internal Validity

Internal validity is a theoretical concept that refers to the rigor in an experiment or research design. The degree of internal validity depends on the extent to which the investigator has controlled all variables that can potentially affect the results. If an experiment or research design is judged to have good internal validity, then the experimenter has been able to control for factors that could potentially distort the results. High internal validity is demonstrated by:

▶ A double-blind study in which the investigator eliminates researcher bias and subject influence
▶ Control of the placebo effect whereby the subject's suggestibility and personal influence are eliminated

▶ Inclusion of a control group to eliminate the Hawthorne effect
▶ Matching comparative groups to ensure that all groups compared are not different in variables such as age, gender, degree of disability, intelligence, and socioeconomic status
▶ Baseline measures of pretest to ensure that comparative groups are equivalent
▶ Posttest measures that are compared with pretest measures
▶ High reliability and validity of outcome measures or tests to ensure that variables are accurately measured
▶ Regard for maturational factors that could distort results
▶ Random selection of subjects to reduce bias in samples
▶ Standardization of administering test and research procedures
▶ Control for practice effect in test taking to ensure that gain in scores is not attributable to the participant's familiarity with test.

Some ways to increase internal validity are listed in Table 7–3.

7.8 Methodology Section

The methodology section of a study includes the following components: the method of selecting subjects, location of study, description of tests and apparatuses used in measuring variables, procedure for collecting data, statistical techniques used for analyzing data, computer use (if applicable), projection of time for completing the study, and the procedure of obtaining informed consent from human subjects. Pragmatic as well as rational considerations guide the investigator in finding the answers to the following questions:

▶ How many subjects should be included in the study?
▶ Should subjects be randomly selected, or should they be volunteers or a convenience sample?

Table 7–3. Increasing Internal Validity

Problem	Solution
Hawthorne effect	Ensure that control and experimental groups receive equal treatment time.
Honeymoon effect	Do a follow-up study.
Placebo effect	Use motivational techniques to help clients self-improve.
Bias of researcher	Have objective test administrator collect pre-post data.
Unreliability of test	Design new instrument with the goal of high reliability and validity. Use triangulation (e.g., clinical observation, client report, physiological measure).
Insensitivity of test to detecting changes in behavior	Use criterion-referenced testing. Use triangulation.
Unsubstantiated validity	Do a pilot study to test validity with an established test instrument.
Sample is not representative of target population	Use striated samples. Examine characteristics of sample group for similarities with target population (e.g., age, gender, severity of illness).
Maturational factors affect results	Use covariance in statistical analysis (ANCOVA) to control for differences in pre- and postmeasures.
Differences in cognitive abilities of individuals	Use covariance (ANCOVA) to control for cognitive levels.
Comparative groups are not equal	Set up selection criteria for selection inclusion (e.g., age, gender, SES, intelligence, ethnicity).
Treatment method is not stated clearly	Operationalize treatment method so that it can be replicated.

▶ Where should the study take place?
▶ What tests, diagnostic procedures, questionnaires, or rating scales should be employed in the study?
▶ What are the procedures and time sequence for data collection?
▶ What are the costs of the study?

The process for the research methodology is shown in Figure 7–8.

7.9 Selection of Participants

One primary purpose of research is to discover relationships between variables in sample groups and to generalize these relationships to a larger population. The ability to generalize results establishes the *external*

validity of a study. Because research usually involves sample groups from populations rather than the total population, the selection of a representative sample is crucial when generalizing results.

In selecting a sample, the first step is to identify a target population. For example, individuals with spinal cord injury, individuals who are juvenile offenders, occupational therapists, graduate students, or administrators of rehabilitation programs are identifiable populations. The target population is narrowed considerably by establishing a screening criteria. A screening criteria contains both *inclusional* and *exclusional* factors. For example, a researcher interested in cardiac rehabilitation may want to select a specific population within the area of cardiovascular disease (e.g., individuals

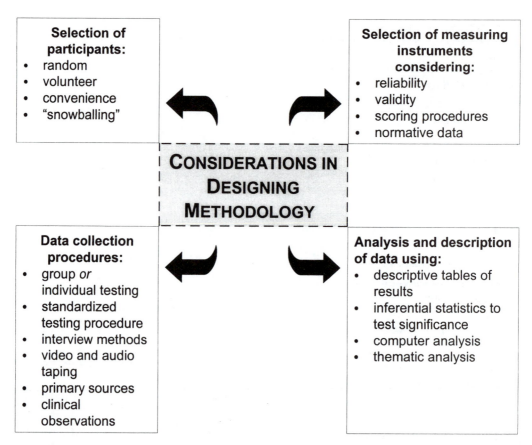

Figure 7–8. Sequential process of research methodology. Notice that there are four basic steps and, within those steps, questions that must be answered.

who have had heart transplants). The screening criteria will enable the investigator to identify a specific population and to control the variables that could potentially affect the results. In setting up a screening criteria for patients with cardiac disease, variables such as age, gender, socioeconomic status, occupation, body type (endomorph, ectomorph, and mesomorph), onset of illness, and range of cardiorespiratory function as indicated by pulse rate and blood pressure should be considered.

Refinement of these variables should narrow the population. An example of a target population obtained from a priori criteria is (inclusionary variable): (a) individuals with coronary disease, (b) male, (c) middle-class, (d) living in urban areas, (e) between the ages of 55 and 65, (f) primarily seden-

tary, and (g) with resting pulse rates below 80. In considering exclusional factors, the researcher specifies variables that are screened out of the study. These variables could include the absence of secondary illnesses (as determined by clinical examination), mental retardation, or psychosocial dysfunction.

The example from a double case study by Kopolow and Jensen (1975) shows the extensiveness of criteria employed in selecting two participants with quadriplegia (see Table 7–4). Screening criteria are identified prior to subject selection. The investigator operationally defines the variables identified in the criteria. The rigor in specifying the population to be studied within a narrow domain enables other investigators to replicate the research design by iso-

Table 7–4. Screening Criteria for Study Participant Inclusion (Quadriplegia)

1. The participants were individuals with C_{5-6} traumatic quadriplegia.

2. The participants were male.

3. The participants were 18 to 26 years of age at onset of injury.

4. The participants had at least a high school education.

5. One participant was engaged in either full- or part-time employment, including student and/ or homemaker, while the other participants were unemployed.

6. The participants were residing in nonmedical facilities.

7. The participants were 1 to 2 years postinjury.

8. The participants were Caucasian.

9. The participants were native, English-speaking Americans.

10. The participants had normal cognitive functioning.

11. The participants' medical records were available.

12. The participants were willing to participate in the study and signed an informed consent form.

---

lating specific variables. By specifying the population and operationally defining the variables in the screening criteria, the investigator has identified a target population.

The next step in selecting participants for the study is to locate all of the units in the target population. Studies of the personality characteristics of allied health professionals, for example, would entail obtaining annual directories of members from professional associations, noting that not all practicing therapists are members of their professional associations. (See Appendix A–1 for a list of professional organizations and their Internet addresses.)

Location of populations with disabilities, such as individuals with paraplegia living in the community, may be obtained through consumer organizations that represent geographic areas. By geographically limiting the representativeness of the study, the investigator controls for social and environmental factors that could potentially affect the results. On the other hand, the investigator may want to guide the scope of the study by identifying *stratified samples,* that is, homogeneous subgroups of a population based on variables such as geography, educational level, and treatment setting (com-

munity vs. hospital or disability group). Stratified samples are usually determined by previous evidence implying that the variable identified has a significant effect on a dependent variable. For example, in examining the guiding question, *Does exercise prevent the recurrence of heart disease?* the investigator would control for the variable of smoking because previous evidence has related smoking to heart disease. In using stratified samples, the investigator would separate out populations of smokers who exercise from nonsmokers who do not exercise.

Appendix A–2 provides a selected list of health associations and their Internet addresses. Additional ideas for obtaining participants can be obtained from the *Encyclopedia of Associations: International Organizations,* (Gale Group, 1999). This resource lists addresses and telephone numbers of nearly 21,000 national and international associations, including professional health associations.

7.9.1 External Validity

External validity refers to the researcher's ability to generalize the results of a research study from a sample to a total population. In general, researchers seek to generalize the results from a study to the population at large. For example, if a researcher found in a clinical study that aerobic exercise is effective in reducing depression in a particular sample, he or she would want to test whether the results could be generalized to all individuals with clinical depression. The extent to which an investigator can with confidence generalize the results of a study depends on the number of subjects in the study and whether the study has been replicated, confirming previous results. It is not unusual for government agencies to sponsor extensive clinical trials using large numbers of subjects to test the effectiveness of a new vaccine. These types of studies have a high degree of external validity. The example of the development of the polio vaccine during the 1950s demonstrates the ability to obtain external validity from one extensive clinical trial. External validity is also dependent on internal validity, however. In other words, the results of a study cannot be generalized to a population if internal validity is weak.

7.9.2 Random Sampling

Random sampling and *random assignment* are seen by researchers as methodological virtues. If a study includes a random selection of subjects, it is assumed that the investigator has controlled for researcher bias when selecting a representative sample of the population. The concept of random sampling implies that in a population that includes all the components (e.g., all occupational therapists, all individuals with diagnoses of schizophrenia, all nursing homes), units of subjects or institutions are representative of the total population. Random sampling is a method to select a representative group from the population. Random sampling does not necessarily ensure a representative group; it serves to eliminate researcher bias in selecting a sample. One method used in random sampling is to assign a number to each population unit and

select a representative sample by choosing units from a list of random numbers. For example, an investigator wants to randomly select 40 graduate programs in occupational therapy that are representative of all the programs, totaling approximately 125 in the United States. The investigator would assign a number from 1 to 125 to each school and then from a list of random numbers select 40 schools. Because the schools are dispersed throughout the country, a representative sample of 40 should reflect the geographical distribution. If a check of the 40 schools reveals that the sample is biased in the direction of a single region, then repeated random selections would be obtained until a fair degree of geographical representativeness occurs. At this point, the reader may ask, why bother with obtaining a sample from random numbers? Why not just merely select a school from each geographical region? The reason this is not valid is because the researcher may overtly or inadvertently select schools that are typical of an educational philosophy or teaching model. Random sampling is simply a method to ensure researcher objectivity. In clinical research on human subjects, this method is sometimes difficult because subjects have the option to participate in the study. Another difficulty is in applying random sampling techniques to potentially large populations of individuals with disabilities situated in a wide geographic area. Is it possible to randomly sample all children with spina bifida, all patients with coronary disease, all prison inmates, all adolescents with attention deficit hyperactivity disorder, or all individuals with spinal cord injury in the United States? The complexities and problems in locating every subject in the population do not warrant the errors that will occur by the very nature of the process. If random sampling of large populations is not practical, are there other objective selection methods that a clinical researcher can use? The answer to this question is yes—if the researcher maintains objectivity by devising systematic methods to obtain subjects and by narrowing the study. By delimiting the population, the investigator can apply random sampling techniques. For example, instead of defining the population as all patients with arthritis in the United States, the researcher delimits the population to all patients with arthritis treated in a specific hospital. The title of the study should describe the population sampled. For example, consider these hypothetical titles:

▶ Survey of Hand Function in the Patient with Arthritis
▶ Survey of the Hand Function of Individuals with Arthritis in a General Hospital in the Northeast.

In the first example, the investigator implies that the survey represents all patients with arthritis. In the second example, the investigator has delimited the population to those patients with arthritis receiving treatment in a specific hospital. For most investigators, it is almost impossible realistically to sample a nationwide population of patients with arthritis. The difficulty in locating every member of the population, the cost of the survey, and the extensive time involved in collecting data are practical considerations that would hinder such a study.

7.9.3 Convenience Sample and Volunteers

It is valid to randomly sample from a *convenience population* (i.e., a population readily available to a researcher) as long as the researcher does not generalize the results to that portion of the population that was not sampled. In selecting a random sampling of patients with arthritis from an identified population, the researcher would consider the following factors:

▶ Diagnosis of arthritis operationalized by physician evaluation or by anatomical or physiological evidence

▶ Age groupings separated into designated units
▶ Differentiation of gender
▶ Occupational groupings, such as professional, skilled, unskilled
▶ Socioeconomic status
▶ Level of education
▶ Age of onset
▶ Presence of stress
▶ Other relevant variables that could potentially affect the onset and course of arthritis, such as exercise, diet, physical condition, obesity, and weather

The variables above can be used to establish screening criteria for subject inclusion in the study or in setting up stratified samples that can be statistically analyzed later for differences.

Another method to counteract researcher bias in selecting subjects is *random assignment*. For instance, if an investigator is interested in comparing simultaneously two treatment methods for patients with stroke, random assignment would be applied after a population of patients with stroke in a specific rehabilitation center is identified through screening criteria. The investigator would establish two samples by randomly assigning participants to each group from a list of random numbers. In this hypothetical example, the selection of the specific rehabilitation center where the patients with stroke were treated actually provides a convenience sample.

Another frequently used method of obtaining subjects in clinical research is the use of *volunteers*. The limitation of using volunteers is that they are a self-selected group who may not be representative of a population. The use of screening criteria with volunteers is one method to determine if the volunteers are a representative group in a target population. In many studies, volunteers are used to assess normal physiological function, and it is important that the investigator establish criteria for normality excluding individuals with above or below average vital capacities. In combination with an objective screening procedure, volunteers are acceptable samples in selected studies.

The relationship between the target population and representative sample and statistic is as follows:

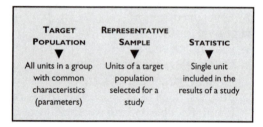

TARGET POPULATION	REPRESENTATIVE SAMPLE	STATISTIC
▼	▼	▼
All units in a group with common characteristics (parameters)	Units of a target population selected for a study	Single unit included in the results of a study

A statistic is the actual subject included in a study. Subjects can be lost in a study through attrition, such as death, change of residence, or voluntarily dropping out of the study. The characteristics of a population such as physiological capacities, personality factors, and demographic information (i.e., social and personal data) are parameters. These values are usually estimated or unknown because most populations are too large to measure in their entirety.

7.10 Size of Sample

Researchers are constantly plagued by the question, *How many subjects should I include in the study?* The often repeated response is: *as many as possible because the higher percentage of subjects from a population, the more the likelihood that the sample is a true representation.* The problem of the sample size can also be analyzed from the statistical point of view, which takes into account statistical significance at a confidence level. If one is familiar with statistical tables for the *t*-test, analysis of variance, and correlation coefficient, then it will become clear that in arriving at a statistically significant result, the number of subjects affects significance because the degrees of freedom are derived from the number of subjects in a study. For example, in applying the Pearson correlation coefficient to a study, a small *r* of .20 can be statistically significant at the .05

level with samples sizes over 100. On the other hand, the researcher needs an *r* of .58 for a sample size of 10 subjects to obtain statistical significance at the .05 level. In summary, if an investigator is interested in using statistics to derive an adequate sample size, he or she must take into consideration the critical values needed at specific levels of statistical significance, such as the .05 or .01 levels, and the difference between means of groups that will be accepted as clinically significant.

Another consideration in determining sample size is the time length of the study and the financial resources available to collect data from participants. For example, if the researcher has only 3 months to collect data, the number of participants is limited to the time it takes within this period. If the researcher assumes that he or she needs as many subjects as possible, then the costs and the time for collecting data for each participant should be calculated as part of the research proposal. Many times these pragmatic considerations are the sole criteria for determining sample size, especially when one is awarded a grant for the research.

7.11 Selection of Measuring Instrument

7.11.1 Selecting a Specific Test for a Research Study

The decision whether to select a published test (i.e., publisher or article) or to construct a new test is a frequent dilemma for the researcher. Figure 7–9 describes this process. Further discussion on this topic is in Chapter 9.

The conceptual definition of a variable should lead the investigator to a specific test that is the most appropriate one when operationally defining a variable. In clinical research, it is critical for the investigator to select a measuring instrument that has high reliability and is a valid measure of outcome. Measuring improvement or change

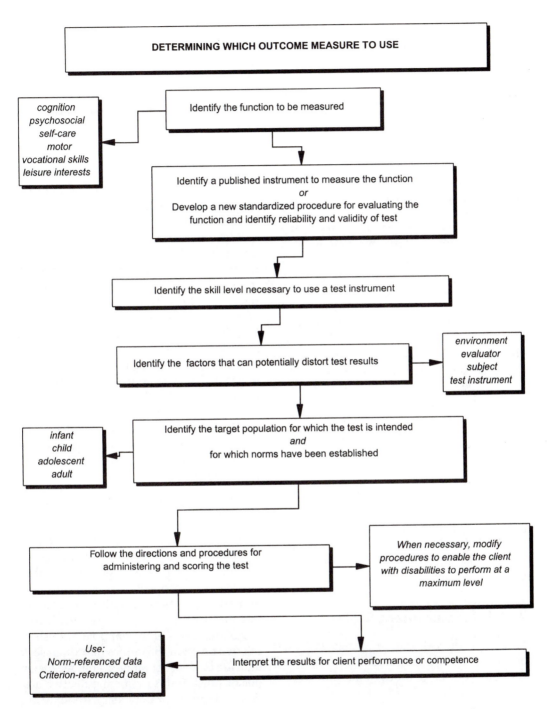

Figure 7-9. Steps in choosing a test instrument and the process of deciding what to use as the outcome measure. The researcher must decide whether to construct a new test or use a previously published test based on a number of factors.

in such areas as cognition, psychosocial, self-care, motor, vocational skills, and leisure interests depends directly on the adequacy and sensitivity of the instrument. A crude measuring instrument that does not have the capacity to detect subtle changes in an individual's functioning or behavior is of limited value to the researcher.

7.11.2 Concept of Measurement and Numbers: Data

Data in statistics are derived from empirical observations. These observations are the result of a standardized measurement procedure, such as simple counting, interviews, psychometrics, or machine monitoring of physiological functions. *Measurement* is the assignment of numbers to objects, persons, or events according to rules. Measurement transforms certain attributes of the world into numbers, which can then be summarized, organized, and analyzed by statistical procedures.

The properties or characteristics of objects, persons, or events are called *variables* (e.g., height, weight, intelligence). A variable will typically assume two or more different values, reflecting the fact that objects, persons, or events vary in characteristics. This concept of *individual differences* is central to most scientific disciplines. One of the purposes of statistics is to reflect and summarize such individual differences in the values of variables.

7.11.3 Measurement Scales

Measurement scales are a system for the numerical representation of the values of a variable. Four basic types of measurement scales are distinguished in statistics:

Nominal Scale Data

Nominal scale measurement is the most discrete and simplest level of data. With nominal scale data, observations are arranged into various classes or categories.

Observations falling into the same class or category are considered qualitatively equivalent, whereas observations in different classes are considered qualitatively different. The classification of eye color, for example, into blue, brown, hazel, or grey, is an example of nominal scale data.

Numbers are assigned usually to each class or category, but these numbers merely reflect differences between the classes. The numbers do not reflect magnitude or order; they only distinguish one class or category from another.

With nominal scale measurement, categories and classes are determined, and a count is made of the number of observations in each category. Because nominal data constitute the most elementary level of measurement, the only arithmetic operation that can be performed on the numbers is counting the number of observations in a category and then analyzing proportional differences between categories. Examples of nominal scale data in health research include diagnostic categories, subspecialization areas, geographic locations, leisure interests, and health care environments (e.g., hospitals, nursing homes, or rehabilitation clinics).

Ordinal Scale Data

Ordinal scale data is the next level of measurement where objects or individuals are not only distinguished from one another, but also are arranged in order or rank. The numerical values of a variable are arranged in a meaningful order to indicate a hierarchy of the levels of the variable or to show relative position. Examples of ordinal scale data are birth order among siblings, the order of finish in a race, or the relative academic standing of university students in a class. The numbers assigned in the above examples not only distinguish between individuals, but also indicate the order or rank of the individuals relative to one another.

The major limitation of ordinal scales is the inability to make inferences about the degree of difference between values on the scale. Numbers assigned in ordinal scale measurement have the properties of both distinctness and order, but the difference between the numbers may not be equal. For example, the difference between 1st and 3rd place in a race may not be equivalent to the difference between 25th and 27th place in the race. There may be wide or narrow differences between each rank. With ordinal scale data, it is only possible to state that one individual or object ranks above or below another. Examples in health care include percentile rank, the degree of improvement, muscle strength categories (e.g., good or fair), self-care index, the severity of illness or injury, and the degree of pain.

Interval Scale Data

Interval scale measurement extends ordinal scales by adding the principle that equal differences between scale values have equal meaning. Thus, the difference between each variable score is equivalent. With interval measurement, numbers serve two purposes: (a) to convey the order of the observations and (b) to indicate the distance or degree of differences between observations. Numbers are assigned so that equal differences in the numbers correspond to equal differences in the property or attribute measured. However, the zero point of the interval scale can be placed arbitrarily and does not indicate absence of the property measured.

Examples of interval scale data are calendar years and the temperature scales of Celsius and Fahrenheit. In a temperature scale, the difference between 10 and 15°C is the same quantitative difference as between 20 and 25°C, but 20°C is not twice as warm as 10°C because there is no true zero point.

Interval scales are important in scientific research. Many human characteristics and attributes, such as intelligence scores, range of motion, dexterity, coordination, and standard scores, are scales with approximately equal intervals. In addition, more sophisticated inferential statistical procedures may be performed with interval scale data compared with the lower level nominal and ordinal data.

Ratio Scale Data

Ratio scale data is the highest level of measurement and includes the maximum amount of information. The ratio scale is named as such because the ratio of numbers on the scale is meaningful. Because there is a genuine zero point, equal ratios between scale values have equal meaning (i.e., the ratio 40:20 is equivalent to 100:50 or 120:60). The zero point on a ratio scale indicates total absence of the property measured. With ratio scale data, all arithmetic operations (addition, subtraction, multiplication, and division) are possible. Measurement of such variables as height, weight, heart rate, and respiratory rate are all ratio scaled. Figure 7–10 illustrates the differences between the four basic types of measurement scales, and Table 7–5 illustrates their characteristics and properties.

Progress in scientific research gained momentum with the design of tests and instruments that measured and recorded human functioning accurately. The measuring instrument is the sine qua non of research. Without an adequate measuring instrument, a problem remains unresearchable. The adequacy of a measuring instrument is determined by its reliability (i.e., consistency in measurement) and validity (i.e., soundness in measurement).

Various examples of measurable variables in health and education research are described in Table 7–6. "In its broadest sense, measurement is the assignment of numerals to objects or parts according to rule" (Stevens, 1951, p. 1).

In the foregoing example (Table 7–6) of measurable variables, numbers can be assigned to indicate the degree of improvement, strength, perceptual ability, and quality of life. Rating scales can also be devised using a continuum of measurement, equal intervals, or item ranking. Likert-type scales

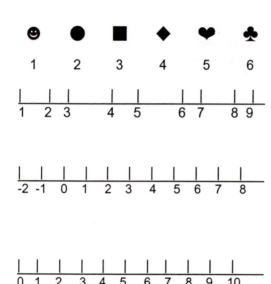

Nominal scale: Numbers act as labels only, indicating differences in kind (e.g., identification numbers).

Ordinal scale: Numbers represent rank ordering. Differences between rank are not equidistant (e.g., grade levels).

Interval scale: Equal differences between values represent equal amounts, but ratios have no meaning because of the arbitrary location of the zero point (e.g., temperature).

Ratio scale: Equal differences between values represent equal amounts. Equal ratios of values are also equivalent because of a genuine zero point (e.g., weight scale).

Figure 7–10. Differences between the four measurement scales are illustrated.

Table 7–5. Classification of Scales of Measurement

Measurement Scale	Type of Variable	Researcher Application	Purposes	Examples
Nominal	Discrete	Sorting of items	Establishing mutually exclusive groups	Occupations, diagnostic groups
Ordinal	Discrete	Rank ordering of items	Determination of greater or lesser	Patient improvement, clinical performance of students
Interval	Continuous	Equal ordering of items	Establishing equal intervals on a continuum	Intelligence, perceptual–motor abilities, work capacities
Ratio	Continuous	Equal ordering of items with an absolute zero point	Establishing continuous measurement with zero point	Range of motion, muscle strength, weight, height, auditory and visual acuity

using descriptor adjectives is another alternative. In this scale, it is not assumed that there are equal intervals between numbers (e.g., 1 to 2 is not assumed to be the same distance as 2 to 3) or that there is an absolute zero. Nonetheless, measurement at this level is an improvement over a clinician subjectively stating, on the basis of treat-

ment, that the patient has either improved or not improved. Measurement enables the clinical researcher to operationally define and objectively evaluate an outcome variable. Without objective measurement, clinicians have no criteria or standards to compare the effects of various treatment modalities.

Table 7–6. Measurable Variables

Variable to Be Tested	Examples of Measuring Instruments
Hand strength:	*Dynamometer*
Range of motion:	*Goniometer*
Attitudes toward individuals with disabilities:	*Attitudes Toward Disabled Persons Scale*
Clinical performance of students:	*AOTA's Clinical Rating Scale*
Psychological improvement:	*Tennessee Test of Self Concept*
Social values and life goals:	*Life Satisfaction Index*
Stress management:	*Stress Management Questionnaire*
Sensory integration:	*Sensory Integration and Praxis Tests*
Cognitive functioning:	*Allen's Cognitive Level*
Self-care:	*Functional Independence Measure*
Developmental levels:	*Miller Assessment Profile*
Eye-hand coordination:	*Developmental Test of Visual-Motor Integration*
Perceptual ability:	*Test of Visual Perceptual Scales (non-motor)*
Social skills:	*Kohlman Evaluation of Living Skills*
Hand function:	*Jebsen Test of Hand Function*

For example, an investigator is interested in comparing two methods of increasing self-care skills in patients who have experienced a stroke. After establishing two groups on the basis of screening criteria and random assignment, the researcher operationally defines self-care skills, such as independence in dressing. The operational definition includes the test and procedure in measuring the dependent variable, *self-care.* In another example involving retrospective research, an investigator is interested in correlating the relationship between disengagement in social decision making and choice of housing for individuals who are older (e.g., nursing home care or independent community living). The presumed independent variables, *housing arrangements,* are hypothesized to affect social decision making. Screening criteria are established in operationally defining the two housing arrangements. The researcher would then select the settings, and subjects would be selected randomly from each institution.

The crux of the research is in operationally defining the concept of social decision making by selecting an objective standardized test.

In selecting a measuring instrument the researcher is faced with two basic questions:

1. Does the instrument measure a variable consistently?
2. Is the instrument a true measure of the variable?

The first question seeks a reliability index, and the second question raises the issues of validity.

7.11.4 Reliability

If one assumes that a specific characteristic of an individual remains stable over time, then a reliable measuring instrument should reflect the stable characteristics through repeated trials. For example, an electron microscope, sensitive enough to enlarge chromosomes so that a researcher can perceive them, maintains a consistency in measurement. In the physical sciences, where comparison dictates the foundation of measurement, the reliability of instruments has evolved progressively. Nonetheless, the individual using a sensitive measuring instrument can affect what is being measured (Heisenberg Uncertainty Principle). For example, astronomers observed that the individual's reaction time in viewing the movement of stars affects calculation of determining distances between the stars. In response to this human factor, astronomers developed automatic means to record distances between celestial objects. The control of the personal equation in measurement is an important factor to consider in every research study where there is an interaction between the object observed and the investigator. This is especially true in qualitative research, such as in interviewing subjects where the investigator's presence affects the behavior of the interviewee.

Researchers strive to reduce the error factor in measurement by increasing the reliability of an objective test or instrument and reducing the variability of extraneous factors in the individual. Instruments, such as the electrocardiograph (EKG or ECG), electroencephalograph (EEG), X-Ray, electromyograph (EMG), positron emission tomography (PET scan), magnetic resonance imaging (MRI), and single-photon emission computed tomography (SPECT) are usually reliable indicators of bodily functions. On the other hand, questionnaires, surveys, rating scales, attitude inventories, interest tests, and objective psychological tests may be less reliable. The nature of the test affects the reliability index. Automatic instruments that record bodily functions need to be mechanically sound or calibrated to be reliable. In devising a reliable instrument, the investigator is concerned with eliminating items that are ambiguous or that can be answered in more than one way. Reliability is not a simple concept that merely reflects the consistency of

the instrument. In any test administered to subjects, individual differences—such as level of reading ability, need to conform, desire to please the examiner, motivation, and test anxiety—are important factors that could potentially increase the error variance and decrease the consistency of response. Because human beings are constantly reacting to internal and external factors, reliability must be interpreted in a relative degree when considering psychological tests, questionnaires, and attitude scales. Most researchers with human subjects accept a reliability coefficient of approximately $r = .80$ or above to be an acceptable level of a test's consistency in measuring a variable.

Techniques for Measuring Test Reliability

Test reliability is usually measured by correlating two sets of scores and arriving at a correlation coefficient. For example, an investigator is interested in devising a test of perceptual-motor ability with school-age children from 8 to 11 years old. In the process of devising the test, the investigator constructs 50 items that measure perceptual-motor ability. The items are screened for clarity in a pilot study with 24 children as subjects. The investigator seeks to determine split half reliability and test-retest reliability. In split half reliability, the test is broken into two equal parts (in this example, 25 items each) and correlated with each other. In test-retest reliability, a test is given twice within a short period of time (usually within 2 weeks) and the scores on the two tests are correlated.

In the following hypothetical example (Table 7–7), there is a perfect positive correlation ($+1.00$) between the scores on the first and second tests. The scores reflect also a practice effect, which is typical of test-retest reliability. A practice effect exists when scores increase consistently as a function of the subject's familiarity with the content of the test and his or her reduced anxiety. In many published tests, the

Table 7–7. Hypothetical Data for Testing Reliability

| | Test-Retest Reliability | |
Subject	Test 1	Test 2
01	69	72
02	34	37
03	71	74
04	20	23
05	95	98
06	10	13
07	99	102
08	81	84
09	92	95
10	49	52
11	97	100
12	63	66
13	86	89
14	9	12
15	96	99
16	81	84
17	20	23
18	69	72
19	81	84
20	24	27
21	97	100
22	55	58
23	54	57
24	97	100
25	68	71

practice effect is controlled when developing normative data.

7.11.5 Item Analysis

When devising a test or assessing students, a researcher may be interested in the effectiveness of individual test items that differentiate between high and low achievers.

The researcher may also be interested in eliminating those items that are ambiguous and have a low discriminative level. Item analysis is a method of gauging the difficulty value and ambiguity of each item. In item analysis, the percentage of passes and failures are calculated for each item. For example, if items 1, 2, and 3 are passed respectively by 80, 60, and 40% of the subjects, we can infer that item 3 is either more difficult or more ambiguous than item 1 or 2. Another method is analyzing items to determine which items were passed by high scorers and failed by low scorers. This analysis will enable the researcher to separate out those items that have discriminative value. Items that are passed in all cases have little discriminative value but may indicate the level at which all members of the group are functioning. This may be particularly important in criterion-reference tests where the test administrator is most concerned with issues related to competency.

7.11.6 Validity

Validity reflects the authenticity of a test. Does the test measure what it purports to measure? A test may measure a concept consistently but it may not, in fact, measure what the researcher identifies as the intent of the test. Psychological tests purporting to measure general intelligence, self-image, body defensiveness, and attitude toward individuals with disabilities may be measuring other concepts. The degree to which a test is valid is the degree of empirical evidence that corroborates the results of a test. Tests or instruments that collect primary data, such as an EMG, X-Ray, goniometer, ergometer, and MRI are easily verified and corroborated. By contrast, tests that collect secondary data derived from multiple factors in the individual, such as visual perception, are more difficult to validate. Personality, attitude, values, perception, and interests are complex variables derived from many facets of the individual's life that are related to genetic, social learning, cultural identification, and physiological factors. The researcher seeking to validate a visual-perceptual test is limited by the ability to corroborate the findings. Traditionally, validity is established on the following bases:

▶ *Content or face validity:* the degree to which the test appears to measure a concept by a logical analysis of the items. Does each item appear to relate to the content being tested?
▶ *Concurrent validity:* the degree of correlation with another standardized instrument. A new test may be derived because it is less time-consuming and less expensive than another established validated instrument. What is the correlation between the established test and the new test?
▶ *Predictive validity:* the degree to which a test can predict success or accuracy over a period of time (longitudinally). For example, a test devised to predict success in a graduate program for occupational therapists or success in a rehabilitation program for patients with stroke are examples of predictive validity. In the examples, follow-up data from longitudinal studies would determine the correlation between the initial test predictor score and subsequent success in a program.
▶ *Construct validity:* considered to be the highest form of empirical evidence that is most sought after by scientific researchers. Construct validity assumes a theoretical rationale underlying the test instrument. In testing an instrument for construct validity, the researcher seeks behavioral data to substantiate the position that the test is in fact measuring a defined variable. For example, an investigator devising a test to measure self-image would first construct a theory that underlies the concept. The theory would include developmental factors, relationships with other variables, and behavioral observations supporting the evidence for construct validity. In another example, the electroencephalogram, which records

brain waves and is used indirectly for diagnosing brain damage, can be checked for construct validity through dissection of an animal brain or through postmortem examination.

7.12 Ethical Principles Guiding Human Research

Boxes 7–1 through 7–6 give examples of documents related to ethical issues guiding clinical research.

7.12.1 The Declaration of Helsinki

The Declaration of Helsinki, which offers recommendations for conducting experiments using human subjects, was adopted in 1962 and revised by the 18th World Medical Assembly, Helsinki, Finland, in 1964. Subsequent revisions were approved in Tokyo (1975), Venice (1983), and Hong Kong (1989). The 1997 version, reprinted in Box 7–1, is available on the Internet at http://bioscience.igh.cnrs.fr //guides/declhels.htm (World Medical Assocation, 1997).

7.12.2 Harvard University Medical School

The guidelines reproduced in Box 7–2 "outline principles that should be followed at Harvard Medical School when conducting research. . . . They are a supplement to the *Guidelines for Investigators in Scientific Research,* first issued in February 1988 (Harvard Medical School, 1996). The full document, *Faculty Policies on Integrity in Science,* is available in hard copy from the Office for Research Issues, Harvard Medical School (1991).

The *Code of Federal Regulations,* published by the Department of Health and Human Services (1991) provides additional information concerning the use of humans in research. This information is available at http://www.fas.harvard.edu/~research/

Box 7–1. Declaration of Helsinki[1]

DECLARATION OF HELSINKI:
RECOMMENDATION FOR CONDUCT OF CLINICAL RESEARCH

INTRODUCTION: It is the same mission of doctors to safeguard the health of people. Their knowledge and conscience are dedicated to the fulfillment of this mission. The declaration of Geneva of the World Medical Association binds the doctor with the words "The health of my patient will be my first consideration" and the International Code of Medical Ethics declares that "Any act or advice which could weaken physical or mental resistance of a human being may be used only in his interest". Because it is essential that the results of laboratory experiments be applied to human beings to further scientific knowledge and to help suffering humanity, the World Medical Association has prepared the following recommendations as guide to each doctor in clinical research. It must be stressed that the standards as drafted are only a guide to physicians all over the world. Doctors are not relieved from criminal, civil and ethical responsibilities under the laws of their own countries. In the field of clinical research a fundamental distinction must be recognized between clinical research in which the aim is essentially therapeutic for a patient, and the clinical research, the essential object of which is purely scientific and without therapeutic value to the person subjected to the research.

I. Basic principles
   1. Clinical research must conform to the moral and scientific principles that justify medical research and should be based on laboratory and animal experiments or other scientifically established facts.
   2. Clinical research should be conducted only by scientifically qualified persons and under the supervision of a qualified medical person.
   3. Clinical research can not legitimately be carried out unless the importance of the objective is in proportion to the inherent risk to the subject.
   4. Every clinical research project should be preceded by careful assessment of inherent risks in comparison to foreseeable benefits to the subject or to others.
   5. Special caution should be exercised by the doctor in performing clinical research in which the personality of the subject is liable to be altered by drugs or experimental procedure.
II. Clinical Research combined with professional care
   1. In the treatment of the sick persons, the doctor must be free to use a new therapeutic measure, if in the doctor's judgment it offers hope of saving life, reestablishing health, or alleviating suffering. If at all possible, consistent with patient psychology, the doctor should obtain the patient's freely given consent after the patient has been given a full explanation. In case

[1]This document is printed in the World Medical Association, Handbook of Declarations, 1997, and is available on the Internet at http://bioscience.igh.cnrs.fr//guides/declhels.htm

continued

of legal incapacity, consent should also be procured from the legal guardian; in case of physical incapacity the permission of the legal guardian replaces that of the patient.

2. The doctor can combine clinical research with professional care, the objective being the acquisition of new medical knowledge, only to the extent that clinical research is justified by its therapeutic value for the patient .

III. Nontherapeutic clinical research

1. In the purely scientific application of clinical research carried out on a human being, it is the duty of the doctor to remain the protector of the life and health of that person on whom clinical research is being carried out.

2. The nature, the purpose and the risk of clinical research must be explained to the subject by the doctor.

3a. Clinical research on a human being can not be undertaken without that person's consent after being informed; if the person is legally incompetent the consent of the legal guardian should be procured.

3b. The object of clinical research should be in such a mental, physical and legal state as to be able to exercise fully the power of choice.

3c. Consent should, as a rule, be obtained in writing. However, the responsibility for clinical research always remains with the research worker; it never falls on the subject even after consent is obtained.

4a. The investigator must respect the right of each individual to safeguard his/her personal integrity, especially if the subject is in a dependent relationship to the investigator.

4b. At any time during the course of clinical research the subject or the subject's guardian should be free to withdraw permission for research to be continued. The investigator or the investigation team should discontinue the research if in their judgment, it may, if continued be harmful to the individual. (p. 1)

45CFR46.html@○46.115. Other federal regulations can be found at the Code of Federal Regulations Web site (http://www.access.gpo.gov/nara/cfr/)

7.12.3 The University of South Dakota Human Subjects Review Protocol (HSRP)

The University of South Dakota Human Subject Approval Request and accompanying instructions have been reproduced in Box 7–3. These are available through the Research Office at the University of South Dakota, Slagle Hall, 414 E. Clark St., Vermillion, SD, 57069 or through the Internet at http://www.usd.edu/oorsch/forms.html.

Box 7–4 is an example of a checklist that can be used by the researcher to conform with Institutional Review Board (IRB) guidelines.

7.13 Data Collection Procedures

The time schedule for collecting data, the costs of the study, the setting for administering group or individual tests, a cover letter to prospective subjects explaining the nature of the study, an individual data collection sheet recording descriptive information and test scores, an informed consent agreement between the researcher and subject, and the statistical techniques used to analyze the data are all factors for the

Box 7–2. Guidelines for Investigators in Clinical Research[1]

INTRODUCTION

These guidelines outline principles that should be followed at Harvard Medical School when conducting research. They are a supplement to the Guidelines for Investigators in Scientific Research, first issued in February 1988. Clinical research may be defined as investigations involving human subjects or the use of patient samples. The scientific practices described here are generally accepted by investigators conducting both multi-center and single-institution clinical studies and help ensure both the quality and integrity of scientific findings in clinical research. The guidelines are not intended to relieve investigators of any ethical obligations that may be imposed by individual Institutional Review Boards overseeing the rights of study subjects in clinical research.

A major component of clinical research consists of either prospective clinical trials or retrospective studies based on medical or administrative records. Of these two types of studies, prospective trials contain fewer chances for investigator bias and for lost or incomplete data than do retrospective studies, and are to be preferred whenever they are feasible. Some phenomena, however, such as rare diseases or diseases requiring exceptionally long follow-up, can only be studied from a case series assembled from medical records. These guidelines address issues that arise in both types of studies.

The implementation of these guidelines rests within each of the affiliated institutions and the department in which the research is conducted. Whenever research is carried out by non-faculty, such as a student or fellow, the supervisor of that individual is responsible for ensuring that these guidelines are followed.

I. EXPERIMENTAL DESIGN

Successful clinical studies acknowledge the complexity of conducting scientific research with human subjects, and are based both on the principles of experimental design and on respect for the rights of study subjects. Experiments in human subjects generally have highly variable outcomes, and efficient designs that lead to unbiased conclusions are critical.

Recommendations

1. Each study, whether it be observations on one or more patients, a randomized trial, or a population based study, should have clearly articulated research objectives that can be achieved from a successful execution of the study design.

2. Whenever some aspects of a study involve clinical or scientific specialties outside the expertise of the investigator, drafts of the protocol or research plan should be circulated to specialists in those areas for review and comment.

3. Every prospective or retrospective clinical study should have a written protocol or research plan that states the goals of the study, provides a

[1]Reprinted with permission from the Office for Research Issues, Harvard Medical School. Copyright 1996, Harvard Medical School. This document is available at http://www.hms.harvard.edu/integrity/clinical.html

continued

background and rationale for the study, specifies the criteria for inclusion or exclusion of cases, outlines the methods and timings of follow-up, gives a precise definition of the types of anticipated outcome measures, and gives the details of the statistical design. The study design should minimize the possibility for investigator bias in the interpretation of the results. The design specification may range from a description of anticipated measurements in an exploratory study to a precise specification of the number of cases that will be registered in a phase III randomized trial. In the case of prospective trials, the protocol should describe in detail how patients are to be treated or managed. Any substantial changes to the conduct of the study, including modifications of the sample size, eligibility criteria, or treatment regimens, should be reflected in amendments made to the protocol or research plan and approved by co-investigators and the Institutional Review Board.

4. In randomized clinical trials, the sequence of treatment assignments should be prepared by a statistician or other experienced investigator associated with the trial and kept confidential. In no instance should an investigator treating patients on the trial know the sequence of potential treatment assignments.

5. Clinical studies all require approval of local Institutional Review Boards. Every prospective clinical study should contain an Informed Consent form that explains in clear, non-technical terms the possible risks and benefits for subjects participating in the trial.

II. DATA MANAGEMENT AND TRIAL MONITORING

Complete and accurate data are an essential part of the record of any clinical research. Since serious problems can occur when data are missing or are not consistent with source medical records, each study should include a plan for the keeping of accurate and well documented data not subject to loss through computer failure or insecure storage.

Recommendations

1. In prospective trials, data should be abstracted from source medical records as the trial proceeds, using data collection forms designed at the outset of the study. Data collection forms should also be used in retrospective record studies.

2. The criteria for the evaluation of study subjects (including the classification of outcome and any treatment side effects) should be specified in the protocol or research plan.

3. Interim review of the data from an ongoing trial should make use of statistical methods that guard against increased false-positive or false-negative reporting rates caused by inappropriate conclusions from preliminary analyses.

4. For research involving primary data collection, the principle investigator should retain original data for as long as practically possible, but never for less than five years from the first major publication or from the completion of an unpublished study. All data should be kept in the research unit responsible for conducting the study. Copies of computer programs and the results from statistical calculations used in research involving nationally gathered survey data should also be kept by research units for a minimum

of five years from publication based on these results. After notification to responsible departmental officials, principal investigators may make copies of original data or computer programs for personal use or when moving to another research unit or institution.

5. If primary data are kept on a computer file, backup files should be maintained, preferably at a second site, to prevent loss from computer failure.

III. SCIENTIFIC REPORTING

Writing a manuscript reporting the results of a clinical study is a complex and demanding task. Unclear or ambiguous reports reduce the value of a study and may lead to a discrediting of the research.

Recommendations

1. The statistical analysis used in reporting the results should coincide with the planned analysis used to design the study. Reasons should be given in the manuscript for any different analyses that are used.
2. All cases registered in a clinical trial or records reviewed in a retrospective study must be accounted for in any manuscript reporting the results. Any case not used in the analysis of outcome data should be identified (by case number) and the reason for exclusion noted.

IV. AUTHORSHIP

Clinical studies often involve investigators from several subspecialties, and it may not always be possible for a single investigator to confirm each piece of data used in the report of a trial. While each participating investigator must be actively involved in verifying the sections of a manuscript that discuss his/her specialty area, there must nevertheless be a primary author who is responsible for the validity of the entire manuscript.

Recommendations

1. Criteria for authorship of a manuscript should be determined and announced by each department or research unit. The committee considers the only reasonable criterion to be that the co-author has made a significant intellectual or practical contribution. The concept of "honorary authorship" is deplorable.
2. The first author should assure the head of the research unit or department chairperson that he/she has reviewed all primary data on which the report is based and provide a brief description of the role of each co-author. (In multi-institutional collaborations, the senior investigator in each institution should prepare such statements.)
3. Appended to the final draft of the manuscript should be a signed statement from each co-author indicating that he/she has reviewed and approved the manuscript to the extent possible, given individual expertise.

investigator to consider in the prospectus for the study.

The checklist in Table 7–8 should guide the investigator in preparing a data collection procedure. The reader should review this frequently to ensure that all parts of the data collection have been considered.

7.13.1 Informed Consent and Forms

The informed consent is a legal document that informs participants about the procedures that are to occur, the place in which the data collection will occur, the amount

Box 7–3. The University of South Dakota Human Subjects Review Protocol (HSRP)[1]

THE UNIVERSITY OF SOUTH DAKOTA
HUMAN SUBJECT APPROVAL REQUEST

1. PROJECT DIRECTOR: _____ PHONE #: _____
   COLLEGE/SCHOOL: _____ DEPARTMENT: _____

2. PROJECT TITLE: _____
   _____

3. SPONSORING AGENCY: _____

4. PROJECT PERIOD: FROM __/__/__   TO __/__/__
5. LOCATION OF STUDY: _____

6. TYPES OF SUBJECTS TO BE SELECTED:
   ___ Normal Adults ___ Minors   ___ Prisoners
   ___ Fetuses   ___ Pregnant Women ___ Mentally Disabled or Retarded
7. IS EXEMPTED STATUS REQUESTED?   ___ Yes   ___ No
   Exemptions are granted by the compliance officer after review of the approval
   request. If "yes", indicate basis for exemption:
   ___ Common Educational Setting   ___ Educational Tests
   ___ Survey/Interview Research   ___ Observational Research
   ___ Study of Existing Data
8. Are any drugs or chemical or biological agents to be administered to human
   subjects?
   ___ Yes   ___ No
9. Are specimens or samples of tissues, body fluids, or other substances to be
   collected from participants?
   ___ Yes   ___ No
10. RESEARCH PROTOCOL: Complete a description of the proposed study in the
    format shown on the reverse side of this form, following instructions. If a more
    complete description is provided, a brief summary, in the format given, is still
    required.

11. INFORMED CONSENT: Attach copies of all forms which will be used to ob-
    tain the legally effective informed consent of human subjects or their legal
    representatives.
12. Instruments: Attach copies of any questionnaires or survey instruments.
AUTHORIZING SIGNATURES:
    PROJECT DIRECTOR: _____   __/__/__
    ADVISOR (If student Project): _____   __/__/__
    CHAIRPERSON: _____   __/__/__
    DEAN: _____   __/__/__

[1]Revised: 9/9/98. Reproduced from the University of South Dakota and available through the Research Office at the University of South Dakota, Slagle Hall, 414 E. Clark St., Vermillion, SD, 57069 or
through the Internet at http://www.usd.edu/oorsch/forms.html.

The signed original of this form and one copy and two copies of the consent form(s) must be submitted for review. Single copies of any other appropriate materials, such as a fuller protocol description, letter to subjects, etc., must also be provided. Eight (8) additional copies of this form and attachments will be requested if the project needs to go to the full Committee for review. Additional copies of commercial survey insstruments are not required.

RECEIVED - RESEARCH COMPLIANCE OFFICE ___ / ___ / ___
EXEMPT: ___ EXPEDITED: ___ COMMITTEE: ___

RESEARCH PROTOCOL
A. Objectives:
B. Participants (number and selection criteria):
C. Time required of human subjects:
D. Financial compensation of subjects (if any):
E. Benefits to subjects:
F. Importance of the knowledge to be gained:
G. Research protocol:
H. Confidentiality:
I. Risks and efforts for their reduction:

THE UNIVERSITY OF SOUTH DAKOTA
INSTRUCTIONS FOR COMPLETING THE
HUMAN SUBJECTS APPROVAL REQUEST FORM
All proposals for research projects involving human subjects are subject to review according to Federal Regulation 45 CFR 46 Protection of Human Subjects. The following instructions will assist you in completing the Approval Request Form on a step by step basis.

1. PROJECT DIRECTOR: The faculty or staff member who will be primarily responsible for the conduct of the proposed research, including supervision of the use of human subjects in the research. In the case of student-originated studies, give the names of both the student and his or her faculty sponsor.

2. PROJECT TITLE: A brief descriptive title for the proposed research. If the project represents a grant or contract application the title should be the same as that used on the formal proposal.

3. SPONSORING AGENCY: If no external sponsor is sought for the research, please indicate "NONE."

4. PROJECT PERIOD: Indicate the period from initiation of interaction with the human subjects until all interaction as subjects is completed.

continued

5. <u>LOCATION OF STUDY</u>: Specify the location(s) where the testing, etc. of human subjects will take place.

6. <u>TYPES OF SUBJECTS</u>: Normal adults are those individuals 18 years of age or older who have the capacity to render legally informed consent for their own participation in the study. The participation of minors requires the signature of at least one parent or guardian as well as the assent of the minor. Special care must be taken to exclude minors from projects involving college students when parental permission has not been obtained.

7. <u>EXEMPTION FROM COMMITTEE REVIEW</u>: University policy, in conformity with US Department of Health and Human Services regulations, provides for the exclusion of certain low-risk, human subjects research from the requirements for full Human Subjects Committee review. Such exemptions will be determined on a case-by-case basis by the Compliance Office. The criteria for exemption are as follows:

<u>Common Educational Settings</u>: Research is exempt if conducted in established or commonly accepted educational settings, involving normal educational practices, such as (1) research on regular or special education instructional strategies; or (2) research on the effectiveness of or the comparison among instructional techniques, curricula, or classroom management methods.

<u>Educational Tests</u>: Research involving the use of educational tests (cognitive, diagnostic, aptitude, achievement) is exempt if information taken from these sources is recorded in such a manner that subjects cannot be identified, directly or through identifiers linked to the subjects.

<u>Survey/Interview Research</u>: Research involving survey or interview procedures is exempt, except where responses are recorded in such a manner that human subjects can be identified, directly or through identifiers linked to the subjects' <u>and</u> (1) the subject's responses, if they became known outside the research, could reasonably place the subject at risk of criminal or civil liability or be damaging to the subject's financial standing or employability; or (2) the research deals with sensitive aspects of the subject's own behavior, such as illegal conduct, drug use, sexual behavior, or use of alcohol.

All research involving survey or interview procedures may be exempt when the respondents are elected or appointed public officials or candidates for public office.

<u>Observational Research</u>: Research involving the observation (including observation by participants) of public behavior, is exempt except where observations are recorded in such a manner that the human subjects can be identified, directly or through identifiers linked to the subjects; and (1) the observations recorded about the individual, if they became known outside of the research, could reasonably place the subject at risk of criminal or civil liability or be damaging to the subject's financial standing or employability; or (2) the research deals with sensitive aspects of the subject's own behavior such as illegal conduct, drug use, sexual behavior, or use of alcohol.

Study of Existing Data: Research involving the collection or study of existing data, documents, records, pathological specimens, or diagnostic specimens, is exempt if these sources are publicly available or if the information is recorded (visual scanning of records, listening to audio tapes or viewing video tapes does not constitute recording) by the investigator in such a manner that subjects cannot be identified, directly or through identifiers linked to the subjects.

8. <u>DRUGS</u>: Indicate whether any drugs or chemicals or biological agents will be used in the treatment or testing of human subjects. If "yes" complete drug form.

9. <u>SPECIMENS</u>: Indicate whether the study will require the collection of tissue, body fluids, or other specimens from the human subject participants.

10. <u>RESEARCH PROTOCOL</u>: A concise but complete narrative description must be included with the Human Subjects Approval Request. This narrative should include the following:

a) a concise statement of the objectives (including therapeutic intent, if any) of the study.

b) the specific selection procedures which will be used to select human subject participants for this study, including an enumeration of the specific criteria for eligibility. The number of participants (at least approximate).

c) the time required of each subject (the number of hours of direct participation and the calendar period or participation).

d) a description of compensation, remuneration, or other rewards which will be provided to subjects for their participation.

e) a description of the expected benefits, if any, which may reasonably be expected to accrue to individual participants (apart from remuneration described under (d) above).

f) explicit description of the methods, procedures and design of the study, including a review of all treatments, tests, or other procedures involving the human subject participants.

g) identification of any potential risks and hazards to human subjects associated with participation in the study, including both physical and mental or psychological risk and hazard.

h) a description of procedures which will be followed to minimize or reduce the potential risks and hazards associated with the study and identification of the provisions which will be made to provide care, treatment, or remedy for injury resulting from participation in the study.

i) a description of the procedures which will be followed to secure the legally effective informed consent of participants and/or their legal representatives.

11. <u>INFORMED CONSENT</u>: Informed consent requirements are stringent. The check list used for review of consent forms is appended. Exempt human-subject

continued

projects do not require the use of consent forms, but they remain good professional practice. A less detailed consent form is often appropriate. Example consent forms will be provided on request.

12. <u>INSTRUMENTS</u>: Copies of any questionnaires or survey instruments.

DEFINITIONS

The wording of the following definitions is taken directly from the federal regulations.

<u>RESEARCH</u>: means a systematic investigation designed to develop or contribute generalizable knowledge.

<u>HUMAN SUBJECT</u>: means a living individual about whom an investigator conducting research obtains (1) data through intervention or interaction with the individual, or (2) identifiable private information.

<u>INTERVENTION</u>: includes both physical procedures by which data are gathered (for example, venipuncture) and manipulations of the subject or the subjects' environment that are performed for research purposes.

<u>INTERACTION</u>: includes communication or interpersonal contact between investigator and subject.

<u>PRIVATE INFORMATION</u>: must be individually identifiable in order for obtaining the information, to constitute research involving human subjects.

<u>ASSENT</u>: means affirmative agreement to participate in research.

<u>MINIMAL RISK</u>: means that the risks of harm are not greater than those ordinarily encountered in daily life during the performance of routine physical or psychological examinations or tests. (Significant risk is all other risk.)

of time required for participation, and the potential risks or hazards of the study. Informed consent must be documented (United States Department of Health and Human Services, National Institutes of Health, Office for Protection from Research Risks, 1991). A copy of the signed informed consent form must be obtained for the principal investigator's files from each participant, or in the case of a minor, the parent, guardian or surrogate parent. A copy should be given to each participant. The participant's copy should include the name, address, telephone number, and E-mail address of the person to whom requests for information or

results may be addressed. It must also include the name, address, telephone number, and E-mail address of the person to whom complaints may be addressed. The informed consent form should be written in language that is easily understood by all participants.

The following is described in detail in the informed consent form:

▶ The procedure for obtaining informed consent
▶ A brief statement regarding the objectives of the study
▶ The amount of time each subject will be asked to participate in the study

Box 7–4. Checklist for Conforming to the Guidelines for IRBs[1]

TITLE
- Does the title of the study appear and match the title used on the Request for Approval Form?

INVITATION TO PARTICIPATE
- Does the consent form begin with a clear invitation to participate?
- Is there a description of who participants will be, how they were selected?

PURPOSE
- Is there a clear statement of the purpose of the research?
- Does it state who is conducting the research?
- Does the consent form state that participation is voluntary?
- Is it stated that the participant may withdraw without penalty?

PROCEDURES
- Is the explanation of procedures adequate?
  - Type of research (e.g., survey/instruments, experiment, interview)
  - Type of questions being asked (e.g., sensitive, innocuous)

BENEFITS
- Is the statement of potential benefits adequate?

COMPENSATION
- Is the availability of compensation stated?
- Is there a cost/no cost to the participants?
- Is there compensation in case of injury?
- Is there alternative treatment available?
- Is there a statement on emergency medical treatment? (for more than minimal risk studies)

RISKS
- Is the description of the potential risks and discomforts adequate?
- Are methods of risk reduction in place? (i.e., referral in case of upset due to questions asked)
- Does it state that the investigator may withdraw participant if it is in his or her best interests?

CONFIDENTIALITY
- Is the assurance of confidentiality clear and complete?
- Is the FDA access (or other access) to research records statement included?
- Is there an offer to answer all questions, now and later?

[1]Adapted from the Human Subjects Committee, University of South Dakoka

continued

- Is statement concerning questions about participants rights included?
- Does it state that participants will receive a copy of his or her consent form?

SIGNATURES
- Is standard concluding statement included?
- Are there dated subject and investigator blanks?
- Is there a witness signature blank? (for more than minimal risk studies)

GENERAL QUESTIONS
- Is the investigator's name, phone number and E-mail address on the form (i.e. signature block)
- Is the consent form written in "lay language?"
- Is the consent form free of any threatening language?
- If children are included as subjects, is provision made for securing the assent of the child and the consent of the parent/guardian?
- Has permission been obtained from schools, agencies involved?
- What is the overall risk classification (e.g., minimal, greater than minimal)?

Table 7–8. Checklist for Guiding Data Collection

Time Schedule
- Have you determined the length of time needed for administering individual or group testing?
- Have you considered travel time and time for interviewing?
- Have you determined the length of time for scoring tests?

Informed Consent
- Have you prepared a form describing to the subject the procedure, tests, information, and length of time involved?
- Have you informed the participant that he/she may decline from the study without any implied penalty?
- Does the participant have a signed form in his/her possession?

Data Collection Sheet
- Have you prepared a data collection sheet for each subject, coding the name to guarantee anonymity and providing room for every datum item collected?

Computer Analysis
- Have you considered using computer time in analyzing the data?

Statistical Techniques
- Does the study meet the assumptions of a parametric statistic?
- If not, what specific nonparametric statistics will be used to analyze the data?
- Have you done a statistical analysis of the hypothetical data?

Cost Analysis
- Have you considered costs of purchasing tests or instruments?
- Have you considered costs of postage, address labels, and mailings?
- Have you considered costs of analyzing data?
- Have you considered costs of travel?
- Have you considered costs of telephone calls?
- Have you considered payment for participants?

▶ The compensation, remuneration, or other awards, if any, to be received by the subjects

▶ A description of any expected benefits that may be obtained by the participant

▶ A description of the procedures and methods to be used in the study

▶ The identification of potential risks or hazards that might occur during the study

▶ The procedures that will minimize any identified risks or hazards

▶ The procedures that will ensure confidentiality of the participants.

When children are used in research, additional procedures must be used According to the *Code of Federal Regulations* (United States Department of Health and Human Services, National Institutes of Health, Office for Protection from Research Risks, 1991, Sect. 46.408), permission must be obtained from the parents, guardians, or surrogate parents to use the child **and** assent must be obtained from the child

> when in the judgment of the IRB the children are capable of providing assent. In determining whether children are capable of assenting, the IRB shall take into account the ages, maturity, and psychological state of the children involved. This judgment may be made for all children to be involved in research under a particular protocol, or for each child, as the IRB deems appropriate. If the IRB determines that the capability of some or all of the children is so limited that they cannot reasonably be consulted or that the intervention or procedure involved in the research holds out a prospect of direct benefit that is important to the health or well-being of the children and is available only in the context of the research, the assent of the children is not a necessary condition for proceeding with the research. Even where the IRB determines that the subjects are capable of assenting, the IRB may still waive the assent requirement under circumstances in which consent may be waived in accord with Sec. 46.116 of Subpart A. (p. 124)

Although not required, the investigator may want to develop a written assent for children rather than just asking the child to verbalize assent. Care should be taken to ensure that the reading level is appropriate for the age and ability level.

7.13.2 Example of an Informed Consent Form

Box 7–5 depicts a model for an informed consent form and Box 7-6 displays a sample of a cover letter. These forms have been developed by the Human Subjects Committee at the University of South Dakota and available on-line at http://www.usd.edu/oorsch/forms.html.

7.14 Methodological Limitations of a Study

Researchers can assume that most studies have limitations in selecting a sample, using a measuring instrument, collecting data, or analyzing results. A section devoted to the limitations of a study is an objective means for discussing flaws in research methods. This section is not meant to be an excuse or rationalization for not obtaining acceptable results or confirming predicted hypotheses, but rather an unbiased analysis of shortcomings in the research. These flaws in methodology do not necessarily mean that the research is worthless or inadequate; on the contrary, it serves to guide future researchers in avoiding the same mistakes when the research is replicated or another research design is proposed. Research often involves trial-and-error methods with factors of risk and uncertainty. Results are significant if the researcher has been objective and unbiased. The honesty and integrity of the researcher are enhanced when both the merits and deficiencies of a study are objectively reported. Likewise, the limitations of a study can serve as the basis for recommending further research.

BOX 7–5. MODEL CONSENT FORM FOR PARTICIPATION IN A NONMEDICAL RESEARCH PROJECT[1]

The University of South Dakota
Vermillion, SD 57069
Department of _____
Project Director: _____ Phone # _____

Please read (listen to) the following information:

1. You are invited to be one of (approximate number) participating in a research project under the direction of the Department of _____ of the University of South Dakota. _____ is the Project Director. You have been invited because (. . . selection criteria).
2. The project is entitled:
   _____
3. The purpose of the project is to
   _____
4. If you consent to participate, you will be involved in the following process which will take about _____ minutes of your time over a period of _____ months.
5. Participation in this project is voluntary. You have the right to withdraw at any time without penalty (i.e., affecting your care, grades, etc.). If you have any questions, you may contact the project director at the number listed above. If you have any questions about your legal rights as a human subject, you may contact the Human Subjects Committee Chair, Dr. _____.
6. (There are no known risks) or (the risks are . . .) to your participation in the study. (If questions are of a sensitive nature, you need to indicate how you will handle someone becoming upset, i.e., referral).
7. (The benefits to you are) . . . (there are no direct benefits) . . . (personal, extra credit, etc.)
8. There (is) (is no) monetary compensation for your participation in this study.
9. Your responses are confidential. When the data are presented in the written report, you will not be linked to the data by your name, title or any other identifying item.
10. I have read the above, have had any questions answered and agree to participate in the research project. I will receive a copy of this form for my information.

_____   _____
Participant's Signature   Project Director's Signature

_____   _____
Date   Date

[1]Developed by the Human Subjects Committee at the University of South Dakota and available on-line at http://www.usd.edu/oorsch/forms.html. (Reproduced from the University of South Dakota Web site at http://www.usd.edu/oorsch/forms.html)

BOX 7–6. MODEL OF A COVER LETTER[1]

Model Cover Letter

Dear _____ :

I/we are conducting a study entitled "_____" as a part of a _____ (i.e., dissertation, class project, etc.) at the University of South Dakota.

The purpose of the study is _____
_____
_____
_____ .

You as a _____ (student, teacher, etc.) are invited to participate in the study by _____ (completing the attached survey, taking part in an interview, etc.). **(The types of questions being asked should be included)** It will take approximately ____ minutes of your time.

Your participation in this project is voluntary. You have the right to withdraw at any time without penalty (i.e., status, grades, care, etc.) We realize that your time is valuable and have attempted to keep the requested information as brief and concise as possible.

There are no known risks . . . (the risks are) to your participation in the study. (If the questions are of a sensitive nature, you may wish to give them the option of not answering the ones they find upsetting).

The benefits to you in participating in the study are . . . (There are no direct benefits).

Your responses are confidential. When the data are presented in written report, you will not be linked to the data by your name, title or any other identifying item.

Please assist us in our research and return the completed survey (. . . enclosed envelope, box, etc.). Your consent is implied by the return of the completed questionnaire.

If you have any questions, now or later, you may contact us at the number below. If you have any questions about your rights as a human subject, please contact the Human Subjects Committee chair, [name of chair] at [phone number], or [e-mail address]. Thank you very much for your time and assistance.

Sincerely,

Project Director
Address
Phone #

[1]Developed by the Human Subjects Committee at the University of South Dakota and available on-line at http://www.usd.edu/oorsch/forms.html. (Reproduced from the University of South Dakota Web site at http://www.usd.edu/oorsch/forms.html)

CHAPTER

Data Analysis and Statistics

> *Statistical interpretation depends not only on statistical ideas, but also on "ordinary" thinking. Clear thinking is not only indispensable in interpreting statistics, but is often sufficient even in the absence of specific statistical knowledge.*
> —W. A. Wallis and H. V. Roberts,
> *The Nature of Statistics* (p. 29)

Operational Learning Objectives
At the end of this chapter the learner will

1. Define statistics
2. Describe the importance of statistics in contemporary society
3. Understand the difference between descriptive and inferential statistics
4. Understand the concept of measurement and data
5. Understand the difference between discrete and continuous data
6. Identify seven statistical models for analyzing clinical research data
7. Distinguish between parametric and nonparametric statistical tests
8. Understand when to apply specific statistical tests to clinical research designs

8.1 Definition and Meaning of Statistics

Statistics, as a practical discipline, is defined as the application of statistical tests and procedures for organizing, analyzing, and interpreting results or data according to mathematical formulas. Statistics is taught in almost every university and college in the United States. Although statistics is derived from mathematics, it is taught in many academic departments with application to economics; agriculture; medicine; natural, physical, and social science; nursing; the allied health professions; and education. The rapid evolution of mainframe and personal computers has expanded the role of statistics to almost every aspect of our lives including banking, retailing, education, manufacturing, farming, politics, communication, transportation, and health care. Through the availability of modems and electronic mail, statistical programs and databases are easily accessible to researchers. Computer programs using sophisticated statistical models have enabled poll-sters to predict election results based on representative sampling procedures and insurance companies to set up actuarial tables based on the presence or absence of risk factors for morbidity and mortality.

Statistics is also an essential component of clinical research, enabling the investigator to objectively describe and infer logical conclusions from the results. In general, statistical analysis of the data strengthens the impact of the results and allows the investigator to compare current findings with previous research. The researcher in occupational therapy should have a basic understanding of descriptive statistics and the most frequently used inferential statistical tests and procedures. Inferential statistics include *t* test and analysis of variance for comparing sample means, Pearson correlation coefficient and Spearman rank order correlation for testing relationships between variables, and Chi-square for testing the differences between observed and expected frequencies. The researcher should be able to calculate the incidence (initial occurrences) and prevalence (prevailing rates) of diseases and be able to read and interpret vital statistics related to morbidity and mortality. Quantifiable or measurable data are counted as statistics. For example, the total number of individuals with a spinal cord injury, number of workers with disabilities, or the number of occupational therapists working in public schools are identifiable statistics.

Historically, the earliest statistics amassed by local authorities were census counts. Sta-tistical occurrences also replaced subjective descriptions of populations, such as "abun-dant," "flourishing," and "enormous," to describe epidemics and population density. The first use of statistics recorded factual information, such as the annual rate of births, deaths and marriages. During periods of epidemics, such as the "black death" (bubonic plague) in London during the 16th and 17th centuries, statistics were used to tabulate the number of deaths and their presumed causes. Also, tax collectors used statistics in Europe before the Middle Ages to assess wealth and agricultural holdings. In the latter half of the 18th century, census taking became a systematic governmental function. The U.S. Constitution of 1790 includes provision for a regular population census every 10 years. The application of probability theory to the prediction of death rates (actuarial tables among populations) and the use of sampling procedures advanced the science of statistics. In the mid-19th century, statistical societies were founded (e.g., the American Statistical Association was organized in Boston in 1839). Vital statistics became more accurate, and methods were developed to analyze health data and to correlate injuries and diseases with occupation and social class. The emergence of modern statistics based on probability theory led to the application of statistical methods in laboratory and clinical research. R. A. Fisher, a geneti-cist, extended statistics from small samples where inferences were made to large popula-tions. The work of Fisher and his colleagues in the early part of the 1900s led the way to quantifiable analysis of research data in the biological, physical, and social sciences. Cur-rently, hundreds of textbooks are published on the application and theory of statistics in a wide range of professional disciplines. In spite of this, the field of statistics is as much of an art as an empirical science. There are many points of disagreement on the correctness of applying specific statistical tests to research data. The student learning and applying statis-tics must decide which statistical tests are most appropriate for analyzing the results. How the variable is measured (e.g., continuous or discrete), the probability level required, and the direction of the hypothesis stated will help the researcher to select a specific statistical test. The material presented in this chapter is organized to aid the student in reading and understanding statistics presented in research articles and to follow a step-by-step proce-dure in calculating statistical results. Each step in the process of deciding on the statistical test to be employed, the analysis of the raw data, and the interpretation of the statistical results should be carried through in a problem-solving, reflective manner.

8.2 Relationship of Statistics to Clinical Practice

Statistics as a methodology enables the researcher to organize, analyze, and interpret data. In the context of a research design, statistical application does not change the quality of the data or influence the validity of the results. In conducting research, the investigator should have an overall concept of the meaning of the projected results and how a statistical test will be used to accept or reject a hypothesis. For example, an investigator wishes to compare attitudes of health professionals and nonhealth professionals toward individuals with disabilities utilizing a survey questionnaire. He or she has hypothesized that health professionals will have more positive, realistic attitudes toward individuals with disabilities than will nonhealth professionals. Then the researcher would apply a statistical test, such as an analysis of variance, to accept or reject the hypothesis.

The process of statistical analysis and its relationship to clinical practice is illustrated in Figure 8–1. In this example a clinician proposes to test the effectiveness of a specific treatment method. Six stages may be distinguished in this process:

1. A hypothesis is conceived.
2. A research plan is devised to study the effects of a treatment method or procedure traditionally used by clinicians.

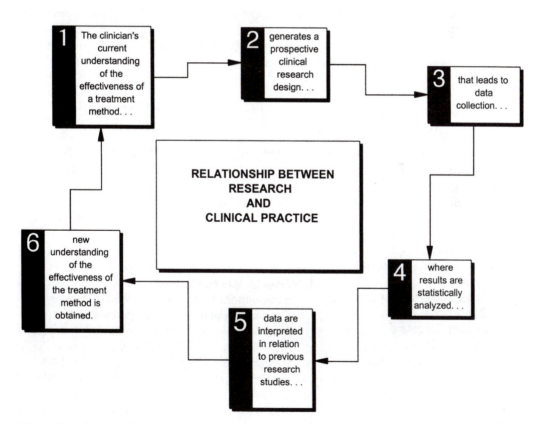

Figure 8–1. Relationship between research and clinical practice. Notice that the relationship is continuous; the completion of Step 6 leads back to Step 1. A clinician should be continually involved in practices that lead to research that can be applied to clinical practice.

3. Quantifiable data are collected from a patient group.
4. The data are statistically processed and analyzed.
5. The results are interpreted.
6. Conclusions are drawn, and the information is disseminated back to the scientific community and clinical practitioners.

The cycle continues with new treatment methods introduced and ineffective methods discarded. Hopefully, the process leads to the evolution of clinical efficacy.

This example demonstrates the importance of statistics to clinical research. What are the most common statistical procedures employed in clinical research?

Statistical procedures employed in clinical research are based on descriptive and inferential statistics. Figure 8–2 outlines the specific descriptive and inferential statistical tests.

Descriptive statistics are procedures for reducing, summarizing, and describing results or data. In descriptive statistics, for example, a large set of data are reduced to summary values, graphs, frequency polygons and scatter diagrams, measures of central tendency (mode, median, and mean), measures of variability (range, standard deviation, and variance), and incidence and prevalence rates.

Inferential statistics are methods for generalizing data collected from a representative sample to a larger target population that includes all subjects or observations. The essence of inferential statistics is to sample a representative portion of a population to infer information representative of the whole population. Inferential statistics are applied for two main purposes: (a) to estimate the characteristics of a population (parameters) and (b) to test hypotheses about populations. In inferential statistics a sample is drawn from the target population, the characteristics of this sample are measured, and inferences or estimates about the corresponding characteristics are made to the population at large.

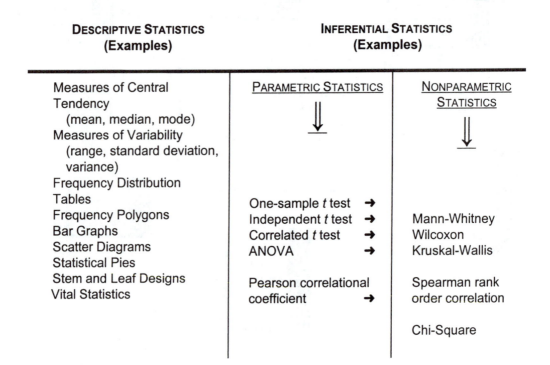

Figure 8–2. Statistical procedures and tests used in the analysis of data.

A *parameter* is a descriptive value attributed to population. Parameters are usually unknown. For example, in the population of individuals with spinal cord injury in North America, the parameter value of age would be inferred or estimated because it would be almost impossible to survey all individuals in North America who have spinal cord injury. The parameter value is usually estimated through descriptive studies of representative samples in more than one geographical area. The data from a representative sample are extrapolated to the target population. The reliability of the estimate increases with the number of descriptive studies that show concurrence.

A *statistic* is a quantitative measure of a sample. For example, the average heart rate of a sample of college students is 72 beats per minute. This is a statistic with a summary value representing the average heart rate in the sample. When a total population is available and every individual is measured, a parameter value may be computed directly. Population data usually are not available, so that researchers use a representative sample drawn from a population to compute a statistic and employ inferential statistics to estimate or extrapolate parameter values. Vital statistics are used to estimate the incidence or prevalence rates of a specific disability in a population. For example, if an investigator is interested in determining the number of individuals with a diagnosis of muscular dystrophy in the United States, he or she can carry out epidemiological studies with representative samples in specified geographic areas such as in the Midwestern states. Frequently, epidemiological studies are replicated in other geographical areas to test the validity of previous results and to monitor trends in the incidence and prevalence rates of specific diseases.

8.2.1 The Process of Statistical Analysis

The important steps for researchers are to develop a hypothesis, select the appropriate statistical test, calculate the results, and finally interpret the data. The decision process in applying statistics and interpreting the results is shown diagrammatically in Figure 8–3.

8.3 Key Definitions of Statistical Concepts

The first step in understanding statistics is to understand the definitions of statistical terms. With a conceptual understanding of statistics, one can critically understand published studies that use statistical designs. The bases on which hypotheses are substantiated or rejected and on which conclusions are generated are derived from a statistical analysis of the results. The following definitions are essential to understand statistics. They are listed alphabetically and are intended to be used as a reference aid.

▶ *Continuous variables* are examples of interval or ratio scale measurement. Weight, height, age, muscle strength, blood pressure, and hearing acuity are all examples of continuous variables. It is assumed that, in measuring continuous variables, there are an infinite number of values between each pair of scores.

▶ *Data* are the numerical results of a study. In a descriptive study of a population, data are enumerated totals, such as the number of emergency patients in a hospital clinic or the number of health care workers in a rural area. Descriptive statistics of populations, such as the mean and median, are data. In small sample research in which inferential (probability) statistics are used, data represent comparative results derived from the research. These results are the bases of discussion and interpretation. The singular of data is datum or statistic.

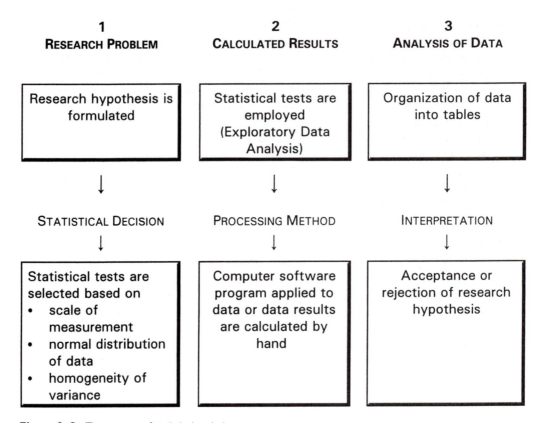

Figure 8–3. The process of statistical analysis.

▶ *Degrees of freedom (df)* is a mathematically derived value used in reading statistical tables. It is *usually* calculated by subtracting 1 from the total number (N) of subjects in a group. It is defined as the number of observations in the calculation of a statistic that are free to vary.

▶ *Dichotomous variables* contain only two subsets, such as male and female subjects, improvement or no improvement, experimental and control group, or any other two variable sets created by the investigator or found naturally.

▶ *Discrete variables* identify separate categories, such as diagnostic groups, allied health professions, occupations, vitamins, pharmaceutical drugs, and treatment methods. Discrete variables belong to a set of objects sharing some trait or characteristic. They are examples of nominal scale measurements.

▶ A *directional hypothesis* predicts that:
   1. there will be a statistically significant difference in a specified direction between two groups after applying a treatment in experimental research, or
   2. there will be a statistically significant relationship (positive or inverse) between two variables.

▶ *Frequency* is the number of times that a result occurs. A frequency distribution table of results describes the number of times a variable falls into a discrete category.

▶ *Measures of central tendency* are descriptive statistics—such as the mean, median, and mode—that measure the center or location of a data distribution.

▶ *Measures of dispersion or variability* are descriptive statistics that indicate the spread of scores in a data distribution. The range, variance, and standard deviation scores are measures of dispersion. Factors such as the difference between the highest and lowest scores and the number of scores that deviate from the mean influence measures of dispersion.

▶ *Nonparametric statistics* are sometimes referred to as "distribution-free" statistical tests because they are applied to data for which no assumptions are made regarding the normal distribution of the population and interval scale measurement. The advantages of nonparametric statistics are that they can be applied to small sample data without having to meet the stringent assumptions of parametric statistics. Examples of nonparametric tests include Chi-square, Spearman rho, Mann-Whitney test, Wilcoxon test for correlated samples, and Kruskal-Wallis test.

▶ The *normal curve or bell-shaped distribution* represents a theoretical distribution that approximates the range and frequency of many normal human functions and anatomical descriptions, such as blood pressure, lung capacity, height, and weight. The major assumption underlying the concept of a normal curve is that variables are distributed along a continuum with the greatest frequency in the middle and the least frequency at the outer edges of the distribution. Figure 8–4 indicates the percentage of cases found within each area of the normal curve. For example, 68% of cases are distributed toward the center of the curve in a symmetrical pattern. The basis of inferential parametric statistics rests on the assumption that the sample data are derived from a population that is normally distributed.

▶ A *null hypothesis* predicts that there will be no statistically significant difference or correlation between two or more specified groups, that is, after experimentally manipulating a variable or when testing the relationships between variables.

▶ *Parametric statistics* are applied to data in which certain underlying assumptions have been made. These are:
  1. The variables measured approximate a normal distribution curve in the target population sampled.
  2. The sample is a random selection or is representative of the target population.
  3. The variables are measured by an interval scale; that is, there is equal arithmetical distance between each value or scores.
  4. The variance, such as the standard deviation, within the compared groups are approximately the same.

  Examples of parametric statistics are *t* test, analysis of variance (ANOVA), and Pearson product-moment correlation coefficient.

▶ A *research hypothesis* is a prediction of results.

▶ *Standard deviation* is a statistical measure of the dispersion of scores from the mean.

▶ *Standard error of measurement (SEM)* is a statistical value that indicates the band of error surrounding a test score. For example, a raw score of 90 with a *SEM* of 4 represents a score ranging from 86 to 94.

▶ *Statistical assumptions* are preconditions that are required before a specific statistical test can be applied. These assumptions usually involve the following factors:
  1. The variable distributed in a population approximates the normal curve. For example, muscle strength, intelligence, systolic blood pressure, and height are variables that are assumed to approximate a normal curve in a standard population.

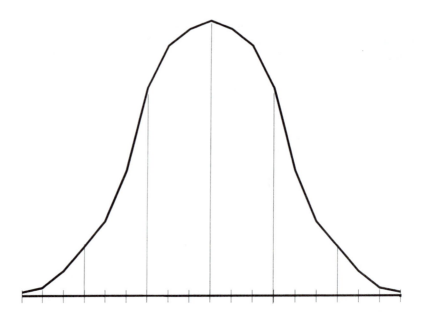

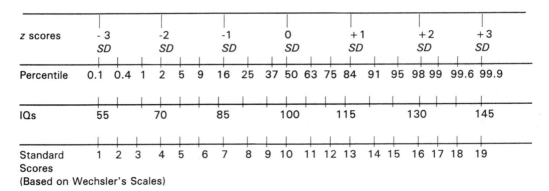

| z scores | -3 SD | -2 SD | -1 SD | 0 SD | +1 SD | +2 SD | +3 SD |

Percentile   0.1 0.4 1   2   5   9   16   25   37 50 63 75 84   91   95 98 99 99.6 99.9

IQs   55   70   85   100   115   130   145

Standard Scores
(Based on Wechsler's Scales)   1 2 3   4 5   6 7   8 9 10 11 12 13 14 15 16 17 18 19

Figure 8–4. The bell-shaped curve, which illustrates the percentage of population at each level. Included in this figure are the relationships between the standard deviations (*z* scores), percentiles, IQ scores, and standard scores (based on Wechsler's scaled scores).

2. The data collected are measurable. Some statistical tests require interval scale data, whereas other tests allow for ordinal or nominal scale data.
3. There is a homogeneity of variance within the group scores. Large differences in standard deviations of two groups present some difficulty, although it is unclear what constitutes a large difference. Some statisticians (Welkowitz, Ewen, & Cohen, 1971) have recommended ignoring this assumption if the two sample sizes are equal (and there are no vast differences between the standard deviations) when applying the *t* test.
4. The sample is randomly selected from a population. The object of random sampling is to obtain an unbiased sample that is to be truly representative of a population. The difficulty in obtaining a true random sample when applied

to clinical research is that it is almost impossible to identify and locate a population, such as all individuals diagnosed with diabetes, arthritis, or schizophrenia and then select a random sample from this population. The most prevalent sample in clinical research is the convenient sample accessible to the researcher, such as in a teaching hospital, university, public school, or outpatient clinic. It is possible, however, to assign random samples from a convenient population, such as hospital patients, who can be randomly assigned to experimental and control groups.

5. The groups compared are independent of each other.

▶ *Statistical tables* contain critical levels and values of probability for accepting or rejecting a hypothesis. By using a statistical table, the investigator determines whether the statistical value obtained is significant compared with the critical value. Using statistical tables, the investigator decides the level of significance, such as .05 or .01.

▶ *Statistically significant results* means that there are differences between two or more groups that are not due to chance. In every statistically significant result, there is a comparison between the effects on two or more groups.

• *Experimental Clinical Research:* In clinical research, statistically significant results are traditionally accepted at the .05 level or .01 level, which means that the results are not due to chance in 95 out of 100 cases or 99 out of 100 cases. In using the concept of statistical significance, the investigator performing experimental clinical research assumes an explanation that is sometimes confusing to students who think that statistics is an exact science that can be used to determine cause-and-effect relationships. Conclusive cause-and-effect relationships are only meaningful when an investigator can control every variable that may affect the results. The closest that medical research comes to the control of extraneous variables is in experimental animal research where environmental and sometimes genetic factors can be rigorously controlled. In clinical research with human subjects, it is almost impossible to attain results that are 100% conclusive because of the interactional effects between the therapist, patient, treatment method, and environment. Inferential statistics, which are based on probability theory, are applied to data derived from samples of populations so that everyone in a population is not tested or measured. Samples per se indicate inconclusive data and an uncertainty even if a representative sample has been selected. In summary, a statistically significant result in experimental clinical research implies the following:

1. Probability theory is assumed in interpreting the data.

2. A sample of population is used rather than the entire population.

3. There is an allowance for error based on a researcher's inability to control all variables that may possibly influence the results.

4. Conclusiveness of results is not assumed, and the investigator can only suggest that a cause-effect relationship exists.

▶ *Test of statistical significance* is based on the characteristics of the normal curve and probability theory.

1. *Two-tailed tests of statistical significance* are used in analyzing data if the researcher has stated the hypothesis in a null form.

2. *One-tailed tests of statistical significance* imply that the researcher has predicted a directional hypothesis, and there is prior evidence, either through a literature review or clinical observation, that there will be a statistically significant difference between the groups or a statistically positive correlation between variables.

▶ *Variables* are factors that can be operationally defined, categorized, and measured. Variables can be homogeneous groups, such as undergraduate university students, patients with hemiplegia, or hospital administrators. Variables are also conditions or behavior such as group therapy, cardiovascular disease, or ADL training. In experimental research, the *independent variable*, which is manipulated by the investigator, is the direct cause of the *dependent variable*, which is the resultant effect. Variables can be discrete, dichotomous, rank order, or continuous. (Also refer to Chapter 7, Research Design and Methodology, for further discussion about variables.)

▶ *Variance* is a measure of the average of each score's deviation from the mean. Variance is an intermediate value used in calculating the standard deviation.

8.3.1 Universal Symbols Used in Statistics

α alpha, associated with hypothesis testing, the probability of a Type I error

β beta, associated with hypothesis testing and the chance of a Type II error

χ^2 Chi-square statistical test

df degrees of freedom

f frequency of cases in a distribution

F statistic associated with analysis of variance (ANOVA)

μ mu, the population or parameter mean; oftentimes, this value is unknown and estimated by the mean

H_0 null hypothesis or the concept that there is no statistically significant relationship between two or more variables (e.g., $\mu_1 = \mu_2$)

H_1 alternative hypothesis, opposite of null hypothesis (e.g., $\mu_1 \neq \mu_2$)

n number of subjects within a designated sample

N total of number of subjects in a group or population

p probability of a chance occurrence

$p\text{-}value$ obtained or observed significance value; for example, if $p < \alpha$, H_0 is rejected

r the Pearson product-moment correlation coefficient indicating the degree of relationship between two variables or two sets of data

r_s the Spearman rank order correlation for ordinal data (formerly rho [ρ])

s the standard deviation of a sample (SD)

σ lowercase sigma, the standard deviation of a population, usually estimated by s

Σ uppercase sigma, sum of an arithmetic calculation

t t test statistic

t_{obs}	*t* observed, *t* value derived from the *t* test
t_{crit}	*t* critical, the value derived from a statistical table of values found through α levels
z	standard score measured in standard deviation units
$\neq$	not equal to
$\geq$	more than or equal to
$\leq$	less than or equal to
$\overline{X}$	the mean value of a sample

8.4 Seven Statistical Models for Clinical Research

Seven statistical models for analyzing data are outlined in Table 8–1. These models represent the most frequently used statistical tests for clinical researchers. The format in presenting each model is to define the model and the statistical tests that the models represent, analyze an example of the statistical test from the literature, outline sequential steps in calculating the statistical results, and follow through with a hypothetical stepwise example. Many statistical tests are not covered in these models. References to textbooks on statistics are provided throughout the chapter as a guide for those researchers inspired to further explore the world of statistics. As one becomes adept in using statistical software programs for personal computers, the options for selecting statistical tests broaden. First it is important for the clinical researcher to understand the concepts underlying the statistical applications, however. Doing statistical tests with a hand calculator and doing exploratory data analysis aids the researcher to better understand statistical processes that are done later through computer software programs.

8.4.1 Model I: Descriptive Statistics

In this model, the researcher calculates descriptive statistics based on data collected from a representative sample or the total population. The statistical procedures include:

► Frequency distribution tables
► Frequency polygons
► Histograms and bar graphs
► Scatter diagrams
► Statistical pies
► Stem and leaf
► Measures of central tendency
► Measures of variability
► Vital statistics

8.4.2 Model II: One-Sample Problems

The purpose of this statistical model is to compare data collected from a representative sample of a population and then to compare the obtained value with a parameter value that is known or estimated or to a standard value. Examples include comparing air

Table 8–1. Seven Statistical Models

	Statistical Model	Purpose	Examples of Statistical Tests or Procedures
I.	**Descriptive Statistics**	Describe the statistical characteristics in samples or populations	Measures of central tendency (mean, mode, median), measures of variability (range, standard deviation, variance), frequency distribution table, frequency graph, scatter diagram, statistical pie, stem and leaf, vital statistics
	Inferential Statistics		
II.	One-sample	Test the difference between a sample mean and a parameter mean	One-sample *t* test
III.	Two independent samples	Test the differences between sample means from two independent groups	Independent *t* test (parametric statistic) Mann-Whitney *U* test (nonparametric statistic)
IV.	Paired-data sample	Test the differences between two conditions (means) in the same sample	Correlated *t* test (parametric statistic) Wilcoxon signed rank test (nonparametric statistic)
V.	*k*-independent samples	Test the differences between means from two or more independent groups	ANOVA (parametric statistic) Kruskal-Wallis (nonparametric statistic)
VI.	Correlation	Test the relationship between two variables	Spearman rank order (nonparametric statistic), Pearson correlation coefficient (parametric statistic), regression line, correlation matrix
VII.	Observed frequencies	Test the differences between observed minus expected frequencies	Chi-square (nonparametric statistic)

Note. Adapted from *Statistics for the Allied Health Sciences* by R. J. Larson, 1975, Columbus, OH: Merrill Publishing. Copyright 1975 by Merrill Publishing.

samples from a metropolitan area to a standard accepted for clean air. The research question that this model answers is whether the mean of the representative sample and the established parameter mean value are statistically significantly different. The statistical procedure for this model is the one-sample *t* test.

8.4.3 Model III: Two Independent Samples

The purpose of this statistical model is to test whether the means for two representative samples are statistically significantly different. An example in clinical research is determining whether one treatment method (such as sensory integration therapy) is more effective in reducing hyperactivity than a comparable treatment method (such as relaxation therapy) in two independent groups. The statistical test (independent *t* test) is applied to determine whether there is a statistically significant difference between the two treatment methods. The Mann-Whitney nonparametric statistical test is another example used to evaluate data using this model.

8.4.4 Model IV: Paired-Data Sample

The primary purpose of this statistical model is to examine the difference between mean values in one sample group with two data points, such as pretest and posttest. This statistical model employs the correlated *t* test to test whether there will be a statistically significant difference between the means in two conditions. This statistical model is frequently used in clinical research to determine if a treatment method is effective when compared to a baseline measure of a dependent variable. The Wilcoxon nonparametric statistical test is an alternative to the parametric one-sample correlated *t* test.

8.4.5 Model V: Independent Samples

If the researcher is comparing the means of more than two independent samples, then he or she applies an analysis of variance (ANOVA). The ANOVA is similar to the independent test when two independent samples are compared. If the results of the ANOVA are statistically significant, then the researcher employs post-hoc tests to determine which groups are statistically different from each other. These post-hoc tests (similar to *t* tests) include the Scheffé, Duncan multiple analysis, or Tukey tests. The nonparametric alternative to ANOVA is the Kruskal-Wallis statistical test.

8.4.6 Model VI: Correlational Sample

In this statistical model, the researcher measures the degree of relationship between two variables, such as in a study examining the relationship between perceptual motor skills and functional abilities in self-care. The relationship can range from zero, indicating that the two variables are completely independent and do not affect each other, to 1.00, indicating a perfect relationship between two variables. An example of a perfect correlation is the effect of temperature on the expansion of the chemical element mercury. As the temperature goes up, mercury expands; as the temperature goes down, mercury contracts. A perfect correlation can be positive ($+1.00$) when both variables change in the same direction, or it can be negative or inverse (-1.00) when the variables change in inverse directions (i.e., as one variable goes up, the other variable goes down). An example of an inverse relationship is the presence of serotonin, a neurotransmitter, and symptoms of depression. As serotonin is depleted in the blood, the symptoms of depression increase.

The relationship between two variables can be described in a scatter diagram. The Pearson correlation coefficient for interval scale data and the Spearman rank order correlation for ordinal scale data are applied to evaluate the degree of relationship (r) between two variables. A regression line can be calculated when there is a high correlation between two variables. The regression line is calculated by using the results of the Pearson correlation coefficient and plugging the values into a formula for the regression line. In this formula, variable values are estimated from known X variable values. This is illustrated in Figure 8–5.

8.4.7 Model VII: Observed Minus Expected Frequencies

In this model, the investigator compares groups or conditions on the basis of frequency or nominal data. Chi-square is the statistical test used when comparing the differences between observed frequencies and expected frequencies based on probability. Chi-square is used frequently, for example, in drug research to compare the differences in the number of patients who have improved with an experimental drug as compared with the number of patients taking a placebo who have improved.

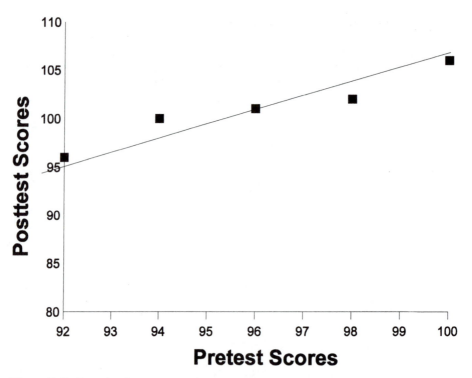

Figure 8–5. Example of a scattergram showing the relationship between two variables. When the value of X is known, then the value of Y can be predicted by the use of the regression line.

8.5 Model I: Descriptive Statistics: Organization and Tabulation of Descriptive Data

8.5.1 Table of Percentage

Statistical analysis begins with organizing data into summary tables and diagrams. In descriptive studies as in survey research, tabular summaries of data provide the results. For example, Table 8–2 summarizes data from interviews with 115 elderly residents in a nursing home regarding their risk for falling.

The table reports the percentage of the 115 residents who replied "yes" to the interview questions. An alternative way of describing data is to list the actual frequency of responses rather than convert the frequency to percentages. For example, 96% or 110 of the residents use eyeglasses and only 6% or 7 of the subjects always or most of the time are dizzy on arising.

Another method of displaying data is to compare results between periods of time, distances, or events. In Table 8–3, the researchers examine the relationship between the stage of illness at diagnosis (whether the cancer is localized or has spread throughout the body) and the distances in kilometers (k) that a patient lives from the Three Mile Island nuclear plant. Data were collected from a review of patient charts at all local and regional hospitals.

In examining the results, one notes that pre- versus postpercentages of selected cancers are listed at three categories of distance from the patients' homes to the nuclear plant, (i.e., 0–6 k, 6–12 k, and more than 12 k). Data were collected from 1975 to 1979 (prenuclear

Table 8–2. Subjects' Reported Fall Risk Factors

Fall Risk Factor	% of Subjects Reporting
Health compared with peers	
Excellent	7
Good	57
Fair	28
Poor	8
Use eyeglasses	96
Always/Most of the time	55
Use walking aid	38
Always/Most of the time	20
Dizzy on arising	31
Always/Most of the time	6
Pain in muscles, bones, joints	80
Always/Most of the time	45
Hold on for support	30
Always/Most of the time	13
Difficult to get in and out of bed	16
Always/Most of the time	4
Use prescription medication	80
Use alcohol	43
One a week or more	7
Stand on chair to reach	56
Have grab bars in bathroom	85
Breathless	54
Always/Most of the time	23

Note. From "Falls and Fear of Falling among Elderly Persons Living in the Community" by J. E. Walker and J. Howland, 1991, *American Journal of Occupational Therapy, 45*, p. 120. Copyright 1991 by *American Journal of Occupational Therapy.* Reprinted with permission.

accident) and 1979 through 1985 (postnuclear accident). Based on the data presented in Table 8–3, the authors concluded that a modest postaccident increase in cancer was observed. The reader will note that of the 36 possible results (12 cancer sites × 3 distance categories), there were 21 increased percentages from pre to post, while 15 of the results showed decreased percentages from preaccident to postaccident.

The above examples demonstrate the importance of descriptive statistics in summarizing results from a research study. A number of methods can be used to describe data. The most frequently used descriptive methods for organizing data are discussed in the following section.

8.5.2 Frequency Distribution Table

A *frequency distribution table* is organized into columns of data that include the number or frequency of cases (and the equivalent percentages) that fall into a designated category. In the research study in Table 8–4, a frequency distribution table describes the age and gender of the population sampled in the study.

The first column of a frequency distribution table includes the class intervals (in this example, age group by years). It could also represent data such as range of motion in degrees, scores on perceptual tests, or diastolic blood pressure. The class intervals are separated into equal 10-year intervals in the above example (e.g., 15–24 and 25–34). The second column of a frequency distribution includes the number of classes tallied within the class intervals as with 36 males between the ages of 5 and 14. The third column includes the percentage of cases within a class interval. For example, there are 52 females in the class interval of 25 to 34, which represents 52 over a total of 228 females in the study of 22.8%, which is rounded to 23%. We can also determine the *cumulative frequency* of each class interval and the *cumulative relative frequency* with the data provided in the study. The following data are reorganized into a frequency distribution table to include relative frequency and cumulative relative frequency for males only:

Class Interval	Frequency (f)	Relative f (%)	Cumulative f	Cumulative rf (%)
5–14	36	6	36	6
15–24	147	24	183	30
25–34	200	33	383	63
35–44	105	17	488	80
45–54	60	10	548	90
55–64	41	7	589	97
>65	21	3	610	100
Unknown	4	.006	614	100
Total	**614**	**100%**	**614**	**100%**

Frequency Distribution Table for Males

In summary:

▶ *Class interval* is the category of score values in a distribution. The number of class intervals is determined by the number of subjects in the study and the range of values or scores.
▶ *Frequency of cases* include the total number of cases within an assigned class interval.
▶ *Relative frequency* or *percentage* is the percentage of cases falling within the class interval and is calculated by dividing the number of cases within the class interval by the total number of cases in the distribution.
▶ *Cumulative frequency* represents the total number of scores within a class interval that is added cumulatively from the lowest to the highest class interval. The

Table 8–3. Example of a Frequency Distribution

Stage of Diagnosis	0–6 k pre vs. post		> 6–12 k pre vs. post		> 12 k pre vs. post	
Breast Cancer						
Local	39.3	40.4	39.4	51.8	46.0	48.5
Regional	52.6	42.5	31.3	30.7	32.2	36.5
Distant	8.2	17.0	29.1	17.8	21.7	15.0
Prostate Cancer						
Local	62.2	41.7	56.1	59.8	53.3	60.9
Regional	9.0	13.5	20.2	10.7	17.7	15.6
Distant	29.8	44.9	23.7	29.5	29.0	23.5
Lung Cancer						
Local	30.7	36.9	37.5	24.0	23.6	26.7
Regional	23.9	16.9	13.6	26.2	29.4	25.5
Distant	45.4	46.4	48.9	49.8	47.0	47.9
Colon Cancer						
Local	29.7	39.3	30.9	29.1	27.0	30.8
Regional	43.9	29.9	31.7	34.7	35.9	36.2
Distant	26.4	30.8	37.4	36.2	37.1	33.0

Note: From "Cancer Rates after the Three Mile Island Nuclear Accident and Proximity of Residents to the Plant" by M. C. Hatch, S. Wallenstein, J. Beyen, J. W. Nieves, and M. Susser, 1991, *American Journal of Public Health, 81,* p. 723. Copyright 1991 by *American Journal of Public Health.* Reprinted with permission.

Table 8–4. Age and Sex Distribution of Migrant Survey Population

Age Group (Years)	Male No.	Male (%)	Female No.	Female (%)	Total No.	Total (%)
5–14	36	6	31	14	67	8
15–24	147	24	75	33	222	26
25–34	200	33	52	23	252	30
35–44	105	17	29	13	134	16
45–54	60	10	24	11	84	10
55–64	41	7	10	4	51	6
65+	21	3	6	3	27	3
Unknown	4	0	1	0	5	0
Total	**614**	**100**	**228**	**(101)***	**842**	**99**

*totals differ from 100% due to rounding

Note. From "Tuberculosis Risk among Migrant Farm Workers on the Relmarva Peninsula" by M. L. Jacobson, M. A. Mercer, L. K. Miller, and T. W. Simpson, 1987, *American Journal of Public Health, 77,* p. 30. Copyright 1987 by *American Journal of Public Health.* Reprinted with permission.

grand total of the cumulative frequency equals the total number of scores or cases in the distribution.

▶ *Cumulative relative frequency* or *cumulative percentage* is the percentage of cases added from the lowest class interval through the highest class interval. The percentage should total 100%.

Constructing a Frequency Distribution Table

The table below displays hypothetical ungrouped raw scores on resting heart rate for 50 healthy young adults.

Step 1. Record raw scores from ungrouped data.

Subject	Score	Subject	Score	Subject	Score	Subject	Score
01	54	14	67	27	54	40	79
02	72	15	74	28	73	41	85
03	80	16	76	29	72	42	52
04	53	17	79	30	78	43	56
05	75	18	77	31	78	44	67
06	53	19	48	32	56	45	55
07	78	20	76	33	80	46	79
08	47	21	47	34	84	47	81
09	72	22	50	35	72	48	72
10	54	23	65	36	68	49	67
11	66	24	83	37	57	50	71
12	68	25	55	38	57		
13	68	26	76	39	63		

Step 2. Identify the highest and lowest values in the distribution. Subjects 08 and 21 have heart rate scores of 47 (lowest score). Subject 41 has a heart rate score of 85 (highest score).

Step 3. Calculate the range (highest score to lowest score). In our example, the range is 85 − 47 = 38.

Step 4. Determine the number of class intervals. The determination of the number of class intervals depends on the number of scores in the frequency distribution and the range of scores. Too many or too few class intervals may not give adequate information to describe the distribution. Determining the number of class intervals is a trial-and-error process. For example, compare three frequency distributions using the same scores but with class intervals of too many, too few, and approximately correct. These data are shown in Table 8–5. Most researchers constructing frequency distributions establish 6 to 15 class intervals as a general rule.

Step 5. Determine the size of a class interval. The size of the class interval is determined through estimation by dividing the range of scores by the number of class intervals. Using the same example, the range of 38 is divided by 13 (the number of class intervals) to yield a class interval size of 3. It is recommended that an odd number be selected for the class interval so that the midpoint of the class interval is a whole number. For example, the midpoint of the class interval of 83–85 is 84. Later, in calculating group means from a

Table 8–5. Intervals for Class Data

Number of Class Intervals (CI)		
Too Many (20 CI)	**Too Few (4 CI)**	**Approximate Correct (13 CI)**
84–85	75–85	83–85
82–83	65–74	80–82
80–81	55–64	77–79
78–79	45–54	74–76
76–77		71–73
74–75		68–70
72–73		65–67
70–71		62–64
68–69		59–61
66–67		56–58
64–65		53–55
62–63		50–52
60–61		47–49
58–59		
56–57		
54–55		
52–53		
50–51		
48–49		
46–47		

frequency distribution table, the reader will find that it is easier to work with whole numbers than with fractions in calculating values.

On the other hand, if we determine that the size of a class interval in the previous example is 5, how many class intervals would be established? In this case the range of scores (38) is divided by the size of the class intervals (5) to arrive at 8 class intervals.

CI	Midpoint
81–85	83
76–80	78
71–75	73
66–70	68
61–65	63

(continued)

CI	Midpoint
56–60	58
51–55	53
46–50	48

Step 6. Tally the number of scores within each class interval. Check to determine if the number of tallies total up to the number of scores in the frequency distribution.

Class Interval	Real Limits*	Midpoint	Tally	f	cf
83–85	82.5–85.5	84	|||	3	50
80–82	79.5–82.5	81	|||	3	47
77–79	76.5–79.5	78	|||||||	7	44
74–76	73.5–76.5	75	|||||	5	37
71–73	70.5–73.5	72	|||||||	7	32
68–70	67.5–70.5	69	||	2	25
65–67	64.5–67.5	66	||||||	6	23
62–64	61.5–64.5	63			1	17
59–61	58.5–61.5	6	0	0	16
56–58	55.5–58.5	57	||||	4	16
53–55	52.5–55.5	54	|||||||	7	12
50–52	49.5–52.5	51	||	2	5
47–49	46.5–49.5	48	|||	3	3
Total				**50**	**50**

*Defining the upper and lower real limits of the class intervals is described below.

The upper real limit of a class interval is the highest value contained in the interval. Conversely, the lower real limit of a class interval is the lowest value contained in the interval. In dealing with numbers having at least two decimals, round the number up to include it in the nearest class interval. For example, 82.50 or above would be tallied in the class interval 83–85. On the other hand, 82.44 would be tallied into the class interval 80–82 as shown in the example.

Step 7. Determine the relative frequency or percentage. Calculate the relative frequency of the scores in each class interval by dividing the number of cases or scores in the class interval by the number of cases in the frequency distribution. This is illustrated in Table 8–6.

$$\text{Percentage} = \frac{\text{Frequency of cases in the class interval}}{\text{Total cases in the frequency distribution}}$$

Step 8. Determine cumulative frequency. Calculate the cumulative frequency by adding the total frequency in each class interval consecutively from the highest class interval to the low-

Table 8–6. Calculation of Cumulative Frequency

Class Interval	Frequency	Percentage	Cumulative Percentage
84	3	3/50 = 6%	100%
81	3	3/50 = 6%	94%
78	7	7/50 = 14%	88%
75	5	5/50 = 10%	74%
72	7	7/50 = 14%	64%
69	2	2/50 = 4%	50%
66	6	6/50 = 12%	46%
63	1	1/50 = 2%	34%
60	0	0/50 = 0%	32%
57	4	4/50 = 8%	32%
54	7	7/50 = 14%	24%
51	2	2/50 = 4%	10%
48	3	3/50 = 6%	6%
Total	50	50/50 = 100%	100%

est. In the previous example, the number of cases in the class interval 83–85 is 3. This number is added to the number of cases in the class interval 80–82, which is also 3, giving a cumulative frequency of 6. The completed frequency distribution table is shown in Table 8–7.

Summary of Construction of Frequency Distribution Table

1. Organize raw scores from ungrouped data by arranging values from the lowest to the highest scores.
2. Identify the lowest and highest scores in the distribution.
3. Calculate the range, which is the difference or distance from the lowest to the highest scores in the distribution.
4. Determine the number of class intervals, using the rule of thumb of selecting within a range of six to fifteen categories of intervals.
5. Determine the size of each class interval. First estimate the size of class intervals by dividing the range by the number of class intervals. Try to select an odd number so that the midpoint of the class interval will be a whole number.
6. Count or tally the number of scores within each class interval.
7. Calculate the relative frequency or percentage of scores in each class interval.
8. Calculate the cumulative frequency by adding in succession the frequencies in each class interval. Check that the number of cases counted in succession is equal to the total number of cases or scores in the distribution.
9. Determine the cumulative relative frequency, which is the percentage of cumulative frequency sitting in each class interval. It is customary to start from the lowest class interval when calculating cumulative values.

Table 8–7. Frequency Distribution of Heart Rate Scores for Hypothetical Population

CI	Midpoint	f	cf	rf %	crf %
83–85	84	3	50	6	100
80–82	81	3	47	6	94
77–79	78	7	47	14	88
74–76	75	5	37	10	74
71–73	72	7	32	14	64
68–70	69	2	25	4	50
65–67	66	6	23	12	46
62–64	63	1	17	2	34
59–61	60	0	16	0	32
56–58	57	4	16	8	32
53–55	54	7	12	14	24
50–52	51	2	5	4	10
47–49	48	3	3	6	6

8.5.3 Graphs and Other Pictorial Representations

In addition to presenting data in tables, many researchers use pictorial presentations to display results and describe data. These presentations can be in the form of frequency polygons, histographs, bar graphs, pie graphs, and stem and leaf.

8.5.4 Frequency Polygon

A frequency polygon is a line graph displaying the frequency of data by categories. The categories compared are on the horizontal axis (abscissa), and the frequencies of occurrences are on the vertical axis (ordinate).

The frequency polygon in Figure 8–6 shows the number of coronary artery bypass surgeries performed in Ontario for the years 1979, 1981, 1983, and 1985. The age group categories are listed on the X axis, the abscissa. Note that usually the midpoint of the category is used as a reference point for plotting the frequencies within each category. In this example, the age categories range from 20 to 49, through 70 and above. The age groups of 50–54, 55–59, 60–64, and 65–69 have an interval of 5 years, and the first age grouping includes those from 20 to 49, an interval of 30 years. The investigators collapsed the data for this age group because so few bypass surgeries were performed on persons of 20 through 49 years. Surgeries were also infrequent for those age 70 and above. The frequency of cases is shown on the ordinate, or Y axis. In this example, the investigators transformed the actual numbers into rates per 100,000 of the population. For example, in the age group 55–59, 150 per 100,000 of this population in Ontario had artery bypass surgery in 1981. Equal intervals of 50 per 100,000 were selected by researchers to indicate categories of frequency.

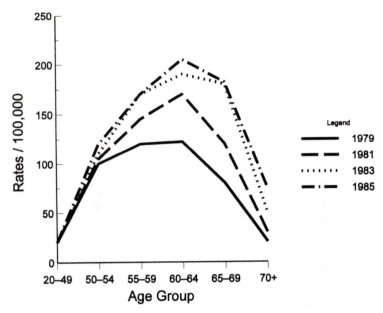

Figure 8–6. Age-specific rates of coronary artery bypass surgery illustrated in a frequency polygon. From "Monitoring the Difusion of Technology: Coronary Artery Bypass Surgery in Ontario" by G. M. Anderson and J. L. Lomas, 1988, *American Journal of Public Health, 78*, p. 252. Copyright 1988 by *American Journal of Public Health*. Reprinted with permission.

8.5.5 Histograms and Bar Graphs

Histograms and bar graphs are often used by investigators to display frequency of data within categories, similar to frequency polygons. In histograms, the bars are attached to each other as in Figure 8–7, whereas in bar graphs, each bar is detached from one another. The distinction sometimes is based on aesthetic reasons. The histogram shown in Figure 8–7 describes the type of activities in which occupational therapy students participated while completing their level 1 fieldwork experiences. On the abscissa is the type of fieldwork experience and on the ordinate, the relative frequency or percentage of time spent in a specific activity, such as passive observer, is plotted.

Constructing a Frequency Polygon, Histogram, or Bar Graph

A frequency polygon, histogram, or bar graph graphically depicts the data provided in a frequency distribution table. The data provided in the *Frequency Distribution of Heart Rate Scores* in Table 8–7 will be used in the following examples.

    Step 1. Identify the X axis (abscissa) and the Y axis (ordinate). This is illustrated in Figure 8–8.

    Step 2. Label the abscissa descriptively. In the example in Table 8–7, the heart rate values range from the lowest score of 47 to the highest of 85. The midpoints of each class interval are located on the abscissa (Figure 8–9). The class intervals are extended on both ends to include zero frequency intervals. The lowest class interval with zero frequency is 44–46 with a midpoint of 45. The highest class interval with zero frequency is 86–88 with a midpoint of 87. There are now 15 class intervals including the zero frequency intervals.

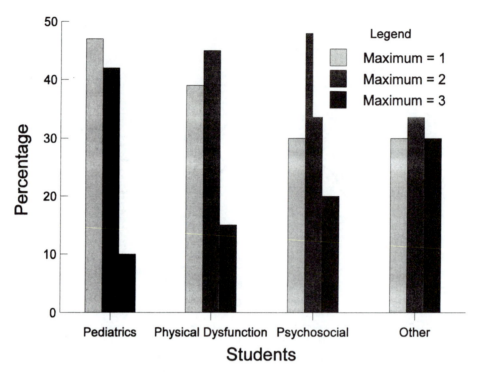

Figure 8–7. Example of a histogram depicting the maximum number of Level I fieldwork students supervised at one time in each type of facility. From "The Level I Field Work Process" by L. D. Shalik, 1990, *American Journal of Occupational Therapy, 44*, p. 702. Copyright 1990, *American Journal of Occupational Therapy.* Reprinted with permission.

Step 3. Organize the ordinate into frequency of occurrence. In the previous example, frequencies of occurrence range from 0 to 7. As a rule of thumb, the number of class intervals for frequency should be between 8 and 15. In this case, there will be 8 class intervals including 0.

The frequency polygon is depicted in Figure 8–9 with the data from Table 8–7. The histogram is depicted in Figure 8–10 with the same data used in constructing the frequency polygon. Bar graphs are similar to histograms, differing only in that the bars are detached (McCall, 1986).

8.5.6 Cumulative Frequency Distributive Polygon

A cumulative frequency distribution polygon is a line graph that shows the total number of observations or cases up to the upper real limit of a given class interval. For example, in Section 8.5.2 Step 8, determining cumulative frequency, the data for the heart rates for 50 subjects are displayed. In Figure 8–11, the cumulative frequency distribution polygon is constructed from the previous table of hypothetical heart rate values (Table 8–7).

Cumulative frequency curves are useful in specifying the individual subject's relative position or standing in a total distribution of scores. For example, someone with a heart rate of 80 in the above distribution is in the 94th percentile or upper 6% of the distribution. Cumulative frequency curves often are useful in plotting group test data, such as grip strength, range of motion, blood pressure, and achievement test scores. Individual test data plotted on a cumulative frequency curve can be used to evaluate an individual's function and diagnosis.

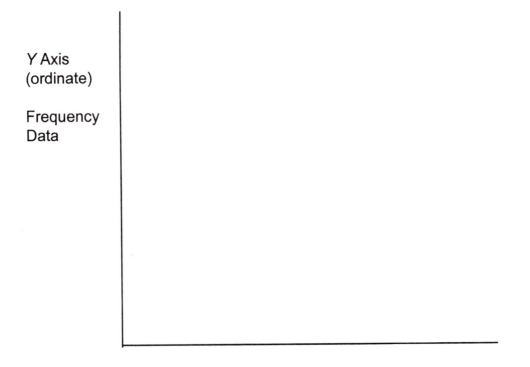

Y Axis
(ordinate)

Frequency
Data

X Axis (abscissa)
Class Intervals or Time Data

Figure 8–8. Parts of a frequency polygon, histogram, or bar graph. The frequency data are plotted along the vertical axis or ordinate (*Y* axis), while the class intervals or time data are plotted along the horizontal axis or abscissa (*X*).

In designing a cumulative frequency curve, the ordinate axis is used to display cumulative frequencies, cumulative percentages, or cumulative proportions. The abscissa shows the score values as midpoints or individual scores.

The shape of the cumulative frequency curve reflects the form or shape of the original frequency distribution. As a general rule, the cumulative frequency curve will have the greatest slope or most rapid rate of rise at the point where there is the greatest accumulation of the scores in the original frequency distribution. The cumulative frequency curve levels off and shows the lowest slope for the class intervals when there are fewer scores. Cumulative curves do not describe variations in the data as well as histograms and should not be used to draw conclusions about the form or shape of the data. The original frequency distribution is best used for this purpose.

8.5.7 Statistical Pie

A statistical pie is a pictorial representation of the relative percentage of discrete variables or nominal categories, such as health professions, distributions of disease, occupational role functions, types of work injuries, or treatment techniques applied. It is particularly useful to quickly assess the relative percentage of each category. In Figure 8–12, the

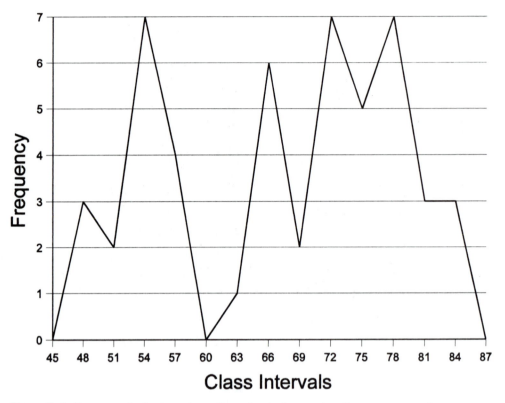

Figure 8–9. Frequency distribution polygon illustrating the frequencies of heart rate scores for a hypothetical population. The data used to plot this polygon are from Table 8–7.

percentage of placement of students with special needs in each type of educational placement is graphically displayed in a statistical pie.

Constructing a Statistical Pie

Step 1. Make sure the statistical pie is relevant for describing data. The statistical pie is appropriate when there are between 3 and 10 discrete categories. If there are more than 10 categories, the data will be better presented in a frequency distribution table. The data collected should be categorical and inclusive. For example, data collected regarding the cause of death should include all major causes for a designated population and should add up to 100%. Unknown causes should be included in the statistical pie.

Step 2. First organize data into a frequency distribution table deriving relative percentages for each category. In the hypothetical example below, specialty areas for female physicians are described. A sample of 250 female physicians were surveyed.

Medical Specialty	*Frequency*	*Relative Percent*
Pediatrics	84	33.6
Psychiatry and Neurology	34	13.7
Internal Medicine	25	10.0
Anesthesiology	23	9.1

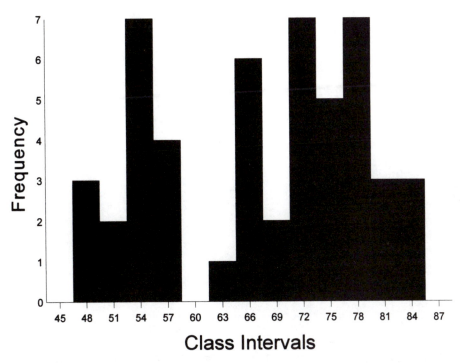

Figure 8–10. Histogram of heart scores in a hypothetical population. The data from Table 8–7 and depicted in Figure 8–9 in a frequency polygon are depicted in a histogram here.

Medical Specialty	Frequency	Relative Percent
Pathology	22	8.6
General Surgery	4	1.6
Other	58	23.4
Totals	**250**	**100**

Step 3. Transform relative percent into the degrees of a circle, which is the proportion of 360 degrees. The relative percent is multiplied by 360 degrees.

Step 4. Use a protractor and compass to construct the statistical pie. Divide the statistical pie with a protractor into seven segments running clockwise starting with the largest category at 12 o'clock, which in this example, is pediatrics (33.6% or 121°), other (23.4% or 84°), and psychiatry and neurology (13.7% or 49°). Continue with the other specialty areas in completing the 360° circle.

Step 5. Label each segment category with the relative percent rather than the degrees of arc. The completed statistical pie is shown in Figure 8–13.

8.5.8 Scatter Diagrams

A scatter diagram is a graphic representation of the relationship between two variables. In this example, the researchers graphically depict the relationship between age (presumed

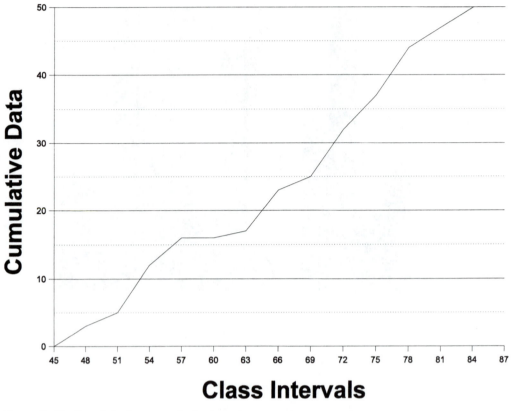

Figure 8–11. Cumulative frequency distribution polygon using data from Table 8–7.

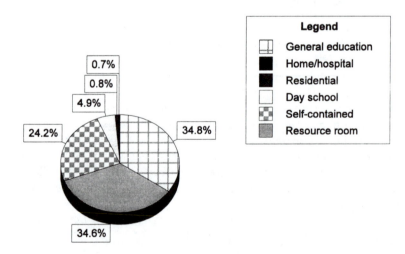

Figure 8–12. An example of a statistical pie graph that illustrates the percentage of students with special needs in different types of educational placements. Data for this graph are adapted from the *Fifteenth Annual Report to Congress on the Implementation of the Education of the Handicapped Act*, USOE, 1993. The data reflect information collected in 1990.

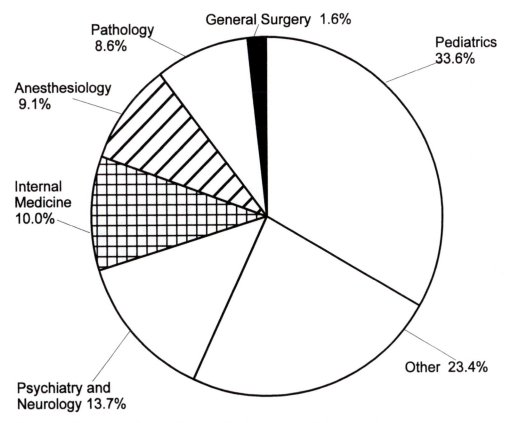

Figure 8–13. Statistical pie graph illustrating data from the hypothetical data of women physicians.

independent variable) and heart rate (presumed dependent variable) in boys and girls between the ages of 2 and 18 (Figure 8–14). The size of the class interval for age is 2 years, and the size of the class interval for heart rate is 10 beats per minute with a range of 60 to 110. The highest heart rate score observed in the sample of 24 subjects was approximately 105, and the lowest was 60. Note that the researcher set up the graph with a break line (//) on the ordinate to indicate there were no heart rate scores below 60. This is a convenient way of preparing scatter diagrams where ranges begin above zero.

The points located on the scatter diagrams are coordinates in which the two variables intersect. For example, the 10-year-old boy had a heart rate of approximately 70 beats per minute. Each use of the coordinate points indicates the relationship between the two variables for each subject.

Visual examination of the scatter diagram (Figure 8–14) often reveals a trend. In this example, heart rate scores became lower as the age increased from 2 to 17. Gender differences are noted starting at age 10.

Constructing a Scatter Diagram

In a hypothetical example a researcher collects the following data, examining the relationship between grip strength as measured by a Jamar dynamometer and Functional Activities of Daily Living (ADL) scores as measured by the Klein-Bell Test for patients with muscular dystrophy.

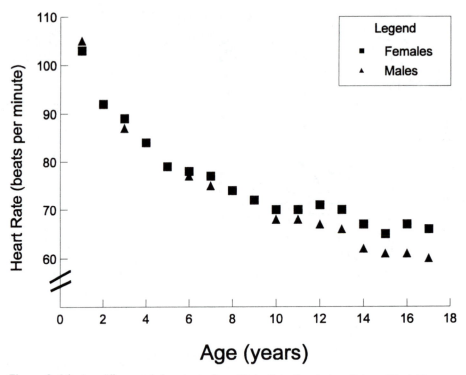

Figure 8–14. Age differences in heart rate. From "Pulse Rate, Respiratory Rate and Body Temperature of Children Between Two Months and Eighteen Years of Age" by A. Iliff and V. A. Lee, 1952, *Child Development, 23,* 237–245. Copyright 1952 by *Child Development.* Reprinted with permission.

Step 1. Record raw data for hypothetical example of grip strength and ADL scores in patients with muscular dystrophy.

Subject	Grip Strength (abscissa)	ADL Score (ordinate)
01	15	20
02	40	95
03	30	50
04	30	80
05	10	20
06	25	15
07	10	15
08	20	42
09	20	15
10	15	75
11	40	70
12	30	60

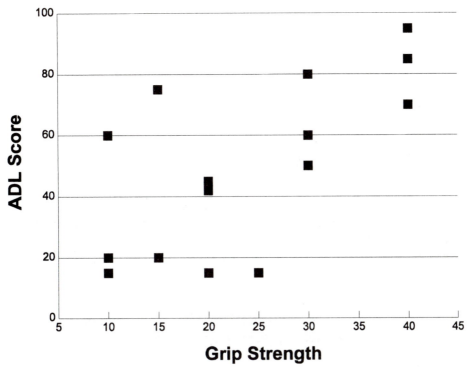

Figure 8–15. Example of a scattergram. Hypothetical example showing the relationship between grip strength and ADL scores in patients with muscular dystrophy.

Subject	Grip Strength (abscissa)	ADL Score (ordinate)
13	20	45
14	10	30
15	40	85

Step 2. Determine the range along the abscissa (grip strength) and ordinate (ADL scores). The range for grip strength is 30 (highest value, 40, minus lowest value, 10). The range for ADL scores is 80 (highest value, 95, minus lowest value, 15).

Step 3. Determine the number of the class intervals for each variable. Using the convention of 6 to 15 class intervals, we would establish 8 class intervals for grip strength with the size of the interval being 5. The actual score values are 5, 10, 15, 20, 25, 30, 35, 40 (along the abscissa). For ADL scores, the class interval is 20 with a range from 15 to 95. The actual score values plotted along the ordinate are 0, 20, 40, 60, 80, and 100.

Step 4. Design the scatter diagram (illustrated in Figure 8–15) with the score value on the abscissa (grip strength) and ordinate (ADL scores). For example, Subject 01 had a grip strength score of 15 and an ADL score of 20. The investigator plots the coordinates for all 15 subjects.

In the above example, a *positive relationship* is noted because as scores on one variable increase, scores on the other variable increase correspondingly. A negative or inverse relationship is obtained when scores on one variable increase while the corresponding scores on the other variable decrease. The degree of relationship between the two variables of the *correlation coefficient* will be discussed later in this chapter (Section 8.11).

8.5.9 Measures of Central Tendency

The first step in organizing data is usually to design a frequency distribution table or graph. The table or graph provides information concerning the form of the data. The properties of a set of data can be further described by calculating a summary statistic, such as a measure of central tendency. Measures of central tendency describe "typical" or "average" values in a distribution of data. An index of central tendency provides one value that best captures the distribution as a whole. There are generally three ways to do this:

1. *Mode:* The most frequent score in a distribution
2. *Median:* The point halfway between the top and bottom halves of a distribution (50th percentile)
3. *Mean:* The arithmetic average of all the scores

Mode

The mode is the easiest measure of central tendency to compute and the simplest to interpret. It may be used to describe any distribution, whether the data is nominal, ordinal, interval, or ratio.

Definition The mode is the most frequent score (raw or ungrouped data) or the midpoint of the interval containing the most scores (grouped data). In a frequency distribution graph, the mode is the highest peak in the graph. Figure 8–16 illustrates the mode using the following data on a distribution of scores in which there is only one mode:

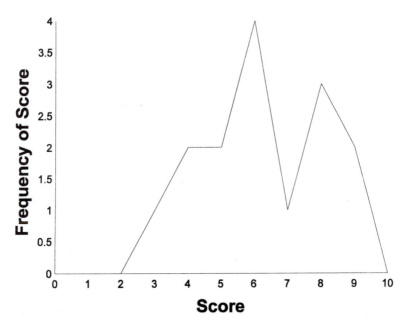

Figure 8–16. Illustration of a mode. The highest point is the mode.

Score (X)	Frequency of Score (f)	
3	1	
4	2	
5	2	
6	4	Mode = 6
7	2	
8	3	
9	2	

There is no mode in a distribution of scores if all the scores occur with the same frequency (Figure 8–17). For example:

Score (X)	Frequency of Score (f)
1	2
2	2
3	2
4	2

When two adjacent scores have the same frequency and this frequency is higher than any other scores in the distribution, the mode is the average of the two adjacent scores (Figure 8-18). For example:

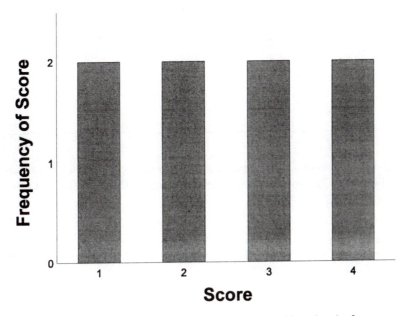

Figure 8–17. Example of data where there is no mode. Note that the frequency of each score is the same.

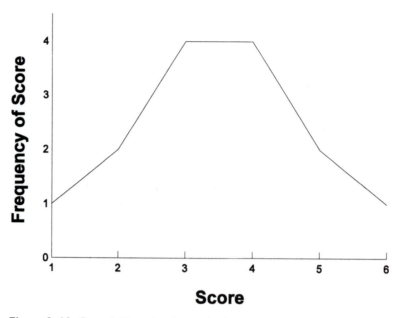

Figure 8–18. Example illustrating the mode when the data has two adjacent numbers with the same frequencies. In this case, the mode is equal to the average of the two adjacent numbers.

Score (X)	Frequency of Score (f)	
1	1	
2	2	
3	4	
		Mode = 3.5
4	4	
5	2	
6	1	

For grouped data, it is necessary to first calculate the midpoint of each class interval before computing the mode. The mode is then the midpoint of the interval containing the most scores (Figure 8-19).

Class Interval	Midpoint	Frequency of Scores (f)	
10–12	11	2	
13–15	14	2	
16–18	17	3	
19–21	20	5	Mode = 20

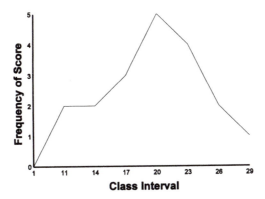

Figure 8–19. Example of a mode when grouped data are used.

Class Interval	Midpoint	Frequency of Scores (f)
22–24	23	4
25–27	26	2
28–30	29	1

The mode is the simplest measure of central tendency but it has two primary limitations:

1. Frequency distributions may have more than one mode, such as a bimodal or even trimodal distribution. In this case, there may be ambiguity about which mode to report, especially if the two (or more) peaks in the distribution are nearly equal. Often one mode is reported as the *primary* or major mode (slightly higher peak), and the other peak reported as the *secondary* or minor mode (Figure 8–20).
2. When data are grouped, the mode is sensitive to the size and number of class intervals. By changing the class intervals for a distribution, the mode will change—sometimes drastically.

Median

A second and more sophisticated measure of central tendency is the median. The median is appropriate as a measure of central tendency for ordinal, interval, or ratio data but not for nominal or categorical data from which the mode is the only measure of central tendency that can be calculated.

Definition. The median is the 50th percentile in an ordered group of scores, that is, the point in an array of scores that has 50% of the cases below it and 50% of the cases above it. The median divides the ranked scores into halves, with one half of the scores below the median and one half of the scores above the median.

The calculation of the median is a simple procedure for raw or ungrouped data:

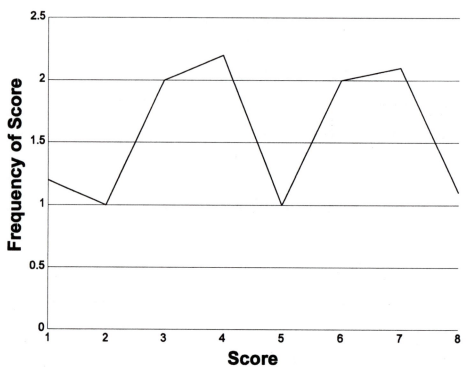

Figure 8–20. Example of scores with an ambiguous mode. The slightly higher peak is considered the primary or major mode, while the next highest peak is considered the secondary or minor mode.

Step 1. When the number of cases, N, is odd, the median is the score of case (N+1)/2 after scores are ranked (either in ascending or descending order). For example, consider the following array of nine scores:

$$6, 2, 17, 5, 11, 8, 3, 13, 10$$

To calculate the median, the nine scores are ranked in order as follows:

Rank of Score	Score	Frequency	
1	2	1	
2	3	1	4 scores below median
3	5	1	
4	6	1	
5	8	1	Median = 8
6	10	1	
7	11	1	
8	13	1	4 scores above median
9	17	1	

$$\text{Median} = (\text{score for rank } N + 1) / 2$$
$$= (\text{score for rank } 9 + 1) / 2$$
$$= \text{score for rank } 5.$$

Therefore the median is equal to the score for rank #5, which is equal to the score of 8.

Step 2. When N is even, the median is the score midway between the scores after all scores are ranked. For example, consider the following $N = 8$ scores:

$$2, 1, 10, 7, 0, 15, 8, 5$$

The first step in calculating the median is again to rank order the scores.

Rank of Score	Score	Frequency of Score	
1	0	1	
2	1	1	3 scores below median
3	2	1	
4	5	1	Median = 6
			midpoint of 5 and 7
5	7	1	
6	8	1	
7	10	1	3 scores above median
8	15	1	

For *grouped data,* the median is the point in a distribution at or below which exactly 50% of the cases fall. The median is calculated by constructing a cumulative frequency distribution. The median is then calculated from the cumulative frequency distribution with the following formula:

$$\text{Median} = LL + w_i \{ [(N / 2) - cf] / f_i \}$$

where LL = lower real limit of the median interval

$\quad\quad w_i$ = width of class interval

$\quad\quad N$ = number of cases

$\quad\quad cf$ = cumulative frequency up to the median interval

$\quad\quad f_i$ = frequency within the median interval

The first stage in calculating the median is to construct a cumulative frequency distribution beginning with the lowest class interval and proceeding in ascending order to the highest class interval. The next step is to locate the interval that contains the 50th percentile or the median by examining the cumulative frequency column. For example:

Class Interval	Real Limits	f	cf	Cumulative Percentile	
12–14	11.5–14.5	2	2	10	
15–17	14.5–17.5	4	6	20	
18–20	17.5–20.5	3	9	45	
21–23	20.5–23.5	5	14	70	The median is in the class interval in which the 50th percentile rests.
24–26	23.5–26.5	3	17	85	
27–29	26.5–29.5	2	19	95	
30–32	30.5–32.5	1	20	100	

Inspection of the above cumulative frequency distribution shows that the median or 50th percentile must fall in the class interval of 21–23 because the previous interval of 18–20 has cumulated only 9 of the 20 total cases, that is, 45% or 45th percentile.

$$LL = \text{lower real limit of median interval} = 20.5$$

$$w_i = \text{width of class interval} = 3$$

$$N = \text{total number of cases in the frequency distribution} = 20$$

$$cf = \text{cumulative frequency } up\ to \text{ median interval} = 9$$
(starting from the lowest to the highest score)

$$f_i = \text{frequency within median interval} = 5$$

Therefore,

$$
\begin{aligned}
\text{Median} &= LL + w_i \{ [(N / 2) - cf / f_i\} \\
&= 20.5 + (3) \{[(20 / 2) - 9] / 5\} \\
&= 20.5 + 3 (1 / 5) \\
&= 20.5 + 3 (.20) \\
&= 20.5 + .6 \\
&= 21.1
\end{aligned}
$$

The above formula can be used to calculate the median for any grouped frequency distribution, as well as for ungrouped distributions (with or without tied scores).

Calculation of the Raw Score From the Percentile Rank. A modification of the formula allows a generalized method for calculating raw scores corresponding to a given percentile rank (PR).

$$\text{Score at PR} = LL + w_i \frac{[(PR)(N) / 100] - cf}{f_i}$$

where

LL = lower real limit of the interval containing the given raw score, that is, (PR)(N) / 100

w_i = width of the class interval

PR = percentile rank

N = number of cases in the distribution

cf = cumulative frequency up to the given class interval containing the raw score

f_i = number of cases within the class interval containing the raw score

In the next example, what is the raw score corresponding to the 90th percentile rank?

$$\text{Raw score } (rs) \text{ at 90th percentile rank} = LL + w_i \frac{[(90)(N) / 100] - cf}{f_i}$$

where

LL = 26.5	cf = 17
w_i = 3	f_i = 2
N = 20	PR = 90

$$rs = 26.5 + (3) \frac{[(90)(20) / 100] - 17}{2}$$

$$rs = 26.5 + (3) \{[(180 / 100) - 17] / 2\}$$

$$rs = 26.5 + 3 [(18 - 17) / 2]$$

$$rs = 26.5 + 3 (1 / 2)$$

$$rs = 26.5 + 1.5$$

Therefore, a percentile rank of 90 corresponds to a raw score of 28.

Calculation of the Percentile Rank (PR) From the Raw Score. A researcher may also want to calculate the PR from the raw score. For example, given a raw score of 19 in a group distribution (see above data), what is the PR?

$$PR = \{f_i(rs - LL) + [(w_i) (cf)]\} / [(N) (w_i)]$$

where f_i = 3	rs = 19
LL = 17.5	w_i = 3
cf = 6	N = 20

$$PR = \{3(19 - 17.5) + [(3) (6)]\} / [(20) (3)]$$

$$= (4.5 + 18) / 60$$

$$= 22.5 / 60$$

$$= 37.5 \text{ PR}$$

Therefore, a raw score of 19 equals a percentile rank of 37.5.

Mean

The mean is the most widely used and familiar index of central tendency. The mean is the arithmetic average of all the scores in a distribution and is calculated by summing all scores and dividing by the total number of scores.

The general formula for the mean $\bar{x}$ is:

$$\bar{x} = [X_1 + X_2 + X_3 \ldots X_n] / N$$
$$\bar{x} = \Sigma X / N$$

where

X_1 = first raw score

X_2 = second raw score

X_3 = third raw score

X_n = nth raw score

Σ = summation or sum of

N = number of subjects in the distribution

The mean may be conceptualized as a "center of gravity" or "balance point" in which the scores or "weights" on one side exactly balance the scores or weights on the other side. Each weight represents a score from a distribution of scores. The arithmetic mean of all the scores or weights is the center of gravity or balance point. The deviation of scores in one direction exactly equals the deviation of scores in the other direction.

Calculating the Mean With Raw or Ungrouped Data. The mean is readily calculated for a distribution of raw scores in which each score occurs only once. The mean is simply the sum of the raw scores divided by the number of scores. For example, consider the following distribution of eight scores:

$$3, 6, 7, 8, 11, 15, 16, 22$$
$$\Sigma X = 88$$
$$N = 8$$
$$\bar{X} = \Sigma X / N$$
$$\bar{X} = [3 + 6 + 7 + 8 + 11 + 15 + 16 + 22] / 8$$
$$= 88 / 8$$
$$= 11.0$$

The mean or average value is calculated as 11.0.

For ungrouped data with a small sample of scores, the above procedure may be used to calculate the mean. Alternatively, for grouped data, a frequency distribution should be set up. Then the mean is calculated from the frequency distribution table by multiplying each score by the frequency of occurrence and summing the total across all scores before dividing by the total number of scores.

In the following example, several scores occur more than once:

$$2, 3, 3, 4, 5, 5, 6, 6, 6, 7, 8, 8, 9, 9, 9$$

Step 1. The first stage in computing the mean is to form a frequency distribution table.

X	f	fX
2	1	2
3	2	6
4	1	4
5	2	10
6	3	18
7	1	7
8	2	16
9	3	27
		$\Sigma (fX) = 90$

The number in the third column is obtained by multiplying each each raw score by the frequency of occurrence. The symbol fX represents the product of the scores multiplied by the frequency of scores. This column is then summed and divided by the total number of scores, in this example, 15 scores.

$$\bar{X} = \Sigma fx / N$$
$$\Sigma fX = 90$$
$$N = 15$$
$$\bar{X} = 90 / 15$$
$$= 6.0$$

Calculating the Mean for Grouped Data. When working with grouped data, first find the midpoint of each score interval before calculating the mean.

The general formula to determine the mean for grouped data is:

$$\bar{x} = \Sigma fX / N$$

As an example, consider the following scores grouped into six class intervals:

Class Interval	Midpoint (X)	f	fX
3–5	4	2	8
6–8	7	1	7
9–11	10	4	40

(continued)

Class Interval	Midpoint (X)	f	fX
12–14	13	6	78
15–17	16	3	48
18–20	19	4	76
		$\Sigma f = 20$	$\Sigma fX = 257$

Therefore, the

$$\bar{x} = 257 / 20$$
$$\bar{x} = 12.85$$

In the above example, the midpoint of each class interval (X) was multiplied by the frequency in each interval. This product was summed over all the class intervals to give a value equal to 257. This value (ΣfX) is then divided by the total number of scores or the sum of the frequencies (i.e., $\Sigma f = 20$) to yield the final calculated mean of 12.85.

The mean calculated from a grouped frequency distribution will differ slightly from the mean calculated from raw scores. When scores are grouped, information is lost and a certain amount of inaccuracy introduced. As a general rule, the coarser the grouping of scores, the more the grouped mean will differ from the raw score mean. Nonetheless, for most situations in which 10 to 20 class intervals are typically used, the agreement is close enough between the two calculated means.

Comparing the Mode, Median, and Mean

1. As a measure of central tendency, the mean takes into account all the scores of distribution and is affected by each single value. One extreme score or "outlier" can influence the mean to a large degree, especially with small samples. For example, in the following distribution of 10 scores, both the mean and median have a value of 6.0; when an extreme score of 50 is added as the eleventh score, the mean dramatically increases to 10.0, while the median changes only to 7.0:

   Scores: 2, 3, 4, 4, 5, 7, 8, 8, 9, 10

   Mean = 6.0   Median = 6.0

   The mean is changed when an extreme score of 50 is added:

   Scores: 2, 3, 4, 4, 5, 7, 8, 8, 9, 10, 50

   Mean = 10.0   Median = 7.0

   Therefore, when extreme scores or outliers are present in a frequency distribution of scores, the median may be a more appropriate measure of central tendency than the mean.

2. In distributions that are symmetrical in shape, the mean equals the median, and both are equal to the mode if the distribution is unimodal. This is illustrated in Figure 8–21.

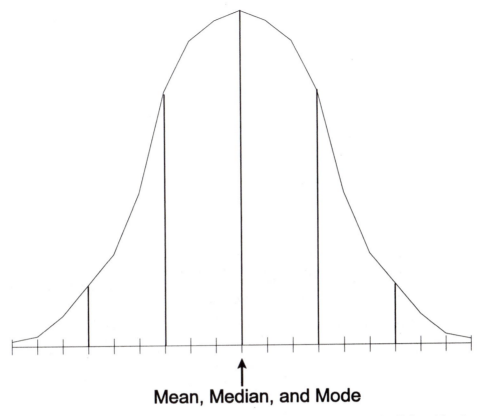

Mean, Median, and Mode

Figure 8–21. The normal unimodal curve depicting the mean, median, and mode. All three fall at the same place on a bell-shaped curve.

3. In distributions that are symmetrical but not unimodal, it is important to report the mode, mean, and median to provide a clearer picture of the shape and central tendency of the distribution. In Figure 8–22, which depicts a bimodal distribution, there are two modes (at 28 and 40) that should be noted: The mean equals the median and both equal 34.

4. In distributions that are skewed to the left or right, the mode, median, and mean will have different values. Note that the mean is pulled either to the right or to the left by the outliers or extreme scores on one end of the skewed distribution. The median is the preferred measure of central tendency for skewed distributions, especially when the degree of skewness increases. Figures 8–23 and 8–24 illustrate the locations of the three measures of central tendency for right- and left-skewed distributions.

8.5.10 Measures of Variability

Measures of variability are descriptive statistics that indicate how scores in a distribution differ from each other and from the mean. For example, in a distribution with the scores 7, 7, 7, 7, the measure of variability is 0 because the scores do not differ from each other and from the mean of 7. The measure of variability increases from zero as the scores vary from

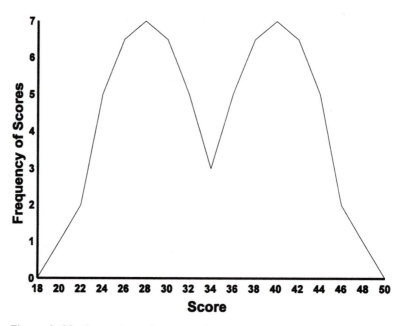

Figure 8–22. Comparison of mean, median, and mode in a bimodal distribution. The two modes have the value of 28 and 38. The median and the mean have the same value, 34.

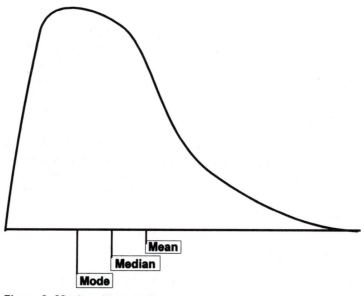

Figure 8–23. A positively skewed distribution. Notice that the figure is pulled to the left, indicating that the scores with the largest frequencies are at the lower end of the distribution.

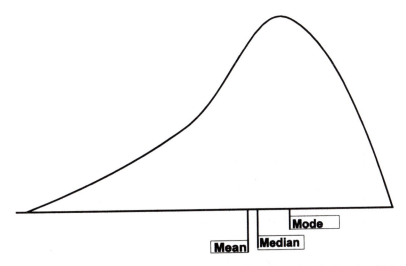

Figure 8–24. A negatively skewed distribution. The figure is pulled to the right, indicating that the scores with the largest frequencies are at the upper end of the distribution.

each other and from the mean. The *measures of variability* are the range, variance, and standard deviation.

Range

The *range* is the value derived from subtracting the largest score in the distribution from the smallest scores. In the distribution 21, 23, 24, 26, 28, 30, the range is 9. The range is a crude measure of variability because only the highest and the lowest scores of a distribution are used.

Variance

The *variance* is a measure of the variability of scores in a distribution that takes into account all the scores in that distribution. The computational formula for the variance is:

$$s^2 = [N \Sigma X^2 - (\Sigma X)^2] / [N (N - 1)]$$

where N = total number of subjects or scores in the distribution

ΣX^2 = raw scores are squared and then the values are totaled

$(\Sigma X)^2$ = the value which equals the square of the summation of the scores.

Example of Calculating the Variance.

Subject	Score (X)	X^2
01	2	4
02	4	16
03	7	49

(continued)

Subject	Score (X)	X²
04	9	81
05	10	100
06	12	144
07	14	196
N = 7	ΣX = 58	ΣX² = 590

Computational Formula for the Variance.

$$s^2 = [N \, \Sigma \, X^2 - (\Sigma X)^2] \, / \, [N(N-1)]$$
$$s^2 = [(7)(590) - (58)^2] \, / \, [7(7-1)]$$
$$s^2 = [4130 - 3364] \, / \, 42$$
$$s^2 = 766 \, / \, 42$$
$$s^2 = 18.238$$

Standard Deviation

The *standard deviation* is the square root of the variance. In the example above, the variance equals 18.23. Therefore, the standard deviation equals 4.27. The standard deviation is an important value that is analogous to the mean. It is used in inferential statistics, such as the *t* test.

8.5.11 Stem and Leaf

Stem and leaf is a method of displaying data developed by Tukey (1977) and is an alternative to the frequency distribution. It derives its name from its display: Any given number is divided into two parts, a stem and a leaf. The first part, the stem, represents a large class into which the number falls, while the second number, the leaf, designates the actual placement in the larger class. For example, the number 15 can be divided into 1 (the stem) and 5 (the leaf), while the number 216 can be divided into 2 or 21 (the stem) and 16 or 6 (the leaf). When the stem and leaves are displayed in a column, the researcher can easily visualize the organization of the data. The researcher is able to identify the specific scores obtained, as well as the frequency of the class of scores. Once the data have been organized into a stem and leaf display, a graph is drawn, allowing the researcher to visualize the structure of the data.

An example of unpublished data helps to explain the concept. Pre- and posttest data were collected to determine the change in understanding of collaboration techniques. The pre- and posttest scores, as well as the ranks for each of the scores, are reproduced in Table 8–8. The stem and leaf display is as follows:

Pretest Scores	Pretest Leaf	Stem	Posttest Leaf	Posttest Scores
59	9	5*		
63, 62	32	6	53	65, 63
71	1	7	16	71, 76

Table 8–8. Pretest and Posttest Scores on Collaboration Data

	Pretest		Posttest	
Subject	Score	Rank	Score	Rank
1	118	13	102	11.5
2	59	1	94	8
3	140	16	114	13
4	99	9	96	9
5	96	8	102	11.5
6	63	2	159	16
7	100	10	71	3
8	136	15	76	4
9	152	18	186	18
10	133	14	198	19
11	92	6	65	2
12	62	3	63	1
13	82	5	148	15
14	192	19	222	20
15	106	11	87	7
16	71	4	82	5
17	—	—	101	10
18	108	12	175	17
19	151	17	140	14
20	95	7	84	6

Note. From S. K. Cutler, D. W. Keyes, and M. Urquhart, 1993, unpublished raw data.

Pretest Scores	Pretest Leaf	Stem	Posttest Leaf	Posttest Scores
82	2	8	724	87, 82, 84
99, 96, 92, 95	9625	9	46	94, 96
106, 108, 118, 136, 133, 140 100	06, 08, 18, 36, 33, 40, 00	1**	02, 02, 01, 14, 48, 40	102, 102, 101, 114, 148, 140
152, 151, 192	52, 51, 92	1	59, 75, 86, 98	159, 175, 186, 198
		2	22	222

The asterisks that follow the number in the stem indicate the number of digits that are included in each leaf. For example, 5* means one digit is added to the stem while 1** means two digits are added to the stem. Although commas are not necessary between the leaves, we have chosen to use them. Notice that the number of digits in the leaf can change within a single display. The use of asterisks indicates a change in digits. In this display, the pretest leaves are displayed on the left, and the posttest leaves are displayed on the right. The stem is placed in the center with the leaves on either side. This allows the researcher to compare sets of data easily. For the reader's convenience, the pre- and posttest scores have been listed.

This system has advantages. First, the leaves do not have to be placed sequentially beside the stems. When the numbers are ranked later (necessary for the graph), the researcher will want to put them in sequential order, however. Second, not only is the researcher able to tell the shape of the data, but he or she can obtain the specific scores. This is not possible in a frequency distribution graph.

When building a stem-and-leaf display, the number of stems is only limited by the data. The researcher does not want to use so many stems that the data are too spread out or too few lines so that the data are too crowded. Trial and error may be necessary to determine the appropriate number of stems. In general, the last digit of a given number becomes the leaf, while the first digit(s) will be used as the stem. Sometimes, when there are too many leaves on one stem, the stem may be split into parts. By splitting the stem, the leaves may be divided. An example of a split stem can be seen by the repetition of the digit 1.

Once a stem and leaf display has been produced, the researcher needs to make a graph. The graph is called a box and whisker plot because of the way in which it is drawn. The graph consists of a box that has lines connected to either side (the whiskers). A box and whisker plot makes use of the ranks of median or middle score, the ranks of the extremes, and the ranks of the hinges. An examination of Table 8–8 shows the median for the pretest to be 100 (rank of 10) and the median of the posttest to be 101.5 (rank of 10.5). The extremes are the ranks of the highest and lowest scores. The pretest extremes are 59 and 192, ranked at 1 and 19. The posttest extremes are 63 and 222, ranked at 1 and 20. The hinges or quartile ranks lie halfway between the median and the extremes. They are obtained by the following formula:

Lower hinge = ½ (lower extreme + median)

Upper hinge = ½ (upper extreme + median)

When the rank of a median is not a whole number, drop the decimal (e.g., 10.5 becomes 10). The upper and lower hinges become the upper and lower limits of the box. The whisker is a line that connects the hinges to the extremes. An example of this is seen in Figure 8–25. An examination of the two box plots in this figure reveals that there is little difference between the two scores. Although the upper extreme and the upper hinge is higher on the posttest, the medians, lower extreme, and lower hinge are similar. There is more variability on the posttest.

Construction of a Stem and Leaf Display and Box Plot

Step 1. Make a stem and leaf display. The following scores have been collected from posttests. Because the scores are between 72 and 97, both the stem and leaf will consist of a single digit. Because of the number of scores that fall between 80 and 89, the stem will be divided into two.

Scores: 88, 82, 75, 93, 96, 81, 83, 82, 97, 96, 87, 88, 72, 75, 95, 82, 80, 87, 89, 88

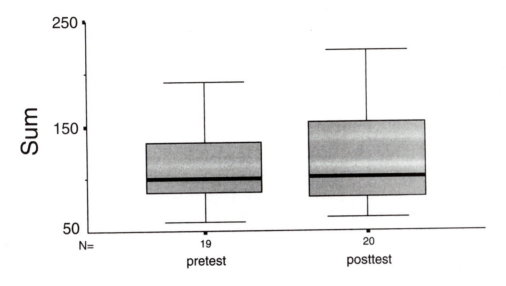

Figure 8–25. An example of a box and whisker plot using the data from Table 8–8. The data are from an unpublished study by Cutler, Keyes, and Urquhart, 1993.

Stem	Leaf	Cumulative Rank	Scores Repeated	No. of Leaves
7*	525	3	75, 72, 75	3
8	213220	9	82, 81, 83, 82, 82, 80	6
8	878798	15	88, 87, 88, 87, 89, 88	6
9	36765	20	93, 96, 97, 96, 95	5

The asterisk is placed after the 7 to denote that only one digit is used in the leaf.

Step 2. Find the median score. Because there are 20 scores, the median rank will be 10.5. The score that falls at this rank is 87.

Step 3. Find the extremes. The extremes are the ranks of the highest and lowest scores or, in this case, those scores with a rank of 1 and 20. The scores for rank 1 and rank 20 are 72 and 97, respectively.

Step 4. Calculate the hinges. The hinges or quartile ranks lie halfway between the median and the extremes. They are obtained by adding the rank of the extremes to the rank of the median and dividing by 2. When the median rank has a decimal, drop the decimal.

Lower hinge = (1 + 10) / 2 = 11 / 2 = 5.5. The rank for the lower hinge is at 5.5. The score that would fall at this rank is 81.5, obtained by finding the halfway point between the scores that rank at 5 and 6, respectively (e.g., 81, 82).

Upper hinge = (20 + 10) / 2 = 15. The score at this rank is 89.

Step 5. Draw a box using the lower and upper hinges as the outer limits of the box and connect the extremes to the box with a solid line. Notice that the box can be drawn horizontally or vertically.

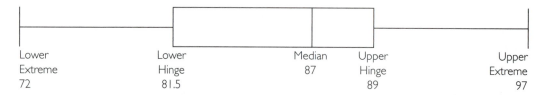

| Lower Extreme 72 | Lower Hinge 81.5 | Median 87 | Upper Hinge 89 | Upper Extreme 97 |

An examination of this box plot suggests that the scores are negatively skewed; that is, more scores are at the upper end of the distribution than the lower end.

Reference: J. W. Tukey, (1977). *Exploratory Data Analysis.* Reading, MA: Addison-Wesley Publishing Company.

8.5.12 z-Scores and the Normal Curve

The z scores are summary values that indicate the distance between a raw score and the mean, using standard deviation units. For example, a z score of 0 (zero) is equal to the mean. The z scores are important to describe the relative standing of a raw score. For example, a raw score of 40 is equal to a z score of +1 in a normal distribution with a mean equal to 30 and one standard deviation equal to 10. Figure 8–26 illustrates the z score for a raw score of 40.

In this example, a raw score of 40 is equal to a percentile rank of 84, which means that an individual with a z score of +1 did better than, or is above, 84% of the individuals in that distribution.

The formula for calculating z -scores is:

$$z = \frac{\text{raw score} - \text{mean}}{\text{standard deviation}}$$

In the above example:

$$z = [40 - 30] / 10$$
$$z = 10 / 10$$
$$z = +1$$

The z scores can be positive or negative depending on whether the raw score is above or below the mean. These scores are widely used in psychometric testing and are helpful in interpreting raw scores.

Normality and the Normal Curve

For the occupational therapist, one of the most difficult decisions is to decide whether a physiological or psychological function is within normal limits. What is normal blood pressure, heart rate, muscle strength, height, visual-perceptual function, or intelligence? Is normality a function of personality or behavior or it is a statistical value?

When an individual goes to a physician for a physical examination, the physiological and neurological functions are tested to determine whether they are within normal limits. Predetermined values are used by the physician to compare with the patient's results. Individual differences within a range of normality are accepted by the physician to deter-

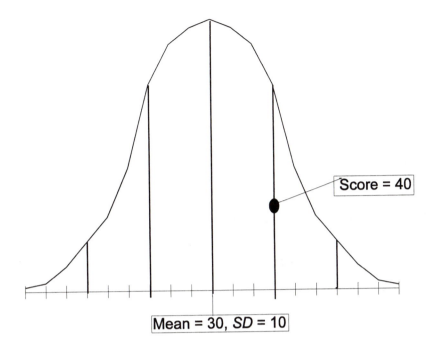

Score = 40

Mean = 30, *SD* = 10

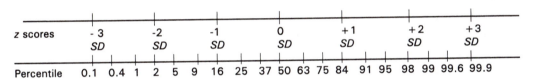

z scores	- 3 *SD*	-2 *SD*	-1 *SD*	0 *SD*	+ 1 *SD*	+ 2 *SD*	+ 3 *SD*

| Percentile | 0.1 | 0.4 | 1 | 2 | 5 | 9 | 16 | 25 | 37 | 50 | 63 | 75 | 84 | 91 | 95 | 98 | 99 | 99.6 | 99.9 |

Figure 8–26. Normal curve depicting raw score of 40, mean of 30, *SD* of 10. Notice that a raw score of 40 lies one standard deviation above the mean (e.g., z score of +1) and at a percentile of 84.

mine whether a function is abnormal. The same judgments are made by the occupational therapist in testing range of motion in a specific joint or evaluating muscle strength.

On the other hand, the statistician's definition of normality and abnormality will depend on the frequency of occurrences within designated class intervals. Abnormality is interpreted by the statistician as a variance from the mean value, such as 1 or 2 standard deviation units from the mean of a normally distributed variable. In research, scores or values that are abnormal are considered to be outliers or scores that vary widely from expected values. Many times those outliers or abnormal scores are considered at variance with the test of values in a distribution. Consider the scatter diagram in Figure 8–27. Four of the five scores are consistent with a positive relationship with the X and Y variables. However, one coordinate (50,5) seems to be an outlier and does not fit into the pattern. The outlier or abnormal score should be discussed separately by the researcher.

The normal curve (Figure 8–26) is the statistician's guide for examining the relationship between normal values and outliers. In the normal curve it is expected that 68% of the cases will lie within −1 to +1 standard deviation units and 96% of the cases will lie within −2 to +2 standard deviations units. If we know that a characteristic is normally distributed, then by calculating the mean and standard deviation of a population, we will be able

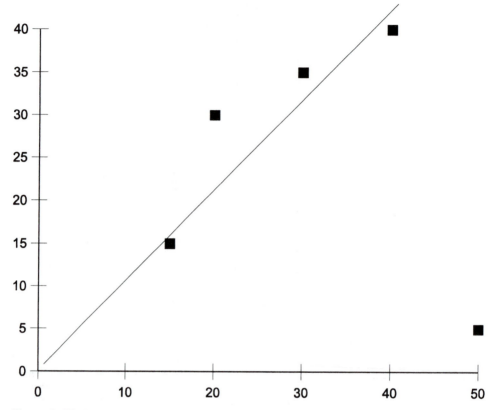

Figure 8–27. Scattergram showing an outliner at the coordinates of 50, 5. The outliner is the score that appears to be significantly different from the other scores.

to determine how many of the cases will be within −2 to +2 standard deviation units from the mean. For example, if we know that the resting heart rate is normally distributed and that the mean value for adults is 72 beats per minute with a standard deviation of 5, then we can determine the percentile ranks (PR) from the raw scores. For example, what is the percentile rank of an individual with a resting heart rate score of 78?

The normal curve in Figure 8–28 shows the relationship between the raw score of 78 and the normal values for resting heart rate. We estimate that, based on the diagram, the PR for a raw score of 78 will be slightly above the 84th PR.

Calculation of PR. First calculate z scores from raw scores:

$$z = (rs - \bar{x}) / SD$$
$$z = (78 - 72) / 5$$
$$z = 6/5 = 1.2$$
$$z = 1.2$$

Look up the percentile rank from the statistical table for the z score of 1.2. Note that in Table C–2 in the Appendix, a z score of 1.2 is equal to the percentile rank of .8849.

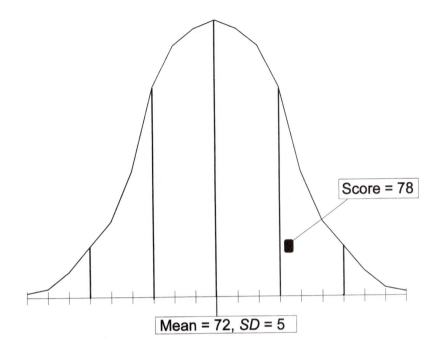

Score = 78

Mean = 72, *SD* = 5

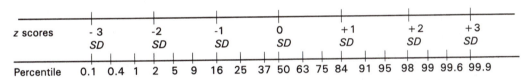

z scores	- 3 SD	-2 SD	-1 SD	0 SD	+ 1 SD	+ 2 SD	+ 3 SD

Percentile   0.1   0.4   1   2   5   9   16   25   37 50 63 75 84   91 95   98 99 99.6 99.9

Figure 8–28. Normal curve depicting the relationship between the heart beat rate of 78 when the mean is 72 and the standard deviation is 5. What is the *z* score of this heart beat? Is it above or below normal?

8.5.13 Vital Statistics

The quality of a health care system in a country is usually described by vital statistics such as the infant mortality rate, rates of illnesses and diseases, life expectancy, and mortality rates from specific diseases. In justifying the need for a research study in a clinical area, the researcher first reports the incidence and prevalence rates of a disability or illness to establish the significance of the study. What are some of the most common vital statistics?

Crude Mortality (Death) or Morbidity (Disease) Rates

The crude mortality or morbidity rate is calculated by dividing the frequency of deaths or illnesses by the total number of individuals in the population. This number is then multiplied by 1,000, 10,000, or 100,000 so it can be used as a comparative figure. For example, if a certain population has a mortality rate of 9.3 per 1,000 population per year, how does this compare with another population where there are 180,000 deaths in a population of 24,000,000?

Calculation of Crude Mortality Rate.

$$\text{Crude death rate} = (180{,}000 / 24{,}000{,}000)\,(1{,}000)$$
$$= .0075 \times 1{,}000$$
$$= 7.5 \text{ per } 1{,}000 \text{ population}$$

In this hypothetical case, the investigator would conclude that there is a lesser mortality rate in the sample of 180,000 deaths per 24,000,000 population than in the 9.3 per 1,000 population.

Prevalence and Incidence Rates of Disability or Disease

How do we determine the incidence rate of a disease? For example, in 1991, there were 43,000 new cases of individuals with AIDS in the United States. At that time, the total population was about 240,000,000. What is the incidence rate of AIDS per 100,000 population for 1991?

Calculation of Incidence Rate.

$$\text{incidence rate} = (43{,}000 / 240{,}000{,}000)\,(100{,}000)$$
$$= (.0001791)\,(100{,}000)$$
$$= 17.91 \text{ per } 100{,}000 \text{ population}$$

Adjusted Rate

Researchers are also interested in obtaining statistics for specific populations. In these examples, the calculation of rates are adjusted. For example, an investigator is interested in comparing infant mortality rates adjusted for gender. In a hypothetical population there are 40,000 births of males and 35,000 births of females. In this population, 150 males and 180 females die at birth. What are the adjusted infant mortality rates for females compared with the total crude rates per 1,000 population?

Calculation of Crude Rate.

$$\text{crude rate} = [(150 + 180) / (40{,}000 + 35{,}000)]\,[1{,}000]$$
$$= (330 / 75{,}000)\,(1{,}000)$$
$$= (.0044)\,(1{,}000)$$
$$= 4.4 \text{ per } 1{,}000 \text{ (for both males and females)}$$

Adjusted Rate—Females.

$$\text{adjusted rate} = (180 / 35{,}000)\,(1{,}000)$$
$$= .0051 \times 1000$$
$$= 5.14 \text{ per } 1{,}000$$

For this hypothetical example, it appears that the infant mortality rate is higher in females compared with the total population.

8.6 Inferential Statistics and Testing a Hypothesis

8.6.1 Probability and Clinical Research

When an investigator predicts a statistically significant relationship between two variables, it is assumed that the relationship will not exist by chance alone. In other words, the researcher is predicting that X factor is related to Y factor, or that the independent variable, whether manipulated or not, is related to the dependent variable. In clinical research, however, it is difficult to control for all possible factors that could affect the dependent variable. For example, if a researcher discovers through a thorough search of the literature that arthritis is a psychophysiological disorder, then a set of research investigations would be generated based on this assumption. In a retrospective correlational study, the researcher could select a group of patients with arthritis and investigate personality relationships and the incidence of arthritis. If a statistically significant relationship is found between the incidence of arthritis and personality relationships, it will be beyond a certain probability level but not necessarily a one-to-one relationship. This means that not all individuals with a certain described characteristic are arthritic. This leads us to the question, why do we accept a partial relationship rather than a 100% probability in clinical research? A number of factors in clinical research impinge on statistically significant results that prevent the perfect 100% probability relationships. They are:

- ▶ Complex interrelationships among variables in which more than one factor contributes to a disability can affect results in clinical research. For example, in arthritis a multifactorial etiology is assumed. In clinical research, however, we may be able to identify only some portion of the variance associated with the onset of arthritis.
- ▶ Diseases in which genetics, age, diet, and numerous other factors influence the course of a disorder can affect research results. There may be individual factors occurring in the individual that are difficult to identify in clinical research during a study.
- ▶ The problem of accurately formulating a diagnosis in chronic disabilities such as arthritis, diabetes, multiple sclerosis, cardiovascular disease, schizophrenia, or ulcerative colitis may affect the results in clinical research. Moreover, the sample may not be a homogeneous group, which could contaminate results.
- ▶ The error variance existing in all clinical research, such as measurement of variables, control of experimental conditions, uniformity of subjects, and data collection procedures, that could affect results.

In short, all statistical analysis using hypothesis testing is based on probability. When inferential statistics are applied in a clinical research study, the investigator bases results and conclusions on the probability that any differences between the experimental and control groups are either attributable to chance or are statistically significantly different.

8.6.2 Procedure for Statistically Testing a Hypothesis

Step 1. State the hypothesis. A null hypothesis is stated unless the researcher is replicating a previous study or has research evidence to support a directional hypothesis.

Null hypothesis is $\mu_1 = \mu_2$ or $r = 0$. Stated in clinical research study: There is no statistically significant difference between means or no significantly statistical relationship between variables.

Directional hypothesis is $\mu_1 > \mu_2$ or r is statistically significant. This is the reverse of the null hypothesis.

Step 2. Select a level of significance. The researcher usually selects the .05 level of significance in the social sciences. This means that the researcher accepts an error level of 5%. The researcher can also state that at $\alpha = .05$, there is a 95% confidence level that results are not due to chance.

Step 3. Apply inferential statistics and select a procedure or parametric or nonparametric statistical test based on the assumptions underlying the test such as randomness, normal distribution of data, and homogeneity of variance.

Step 4. Obtain the critical value from the appropriate table for statistical tests based on whether it is one-tailed or two-tailed test, level of statistical significance, and degrees of freedom.

Step 5. Calculate the value of test statistics, such as t-observed, F-observed, chi-square or correlation coefficient through a mathematical formula.

Step 6. Accept or reject the research hypothesis (null or directional).

8.6.3 Potential Sources of Research Errors Affecting Statistical Significance

One important aspect of clinical research is to reduce the possible errors in an experiment that could impact on the results. These errors include:

▶ *Hawthorne effect:* attention given to subjects may increase positive outcome and camouflage the true effects of the independent variable or treatment method. When a Hawthorne effect is present, the subjects' improvement is caused by the attention received from the researcher rather than the direct result of the treatment intervention.

▶ *Placebo effect:* the suggestion that subjects receiving a treatment, such as medication or a procedure, may produce positive expectations that the treatment will be effective. The subjects may will themselves to improvement. The placebo produces in the subject a desire for improvement. There is some evidence that a psychophysiological effect occurs from the placebo effect.

▶ *Honeymoon effect:* a short-term effect of a new treatment procedure that subjects hope will impact on a disease. The initial enthusiasm disguises the true effects of the treatment procedure.

▶ *Researcher bias:* the researcher carrying out a clinical treatment program affects the results through his or her enthusiasm and desire for the treatment to be effective. The researcher's knowledge of the study may affect its outcome.

▶ *Test administrator bias:* the individual testing the outcome of treatment method is aware of which subjects are in the experimental group and which are in the control group.

▶ *Sampling errors:* if the researcher's results are based on a sample from a population that is not representative, the results will be skewed or biased to the research sample selected.

▶ *Systematic variance:* the researcher fails to control for extraneous variables that could possibly affect the results such as age, gender, intelligence, education, socioeconomic status, or degree of disability.

▶ *Error variance:* the researcher overlooks or minimizes the effects of anxiety, lack of motivation, inattention, distractive environments, and other unexpected problems in the test environment.

Type I and Type II Errors

All of the above factors and other sources of error in an experiment can potentially affect the results of research. The errors in testing a hypothesis are identified as either a Type I or Type II error and result from the researcher accepting or rejecting a hypothesis based on the statistical results. The probability of a Type I error in hypothesis testing is typically accepted at the .05 or .01 level. The researcher has confidence that the results are not attributable to chance in 95 or 99% of the time. Nonetheless, it is possible that the results are false in 5 out of a 100 tries or 1 out of a 100 tries purely on the basis of chance errors. Table 8–9 summarizes the relationship between decision errors and hypothesis testing. The concept in medicine of a false positive or false negative is analogous to describing a Type I or Type II error. A false positive in medicine occurs when a disease is falsely detected, whereas a false negative exists when a disease is overlooked or not detected. Errors in

Table 8–9. Testing the Null Hypothesis, Decision Errors, and Clinical Analogy in Medicine

Null hypothesis H_o predicts that there is no statistically significant differences between means $(\bar{x}_1 = \bar{x}_x)$ or no statistically significant relationship between variables ($r = 0$).

Decision by Researcher	True Situation	Analogy in Medicine
1. Reject Null Hypothesis: • $\mu_1 \neq \mu_2 \neq \mu_3 \neq \mu_4 \ldots$ • $r \neq 0$	**Type I Error (α):** Researcher rejects the null hypothesis when it should be accepted. In reality, there is no statistically significant difference between means or relationship between variables. • $\mu_1 = \mu_2$ • $r = 0$ Researcher should accept the null hypothesis	**False Positive:** Clinician falsely detects the presence of disease or condition when in reality no disease exists. For example, falsely diagnosing breast cancer through mammography screening when in reality breast cancer is not present.
2. Reject Null Hypothesis: • $\mu_1 \neq \mu_2 \neq \mu_3 \neq \mu_4 \ldots$ • $r \neq 0$	**No Error:** Researcher rejects null hypothesis and concludes that there is a statistically significant difference between the means or that r is greater than zero.	**Correct Diagnosis:** Clinician correctly detects presence of disease and concludes a correct positive diagnosis of a pathological condition.
3. Accept Null Hypothesis: • $\mu_1 = \mu_2 = \mu_3 = \mu_4 \ldots$ • $r = 0$	**Type II Error (β):** Researcher accepts null hypothesis when it should be rejected. In reality, there is a statistically significant difference between means or a statistically significant relationship between variables. • $\mu_1 \neq \mu_2$ • $r \neq 0$ Researcher should reject null hypothesis.	**False Negative:** Clinician falsely concludes that based on test results, no disease is present when in reality a disease exists.
4. Accept Null Hypothesis: • $\mu_1 = \mu_2 = \mu_3 = \mu_4 \ldots$ • $r = 0$	**No Error:** Researcher accepts null hypothesis.	**Correct Diagnosis:** Clinician correctly concludes that no disease is present.

clinical medicine can occur because of human error because of mistaken judgments in interpreting results, the unreliability of the test equipment or procedure, or unexplained or temporary variables in the patient's condition that can lead to a false diagnosis. Often, clinicians will use more than one test, as well as repeat tests, to confirm or validate a diagnosis. Researchers, on the other hand, try to reduce Type I and Type II errors by replicating experiments with representative samples from different geographical areas.

In summary, a Type I error is when a researcher rejects a null hypothesis when it should be accepted. A Type II error is when a null hypothesis is accepted when it should be rejected.

8.6.4 Exploratory Data Analysis

John Tukey (1977) stated, "It is important to understand what you CAN do before you learn to measure how WELL you seem to have **done** it" (p. v). In clinical research the question that is usually raised is, how effective is a treatment procedure? For example are sensory integration techniques more effective than neurodevelopment treatment? The researcher has to determine at what level of significance the hypothesis would be accepted. If the researcher is using a standardized test, such as the Sensory Integration and Praxis Tests (SIPT; Ayres, 1989), then a definition of significance should be decided in advance. Guidelines for the degree of differences between the mean at posttest after intervention should be established. For example, one standard deviation above the mean will show significance. If group 1 had a mean of 100 and group 2 had a mean of 85, on a test in which one standard deviation equaled 15, significance has been demonstrated before a *t* test or ANOVA was been applied to the data. This exploratory data analysis is a method of "eyeballing the data" before applying a statistical test to the results. Exploratory data analysis involves:

1. Calculating group means and standard deviations to determine if the results are clinically significant
2. Screening results by collapsing data in nominal categories and performing a chi-square test
3. Describing results in scatter diagrams showing the relationship between variables
4. Using stem and leaf displays and box plots to tally the frequency count within designated categories

Reference: For a more detailed account of exploratory data analysis, see C. C. Hoaglin, F. Mosteller, and J. N. Tukey, (1991), *Fundamentals of Exploratory Analysis of Variance*. New York: John Wiley and Sons; and J. W. Tukey, (1977), *Exploratory Data Analysis*. Reading, MA: Addison-Wesley Publishing Company.

8.6.5 The Concept of Statistical Power and Effect Size

Statistical power is the ability of a statistical test to accurately reject the null hypothesis and to detect a difference between groups when one exists. Statistical power is related to the occurrence of a Type II error when the researcher finds that there is no statistically significant difference between the groups when, in reality, there is a significant difference. It is affected by the size of the sample, the probability level of significance such as .05 or .01, and the magnitude of the relationship between the variables measured. When large samples are used in a clinical study, any statistical analysis will be powerful. For example, a sample of 100 subjects in a clinical study will be more powerful than a sample of 25 subjects. The researcher will have more confidence in rejecting the null hypothesis with a larger number of subjects than with small size samples. However, statistical significance at a .05 level with large numbers of subjects may or may not demonstrate clinical significance. The power of a test, indicating the ability to reject the null hypothesis, also increases when the researcher is willing to accept a higher probability of error such as .05 (has more power) than the .01 level. What this means is that the researcher is willing to accept more error in interpreting the statistical results. Some researchers recommend a power level of .80 (Ottenbacher & Barrett, 1990). Nonetheless, a major question for a clinical researcher still remains: Is this treatment method effective? Statistical power should not be manipulated to camouflage clinical results. Clinical research study results should be analyzed to determine if the treatment method is promising, if it is effective with specific patients, and if it can be refined to improve its effectiveness. Statistical confidence should not be compromised to justify the use of treatment methods when they have not demonstrated effectiveness.

Effect Size

In clinical research, the effect size is presented by researchers to demonstrate the difference between treatment methods and their impact on improvement. For example, if a researcher is comparing the effectiveness of two types of hand exercise programs to increase grip strength, the researcher should apply an independent t test to evaluate statistical significance. The researcher also may be interested in looking at the clinical impact of the two treatment techniques. Effect size is an important concept that reflects both the variance between the groups and the variance within the groups.

The formula for effect size (ES) is:

$$ES = (\overline{X}_1 - \overline{X}_2) / s$$

where s is the pooled standard deviation of both groups

The effect size is zero when the null hypothesis is true (Cohen, 1977). The effect size also serves as an index of the degree of departure from the null hypothesis. For example, a relatively large effect size can be interpreted to mean that the study has high statistical power in accurately rejecting the null hypothesis. Most researchers have defined small, medium, and large effect sizes. Small effect sizes are about .2, medium effect sizes are about .5, and large effect sizes are about .8.

8.7 Model II: One-Sample Problems
(One-Sample *t* Test)

One-sample t tests are applied to research studies in which the investigator is testing whether a sample mean is equal to, less than, or greater than a given value. An example from environmental science is the sampling of air or water to determine if the air or water is polluted. Scientists concerned with the quality of air and water use one-sample t tests to compare samples with parameter values. These parameter values are health standards that have been predetermined by scientific evidence to be at acceptable health levels. At which point is the air considered to be polluted? What are the accepted levels of bacteria for water consumption? These are problems for one-sample t tests. We can also use one-sample t tests for screening populations. For example, is a group sample above or below normal values in height, weight, cholesterol level, blood pressure, heart rate, and hearing acuity? The procedure for applying a one-sample *t* test is to compare the sample mean with a hypothetical parameter value.

8.7.1 Hypothetical Example for Testing for Statistically Significant Differences Between Sample Mean and Parameter Mean Values

Step 1. State the research hypothesis.

a. *Null Hypothesis:* There is no statistically significant difference between the height (μ) of adult Japanese-American men and the standard height (μ_0) of all adult American men.

$$\mu = \mu_0 \text{ (mu, parameter mean value)}$$
$$N = 10{,}000$$

b. *Alternative Hypothesis:* There is a statistically significant difference between the height (μ) of adult Japanese-American men and the height (μ_0) of all adult American men.

$$\mu \neq \mu \text{ (mu, parameter mean value)}$$

Step 2. Select the level of statistical significance: $\alpha = .05$
Step 3. Select test statistics. Use t test.
Formula for a *t* test

$$t = \frac{\overline{X} - \mu_0}{s / \sqrt{N}}$$

(Note: *s* divided by square root of *n*)

Step 4. Identify the t_{crit} from the t distribution table.

a. significance level: $\alpha = .05$
b. two-tailed test of significance
c. $df = N - 1$, $10{,}000 - 1 = 9{,}999$, $t_{crit} = .196$[1]

Step 5. Calculate the test statistic value. From a random sample of 10,000 adult Japanese-American men living in the United States, the following data were collected. A $\overline{X}$ is used rather than a μ because only a sample of the total number is used. In this case, the $\overline{X}$ is a value obtained from a representative sample of the population (μ).

$$\overline{X} = 64 \text{ in.} \qquad sd = 1.8 \text{ in.}$$

Step 6. Identify parameter values. The parameter *values*[2] for the average adult American men are:

---

[1]Because *df* = 9999, which is larger than 120, t_{crit} may be obtained from Table C–2 Normal Curve.
[2]These are hypothetical values set to explain concepts.

$$\mu_0 = 69 \text{ in.} \qquad sd = 1.9 \text{ in.}$$

Step 7. Graph normal curve for parameter value. Because the parameter values are a constant, we can use the normal curve to describe the distribution of parameter values. This is shown in Figure 8–29. For a normal distribution with a mean of 69 and a standard deviation of 1.9, we will expect 68% of adult American men to have heights between 67.1 and 70.9 inches.

Step 8. Graph normal curve for sample. This is shown in Figure 8–30. For the sample distribution with a mean of 64 and a standard deviation of 1.8, we will expect 68% of the adult Japanese-American men to have heights between 62.2 and 65.8 inches.

Step 9. Calculate the t_{obs} using the formula for t test. (See Step 3)

$$t = \frac{\overline{X} - \mu_0}{s / \sqrt{N}}$$

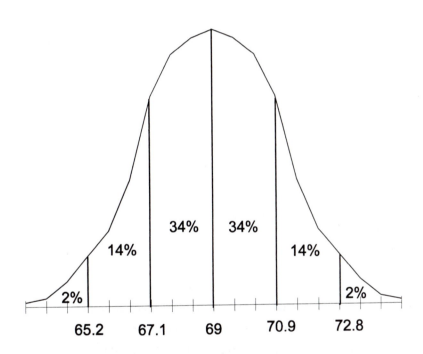

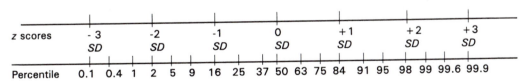

Figure 8–29. Hypothetical data for typical adult American men depicting a normal distribution in which the mean height is 69 inches and the standard deviation is 1.9. Sixty-eight percent of the adult population should fall between +1 and −1 standard deviations, or heights of 67.1 and 70.9 inches.

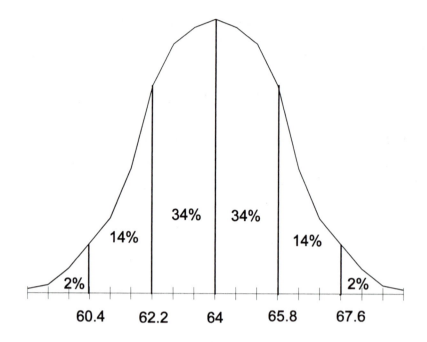

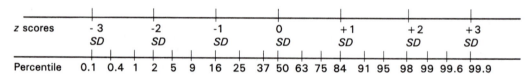

Figure 8–30. Hypothetical data for a sample of 10,000 adult Japanese and American men depicting a normal distribution in which the mean height is 64 inches and the standard deviation is 1.8. Sixty-eight percent of the adult population should fall between +1 and −1 standard deviations, or heights of 62.2 and 65.8 inches.

where $\overline{X}$ = sample mean equals 64

sd = sample standard deviation equals 1.8

μ_0 = parameter mean equals 69

N = sample number of subjects = 10,000

$t_{obs} = (64 - 69) / (1.8 / \sqrt{10{,}000}) = (-5) / (1.8 / 100)$

$t_{obs} = -5 / .018$

$t_{obs} = -277.77$

Step 10. Compare t_{obs} *with* t_{crit}

$$t_{obs} = -277.77 \qquad t_{crit} = 1.960$$

$$t_{obs} > t_{crit}$$

Thus, the researcher rejects the null hypothesis and concludes that there is a statistically significant difference between the height of adult Japanese-American men compared with the average heights of all adult American men.

8.8 Model III: Two Independent Groups

8.8.1 Independent *t* Test

The purpose of this statistical model is to test whether there is a statistically significant difference between the means of two independent samples. This frequently is used to test the differences between two clinical techniques applied to an experimental group and a control or comparative group. For example, if a researcher is examining the comparative effectiveness of two treatment techniques in two independent groups, such as Progressive Relaxation Exercise versus Transcutaneous Electrical Nerve Stimulation (TENS) in reducing pain, then an independent *t* test will be applied to the outcome measure for pain (dependent variable). The *t* test is also applied when the researcher examines whether there is a statistically significant difference in the characteristic abilities of two groups. In the example below from Liu, Gauthier, and Gauthier (1991), the authors compared performances on 12 perceptual spatial orientation tasks in two independent groups: senile dementia of the Alzheimer type (SDAT) and a comparative control group without dementia. Table 8–10 displays the means for both groups on the perceptual variables and the calculated probability level of significance.

Of the 12 variables tested, only 4 did not reach statistical significance at the $p < .05$ level. The researchers used a two-tailed test for determining the critical level of significance with a total n of 30 subjects (15 in each group), at a df of $n - 2$. In a two-tailed test with 28 df, the critical value of t is 2.0484 (see Table C–3 in the appendices). The observed t was above 2.0484 in 8 of the 12 variables tested. The t values reflected the differences between the group means and the comparative homogeneity of the two independent sample standard deviations. In general, a t value is statistically significant when there is a relatively large difference between the group mean and a small difference within the groups. On the other hand, if the differences within the groups are larger than the differences between the groups, then there will likely not be a statistically significant difference between the groups as reflected in the observed t value. For example, in examining the first variable, figure-ground perception (total), the SDAT group mean was 26.33 and the control group mean was 36.47. The mean difference between the groups was 10.14. The standard deviations of 6.61 and 4.63 were comparatively homogeneous. Thus, there was a statically significant difference between the two independent groups. In examining the variable shape (visual), note that the differences between the group means is .33 ($10.00 - 9.67$), while the standard deviation for the SDAT group is .82, thus indicating no statistically significant difference between the two independent group means.

Operational Procedure for Testing for Statistically Significant Differences Between Two Independent Samples

Step 1. State the research hypothesis.

a. *Null Hypothesis:* There is no statistically significant difference between the mean of group 1 versus the mean of group 2:

Table 8–10. Comparison of Performance on Perceptual Spatial Orientation Tasks

Skill	Maximum Score	SDAT Group (n = 15) M (SD)	Control Group (n = 15) M (SD)	p*
Figure-ground perception (total)	48	26.33 (6.61)	36.47 (4.63)	≤ .0001
Figure-ground perception (Part 1)	24	16.00 (3.59)	20.53 (1.19)	≤ .0002
Figure-ground perception (Part 2)	24	10.33 (4.15)	15.93 (3.90)	≤ .001
Shape (visual)	10	9.67 (0.82)	10.00 (0.00)	ns
Shape (tactual)	10	6.13 (2.26)	8.93 (1.34)	≤ .0005
Size (visual)	6	6.00 (0.00)	6.00 (0.00)	ns
Size (tactual)	15	14.33 (1.23)	14.87 (0.35)	ns
Position in space (total)	16	11.93 (4.01)	15.33 (0.82)	≤ .004
Position in space (Part 1)	8	7.20 (1.42)	7.93 (0.26)	≤ .06
Position in space (Part 2)	8	4.73 (2.92)	7.4 (0.74)	≤ .002
Spatial relations	15	11.47 (2.67)	14.73 (0.59)	≤ .0002
Left-right discrimination	10	9.67 (0.72)	10.00 (0.00)	ns

Note. SDAT = senile dementia of the Alzheimer type; ns = not significant. *Two-tailed *t* test for independent samples.

Note: From "Spatial Disorientation in Persons with Early Senile Dementia of the Alzheimer Type," by L. Liu, L. Gauthier, & S. Gauthier, 1991, *The American Journal of Occupational Therapy, 45,* p. 70. Copyright 1991 by *American Journal of Occupational Therapy.* Reprinted with permission.

$$H_0: \mu_1 = \mu_2$$

b. *Directional Hypothesis:* Mean one is significantly statistically different from mean two in a stated direction:

$$\mu_1 > \mu_2$$

c. *Alternative Hypothesis:* Mean one does not equal mean two, and there is a statistically significant difference between the two means (nondirectional):

$$H_1: \mu_1 \neq \mu_2$$

Step 2. Select the level of statistical significance. In social sciences research, the .05 level of significance is traditionally selected.

Step 3. Select statistical test. Use independent *t* test.

Step 4. Decide whether to use a one-tailed or two-tailed test for statistical significance. A two-tailed test is used with a null hypothesis to determine if there are statistically significant differences in either direction of the tail. The model for a two-tailed test are the tails in a normal curve (Figure 8–31). A one-tailed test is used with a directional hypothesis when the researcher predicts that the experimental group mean will be either statistically greater or lesser than a comparison mean.

Step 5. Look up the critical value (t_{crit}) from the published statistical table. The critical value is determined by:

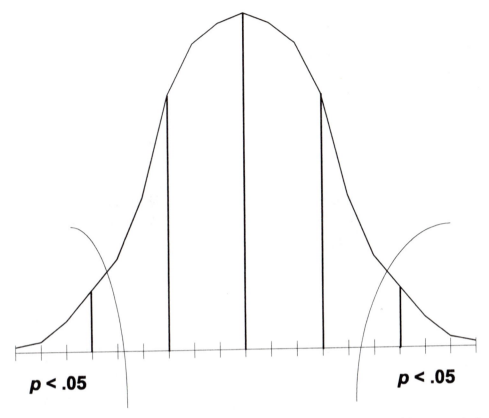

p < .05   p < .05

Figure 8–31. Model for a two-tailed test. A one-tailed test would use only one of the two marked areas.

a. the degrees of freedom (df)
b. the level of significance ($\alpha \leq .05$ or $\leq .01$)
c. the direction of the test (one-tailed or two-tailed)
d. the value of t_{crit} as indicated in the statistical table (see Appendix C–3).

Step 6. Calculate the group means and standard deviations.
Step 7. Do an exploratory data analysis to determine if the differences between the two means are clinically significant and that the standard deviations in both groups are approximately equal.
Step 8. Plot a graph. Use the graph mean and raw scores of group 1 and group 2 to visualize whether there seems to be a statistically significant difference between the group means (see Figure 8–32). If there appears to be a difference between the two group means, then go to Step 8 and calculate the values.
Step 9. Calculate the t_{obs} using the formula.
The formula for t_{obs} is:

$$t_{obs} = \frac{\overline{X}_1 - \overline{X}_2}{\sqrt{\{[(n_1 - 1)\, s_1^2 + (n_2 - 1)\, s_2^2] / [n_1 + n_2 - 2]\}\, \{(1 / n_1) + (1 / n_2)\}}}$$

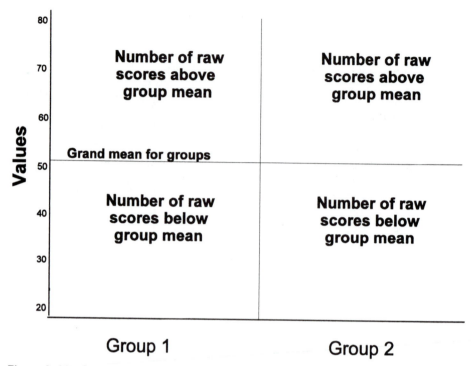

Figure 8–32. Graph to visualize values of scores as a way to estimate possible statistical significance between the group means.

where $\overline{X}_1$ = mean value of group 1

$\overline{X}_2$ = mean value of group 2

n_1 = total number of cases in group 1

n_2 = total number of cases in group 2

s_1^2 = variance (the standard deviation squared) for group 1

s_2^2 = variance for group 2

Step 10. Compare the two values: t_{obs} and t_{crit}.

a. Accept the null hypothesis if t_{obs} is less than t_{crit}.

b. Reject the null hypothesis if t_{obs} is equal to or greater than t_{crit}.

c. Accept the directional hypothesis if t_{obs} is greater than or equal to t_{crit} in the direction that is hypothesized.

d. Reject the directional hypothesis if t_{obs} is less than t_{crit} or if the mean value that is predicted to be greater is less than the mean value of the control or comparative group. For example, a researcher predicts that cognitive training is more effective than behavioral therapy in increasing attention span. The results show a statistically significant difference between the two means, but behavioral therapy demonstrates to be more effective. Because the researcher predicted that cognitive therapy is more effective than behavioral therapy, the directional hypothesis is rejected.

Two Independent Groups Example

Is there a statistically significant difference between stress management and group psychotherapy in reducing anxiety scores in patients with clinical depression?

Hypothetical Posttest Scores on the State-Trait Anxiety Inventory[a]

Stress Management Group			Psychotherapy Group		
Subject	Score	X_1^2	Subject	Score	X_2^2
01	35	1225	01	51	2601
02	41	1681	02	48	2304
03	38	1444	03	52	2704
04	42	1764	04	43	1849
05	43	1849	05	49	2401
06	36	1296	06	54	2916
07	32	1024	07	61	3721
08	40	1600	08	56	3136
09	41	1681	09	54	2916
10	43	1849	10	60	3600
11	42	1764	11	48	2304
12	34	1156	12	46	2116

$\Sigma X_1 = 467$ $\Sigma X_1^2 = 18333$ $\Sigma X_2 = 622$ $\Sigma X_2^2 = 32568$

$\overline{X}_1 = 38.9$ $\overline{X}_2 = 51.8$

Grand Mean $= (\Sigma X_1 + \Sigma X_2) / 24 = (467 + 622) / 24 = 45.37$

[a]Smaller score indicates less anxiety.

Step 1. State the research hypothesis. There is no statistically significant difference between a stress management group and a psychotherapy group in reducing anxiety in a sample of depressed patients. The hypothesis is stated in null form ($\mu_1 = \mu_2$).

Step 2. Select the level of statistical significance. The $\alpha = .05$ level of statistical significance will be accepted.

Step 3. This is a nondirectional two-tailed test for statistical significance because a null hypothesis was stated. Decide the test statistic. Independent t test will be used.

Step 4. Determine the critical value for t from published statistical tables (see Table C–3 in the appendices).

  a. $df = n_1 + n_2 - 2 = 22$
  b. level of significance $\alpha = .05$
  c. $t_{crit} = 2.0739$

Step 5. Calculate the mean and standard deviations.

Stress Management Group	Psychotherapy Group
$\overline{X}_1 = 38.9$	$\overline{X}_2 = 51.8$
$\overline{X}_1 = \Sigma X_1 / n = 467 / 12 = 38.9$	$\overline{X}_1 = \Sigma X_2 / n = 622 / 12 = 51.8$
$s_1 = 3.80$	$s_2 = 5.45$

Computational Formula for Standard Deviation.

$$s = \sqrt{[n \, \Sigma X^2 - (\Sigma X)^2] / [n(n-1)]}$$
$$s_1 = \sqrt{\{[(12)(18333)] - (467)^2\} / [12(12-1)]}$$
$$s_1 = \sqrt{(219996 - 218089) / [12(12-1)]}$$
$$s_1 = \sqrt{1907 / 132}$$
$$s_1 = \sqrt{14.44}$$
$$s_1 = 3.80$$
$$s_2 = \sqrt{\{[(12)(32568)] - (622)^2\} / [12(12-1)]}$$
$$s_2 = \sqrt{(390816 - 386884) / [12(12-1)]}$$
$$s_2 = \sqrt{3932 / 132}$$
$$s_2 = \sqrt{29.78}$$
$$s_2 = 5.45$$

Step 6. Exploratory data analysis.

$$\overline{X}_1 - \overline{X}_2 = 38.9 - 51.8 = -12.9$$
$$s_1 = 3.80 \qquad\qquad s_2 = 5.45$$

The mean difference is greater than the standard deviation for group 1 or group 2. Standard deviation difference between the two groups is 1.65. There is a relative homogeneity of variance for the two groups.

Step 7. Exploratory graph analysis. Figure 8–33 shows the graph obtained from the analysis. There appears to be a significant difference between the two groups.

Step 8. Calculate t_{obs}.

$$t_{obs} = \frac{\overline{X}_1 - \overline{X}_2}{\sqrt{\{[(n_1 - 1)(s_1{}^2) + (n_2 - 1)(s_2{}^2)] / (n_1 + n_2 - 2)\} [(1 / n_1) + (1 / n_2)]}}$$

where

Group 1	Group 2
$\overline{X}_1 = 38.9$	$\overline{X}_2 = 51.8$
$n_1 = 12$	$n_2 = 12$
$s_1{}^2 = (3.80)^2 = 14.44$	$s_2{}^2 = (5.45)^2 = 29.70$

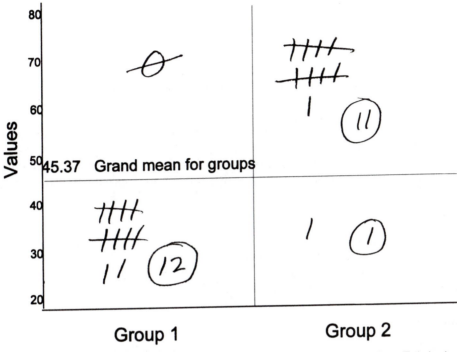

Figure 8–33. Exploratory graph analysis for hypothetical posttest scores on the State-Trait Anxiety Inventory. The graph shows the difference between scores between two independent groups of patients with clinical depression receiving either stress management training or group psychotherapy. The test being performed is an independent *t* test.

$$t_{obs} = \frac{38.9 - 51.8}{\sqrt{\{[(12-1)(14.44) + (12-1)(29.78)] / (12+12-2)\} [(1/12) + (1/12)]}}$$

$$t_{obs} = \frac{-12.9}{\sqrt{[(158.84 + 327.58) / 22] [.1667]}}$$

$$t_{obs} = -12.9 / \sqrt{(486.42 / 22)(.1667)}$$

$$t_{obs} = -12.9 / \sqrt{3.685}$$

$$t_{obs} = -12.9 / 1.9196$$

$$t_{obs} = -6.72$$

Step 9. Compare t_{obs} *and* t_{crit}.

$$t_{obs} = -6.72 \qquad\qquad t_{crit} = 2.0739$$

Examination shows $|t_{obs}|^3 > t_{crit}$. Reject the null hypothesis. There seems to be a statistically significant difference between the two means, indicating that the stress management group was significantly more effective that the psychotherapy group in the reduction of anxiety in patients with clinical depression.

---

[3] $|t_{obs}|$ is an absolute value that disregards the sign. The parallel lines indicate absolute value.

8.8.2 Mann-Whitney U Test

Rationale.

The Mann-Whitney, a nonparametric alternative to the independent *t* test, is used to test whether two independent groups have been drawn from the same population. In practice, the Mann-Whitney is used with ordinal scale data.

1. The null hypothesis states that the two independent groups have the same population distribution.
2. An alternative, directional hypothesis is that there is a significant difference between the group means (when the distributions are approximately the same).

Assumptions

1. Random selection of each group.
2. Two mutually independent groups are compared.
3. The measurement scale is at least ordinal.
4. *n* for each group is less than 20.

Computation

1. Rank order every raw score combining the two groups, (e.g., lowest score in both groups is assigned the rank of 1).
2. When two or more raw scores are the same, average the ranks.
3. Add the ranks for one group, obtaining T_A value.

Formula for Mann-Whitney U Test

$$U_{obs} = [n_A n_B] + [(n_A)(n_A + 1) / 2] - [T_A]$$

where

n_A = number of subjects in 1st group

n_B = number of subjects in 2nd group

Example

Language intelligibility scores were compared between an experimental and control group after a 6-month treatment period. There was no significant difference between the groups on the pretest. (Two-tailed test $\alpha = .05$)
    The following data were collected:

Experimental Group A			Control Group P		
Subject	Score	Rank	Subject	Score	Rank
101	33	12	201	35	13
102	30	10	202	32	11
103	25	8	203	27	9
104	24	6.5	204	24	6.5
105	22	5	205	21	4

Experimental Group A			Control Group P		
Subject	Score	Rank	Subject	Score	Rank
106	19	3	206	18	2
			207	16	1
$T_A = 44.5$			$T_B = 46.5$		
$n_A = 6$			$n_B = 7$		

$U_{obs} = [(6)(7)] + [6(6 + 1) / 2] - [44.5]$

$U_{obs} = 42 + 21 - 44.5$

$U_{obs} = 63 - 44.5$

$U_{obs} = 18.5$

U_{crit}: obtain from table for Mann-Whitney U test (Appendix C–7).

$n_A / n_B = 6 / 7 = U_{crit} = 6 / 36$

If U_{obs} is between 6 and 36, do not reject null hypothesis.

Conclusion

Null hypothesis is not rejected because $U_{obs} = 18.5$, which is between 6 and 36. Thus, the researcher concludes that there is no statistically significant difference in the experimental and control groups in language intelligibility posttest scores.

8.9 Model IV: Paired Data Sample

8.9.1 Correlated t Test

The correlated t test is applied to data when a researcher compares a group's performance or characteristic on two measures. For example, a researcher compares the difference between pretest and posttest scores of an observed variable. Another example is to compare the difference of two variables in one group, such as intelligence and perceptual motor test scores. The difference between the correlated t test and the independent t test is that the correlated t test is applied with one independent group and two variables, whereas the independent t test is applied to scores for two independent groups.

An example of a correlated t test was found in a study by McFall, Deitz, and Crowe (1993) entitled "Test-retest reliability of the test of visual perceptual skills with children with learning disabilities." In that study, the authors compared the difference in the score on the same test between a 1 to 2 week's time period. The table below describes the means, mean differences, and t_{obs}.

Correlated t Tests Between Test and Retest Scores

Subtests	Pretest Mean	Retest Mean	Mean Difference	t Value
Visual Discrimination	11.9	13.01	1.1	−1.89
Visual Memory	9.4	10.5	1.1	−2.41*

(continued)

Subtests (continued)	Pretest Mean	Retest Mean	Mean Difference	t Value
Spatial Relations	10.4	11.1	.7	−1.76
Form Consistency	8.7	9.4	.7	−1.76
Sequential Memory	8.4	8.4	0.0	1.76
Figure Ground	9.2	9.3	.1	−.11
Visual Closure	9.5	11.4	.9	−3.17**

Note. $n = 30$; Critical value for $t_{obs} = 2.0452$; $df = N - 1 = 30 - 1 = 29$; two-tailed test; *$p < .05$, **$p < .01$.

There was a statistically significant difference between test and retest means on the variables of visual memory ($|t_{obs}| = -2.41$) and visual closure ($|t_{obs}| = -3.17$). These t values were above the t_{crit} value of 2.0452. The $|t_{obs}|$ in the other tests were all below 2.045. The minus sign is disregarded in a nondirectional test.

On the basis of a significant statistical difference on these two subtests, the researcher will reject the null hypothesis. The null hypothesis is accepted for the other subtests.

Operational Procedure for Testing for Statistical Significance in a Paired Data Sample

Step 1. State the research hypothesis.

   a. *Null Hypothesis: H_0: $\mu_1 = \mu_2$*
   b. *Alternative Hypothesis: $\mu_1 \neq \mu_2$*
   c. *Directional Hypothesis: H_1: $\mu_1 > \mu_2$*

Step 2. Select the level of statistical significance.

$$\alpha = .05 \text{ or } .01 \text{ level of significance}$$

Step 3. Decide the test statistic and whether to apply a one-tailed or two-tailed test for statistical significance.

Step 4. Look up the critical value for t_{crit} from statistical table.

   a. determine the degrees of freedom: $df = N - 1$
   b. level of significance $\alpha = .05$ or $.01$
   c. one-tailed or two-tailed test
   d. t_{crit} derived from table of values (see Appendix C–3)

Step 5. Calculate the group means and standard deviations for each variable.
Step 6. Do an exploratory data analysis by determining if mean differences are greater than standard deviations for each variable.
Step 7. Plot a graph (see Independent t Test).
Step 8. Calculate t_{obs} using the formula:

$$t_{obs} = \frac{\Sigma D_1}{\sqrt{[N \Sigma D_1{}^2 - (\Sigma D_1)^2 / N - 1}}$$

where ΣD_1 = sum of differences between each subject's score on measured variable

$\Sigma D_1{}^2$ = sum of the squared differences on each score

N = total number of subjects

Step 9. Accept the null hypothesis if $t_{obs} < t_{crit}$.
Step 10. Reject the null hypothesis if $t_{obs} \geq t_{crit}$.

Paired Data Sample

Hypothetical example of correlated t test. Is there a statistically significant difference between performance IQ scores in adults with traumatic brain injury after undergoing an intensive cognitive retraining program?

Performance IQ Scores

Subject	Baseline (Pretest)	X_1^2	After Treatment (Posttest)	X_2^2
01	97	9409	113	12769
02	106	11236	113	12769
03	106	11236	101	10201
04	95	9025	119	14161
05	102	10404	111	12321
06	111	12321	121	14641
07	115	13225	121	14641
08	104	10816	106	11236
09	90	8100	110	12100
10	96	9216	126	15876
	$\Sigma X_1 = 1022$	$\Sigma X_1^2 = 104988$	$\Sigma X_2 = 1141$	$\Sigma X_2^2 = 130715$

Step 1. State the research hypothesis. There is no statistically significant difference between pre- and posttest IQ performance scores in adults with traumatic brain injury who have undergone an extensive cognitive retraining program. This is a null hypothesis ($H_0: \mu_1 = \mu_2$).
Step 2. The level of statistical significance is $\alpha = .05$.
Step 3. Decide whether to use a one-tailed or two-tailed test. This problem requires a two-tailed test because the hypothesis is stated in null form and the researcher is examining statistical significance without direction.
Step 4. Look up t_{crit} (see Appendix C–3).

    a. $df = N - 1 = 9$
    b. $\alpha = .05$
    c. two-tailed test
    d. $t_{crit} = 2.2622$

Step 5. Calculate the group means and standard deviations for the baseline and retest conditions.

Group 1
$\overline{X}_1 = \Sigma X / N = 1022 / 10 = 102.2$
$s_1 = 7.74$

Group 2
$\overline{X}_2 = 1141 / 10 = 114.1$
$s_2 = 7.65$

Standard deviation computation formula

$$s = \sqrt{[N\Sigma X^2 - (\Sigma X)^2] / N(N - 1)}$$

$$s_1 = \sqrt{\{[(10)(104988)] - (1022)^2\} / (10)(10 - 1)}$$

$$s_1 = \sqrt{(10498880 - 1044484) / 90}$$

$$s_1 = \sqrt{5396 / 90}$$

$$s_1 = 7.74$$

$$s_2 = \sqrt{\{[(10)(130715)] - (1141)^2\} / 10(10 - 1)}$$

$$s_2 = \sqrt{(1307150 - 1301881) / 90}$$

$$s_2 = \sqrt{5269 / 90}$$

$$s_2 = \sqrt{58.54}$$

$$s_2 = 7.65$$

Step 6. Exploratory Data Analysis.

$$\overline{X}_1 - \overline{X}_2 = 102.2 - 114.1 = 11.9$$

$$s_1 = 7.74 \qquad\qquad s_2 = 7.65$$

The mean difference between pre- and posttest scores is greater than the standard deviations for pretest and posttest scores. The difference between the standard deviations is relatively small, indicating a homogeneity of variance for the two groups of scores.

Step 7. Exploratory Graph. This is displayed in Figure 8–34.

From the exploratory data analysis, there appears to be a significant difference between the pretest and posttest scores.

Step 8. Calculate t_{obs}.

$$t_{obs} = \frac{\Sigma D_1}{\sqrt{[N\Sigma D^2 - (\Sigma D_1)^2] / (N - 1)}}$$

Subject	Baseline Test	Retest	D_1	D^2
01	97	113	−16	256
02	106	113	−07	49
03	106	101	+05	25
04	95	119	−24	576
05	102	111	−09	81
06	111	122	−11	121
07	115	121	−06	36
08	104	106	−02	4
09	90	110	−20	400
10	96	126	−30	900
	1022	1142	$\Sigma D_1 = -120$	$\Sigma D^2 = 2448$
			$(\Sigma D_1)^2 = 14400$	

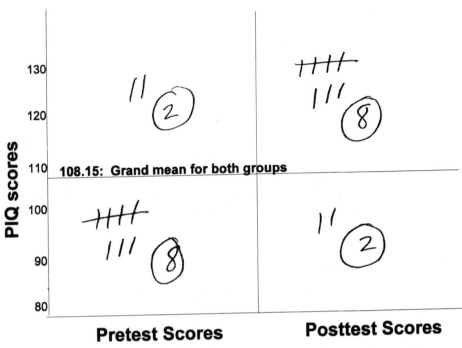

Figure 8–34. Exploratory graph analysis using hypothetical data. The graph shows differences between pre- and post-test performance IQ scores for a group of adults with traumatic brain damage after cognitive retraining. The statistical test being performed is a correlated *t* test.

$$t_{obs} = (-120) / \sqrt{\{[(10)(2448)] - 14400 / 9\}}$$
$$t_{obs} = (-120) / \sqrt{[(24480 - 14400) / 9]}$$
$$t_{obs} = (-120) / \sqrt{10080 / 9}$$
$$t_{obs} = (-120) / \sqrt{1120}$$
$$t_{obs} = (-120) / 33.460$$
$$t_{obs} = -3.586$$

Step 9. $t_{obs} = -3.586$. Using Table C–3 in the appendices, we find that $t_{crit} = 2.2622$. The researcher rejects the null hypothesis and concludes that there appears to be a significant difference between the pre- and posttest scores and that cognitive rehabilitation appeared to be effective in raising Performance IQ scores in this sample of individuals with traumatic brain injury.[4]

8.9.2 Wilcoxon Test for Paired Data Samples

The Wilcoxon signed rank test is a nonparametric alternative to the *t* test for correlated samples.

[4]Note that the negative sign in -3.5 does not affect the value. Both positive and negative values are interpreted equally when compared with the t_{crit} value for the table.

Assumptions in Applying Wilcoxon

  1. Random selection or random assignment of subjects
  2. Measurement scale is at least ordinal.

Example of Applying Wilcoxon

An investigator is interested in comparing the pre- and posttest scores for a group of nine subjects. The null hypothesis is stated with $\alpha = .05$. The data for this example are as follows:

Subject	Pretest Raw Score	Posttest Raw Score	Difference	Rank Difference
01	10	12	−2	(−) 4
02	12	15	−3	(−) 7
03	8	6	2	4
04	6	10	−4	(−) 8
05	14	12	2	4
06	7	6	1	1
07	10	12	−2	(−) 4
08	14	16	−2	(−) 4
09	12	18	−6	(−) 9

Stepwise Procedure for Wilcoxon Signed-Rank Test (Example)

  Step 1. Calculate the difference between the pre- and posttest raw scores, subtracting the posttest raw scores from the pretest raw scores.

  Step 2. Rank order the differences between raw scores from smallest to largest, ignoring the negative or positive signs. Notice that in tied ranks, such as with 2 as a difference, the midpoint of the rank is 4 (2, 3, 4, 5, 6).

  Step 3. Sum the positive rank differences.

  4

  4

  1

  —

  9

  Step 4. Sum the negative rank differences.

  −4

  −7

  −8

-4

-4

-9

———

-36

Step 5. Determine T value. T is the absolute value of the smaller sum of the rank differences.

$$T = 9$$

Step 6. Compare the T_{obs} with T_{crit} from the table for critical values to T (see Appendix C–8).

T_{crit} for $N = 9$, $\alpha = .05$, two-tailed test. $T_{crit} = 5$

Step 7. If the T_{obs} is equal to or less than T_{crit}, then reject the null hypothesis and conclude that there is a statistically significant difference between the pre- and posttest scores. Because $T_{obs} = 9$ is greater than $T_{crit} = 5$, we accept the null hypothesis and conclude that there are no statistically significant differences between the pre- and posttest scores.

References: R. Runyon, (1977). *Nonparametric Statistics.* Reading, MA: Addison-Wesley Publishing Company, pp. 107–110, 181.

8.10   Model V: *k*-Independent Samples

8.10.1   Analysis of Variance

ANOVA is a widely used statistical test equivalent to the independent *t* test when testing for significant differences between two means. ANOVA is applied to statistical data when two or more independent group means are being compared. The statistic for the ANOVA is *F*. (*k* refers to the number of independent groups or conditions in the study.)

$$F = \frac{\text{Variance between groups}}{\text{Variance within groups}}$$

The concept of the ANOVA is that if there are large differences between the group means compared with relatively small differences within the variances or scores within the group, then a statistically significant result, is evident. ANOVA answers the question: Is there a statistically significant difference between the independent groups being tested? For example, does $\mu_1 = \mu_2 = \mu_3 = \mu_k$? ANOVA is always tested by a null hypothesis. When there is a statistically significant result, the researcher then carries out a post hoc analysis, such as the Scheffé, Duncan Multiple Range, Neuman-Keuls and Tukey's procedures. These post hoc tests are similar to *t* tests, applied to the data after attaining a significant *F*.

One-Way ANOVA

A one-way ANOVA simply analyzes the group means for statistically significant differences. The hypothetical table of results that follows is a typical example of a one-way

ANOVA for comparing the effectiveness of three handwriting programs among 19 children with handwriting problems.

ANOVA Summary Table for Comparing Two Treatment Groups

Source of Variance	df	SS	MS	F
Between treatment groups	2	16	8	4.0*
Within treatment groups	16	32	2	
Total	18			

*$p = <.05$, F_{crit} 3.63

> where SS = sums of squares
>
> MS = mean squares
>
> k = number of treatment groups
>
> N = total number of subjects in all groups

F is a derivative value equivalent to F_{obs} that is compared with the F_{crit} derived from a statistical table of values. For example, the F_{crit} for 2 df (treatment groups − 1) and 16 df [number of subjects (19) − number of groups (3)] with 2/16, $\alpha = .05$ is 3.63. Degrees of freedom (df) is derived from between treatment groups ($k − 1$) and within treatment groups ($N − k$).

The result in this hypothetical example shows that there is a statistically significant difference between the three treatment methods for handwriting disorders. F_{obs} 4.00 is > F_{crit} 3.63. Thus, the researcher will reject the null hypothesis.

Example of Two-Factor ANOVA From the Literature

A one-way ANOVA analyzes the group means for statistically significant differences. The two-factor ANOVA looks at the variables from a two-dimensional perspective. It analyzes interactive effects, such as treatment method and therapist personality or treatment method and patient diagnosis. Palmer (1989) studied two methods of bed transfer following back surgery and examined pain experienced by patients preoperative (day 1) and postoperative (day 2). Results are shown in the following table.

Summary Table of Anova on Pain Rating Scores by Transfer Method and Time

Source of Variance	df	F	p Value
Time (pre-post operative)	4	17.196	.000*
Method (2 transfer methods)	1	2.435	.120
Time X method	4	0.911	.458

*$p < .05$ significant

The results show that there was a statistically significant difference between pain ratings during pre- and postoperation time periods. There were no statistically significant differences in the two methods of bed transfer nor in the interactional effects of time and method.

Stepwise Procedures for One-Way ANOVA (Hypothetical Example)

Step 1. State the research hypothesis. The hypothesis is always stated in the null form when using ANOVA. For example, there is no statistically significant difference between electrical stimulation (ES), acupuncture (A), and proprioceptive neuromuscular facilitation (PNF) in improving upper extremity function in patients with chronic hemiplegia.

$$H_0 = \mu_1 = \mu_2 = \mu_3$$

Step 2. Select the level of statistical significance.

$$\alpha = .05$$

Step 3. Identify F_{crit} from table (see Table C–4 in the appendices).

   a. *df* for the numerator = 2 (three treatment groups − 1)
      df for the denominator = 15 (number of subjects minus the number of groups:

$$18 - 3 = 15)$$
$$df = 2 \,/\, 15$$

   b. $\alpha = .05$
   c. $F_{crit} = 3.68$

Step 4. Calculate means and standard deviations.[5]

ES Group			A Group			PNF Group		
Subject	Score	$X_1{}^2$	Subject	Score	$X_2{}^2$	Subject	Score	$X_3{}^2$
01	23	529	01	13	169	01	33	1089
02	31	961	02	19	361	02	42	1764
03	16	256	03	19	361	03	30	900
04	27	729	04	25	625	04	38	1444
05	32	1024	05	18	324	05	44	1936
06	18	324				06	41	1681
07	38	1444						
$\Sigma X_1 = 185$		$\Sigma X_1{}^2 = 5267$	$\Sigma X_2 = 94$		$\Sigma X_2{}^2 = 1840$	$\Sigma X_3 = 228$		$\Sigma X_3{}^2 = 8814$
$\overline{X}_1 = 26.4$			$\overline{X}_2 = 18.8$			$\overline{X}_3 = 38.0$		

$$s = \sqrt{[N\Sigma X^2 - (\Sigma X)^2 \,/\, N\,(N - 1)}$$
$$s_1 = \sqrt{[7(5267) - (185)^2] \,/\, 7(6)}$$
$$s_1 = \sqrt{2644 \,/\, 42}$$

[5]The Fugl-Meyer Poststroke Motor Recovery Test Scores were used for the example. (Range is from 0–60.)

$$s_1 = \sqrt{62.95}$$
$$s_1 = 7.93$$
$$s_2 = \sqrt{[5(1840) - (94)^2] / 5(4)}$$
$$s_2 = \sqrt{364 / 20}$$
$$s_2 = \sqrt{18.2}$$
$$s_2 = 4.26$$
$$s_3 = \sqrt{[6(8814) - (228)^2] / 6(5)}$$
$$s_3 = \sqrt{900 / 30}$$
$$s_3 = \sqrt{30.00}$$
$$s_3 = 5.48$$

Step 5. Exploratory Data Analysis.

$\overline{X}_1 = 26.4$	$s_1 = 7.93$
$\overline{X}_2 = 18.8$	$s_2 = 4.26$
$\overline{X}_3 = 38.0$	$s_3 = 5.48$
$\overline{X}_1 - \overline{X}_2 = 7.6$	$s_1 - s_2 = 3.67$
$\overline{X}_1 - \overline{X}_3 = -11.6$	$s_1 - s_3 = 2.45$
$\overline{X}_2 - \overline{X}_3 = -19.2$	$s_2 - s_3 = -1.22$

There appears to be a statistically significant difference between the means and a relatively homogenous variance.

Step 6. Exploratory Graph Analysis. This graph is shown in Figure 8–35.

$$\text{Group mean} = (\Sigma \overline{X}_1 + \Sigma \overline{X}_2 + \Sigma \overline{X}_3) / (N_1 + N_2 + N_3)$$
$$= (185 + 94 + 288) / (7 + 5 + 6)$$
$$= 507 / 18$$
$$= 28.17$$

There appears to be a statistically significant difference between group 2 and group 3.

Step 7. Calculate F.

Summary Table for One-Way ANOVA

Source of Variance	df	SS	MS	F
Between groups (BG)	2	1039.98	519.99	12.99
Within groups (WG)	15	600.52	40.03	
Total	17			

Formulas for ANOVA:

a.
$$F = \frac{MS \text{ between groups}}{MS \text{ within groups}}$$

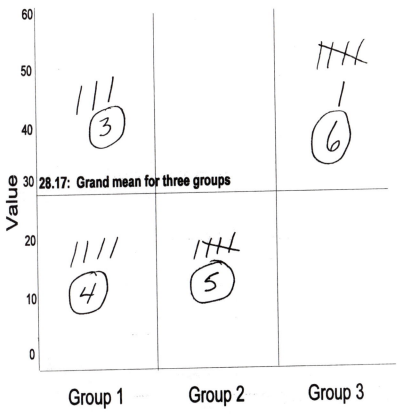

Figure 8–35. Exploratory graph for ANOVA using hypothetical data. The graph shows differences in scores between three different groups.

b. *df* between groups (df_{bg}) = Number of groups minus 1 = (3 − 1) = 2
   df within groups (df_{wg}) = Total number of subjects in all groups minus the number of groups = 18 − 3 = 15
c. Mean Square between groups = SS_{bg} / df_{bg}
   Mean Square within groups = SS_{wg} / df_{wg}
d. Sum of Squares between groups:

$$S_{bg} = \Sigma \left[(\Sigma X_1)^2 / n_1\right] + \left[(\Sigma X_2)^2 / n_2\right] + \left[(\Sigma X_3)^2 / n_3\right] - \left[(\Sigma X_1 + \Sigma X_2 + \Sigma X_3)^2 / \Sigma N\right]$$

Group 1

$$(\Sigma X_1)^2 = (185)^2 = 34225$$
$$n_1 = 7$$
$$(\Sigma X_1)^2 / n_1 = 4889.29$$

Group 2

$$(\Sigma X_2)^2 = (94)^2 = 8836$$
$$n_2 = 5$$
$$(\Sigma X_2)^2 / n_2 = 1767.2$$

Group 3

$$(\Sigma X_3)^2 = (228)^2 = 51984$$

$$n_3 = 6$$

$$(\Sigma X_3)^2 \,/\, n_3 = 8664.0$$

$$\text{Total} = (4889.29 + 1767.2 + 8664.0) = 15320.49$$

$$(\Sigma X_1 + \Sigma X_2 + \Sigma X_3) \,/\, \Sigma N)$$

$$= 257049 \,/\, 18$$

$$= 14280.5$$

$$SS_{bg} = [(4889.29 + 1767.2 + 8664.0)] - [(257049) \,/\, 18]$$

$$SS_{bg} = 15320.49 - 14280.5$$

$$SS_{bg} = 1039.99$$

e. Sums of Squares Within Groups

$$SSwg = \Sigma\,(\Sigma X_2^2 + \Sigma X_2^2 + \Sigma X_3^2) - 15320.49$$

$$SS_{wg} = \Sigma\,(5267 + 1840 + 8814) - 15320.49$$

$$SS_{wg} = 15921 - 15320.49$$

$$SS_{wg} = 600.51$$

$$\text{Mean Square between groups} = SS_{bg} \,/\, df_{bg}$$

$$= 1039.99 \,/\, 2$$

$$= 519.99$$

$$\text{Mean Square within groups} = SS_{bg} \,/\, df_{wg}$$

$$= 600.51 \,/\, 15$$

$$= 40.03$$

$$F = MS_{bg} \,/\, MS_{wg} = 519.99 \,/\, 40.03 = 12.99$$

Step 8. Compare F_{obs} with F_{crit}.

$$F_{obs} = 12.99 \qquad\qquad F_{crit} = 3.68$$

Thus, we reject the null hypothesis and conclude that there is a statistically significant difference between the three groups. This confirms our exploratory data analysis.

Step 9. Conduct a post hoc test. If there is a significant F, meaning that the mean values are statistically significant, then the researcher carries out a post hoc analysis. This analysis is parallel to doing independent t tests and determine which pairs of means have statistically significant differences.

There are a number of post hoc tests that are available to the researcher, such as:

► Tukey's Honestly Significant Differences (HSD)
► Neuman-Keuls
► Duncan Multiple Range
► Scheffé

Example of a Post Hoc Analysis. In the previous example, it was found that F_{obs} is statistically significant when $\overline{X}_1 = 26.4$, $\overline{X}_2 = 18.8$, and $\overline{X}_3 = 38.0$. H_0: Null hypothesis is rejected and we conclude that all the means are not the same. We can now compare each pair of means, such as:

$\overline{X}_1$ compared to $\overline{X}_2$ $\quad\quad$ $\overline{X}_1$ compared to $\overline{X}_3$ $\quad\quad$ $\overline{X}_2$ compared to $\overline{X}_3$

A significant F means that at least one pair of means are significantly different, that is, the highest and lowest mean. Therefore, $\overline{X}_2$ compared to $\overline{X}_3$ has a statistically significant difference. We do not know whether there is a statistically significant difference between $\overline{X}_1$ and $\overline{X}_2$, and $\overline{X}_1$ and $\overline{X}_3$. A post hoc analysis tests for statistical significant difference in these two situations.

In this example the Tukey (*HSD*), a widely used post hoc analysis, was selected. The formula for the Tukey is (Gravette & Wellnau, 1985):

$$HSD = q \sqrt{(MS_{wg} / n)}$$

where

q = a derived table value (see Table C–9 in the appendices: The Student Range Statistic)

MS_{wg} = the value calculated for mean squares within groups and is taken from the ANOVA table. In the above example this value is 40.03.

n = the average of the number of cases in each group. In the above example $n_1 = 7, n_2 = 5,$ $n_3 = 6$. The average is 6.

k = number of groups $(k) = 3$

df for $MS_{wg} = 15$

$\alpha = .05$

$q = 3.67$

$HSD = q \sqrt{(MS_{wg} / n)}$

$HSD = 3.67 \sqrt{(40.03 / 6)}$

$HSD = 9.479$

Therefore, the mean difference between any two group scores must be at least 9.48 to be statistically significant.

1. $\overline{X}_1 - \overline{X}_2 = 26.4 - 18.8 = 7.6$. Therefore, the null hypothesis is accepted and $\overline{X}_1 = \overline{X}_2$.
2. $\overline{X}_1 - \overline{X}_3 = 26.4 - 38.0 = 11.6$. Therefore, the null hypothesis is rejected and $\overline{X}_1 \neq \overline{X}_3$
3. $\overline{X}_2 - \overline{X}_3 = 18.8 - 38.0 = 19.2$. Therefore, the null hypothesis is rejected and $\overline{X}_2 \neq \overline{X}_3$.

In conclusion, a post hoc analysis test determines the pairs of means that have statistically significant differences.

Reference: F. J. Gravette and L. R. Wellnau, (1985). *Statistics for the Behavioral Sciences.* St. Paul: West Publishing Company, pp. 424–425.

8.10.2 Kruskal-Wallis Test for *k* Sample

The Kruskal-Wallis test is a nonparametric alternative to the one-way ANOVA when comparing three or more independent groups.

Assumptions

1. Random selection or random assignment of subjects to each independent group
2. Ordinal scale measurement
3. Each group should have at least five subjects

Example of Applying Kruskal-Wallis

Step 1. The investigator hypothesizes that there is no statistically significant difference between the three groups.

Group I	Raw Score	Group 2	Raw Score	Group 3	Raw Score
Subj 101	10	Subj 201	14	Subj 301	12
102	8	202	12	302	14
103	6	203	10	303	7
104	10	204	8	304	6
105	12	205	9	305	10
106	14				

Step 2. Rank order every raw score, combining all groups (in this example, three groups) with the lowest score assigned a rank of 1. In this example, subject 303's raw score of 4 is assigned the rank of 1.

Subject	Raw Score	Rank	
101	10	8.5	
102	8	4.5	
103	6	2.5	
104	10	8.5	
105	12	12	
106	14	15	$\Sigma_{ranks} = 51$
201	14	15	
202	12	12	
203	10	8.5	
201	8	4.5	
205	9	6	$\Sigma_{ranks} = 46$

Subject	Raw Score	Rank	
301	12	12	
302	14	15	
303	4	1	
304	6	2.5	
305	10	8.5	$\Sigma_{ranks} = 39$

Note. n = 16

Step 3. Sum the ranks for each group.

Group 1	Group 2	Group 3
8.5	15	12
4.5	12	15
2.5	8.5	1
8.5	4.5	2.5
12	6	8.5
15		
$\Sigma = 51$	$\Sigma = 46.0$	$\Sigma = 39.0$
$n_1 = 6$	$n_2 = 5$	$n_3 = 5$

Step 4. Calculate the formula for Kruskal-Wallis (H_{obs})

$$H_{obs} = 12 / [N(N + 1)][(T_1^2/n_1) + (T_2^2 / n_2) + (T_3^2 / n_3)] - [3(N + 1)]$$

where

$$N = n_1 + n_2 + n_3 = 16$$
$$T_1^2 = (\Sigma_{ranks})^2 = 51^2 = 2601$$
$$T_2^2 = 46^2$$
$$= 2116$$
$$T_3^2 = 39^2$$
$$= 1521$$
$$H_{obs} = 12 / [16(17)][(2601 / 6) + (2116 / 5) + (1521 / 5)] - [3(17)]$$
$$H_{obs} = [12 / 272][433.5 + 423.2 + 304.2] - [51]$$
$$H_{obs} = [.044][1160.9] - [51]$$
$$H_{obs} = 51.08 - 51$$
$$H_{obs} = .08$$

Step 5. Calculate H_{crit} for $\alpha = .05$, df = number of groups (k) − 1 = 2.
$H_{crit} = 5.99$ (use Chi-Square table, Appendix C–10, to test for statistical significance).

Step 6. Compare H_{obs} (.08) with H_{crit} (5.991). If H_{obs} is equal to or more than H_{crit}, reject the null hypothesis. In this example the null hypothesis is accepted and we conclude that there is no statistically significant difference between the three groups tested.

8.11 Model VI: Correlation (Pearson and Spearman Correlation Coefficients)

What is correlation? What is the difference between an associational relationship and causality? How do we graph the relationship between variables? What is a correlational matrix? What is a regression line? What is the difference between the Pearson correlation coefficient and the Spearman rank order correlation coefficient? All of these questions relate to the correlational model in statistics.

8.11.1 Definition of Correlation

Correlation is the reciprocal relationship between two variables. It is a general concept that assumes that variables can be measured and correlated. The index of the degree of relationship between two variables is the correlation coefficient. This index can range from zero, which indicates no relationship, to + 1.00 or − 1.00, which indicates a perfect correlation between two variables. For example, a correlation coefficient of .30 indicates a low correlation, whereas .90 is a high correlation. The symbol for correlation is r. A correlational relationship indicates an association between variables; it does not indicate a causal relationship.

8.11.2 Example of a Correlation in the Literature

Table 8–11 displays the the relationship between stress and leisure satisfaction among therapeutic recreation personnel examined by an investigator. The table is a correlational matrix that measures the degree of associations between five variables. Each variable is correlated with each other. The Personal Strain Questionnaire component of the Occupational Stress Inventory, as developed by Osipow and Spokane (1987), and the Leisure

Table 8–11. Correlation Coefficients between Ratings on Personal Strain Questionnaire and Leisure Satisfaction Scale

	Vocational	Psychological	Interpersonal	Physical	Total
Psychological	.65*	—			
Interpersonal	.46*	.57*	—		
Physical	.44*	.61*	.43*	—	
PSQ total	.75*	.87*	.75*	.81*	—
Leisure satis.	−.21	−.30*	−.24*	−.39*	−.37*

Note. * = significant at .05; N = 85.

Note: From "The Relationship Between Stress and Leisure Satisfaction among Therapeutic Recreation Personnel" in P. H. Cunningham and T. Bartuska, 1989, *Therapeutic Recreation Journal*, 23(3), p. 69. Copyright 1989 by *Therapeutic Recreation Journal*. Reprinted with permission.

Satisfaction Scale was administered to 159 individuals who were members of the National Therapeutic Recreation Society. Data were gathered through a mail questionnaire.

Fifteen correlation coefficients (r) were completed to construct the correlational matrix table. The researchers used the $\alpha = .05$ for level of statistical significance. Although statistical significance may be reached at $r = .21$ for 83 df ($N - 2$), ($\alpha = .05$ and a two-tailed test), it is important to note that with correlations, statistical significance is not as important as establishing a clinical level of correlation. For example, in establishing an acceptable reliability for a test, many researchers will accept Pearson correlation coefficients of $r = .80$ or above as acceptable. In the example in Table 8–11, $r = .60$ is considered by some researchers to be low to moderate in clinical significance. In understanding the correlational results, the square of r is the proportion of variance in one variable that is associated with another variable. If $r = .60$, the proportion of variance accounted for is only .36, which means that .64 is that portion of the variance that is not accounted for. Correlation is a measure of predicting the value of one variable Y (unknown) if another variable X is known. If there is a high correlation between the two variables, (e.g., $r = .90$), then the researcher has a high degree of confidence in predicting "if X, then Y." The degree of confidence in the relationship is more important in clinical research than is the statistical r value.

In the example illustrated in Table 8–11, there are comparatively high correlations between the Personal Strain Questionnaire (PSQ) Total and the subscales of the PSQ. Comparatively low-to-moderate correlations exist between the Leisure Satisfaction Scale and the subscales of the PSQ. In other words, clinicians could not predict with confidence that persons with higher levels of leisure satisfaction would experience less stress than persons who have low satisfaction with their leisure. On the basis of these results, the researchers should conclude that there is not a strong relationship between stress and leisure satisfaction even though there is a significant statistical relationship at the .05 level.

8.11.3 Stepwise Procedure for Correlation

Step 1. State the research hypothesis. For example, there is no statistical significant relationship between variable X and variable Y. (Null hypothesis, $r = .00$ or below predetermined level of correlation.)

Step 2. Determine the degree of relationship that will be acceptable for significance.

a. In establishing test-retest reliability, a correlation coefficient of $r = .80$ or above is considered acceptable (Anastasi, 1988).

b. In clinical research, a correlation coefficient of below $r = .60$ is moderate to low.

Step 3. Collect data and arrange raw scores into a table. For example:

Subjects	Variable X Raw Score	Rank	Variable Y Raw Score	Rank	d (difference in ranks between X and Y)	d² (difference squared)
1	31	7	45	5	2	4
2	22	5	58	8	−3	9
3	19	4	57	7	−3	9
4	16	3	48	6	−3	9

(continued)

Subjects	Variable X Raw Score	Rank	Variable Y Raw Score	Rank	d (difference in ranks between X and Y)	d² (difference squared)
5	78	8.5	61	9	−0.5	0.25
6	3	1	36	4	−3	9
7	93	10	18	3	7	49
8	78	8.5	88	10	−1.5	2.25
9	23	6	9	1	5	25
10	15	2	12	2	0	0
	$\Sigma X = 378$		$\Sigma Y = 432$		$\Sigma d = 0$[a]	$\Sigma d^2 = 116.5$

Note. d = difference in ranks between X and Y; d^2 = difference squared.

[a]Note that in computing the differences (d), the sum of the rank differences should equal zero when taking into consideration the negative and positive signs.

Step 4. Rank order each raw score, with lowest score being assigned rank of 1. Note: for tied ranks, take the midpoint of the rank. For example, a raw score of 78 occupies ranks 8 and 9 and becomes rank of 8.5.

Step 5. Do exploratory data analysis. Note in Figure 8–36 that each point in the scatter diagram is a coordinate value. It appears from the scatter diagram that there is a low-to-moderate correlation between the two variables.

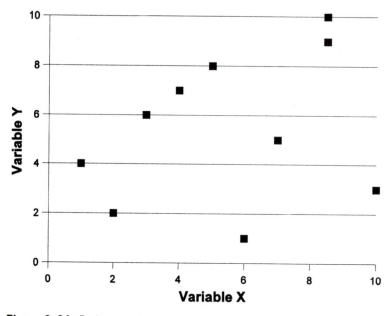

Figure 8–36. Exploratory data on a scattergram using the ranks of the scores. Notice that each point is a coordinate value. There appears to be a low-to-moderate correlation between the two variables.

Step 6. Calculate Spearman rank correlation coefficient and estimate degree of relationship between the two variables (X and Y). The formula for Spearman r_s is:

$$r_s = 1.00 - [(6)(\Sigma d^2) / (N^3 - N)]$$
$$r_s = 1.00 - [(6)(116.5) / (1,000 - 10)]$$
$$r_s = 1.00 - [699 / 990]$$
$$r_s = 1.00 - .71$$
$$r_s = .29$$

The exploratory data analysis indicates that there is a low correlation between the X and Y variables.

Step 7. Calculate the Pearson r correlation coefficient. The Spearman (rank order) is a good screening test for the Pearson (product-moment), which is a more accurate test because the Pearson r computes raw scores, whereas the Spearman r_s computes ranks that are transformed scores. The reader shall note that the Pearson r, which is a parametric test, should be applied to interval or ratio scale data. The Spearman r_s is a nonparametric statistical test that can be used with ordinal scale data. As the reader will note, interval scale data can be transformed to ranks (ordinal scale data).

The formula for the Pearson r product-moment correlation is:

$$r = [N \Sigma XY - (\Sigma X)(\Sigma Y)] / \sqrt{[N \Sigma X^2 - (\Sigma X)^2][N \Sigma Y_2 - (\Sigma Y)^2]}$$

Calculation for Pearson r Product-Moment Correlation

Subject	X	X²	Y	Y²	XY
01	31	961	45	2025	1395
02	22	484	58	3364	1276
03	19	361	57	3249	1083
04	16	256	48	2304	768
05	78	6084	61	3721	4758
06	3	9	36	1296	108
07	93	8649	18	324	1674
08	78	6084	88	7744	6864
09	23	529	9	81	207
10	15	225	12	144	180
	378	23642	432	24252	18313
	$\Sigma X = 378$	$\Sigma X^2 = 23,642$	$\Sigma Y = 432$	$\Sigma Y^2 = 24,252$	$\Sigma XY = 18,313$

$N = 10$	$\Sigma X^2 = 23,642$
$\Sigma XY = 18,313$	$\Sigma Y^2 = 24,252$
$\Sigma X = 378$	$(\Sigma X)^2 = 142,884$
$\Sigma Y = 432$	$(\Sigma Y)^2 = 186,624$

$$r = \frac{[(10)(18313)] - [(378)(432)]}{\sqrt{[(10)(23,642) - 142,884][(10)(24,252) - 186,624]}}$$

$r = (183,130 - 163,296) / \sqrt{(236,420 - 142,884)(242,520 - 186,624)}$

$r = (19,834) / \sqrt{[93,536][55,896]}$

$r = 19,834 / 72,317$

$r = .274$

The Pearson r of .274 is similar to the Spearman r_s of .29. In both computations, the correlation is low and will not be clinically significant because only a small portion of the variance is accounted for.

Step 8. Calculation of Regression Line. A regression line describes the relationship between variable X and variable Y. The formula for the regression line is

$$\overline{Y} = b\overline{X} + a$$

where Y is a predicted variable from the known X value, the b is the slope of the line, and a is the Y intercept. The regression line that is calculated assumes that if a perfect correlation 1.00 exists between two variables, then one could predict the Y value if the X value is known. For example, suppose we derive the formula for a specific regression line to be

$$\overline{Y} = .30X + 1.50$$
$$\text{and } \overline{X} = .500$$
$$\overline{Y} = .30\ (5.00) + 1.50$$
$$\overline{Y} = 1.5 + 1.5$$
$$\overline{Y} = 3.00$$

Therefore, if $X = 5.00$, then $Y = 3.00$ in this example. The calculation of a regression line is useful when there is a high correlation between two variables. On the other hand, a low correlation of $r = .29$ would not warrant constructing a regression line.

The computational formula for the slope is:

$$b = [N(\Sigma\ XY) - (\Sigma\ X)(\Sigma\ Y)] / [N\ \Sigma\ X^2 - (\Sigma X)^2]$$

The formula for the Y intercept is

$$a = \overline{Y} - b\overline{X}$$

Step 9. Identify the critical values for the Spearman Rank Order Correlation Coefficient.

  a. Determine number of subjects (N)
  b. Significance level, such as $\alpha = .05, .01$
  c. Directional or nondirectional hypothesis

For example, with $N = 10$, $\alpha = .05$, nondirectional test, $r_{s(crit)} = .648$ (see Table C–6 in the appendices). In the example above, $r_{s(obs)} = .29$. In this result, the researcher will accept the null hypothesis and conclude that there is no statistically significant relationship between the two variables.

Step 10. Identify the critical values for the Pearson Product–Moment Correlation.

a. $df = N - 2$
b. Significance level
c. Directional or nondirectional hypothesis

In the example as shown, $df = 8$, $\alpha = .05$, nondirectional test, $r_{crit} = .6319$ (see Table C–5 in the appendices). Because $r_{obs} = .27$, the null hypothesis is accepted, and the researcher concludes that there is no statistically significant relationship between the two variables.

The reader should note that as the N increases, the $r_{crit} = $ decreases. For example, for 100 df, $\alpha = .05$ level of significance, $r_{crit} = .1966$, while for 20 df, $r_{crit} = .4227$.

8.12 Model VII: Observed Frequencies (Chi-Square)

When researchers work with nominal data, they frequently are concerned with differences in the number of cases falling into discrete categories such as improved versus not improved or active versus disengaged. The major purpose of this statistical model is to test whether there are statistically significant differences between the observed and the expected frequencies of two independent groups. For example, this model could be applied if a researcher is interested in determining whether there is a gender difference in the distribution of individuals with multiple sclerosis in a population where there are 51% female subjects and 49% male subjects. Is there a statistically significant difference between the number of men as compared with women who have a diagnosis of multiple sclerosis? In this hypothetical example the researcher will compare the observed differences between the number of men and women diagnosed with multiple sclerosis with the expected prevalence, that is, 51% for women and 49% for men.

8.12.1 Example of Chi-Square

In an example from the literature, the investigators examined the factors influencing the successful outcome of tracking individuals with severe psychiatric illnesses in the community compared with those in hospitals. In Table 8–12, the investigators compared the patients treated at home with patients admitted to a hospital in relation to where they were assessed during a psychotic episode.

Formula for Chi-Square

$$\chi^2_{obs} = \Sigma \left[(O - E)^2 \right] / E$$
$$\chi^2_{obs} = [(51 - 42)^2 / 42] + [(3 - 11)^2 / 11] + [(11 - 10)^2 - 10] + [(0 - 2)^2 / 2] +$$
$$[(13 - 22)^2 / 22] + [(13 - 6)^2 / 6] + [(5 - 5)^2 / 5] + [(3 - 1)^2 / 1]$$
$$\chi^2_{obs} = 1.92 + 5.81 + .09 + 2 + 3.68 + 8.16 + 0 + 4$$
$$\chi^2_{obs} = 25.66$$
$$\chi^2_{crit} = 7.82 \ (3 \ df, \alpha = .05)$$

Conclusion

The researchers rejected the null hypothesis and concluded that there is a statistically significant difference where patients are assessed if they are treated at home or admitted

Table 8–12. Location of Assessment During a Psychiatric Episode

Location of Assessment	Patients Treated at Home		Patients Admitted to Hospital		Total Patients
	Observed	Expected	Observed	Expected	
Home	51	42	13	22	65
Hospitals	3	11	13	6	16
Outpatient Clinic	11	10	5	5	16
Police Station	0	2	3	1	3
	65	65	34	34	99

Note: From "Home Treatment for Acute Psychiatric Illness," by C. Dean and E. M. Gadd, 1990, *British Medical Journal, 201*, p. 1023. Copyright 1990 by the *British Medical Journal.* Reprinted with permission.

to a hospital. From the results, the researchers concluded that if patients are assessed at home, they will have significant less probability of hospitalization for a psychiatric illness. The results of the study reinforced their hypothesis that home treatment is a feasible alternative to hospital treatment for many individuals with psychiatric illness. The application of chi-square is an appropriate statistical test when comparing nominal categories of data. It is a simple but powerful statistic that can be applied to outcome studies of clinical populations.

8.12.2 Operational Procedure of Observed Versus Expected Frequencies (Chi-Square)

Step 1. State the research hypothesis. The null hypothesis is: There is no statistically significant difference between the observed versus expected frequencies in normal groups ($\chi^2_{obs} < \chi^2_{crit}$). The alternative hypothesis is: There is a statistically significant difference between the observed versus expected frequencies in nominal groups ($\chi^2_{obs} \geq \chi^2_{crit}$).

Step 2. Select the level of statistical significance. This is usually $\alpha = .05$.

Step 3. Determine the degrees of freedom (df) for the contingency table.

$$df = (r - 1)(c - 1)$$

$$r = \text{number of rows in the table}$$

$$c = \text{number of columns in the table}$$

For example, in a 2 × 2 contingency table, the degrees of freedom is 1. In a 3 × 6 contingency table, $df = 10$.

Step 4. Identify χ^2_{crit} (chi-square critical) from the statistical table of values. The critical value is determined by:

a. Level of significance
b. *df*

For example, α^2_{crit} = 18.307 for α = .05, nondirectional test, with *df* = 10 (see Table C–10 in the appendices).

Step 5. Identify the discrete nominal categories being compared. For example, diagnostic groups, gender, and health care settings.

Step 6. Determine the number of columns and rows in the chi-square contingency table. Chi-square contingency tables are based on the number of columns and rows being compared. Contingency tables range from two rows and columns (2×2 contingency table) to larger number of rows and columns, such as (2×3), (3×5), (6×8).

Step 7. Tabulate the observed number of frequencies within each discrete category or group.

	Nonsmokers		Smokers		
	Observed	Expected	Observed	Expected	
Lung Cancer	500	1,000	1,500	1,000	2,000
No Lung Cancer	4,500	4,000	3,500	4,000	8,000
	5,000		5,000		10,000

The researcher counts the number of individuals with lung cancer who were smokers or nonsmokers in a population.

Step 8. Calculate the expected frequencies based on the probability of chance. The expected frequencies in a cell are computed by multiplying the total frequencies of a row that contains the cell by the total frequencies of the column that contains the cell and dividing this product by the total number of cases in the population. In the example above, the expected frequencies for nonsmokers with lung cancer is equal to:

$$(2000)(5000) / 10,000 = 1,000$$

Step 9. Calculate chi-square (χ^2_{obs}). The formula for chi-square is:

$$\Sigma = (O - E)^2 / E$$
where Σ = grand sum of all the cells
O = observed frequency in each cell
E = expected frequency in each cell

Step 10. Compare the two values: χ^2_{obs} *and* χ^2_{crit} (see Table C–10 in the appendices for critical score).

a. Accept the null hypothesis if χ^2_{obs} is less than χ^2_{crit}
b. Reject the null hypothesis if χ^2_{obs} is equal to or more than χ^2_{crit}

Observed Frequencies, Chi-Square Example

Research Problem. Is cognitive-behavioral treatment as effective as antidepressant medication in treating individuals with clinical depression?

Step 1. Research hypothesis. Null hypothesis: There is no statistically significant difference between the number of individuals with depression who improve with medication (Med) compared to those who receive cognitive-behavioral treatment (CBT).

Step 2. Level of significance: $\alpha = .05$.
Step 3. Determine the df from contingency table.

$$df = (r - 1)(c - 1)$$
$$df = (2 - 1)(3 - 1) = 2$$

Step 4. Identify χ^2_{crit} *from the statistical table of values.*

   a. $\alpha = .05$
   b. $df = 2$
   c. $\chi^2_{crit} = 5.99$ (see Table C–10 in the appendices).

Step 5. The nominal categories are: (a) those individuals treated with CBT who regressed, (b) those individuals treated with CBT who showed no improvement, (c) those individuals treated with CBT who improved, (d) those treated with medication who showed no improvement, and (e) those treated with medication who improved.
   Step 6. There are two rows and three columns: (2 × 3 contingency table).
   Step 7. Enumerate the observed number of frequencies within each nominal category and place in 2 × 3 contingency table.

Treatment	Regressed O	Regressed E	No Improvement O	No Improvement E	Improvement O	Improvement E	Totals
Cognitive-Behavioral	20	24.70	40	57.64	150	127.64	210
Medication	40	35.29	100	82.35	160	182.35	300
Totals	60		140		310		510

In this example, 210 individuals received CBT and 300 individuals received medication. A total of 510 individuals with depression were included in the study. Out of 310 individuals who improved, 160 received medication while the remaining 150 received CBT. The rest of the group (200 individuals) showed either no improvement (remained the same) or regressed.
   Step 8. Calculate the expected frequencies for each nominal category or cell based on the formula. "To complete the expected frequency of any cell, multiply the marginal total for the row that contains the cell by the marginal total for the column that contains the cell, and divide this product by the total number of cases in the table" (McCall, 1986, p. 321).

$$CBT\ (Regressed) = (210)(60) / 510 = 24.70$$
$$CBT\ (No\ Improvement) = (210)(140) / 510 = 57.64$$
$$CBT\ (Improved) = (210)(310) / 510 = 127.64$$
$$Med\ (Regressed) = (300)(60) / 510 = 35.29$$
$$Med\ (No\ Improvement) = (300)(140) / 510 = 82.35$$
$$Med\ (Improved) = (300)(60) / 510 = 182.35$$

Step 9. Calculate chi-square (χ^2_{obs}).

$\Sigma = (O - E)^2 / E$

$\chi^2_{obs} = [(20 - 24.70)^2 / 24.70] + [(40 - 57.64)^2 / 57.64] + [(150 - 127.64)^2 / 127.64] +$
$\quad\quad [(40 - 35.29)^2 / 35.29] + [(100 - 82.35)^2 / 82.35] + [(160 - 182.35)^2 / 182.35]$

$\chi^2_{obs} = .89 + 5.39 + 3.91 + .62 + 3.78 + 2.73$

$\chi^2_{obs} = 17.32$

Step 10. Compare χ^2_{obs} with χ^2_{crit}

$$\chi^2_{obs} = 17.32$$
$$\chi^2_{crit} = 5.991$$

Reject the null hypothesis. There is a statistically significant difference between CBT and medications in the treatment of depression. It appears that CBT is more effective than medication in the improvement of depression in this hypothetical example. Of the 210 individuals, 150 (or 71%) of the CBT group improved, while 160 out of the 300 individuals (or 53%) of the medication group improved.

8.12.3 Kappa

Purpose

To determine the degree of agreement between two or more judges independently ranking a variable. It can be used to measure interrater reliability. Kappa can range from +1.00 to −1.00

Assumptions

1. The units are independent, that is, completed by independent observations.
2. The categories are nominal scale measurements, are fully mutually exclusive, and exhaustive.
3. The judges operate independently.
4. There is no criteria for correctness, choices, clinical judgment, or client attitudes.
5. Judges have equal competence, education, or ability to make ratings.
6. There are no restrictions placed on ranking or rating the variable.

Formula for Kappa

$\text{Kappa} = P_o - P_c / 1 - P_c$

where

P_o = the observed proportion of agreement

P_c = the proportion of agreement expected by chance alone

Example

In a hypothetical observation, two independent observers rate the level of depression indicated by a behavioral scale. One individual is observed by two independent raters during 10 sessions to evaluate the level of depression (i.e., low depression, LD; medium depression, MD; and severe depression, SD). Each category of depression is operationally defined, and each rater has been trained previously using a standardized rating scale. They independently observe a patient on a ward applying a behavior rating scale. Is there a high interrater relationship between the two observers using a standardized rating scale? The data from the observations follow:

Sessions	Observer 1	Observer 2	Agreement
1	LD	MD	no
2	MD	MD	yes
3	LD	LD	yes
4	MD	MD	yes
5	LD	LD	yes
6	LD	LD	yes
7	MD	MD	yes
8	LD	MD	no
9	MD	MD	yes
10	LD	LD	yes
Totals	6 LD, 4 MD, 0 SD	4 LD, 6 MD, 0 SD	Agreements: 8 / 10 = 80%

Stepwise Procedure for Kappa

Step 1. Place data into a 3 × 3 contingency table to display agreements. Use three categories of depression, MD, LD, and SD.

	LD	MD	SD	Marginal Totals
LD	4	2	0	6
MD	0	4	0	4
SD	0	0	0	0
Marginal Totals	4	6	0	(10)

Notice that there were four instances of both observers agreeing on low depression and four instances of both observers agreeing on moderate depression. There were no observations of severe depression. The agreements will always be the numbers in the diagonal cells when there are 2 observers and 1 subject. Also note that when adding frequencies in cells that observer one usually is on the Y axis and observer two is on the X axis of the table. In this example the discrepancy between the two raters occurred in the cell containing 2. This is where observer 1 rated subject twice as LD and observer 2 rates the same subject for sessions 1 and 8 as MD.

Step 2. Calculate for kappa applying the formula.

$Kappa = P_o - P_c / 1 - Pc$

P_o is obtained by adding all the frequencies in the cells that both observers agree.

	Observer 2		
	11	12	13
Observer 1	21	22	23
	31	32	33

Each cell is numbered to represent the rating of each observer. For example, cells 11, 22, and 33 represent agreements of observers 1 and 2. On the other hand, cell 21 represents discrepancy between observers 1 and 2.

P_o = the frequency of agreement over the total number of observations (N). The formula is

$P_o = (n_{11} + n_{22} + n_{33} + n_{ii} \ldots)$

where n_{ii} = and other cells

$n_{11} = 4$

$n_{22} = 4$

$n_{33} = 0$

$P_o = 8 / 10 = .80$

The marginal total is the sum of each row or column.

P_c = marginal totals of observer times marginal totals of observer 2, divided by the total number of observation periods of sessions squared.

$P_c = \{[(6)(4)] + [(4)(6)] + [(0)(0)]\} / 10^2$

$P_c = [(24) + (24) + (0)] / 100$

$P_c = 48 / 100$

$P_c = .48$

$kappa = (.80 - .48) / (1 - .48)$

$kappa = 32 / 52$

$kappa = .61$

A kappa of .70 is considered to indicate an acceptable level of agreement (Sattler, 1988). The results indicate a slightly lower interrater agreement than what statisticians consider acceptable interrater reliability. Note that the percentage of agreement, that is, 80%, is uncorrected for chance. From a pragmatic perspective, kappa should always be interpreted in terms of its value to the clinician. In this example, the clinical researcher would interpret a kappa of .61 as acceptable.

References: For further information see J. Cohen, (1960). "A Coefficient of Agreement for Nominal Scales," *Educational and Psychological Measurement, 20,* 37–46; and J. M. Sattler, (1988), *Assessment of Children* (3rd ed.), San Diego, CA: Sattler.

8.13 Statistical Software Packages

Although the authors have used hand calculations to solve the examples presented in this book, in actuality, many statistical problems can be solved through one of a number of statistical packages available for computers. Three widely used computer programs designed for the health and social sciences are detailed below.

8.13.1 Statistical Product and Service Solutions (SPSS)

This company produces a data analysis package for research scientists. It has been widely used within the social science fields as well as other disciplines. SPSS includes the capabilities to perform basic analyses (e.g., frequencies, correlations) and more advanced analyses (e.g., regression, ANOVA, general linear models, contingency tables, factor and discriminant analysis, nonparametric statistics, and time series. A Graduate Pack, containing the full version of SPSS, is available at a reduced price for students working on an advanced degree (http://www.spss.com/software/education/gradpack/).

The following information was obtained from the SPSS website (http://www.spss.com/software/spss/cando.htm#he):

Healthcare
With escalating costs and increased competition, on-going evaluation of the quality of care and patient satisfaction is essential in order to maintain a high level of performance. SPSS provides all the data analysis tools you need to begin and maintain an effective quality improvement program and make the best decisions. Medical researchers use SPSS sophisticated stats procedures for studies of illnesses and treatments. Whether you're in administration or research, SPSS helps you work more effectively by turning your data into information. Health care professionals use SPSS to:

- ▶ improve patient health outcomes
- ▶ enhance the quality and value of health services
- ▶ provide required data for regulations
- ▶ control costs

Things you can do with SPSS

- ▶ Evaluate treatment effectiveness by DRG code and type of treatment
- ▶ Identify factors influential to positive treatment outcomes
- ▶ Chart the success of current hospital services and programs
- ▶ Identify hospital-wide cost-efficient and inefficient areas
- ▶ Find trends in medical liability cases
- ▶ Compare institution-specific indicators with industry-wide indicators

Sample administration applications

- ▶ patient satisfaction surveys
- ▶ quality improvement studies
- ▶ marketing and planning operations analysis

Sample research applications

▶ outcomes analysis
▶ biomedical research
▶ clinical research
▶ pharmaceutical testing/development (*What People Do With SPSS*, 1999, p. 1)

8.13.2 SAS System

This statistical package is an integrated system of data access, management, analysis, and presentation, which is not limited to a particular computer system. The software is available for mainframes and PCs. Basic and advanced statistics are available, and the analysis can be integrated into a presentation for any type of reporting needs. Training and support are available. Further information regarding SAS can be obtained through the Internet (http://www.sas.com/software/products.html).

Information obtained on the SAS Web site (http://www.sas.com/software/industry/healthcare.html) indicates that it is useful for healthcare statistics:

SAS Software provides extensive statistical tools to handle a wide range of analyses. Corporations, government agencies, research institutes, and universities rely on statistical analyses to make many critical decisions. SAS software provides extensive statistical capabilities that enable analysts to evaluate information from clinical trials of new drugs, database marketing, health surveys, customer preference studies, and stock market trends.

From regression to exact methods to statistical visualization techniques, SAS software provides the tools for both specialized and enterprise-wide analytical needs. In addition, SAS Institute remains committed to its long tradition of enriching its statistical offerings to keep current with evolving statistical methodology. Our statistical software includes capabilities for:

Analysis of Variance

Regression

Categorical data analysis

Multivariate analysis

Survival analysis

Psychometric analysis

Cluster analysis

Nonparametric analysis

The SAS System also provides software for econometrics, quality improvement, and guided data analysis. (*Statistic Analysis*, 1999, p. 1)

8.13.3 SYSTAT

This statistical package is now available through SPSS. More information about the product can be found on the Internet (http://www.spss.com/software/science/systat/systat9.htm). A menu-driven data analysis tool enables data to be analyzed in basic statistics (e.g., descriptive, *t* test, correlation) and more advanced statistics (e.g., ANOVA, multiple regression, and factor analysis). As with most packages, graphics are available.

8.13.4 UNISTAT

This statistical program for Windows® was first made available in 1984. It is described by the company as a "fully fledged spreadsheet for data handling, a wide range of statistics and powerful 2D and 3D presentation quality graphics" (http://www.unistat.com/summary.htm). It can be used alone, or combined with Excel®.

Information obtained from the Web site (http://www.unistat.com/features.htm) indicates that Unistat is able to do the following:

▶ Data Handling: Spreadsheet, Formula editor, Data Import /Export, ODBC, SQL, Wizards and Macros.
▶ Integration with MS Office™: Output to MS Word™ / MS Excel™ and MS Excel add-in mode, Developers' (background) mode.
▶ Data Visualisation: On-screen editing, Interactive graphics, Multiple graphics editor, Exporting and Galleries.
▶ Graphics Procedures: X-Y Scatter Plots, Polar Plots, Spectral Diagrams, X-Y-Z Scatter Plots, X-Y-Z Grid Plots, Spin Plots, Pie Charts, Bar Charts, Area/Ribbon Charts, 3D Bar Charts, High-Low-Close Charts, 2D Functions and 3D Functions.
▶ Descriptive Statistics: Summary Statistics, Confidence Intervals and Quantiles etc.
▶ Distribution Functions: 12 Continuous & 7 Discrete Distributions.
▶ Descriptive Plots: Stem & Leaf Plot, 2D Histogram, 3D Histogram, Log-Probability Histogram, Normal Probability Plot, Plot of Distribution Functions, Box & Whisker Plots, Dot Plots and Ladder Plots.
▶ Statistical Tests: Parametric Tests, Goodness of Fit Tests, One/Two Sample Non Parametric Tests, Multi Sample Non Parametric Tests.
▶ Correlation Coefficients: Pearson, Spearman Rank and Kendall Rank.
▶ Tables: Contingency, Crosstabulation and Breakdown tables.
▶ Power and Sample Size: One Sample, Two Samples, Variance, Correlation, Two Correlations, Proportions, ANOVA, Phi Distribution.
▶ Regression Analysis: Ordinary Least Squares, Polynomial, Stepwise, Non Linear, Logit and Probit Regressions.
▶ Analysis of Variance: Multi-way with interaction selection, General Linear Model (GLM), Homogeneity of Variance Tests, Multiple Comparisons, Regression with Replicates and Heterogeneity of Regression Tests.
▶ Multivariate Analysis: Cluster Analysis, Discriminant Analysis, Multidimensional Scaling, Principal Components Analysis, Factor Analysis, Canonical Correlations and Reliability Analysis.
▶ Multivariate Plots: X-Y Pairs Plots, Rectangle Plots and Icon Plots.
▶ Time Series Analysis: ARIMA Models, Forecasting and Smoothing, Quality Control, Survival Analysis and Fourier Analysis. (*Unistat for Windows: Key features*, 1999, p. 1)

8.14 Summary

In this chapter, the authors have presented the basic statistical concepts and tests that are applied in clinical research. Statistics is both an art and a science. The art of statistics is the decision-making involving the selection of the appropriate statistical test for a research study. There are a number of possibilities in this decision, based on the level of measurement, the probability level for statistical significance, and the number of subjects in the study. The science of statistics is based on mathematical reasoning and use of statistical tables. Mastery of statistics means approaching the subject with an objective attitude and open mind. Statistics should not be applied mechanically such as "throwing data in a computer." The researcher should use statistics in a reflective manner while interpreting and analyzing the results. In this way, statistical analysis is integrated into the research study.

CHAPTER

Selecting a Test Instrument

> *For all such areas of research—and for many others—the precise measurement of individual differences made possible by well-constructed tests is an essential prerequisite.*
> —A. Anastasi, 1988, *Psychological Testing* (p. 4)

Operational Learning Objectives

By the end of the chapter, the learner will:
1. Define key concepts in testing
2. Discuss the early history in the development of testing
3. Identify the major purposes of testing
4. Know where to look for bibliographies of tests in books and in test catalogues
5. Know how to select a test for a specific function and target population
6. Know how to evaluate reliability and validity of tests
7. Know how to incorporate tests into a research proposal
8. Determine the skills necessary in:
   a. administering tests
   b. scoring tests
   c. interpreting results of tests
9. Develop an objective attitude in selecting a test instrument and evaluating its effectiveness
10. Identify the potential sources of error in testing

9.1 Key Concepts in Testing

To understand testing and evaluation, one should be able to define the key concepts. How is a test defined? How does the evaluator determine what is normal behavior and what is atypical behavior? Why are tests used? What are potential sources of error in testing? What is the difference between norm-referenced and criterion-referenced tests? These key concepts, listed in Table 9–1, are elaborated upon in this chapter.

9.2 Early History of Test Development

Tests have been used for generations to make employment and educational decisions. For example, in the 12th century, the Chinese used civil service examinations to make hiring decisions. The ancient Greeks administered physical and intellectual tests as part of the educational process. In Europe, from the time of the Middle Ages, universities gave tests as part of the process of awarding professional degrees and

Table 9–1. Key Concepts in Tests and Measurements

- A **test** is essentially an objective and standardized measure of a sample of behavior (Anastasi & Urbina, 1997).
- A **measurement scale** is a system of assigning scores to a trait or characteristic.
- A **major purpose** of a test is to predict future performance based on a current sample of behaviors.
- An **extremely important quality** of a test is to accurately detect change in an individual's behavior (e.g., improvement).
- The **value** of a test depends on its purposes, ability to predict outcome, and the degree of consistency and precision in defining a variable.
- The **degree of accuracy** of a test is based on its ability to be consistent (reliability) and to test what it claims to measure (validity).
- The **sources of error in measurement** are derived, for example, from the unreliability of the instrument, bias of the test administrator, unreliability of the client, and undesirable test environment.
- **Distributions of data** from heterogeneous populations tend to be normally distributed, while data from homogeneous populations tend to be skewed.
- A **norm-referenced test** is a standardized sampling of behavior that uses data from a heterogeneous group of individuals in interpreting results.
- A **criterion-referenced test** is a standardized sampling of behavior that bases performance on accepted standards of competency.

bestowing honors. In the United States, procedures for testing applicants to the United States Civil Service were introduced in 1883. Not until the 19th century, however, when an interest in providing humane treatment to individuals with mental retardation and mental illness arose, were tests developed that could identify and distinguish between mental retardation and emotional disturbance (Anastasi & Urbina, 1997; Sattler, 1992; see Table 9–2 for a summary of major events in test development).

Traditionally, test theorists have taken the viewpoint that the majority of a population will perform equally on many functions and that there is a normally distributed continuum of abilities. Thus, researchers involved in early test development sought to demonstrate what was normal in an effort to identify those individuals who differed significantly from the normal population. Sir Francis Galton (1822–1911), advocating the importance of individual differences, postulated that differences in physical characteristics such as vision, hearing, reaction time, and physical strength could be used to determine mental capabilities. He tried to validate his beliefs through the use of statistical methods developed by Karl Pearson (1857–1936). Although he was unsuccessful in showing that mental abilities were related to physical characteristics, our use of a normative sample is a direct result of his hypothesis (Swanson & Watson, 1989). James McKeen Cattell (1860–1944), an assistant to Galton, supported Galton's views that "mental tests" measuring sensory and physical abilities differentiated individuals. Although he found no relationship between these abilities and school achievement, he contributed to the understanding of tests and measurement by demonstrating that mental ability could be examined empirically (Sattler, 1992).

Eduardo Séquin (1812–1880) also believed that individuals could be differentiated by sensory and motor-control abilities. Galton had believed that the differences were inherent and unchangeable; however, Séquin believed that training in these areas could improve one's intellectual potential. Currently his materials, such as the form board (a task in which individuals place wooden or plastic shapes into puzzle frames) are used as a part of a test battery for young children (Swanson & Watson, 1989).

Table 9–2. Early History of the Test Movement

Theorist	Occupation	Contribution to Testing
Esquirol (1838)	Physician	Classified individuals with mental retardation into various levels of retardation; believed that language provided the best measure of intelligence.
Paul Broca (1864)	Surgeon	Proposed a relationship between the volume of the brain and intelligence.
Sir Francis Galton (1883)	Biologist	Theorized that physical traits (visual and hearing acuity, muscular strength) and reaction speed could serve as a measure of gauging intellectual abilities.
James McKeen Cattell (1890)	Psychologist	Developed norms in sensory, motor, and simple perceptual processes for comparing individuals, helping to create the concept of mental measurement.
Emil Kraepelin (1895)	Psychiatrist	Developed assessment of daily living skills based on perception, memory, attention, and motor functioning. Interested in the clinical examinations of psychiatric patients: Tests of critical functions were designed to measure practice effects in memory and susceptibility to fatigue and to distraction.
Charles E. Spearman (1904)	Psychologist	Proposed that intelligence was comprised of a primary factor (g) and specific factors (s).
Alfred Binet (1905)	Psychologist	Along with Simon, developed a test that identified children who could not benefit from formal education. This instrument consisted of short tests measuring perception, judgment, comprehension, and reasoning.
Lewis M. Terman (1916)	Psychologist	Popularized and revised Binet's scale by including tasks to identify superior adult intelligence and by assigning age equivalents to items.
H. H. Goddard (1919)	Educator	Introduced Binet's scale in America, adding categories of intellectual ability and identifying "morons" and "idiots."
Robert M. Yerkes (1921)	Psychologist	Instrumental in developing the Army Alpha, a verbal test, and the Army Beta, a visual test, for group testing. He also espoused the idea of point-scales rather than age scales.
Louis L. Thurstone (1938)	Psychologist	Proposed that intelligence was comprised of several different factors, which he called primary mental abilities, all of which could be considered equally important.
David Wechsler (1939)	Psychologist	Developed the Wechsler-Bellevue, the precursor to the Wechsler Scales. This test had a verbal scale and a performance scale.
Raymond B. Cattell (1979)	Psychologist	Along with John Horn, proposed that intelligence was comprised of fluid (nonverbal, novel, relatively culture-free) and crystallized reasoning (acquired skills strongly dependent upon culture).
Jagannath Das (1963)	Psychologist	Used an information-processing model to describe cognitive functioning. Information is obtained through two distinct methods: simultaneously and sequentially.
J. P. Guilford (1967)	Psychologist	Attempted to link theory to test development by proposing a three-dimensional Structure of Intellect with 120 factors that led to a test that measured each factor.
Howard Gardner (1983)	Psychologist	Proposed that there are several autonomous intellectual competencies or multiple intelligences, which are manifested differently in different individuals.

One of the first attempts to classify individuals with mental retardation was made by Jean Esquirol (1772–1840). He recognized that individuals with mental retardation had diverse abilities and concluded that language development was the most important characteristic for distinguishing between degrees of intellectual capacity. His appreciation for the importance of language in the development of intellectual capacity influenced the development of intelligence tests (Anastasi & Urbina, 1997).

While researchers in the United States tried to measure intellectual development through performance on sensory and motor tasks, clinicians in Germany turned toward more complex and abstract tasks as a means of measuring aptitude. Emil Kraepelin (1855–1926), recognizing the importance of measuring skills needed for daily living, developed a battery that measured such skills as perception, memory, motor functioning, and attention. H. Ebbinghaus (1850–1909), after teachers in Germany requested that he develop an aptitude test, produced a timed completion task consisting of reading passages from which words had been left out. This test was a forerunner of group intelligence tests. He also produced tests that assessed arithmetic and memory skills. Carl Wernicke (1849–1905), noted for his work on aphasia and brain localization, investigated individual differences in verbal conceptual thinking and generalization.

9.2.1 Influence of Binet on IQ Testing

In 1905, Alfred Binet, a French psychologist, and a colleague, Theodore Simon, were commissioned by the French government to develop a test that would identify those children who could not benefit from formal education. The content of Binet's test came from educational research and through a deductive analysis of the factors that underlie academic achievement. The Binet-Simon test was developed pragmatically, without a theory of intelligence to guide its contents. Nonetheless, the influence of individuals such as Esquirol and Séquin was apparent in that Binet included items measuring sensory perception, motor control, and language. In addition, the Binet-Simon intelligence test

> had several unique characteristics: (1) questions were arranged in a hierarchy of difficulty, (2) levels were established for different ages (establishment of mental age), (3) a quantitative scoring system was applied, and (4) specific instructions for administration were built into the test. (Swanson & Watson, 1989, p. 9)

The initial test consisted of 30 items related to following simple directions, defining words, constructing sentences, and answering judgmental questions of a psychological nature.

Binet's test was translated into English by H. H. Goddard (1866–1957) in 1910 and Lewis Terman (1877–1956) in 1916 for use in the United States (Sattler, 1992; Swanson & Watson, 1989; Terman & Merrill, 1973). While Binet had perceived his instrument as a way to identify those students who needed to be instructed through alternative methods, Goddard, in the early 19th century, linked intelligence test scores to occupation and social status (Gould, 1996). Terman extended Binet's test by adding additional items suitable for testing adults and by adding the concept of "mental quotient" to that of mental age. Terman's revision became known as the Stanford-Binet, so named because he was a professor at Stanford University in California.

9.2.2 Alternative Tests to the Binet

Binet's test and the revisions by Terman were developed on the premise that one's ability to successfully complete a particular task was related to developmental level. Thus, in a heterogenous set of items arranged in a developmental sequence, age scores could be assigned based on the ability of a majority of children at a given age level to do a particular task. Mental ability was determined by obtaining a ratio between the obtained age score and one's chronological age. Tests that use this format to find mental abilities are said to have an age-scale.

Discontent with age scores lead individuals such as Robert M. Yerkes (1876–1966) and David Wechsler (1896–1981) to develop tests with a radically different scoring format. Rather than using age-score, similar items were put together and points were assigned to each item. Then the raw score, determined by the number of points received, was converted into standard scores and an overall score. Scales with this type of scoring are known as a point-scale. The IQ scores derived in this manner are called Deviation IQs. At this time, most tests developed for school-age children, adolescents, and adults use the point scale, whereas developmental scales, developed for infants, toddlers, and preschoolers, use an age-scale.

Another concern regarding intelligence testing was the emphasis on verbal reasoning seen on the Stanford-Binet. Tests such as the Leiter International Performance Scale (LIPS; Leiter, 1948), the Arthur adaptation of the Leiter International Performance Scale (Arthur, 1949), the Kohs Block Design Tests (Kohs, 1923), and the Culture-Fair Intelligence Scale (Cattell, 1950) were developed to counterbalance the highly verbal influence of the Stanford-Binet. The Wechsler-Bellevue, developed in 1939 by Wechsler, consisted of a verbal and a performance scale. This test, based on Wechsler's conception that intelligence was global, included tasks from various sources (e.g., Kohs Block Design Test, Army Alpha, and Army Beta). Although the items have changed over time, many of the same types of items are included in the present-day Wechsler scales (Sattler, 1992).

9.2.3 Factor Analytical Theories of Intelligence

With the development of computers and more advanced statistical methods (e.g., factor analysis), the concept of intelligence has changed drastically. Although both Binet and Wechsler believed that intelligence was composed of many different abilities, neither one had proposed a theory that identified the components of intelligence. Binet had used items that he believed would assess skills necessary to succeed in an academic setting. Wechsler, on the other hand, had borrowed from a number of available tests, all of which he believed were factors in the construct of intelligence (Sattler, 1992). It fell to theorists like Charles E. Spearman (1863–1936), Edward L. Thorndike (1874–1949), and Louis L. Thurstone (1887–1955) to suggest the components contained in the construct of intelligence. In general, there were three viewpoints regarding the structure of intelligence:

1. Intelligence was composed of a primary factor called *g* made up of complex mental tasks, such as reasoning and problem-solving, and specific factors called *s* that required less complex processes, such as speed of processing, visual-motor, and rote learning (Spearman, 1927)
2. Intelligence was multifactorial and similar abilities clustered to form more complex skills (Thorndike, 1927)
3. Intelligence was comprised of primary factors (e.g., verbal, perceptual speed, inductive reasoning, work fluency, and space or visualization) rather than a single unitary factor (Thurstone, 1938).

More recently, others (e.g., Guilford, Sternberg, Gardner) have proposed alternative theories to account for the nature of intelligence. J. P. Guilford (1897–1987), in an effort to link theory to intelligence tests, proposed in *The Nature of Human Intelligence* (1967) that human intellect could be understood by a three-dimensional model, which he called the Structure of Intellect. This structure contained (a) five operations, which defined the way we process information (e.g., divergent or convergent); (b) four contents, which defined the manner in which the material is presented (e.g., visual or verbal), and (c) six products, which defined the outcome of the mental process (e.g., units or classes). By using combinations of one attribute from each dimension, 120 factors of intelligence can be identified (5 operations × 4 contents × 6 products). Theoretically, if one were to assess a student in each of these 120 factors, one would have a better understanding of how the student learned and could provide an appropriate educational program for that student. Unfortunately, Guilford's model has not been widely accepted, nor has it been used in many research studies.

Raymond B. Cattell and John L. Horn (Cattell, 1963; Horn, 1968) agreed with Guilford that intelligence was not a unitary concept but disagreed in the specific components comprising intelligence. They suggested, instead, that intelligence is made up of two constructs, fluid and crystallized. Tasks considered to be fluid intelligence include unlearned, culture-free, novel experiences in which adaptation or generalization of previously learned tasks is required (e.g., nonverbal analogies, block building, speed of processing, and problem-solving). Crystallized intelligence, on the other hand, is defined as acquired knowledge, such as what is learned in school or in cultural experiences. Examples of tasks measuring crystallized intelligence include vocabulary tests, verbal analogies, rote learning, and rule learning. Two tests that were developed using the concept of crystallized and fluid intelligence are the *Stanford-Binet Intelligence Scale–Fourth Edition* (SBIS:FE; Thorndike, Hagen, & Sattler, 1985) and the *Kaufman Adolescent and Adult Intelligence Test* (KAIT; Kaufman & Kaufman, 1993).

9.2.4 Alternative Theories of Intelligence

Although factor analysis theories of intelligence are still the most widely accepted, two additional approaches to intelligence should be mentioned. One approach, information processing, involves the understanding of the ways in which individuals take in and transform the information so that it can be used. While information processing is frequently linked with memory processes, the concept has been extended by individuals such as Das (Das, Kirby, & Jarman, 1975), and Campione and Brown (1978). Das conceptualized intelligence as having two processes: (a) simultaneous, in which information is processed in a spatial, gestalt manner, and (b) sequential, in which material is sequenced in temporal order. Campione and Brown theorized that intelligence consisted of structures that enabled learning (e.g., memory and efficiency) and an executive system that controlled and managed the components involved in problem-solving (e.g., knowledge, metacognition, and use of learning strategies). The latter theory has led special educators to emphasize the use of strategies in the learning process as a means of improving problem-solving and learning. Continued research is needed to identify ways to teach learning strategies so that learners can benefit from the process.

A second approach to intelligence other than factor analysis is that proposed by Howard Gardner. In *Frames of Mind: The Theory of Multiple Intelligences*, Gardner (1983) proposed that there are several autonomous competencies, each of which can be thought of as separate intelligences. Although he only identified seven of these separate intelligences (linguistic, musical, logical-mathematical, spatial, bodily-kinesthetic, interpersonal, and intrapersonal), he suggested that there may be others. Gardner's theory has taken hold in many educational circles, and curriculums have been developed to encourage development of each of these.

9.2.5 Group Aptitude and Achievement Tests

Although the early IQ tests were administered individually, the advent of World War I resulted in a need for group aptitude (mental ability) testing. In 1917, Yerkes, an

American psychologist and professor at Yale, was appointed by the American Psychological Association to develop group mental tests that could effectively evaluate military recruits. Working with Goddard and Terman, Yerkes developed the Army Alpha, a verbal test, and the Army Beta, a perceptual test, to be administered to recruits who failed the Army Alpha. Although the army made little use of their tests, the major result was the obtaining of normative data on 1.75 million men and the recognition that levels of "intelligence" could be obtained through group testing. What transpired after that was the massive development and the multiplication of group testing for all groups in society. Students and job applicants were routinely administered tests to determine aptitude and achievement. Two factors led to this phenomenon of mass testing: (a) individuals could be tested simultaneously with less time and personnel needed to administer the tests and (b) simplified instructions enabled individuals without professional training in testing to administer the tests. Thus, many professionals working with groups (e.g., teachers, therapists, counselors, personnel directors) are able to administer group tests (Anastasi & Urbina, 1997; Gould, 1996).

Although group testing developed because of the need to determine intellectual ability, issues regarding academic achievement soon became a concern of the nation. Group written examinations were first introduced in the Boston schools in 1845 as a substitute for individual oral examinations. The Stanford Achievement Test, developed in 1923, was the first achievement test to be standardized by using statistical principles of measurement. The practice of mass educational testing continues today at the national level, where students enrolled in public schools are administered a group achievement test during the spring semester. Entrance into postsecondary schools is partially based on the results of the American College Test (ACT) and the Scholastic Aptitude Test (SAT)

tests. Entrance into a profession is routinely accompanied by a test (e.g., Graduate Record Exam [GRE], Graduate Management Admissions Test [GMAT], Law School Admissions Test [LSAT]) developed specifically to evaluate proficiency and knowledge of the profession.

9.3 Outline of Overall Evaluative Process of Testing

The steps in the overall evaluative process of testing are listed in Table 9–3 and are elaborated upon in the following section.

The first step in the process of testing is to determine what will be measured and to operationally define the variable. The researcher must be precise and state clearly what is to be discovered. For example, a clinical researcher is interested in evaluating visual perception. Visual perception consists of a number of different skills, such as discrimination, spatial orientation, form-constancy, memory, figure ground,

Table 9–3. Steps in the Evaluation Process

1. Identify the function to be measured.
2. Identify a published instrument to measure condition, or develop a new standardized procedure for evaluation of function.
3. Identify the skill level necessary to use a test instrument.
4. Identify the possible factors in the environment, tester, subject, or test instrument that can potentially distort the test results.
5. Identify the target population for which the test is intended and for which norms have been established.
6. Strictly follow the directions and procedures for administering and scoring the test, or modifying the test procedure to enable the client with disabilities to perform at a maximum level.
7. Interpret the results based on:
   a. norm-referenced data based on the general population or
   b. criterion-referenced data for client performance or competence.

closure, and visual-motor integration. Although it is possible to evaluate visual perception as a whole, effective treatment necessitates an understanding of the individual's ability in each of the various components.

Once the researcher has identified the function to be measured, he or she selects an instrument to measure that function. Often a published instrument is available. Sometimes published instruments may be better because of the known psychometric properties; however, it may be that there is no instrument, and the researcher has to develop one. This is frequently true when designing an interview or survey questionnaire (see methodological research in Chapter 3).

If the clinical researcher chooses to use a published instrument, then it will be necessary to determine what qualifications are needed to administer the test. Qualification levels are set by the APA Standards for Educational and Psychological Testing, and most test publishers adhere to this policy. Level A requires no special qualification; Level B requires at least a BA in psychology, counseling, or closely related field and relevant training; and Level C requires (a) a graduate degree in psychological education or closely related field and training *or* (b) membership in a professional association that requires training and experience in the ethical and competent use of testing (e.g., APA, NASP), *or* (c) license or certification from an agency that requires training in testing.

The fourth step in the process involves identifying the possible factors in the environment, tester, subject, or test instrument that can potentially distort the test results. These factors are outlined in Figure 9–1. The researcher will want to eliminate as many of these factors as possible.

Once the researcher has identified the variable to be measured, the tests to be used, and the potential error factors that need to be eliminated or reduced, he or she must identify the target population for which the test is intended and for which norms have been established. Sometimes this will seem unclear. For example, a clin-

ical researcher may want to examine the psychological effect and impact or behavior that a child with disabilities has on a parent. The target population may, at first, appear to be the parent; however, the question being asked is how the child with disabilities impacts the parent. Although a questionnaire will be given to the parents, items on the instrument will relate to the child with disabilities. Therefore, the target population is, in reality, the child.

Whether the clinical researcher is administering a standardized test or one that he or she developed, the instrument must be administered the same way every time. An alteration in the test directions or administration will confound the results and make them unreliable. When the directions or procedures are altered or modified, this must be stated in the final report. Keep in mind that the alteration or modification of administering a test will make the norms invalid.

The final step is to interpret the results based on either the typical performance as determined by the norms from a general population or a standard set prior to administration of the test. For example, a researcher wants to see the effect of treatment on reduction of anxiety. The researcher has a choice of measurements: (a) a standardized test that measures the level of anxiety (e.g., *State-Trait Anxiety Inventor* by Spielberger, 1983) and compares the results with the expected level based on the norms for the general population or (b) a custom-designed self-evaluation administered before and after treatment.

9.4 Characteristics of a Good Test in Clinical Research

The accuracy and precision in evaluating a client's performance or improvement in a clinical research study depend on the quality of the test instrument. What are the characteristics of a good test instrument? What are some essential questions in evaluating the purposes and "goodness" of a test?

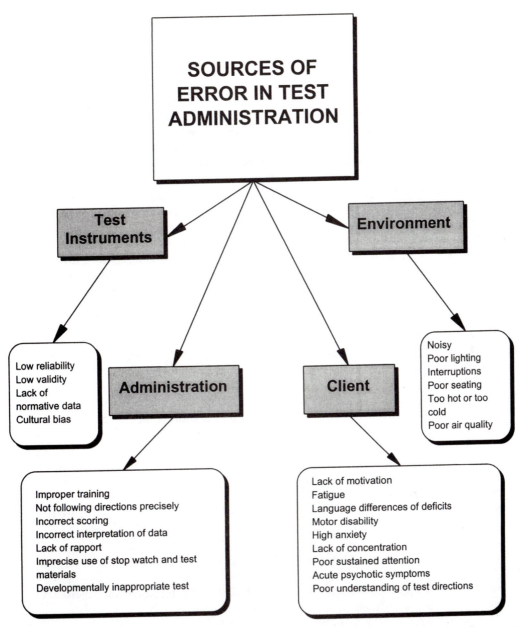

Figure 9–1. Potential sources of error in test administration. Errors come from four main areas: the instrument itself, the administration of the test, the client or subject, and the environment.

► What is the population for whom the test is targeted (e.g., children with learning difficulties, individuals with schizophrenia, persons with muscular dystrophy)?

► What are the specific purposes of the test (e.g., planning treatment goals, determining prognosis, establishing baseline data, or documenting progress)?

► What are the areas of function identified in the test (e.g., social development, prevocational, personality, leisure interests, perceptual-motor abilities, ADL skills, live independently, cognitive level)?

► What are the methods used to evaluate a client? Primary sources for evaluating a client include:

- *medical records:* demographics, previous treatment, and outcomes
- *educational records:* educational attainment, achievement scores
- *clinical observation of performance:* therapists and teacher observations
- *interviews:* formal or unstructured individual interviews
- *objective tests:* objectively scored paper-and-pencil tests, performance scales, and verbal tests
- *survey questionnaires:* group tests, forced choice or open ended
- *self-reports:* evaluation of treatment effectiveness through client's perspective
- *reports from peers, teacher/therapist, or family:* informal reports or observations
- *biomechanical or physiological measurement of human factors:* machine monitoring, test procedures

▶ Is there a standardized procedure or manual of instructions in administering the test and interpreting results? Are there tables of normative data?

▶ Are there special skills or certification that are necessary to administer, score, and interpret results of the test?

▶ Is the scale of measurement used in collecting data identifiable (i.e., continuous, such as interval or ratio, or discrete, such as nominal or ordinal)?

▶ Are error factors controlled that can potentially interfere with obtaining reliable test results?

▶ Are research data reported (such as those derived from previous studies, including reliability, validity, and normative scores?

9.5 Assumptions in Clinical Evaluation

What are some of the assumptions in clinical evaluation that guide a clinician in assessment? The major assumptions are outlined below.

▶ Evaluation is an essential factor in the treatment process. It is used to determine the client's abilities, interests, potentials, and work traits.

▶ Evaluation is used to establish baseline data so as to compare with outcome results.

▶ Evaluation is based on reliable and valid instrumentation. The degree of accuracy in measurement depends on the degree of reliability (consistency) and validity (accuracy).

▶ Error is always present to a degree in evaluation, owing to anomalies in the examiner's presentation of test materials, degree of anxiety or fatigue, client's motivation, less-than-perfect reliability of test, and a less-than-ideal testing environment. Test scores obtained are a sample of the client's performance and represent an approximation of abilities within a given time frame.

▶ The reliability of the test score is increased by eliminating potential error factors that could endanger or distort the test results.

▶ Evaluation can provide data for documentation and the basis for establishing clinical efficacy and quality assurance. Evaluation is an excellent method for objectively determining client progress.

9.6 Major Purposes of Testing in Clinical Research

The major purposes of testing are as follows:

▶ Establish baseline data (experimental research, pretest)
▶ Evaluate outcome or effectiveness of treatment procedure (experimental research, posttest)
▶ Assess the degree of relationship between two variables (correlational research)
▶ Evaluate quality of health care or education progress for accreditation (evaluative research)
▶ Assess developmental landmarks (developmental research)
▶ Assess individual values, interests, or attitudes (survey research)

▶ Evaluate differences between groups (correlational, experimental research)
▶ Evaluate functional assessment (screening target population)

9.7 Conceptual Model for Selecting a Test Instrument for Clinical Research

The decision to select a test from a published source or to construct a new test to measure a defined variable is a frequent dilemma. The measuring instrument is an essential part of a research study and represents the operational definition of a variable. Figure 9–2 shows this process.

The conceptual definition of a variable should lead the investigator to a specific test that is the most appropriate for operationally defining a variable. In clinical research, it is crucial that the investigator select a measuring instrument that has a high reliability and is a valid measurement of outcome. Measuring improvement in such areas as personality, physical capacity, cognitive functions, independent living skills, vocational skills, and perceptual-motor abilities depends directly on the adequacy and sensitivity of the instrument to measure changes. A crude measuring device that does not have the capacity to record subtle changes in an individual's functioning or behavior is of either limited or no value to the researcher.

When deciding on the instrument to use for the outcome measure, the researcher must ask the following questions:

▶ What is the target population?
Examples include:
• normal children, adolescents, adults, elderly
• intellectual deficit
• psychiatric diagnosis
• physically challenged (specify diagnosis)
• social, economic variables
• demographic variables

▶ What are the specific areas of function to be measured?
Examples of these areas include:
• manual dexterity
• intellectual aptitude
• vocational interests
• independent living
• personality
• job readiness
• attitudes toward work
• work experiences
• work tolerance
• social skills
• self-care
• communication
• mobility and transportation
▶ Where will the client be assessed?
Some places for assessment include:
• home
• sheltered workshop
• clinical environment
• school
• office
• hospital
▶ What are the methods for evaluating function?
Some methods include:
• observation of performance
• paper-and-pencil test
• interview
• self-report
• direct measure of function through standardized test instrument
• evaluation by teacher, therapist, or parent
• work samples
▶ Is the test reliable and valid?
• Are there standardized directions for administration?
• Are norm scores available for comparison purposes?
• How many subjects were used in collecting norm values?
• How was reliability of the test established (e.g., test-retest, split half, equivalent forms)?
• How was the validity of the test established (e.g., concurrent, construct, predictive)?
▶ Are the test results easily interpreted?

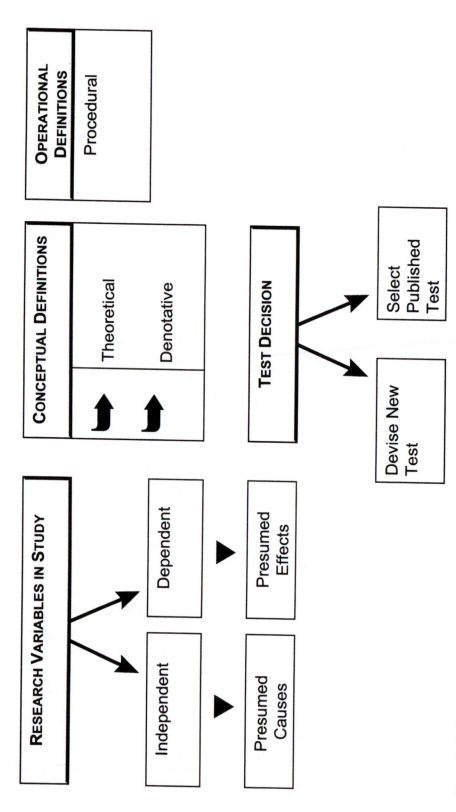

Figure 9–2. Critical steps in determining an appropriate test instrument.

▶ What is the scale of measurement (i.e., ordinal, nominal, interval, or ratio)?

9.8 Bibliographic Sources

Another consideration for testing involves asking the following question: Where can I find the most appropriate test instrument? Examples and names of test instruments can be found in a number of sources, including:

▶ Books on psychological testing, such as the following:

Anastasi, A., & Urbina, S. (1997). *Psychological testing* (7th ed.). Saddle River, NJ: Prentice Hall.

Asher, I. E. (1996). *Occupational therapy assessment tools: An annotated index* (2nd ed.). Rockville, MD: American Occupational Therapy Association.

Bowling, A. (1999). *Measuring health: A review of quality of life measurement scales* (2nd ed.). Buckingham, Great Britain: Open University Press.

Brown, C., McDaniel, R., Couch, R., & McClanahan, M. (1994). *Vocational educational systems and software: A consumer's guide.* Menomonie, WI: Stout Vocational Rehabilitation Institute, University of Wisconsin-Stout.

Cole, B., Finch, E., Gowland, C., & Mayo, N. (1994). *Physical rehabilitation outcome measures.* Toronto, Ontario: Canadian Physiotherapy Association. This text includes 60 outcome measures currently used by physiotherapists in Canada. Each test is described, and reliability and validity data are presented. The tests are organized into four categories: adult motor and vocational activity measures, back and/or pain measures, cardiopulmonary measures, and developmental measures.

Dittmar, S. S., & Gresham, G. E. (1997). *Functional assessment and outcome measures for the rehabilitation health professional.* Gaithersburg, MD: Aspen.

Fischer, J., & Corcoran, K. (1995). *Measures for clinical practice: A sourcebook* (2nd ed.). New York: Free Press.

Hemphill, B. J. (Ed.). (1988). *Mental health assessment in occupational therapy: An integrative approach to the evaluative process.* Thorofare, NJ: Slack.

Hemphill-Pearson, B. J. (Ed.). (1999). *Assessments in occupational therapy mental health: An integrative approach.* Thorofare, NJ: Slack.

Lewis, C. B., & McNerney, T. (1994). *The functional tool box: Clinical measures of functional outcomes.* Washington, DC: Learn.

Lezak, M. (1995). *Neuropsychological assessment* (3rd ed.). New York: Oxford University Press.

Mental measurements yearbook (MMY), Mental measurements supplement, or Tests in print. Published by The University of Nebraska Press. In 1989, the MMY began an alternate-year publication schedule with the Supplement to the Mental Measurements Yearbook or MMY-S. The 12th edition was published in November 1995. (http://www.unl.edu/buros/)

Power, P. (2000). *A guide to vocational assessment* (3rd ed.). Austin, TX: Pro-Ed.

Sattler, J. M. (1992). *Assessment of children* (3rd ed., Rev.). San Diego: Sattler.

Stein, F., & Cutler, S. K. (1998). *Psychosocial occupational therapy: A holistic approach.* San Diego, CA: Singular Publishing Group.

Van Deusen, J., & Brunk, D. (1997). *Assessment in occupational therapy and physical therapy.* Philadelphia: Saunders.

▶ Catalogs of tests, such as the following: (a more complete list is found in Section 9.12)

The Psychological Corporation (TPC), Pro-Ed, and Western Psychological Services (WPS)

▶ Vocational rehabilitation centers
▶ Specialists in work assessment

9.9 Test Instruments

Testing materials and instruments can be found for almost every functional area that one might want to assess. Figure 9–3 diagrams the major categories of tests used in occupational therapy, while the following paragraphs and sections describe the major tests. We have tried to select tests that are commonly used or are important for specific reasons (e.g., they have normative data for populations of individuals with special needs; they are used more frequently by occupational therapists; they have high validity and reliability). We recognize that not all tests are listed. For a more complete list, the reader should refer to one of the books on assessment and testing listed in the previous section or to a publisher's catalog (listed at the end of the chapter in Section 9.12). As a caution, tests are developed or revised yearly, and even the most up-to-date book may not have a description of the test. In case of doubt, it is wise to contact the publisher directly.

9.9.1 Psychosocial Tests

Assessment of psychosocial functioning occurs in several different ways. Observation of a client may occur in a hospital or residential setting. Professionals and paraprofessionals may complete checklists or rating scales as part of the evaluation. Self-report scales used for assessment of self-concept, role identity, stress management, and leisure activities are valuable in the assessment of a client's perceptions. Some of the more widely used psychosocial scales are described in Table 9–4 (Checklists and Self-Report Scales), Table 9–5 (Cognitive and General Assessments), Table 9–6 (In-dependent Living Skills), Table 9–7 (Stress Management), and Table 9–8 (Leisure Interests). Additional tests are described in the following paragraphs. Other examples can be found in the publishers' catalogs.

Behavior Rating Scales

Behavior rating scales are used by therapists, teachers, and clinicians to obtain information about a client's behavior. Usually, the rating scales are paper-pencil instruments filled out by the client's parents or family. Occasionally, rating scales may be completed by a member of the peer group (e.g., another student in the classroom) or as a self-report measuring.

Although rating scales are widely used, there are some disadvantages and cautions to be considered when using them. Because the rating scale is a subjective measurement, response bias is possible. For example, the responder may rate the individual either too harshly or too positively (e.g., Halo effect) than is realistic, or the respondent may restrict the scores to the central range of the scale, leaving the impression that the individual being rated has few strengths or weaknesses. Second, results from rating scales obtained from different settings (e.g., individual therapy and large classroom setting) may show very different scores. This is frequently attributable to the client's varied behavior in different settings. Finally, differences obtained on the scales may occur because of the day on which the rating scale was completed (Martin, Hooper, & Snow, 1986), thereby reflecting the behavioral variability of either the respondent or the client. For these reasons, more than one informant should be used to complete the rating scale. If possible, each informant should complete a couple of rating scales over a short period of time.

Objective Personality Tests

Measurement of personality variables through paper-and-pencil tests are widely

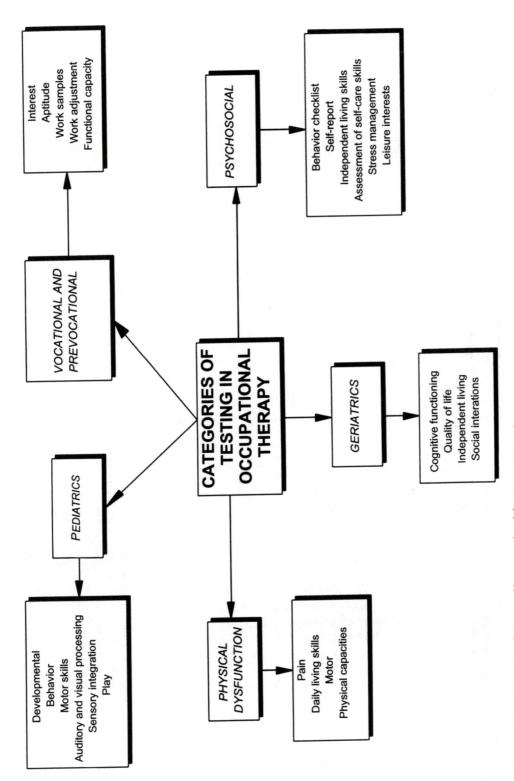

Figure 9–3. Categories of tests used in occupational therapy assessment.

Table 9–4. Psychosocial Assessment in Occupational Therapy: Checklists and Self-Reports

Test	Target Population	Purpose	Variables Assessed	Publisher
Hamilton Depression Inventory (HDI; Reynolds & Kobak, 1995)	Adults	Self-report measure designed to screen for symptoms of depression	Symptoms of depression as defined by the DSM-IV. An overall score defines the level of depression.	Psychological Assessment Resources, Inc. (PAR), P.O. Box 988, Odessa, FL 33556
Health Status Questionnaire (HSQ-12, version 2.0; Health Outcomes Institute, 1995)	Adults	Designed to measure functional status, well-being, and depression	Overall health, functional status, and well-being.	Health Outcomes Institute, 2901 Metro Drive, Suite 400, Bloomington, MN 55425
Magazine Picture Collage (MPC; Lerner & Ross, 1977; Lerner, 1982)	Clients with psychiatric or cognitive impairment	Examine aspects of personality and self, including ego functions and organization; considered to be tangible expression of the client's feelings	Formal, content, and patient-therapist variables based on materials used, placement on page, and interactions	In B. Hemphill (Ed.), 1982, *The evaluative process in psychiatric occupational therapy* (pp. 139–154, 361–362).
Occupational Questionnaire (OQ; Smith, Kielhofner, & Watts, 1986)	Adults and adolescents	Self-inventory of daily activities and volitional issues for those activities	Activity patterns, classification of activities and ranking of activities according to value, interest, and personal causation.	Model of Human Occupation Clearing House, University of Illinois at Chicago, Dept. of OT (M/C 811), College of Associated Health Professions, 191 West Taylor St., Chicago, IL 60623-7250
Occupational Therapy Trait Rating Scale (Clark, Koch, & Nichols, 1965)	Adults with psychosocial dysfunction who are inpatients	Rating scale used by mental health workers; assesses an individual's personality traits	Dominance-manipulativeness; energy or enthusiasm; social isolation; orderliness	In B. Hemphill, 1988, *Mental health assessment in occupational therapy: An integrative approach to the evaluative process*, p. 264–268.
State-Trait Anxiety Inventory (STAI; Spielberger; 1983)	Adults with or without psychosocial dysfunction (other forms are available for adolescents or children)	Assess how anxious an individual feels at a given moment (state) or in general (trait)	State of anxiety (i.e., feeling at a given moment) and trait of anxiety (i.e., how a person generally feels)	Mind Garden, 1690 Woodside Rd., Suite 202, Redwood City, CA 94061 (www.mindgarden.com)
State-Trait Depression Adjective Check Lists (ST-DACL; Lubin, 1981)	Adolescents through adults	Measure state and trait feelings of depression through checklists or adjectives	State of anxiety or trait of anxiety	Psychological Assessment Resources, Inc. (PAR), P.O. Box 998, Odessa, FL 33556

Table 9–5. Psychosocial Assessment in Occupational Therapy: Cognitive and General Assessment

Test	Target Population	Purpose	Variables Assessed	Publisher
Adolescent Role Assessment (Black, 1976)	Adolescents with psychosocial dysfunction	To assess past history and present role development in home, school, and community	Six areas, including childhood play, adolescent socialization, school performance, occupational choice, and work	In American Journal of Occupational Therapy (1976), 30, 73–79
Allen Cognitive Levels (ACL; Allen, 1985; Earhart & Allen, 1988; Allen, Earhart, & Blue, 1992)	Clients with psychiatric or cognitive impairment	Screening tool to classify people into one of six cognitive levels based on Allen's theory	Six cognitive levels: • automatic actions • postural actions • manual actions • goal-directed actions • exploratory actions • planned actions	S & S Arts and Crafts, P.O. Box 513, Colchester, CT 06415-0513
B. H. Battery (Hemphill-Pearson, 1999)	Children and adolescents	Structured instrument to assess the psychological area of human function	Cognitive and psychosocial factors, including problem-solving and abstraction, frustration tolerance, organization and internal structure, and self-awareness	In B. J. Hemphill-Pearson (1999), Assessments in occupational therapy mental health: An integrative approach (pp. 140–155).
Build A City (Clark, 1999)	Adults with psychosocial dysfunction who are in group therapy	Group task or activity that evaluates interactions within a standardized situation and utilizes the constructive, doing process valued in occupational therapy	Communication and work skills within a group; positive and negative interactions between group members	In B. J. Hemphill-Pearson (1999), Assessments in occupational therapy mental health: An integrative approach (pp. 156–169).
Canadian Occupational Performance Measure (COPM; Law et al., 1991, 1994)	Individuals age 7 through adults; individuals with disabilities	Outcome measured designed to detect changes in client's perception of occupational performance. Based on the Model of Occupational Performance	Three subareas are measured (self-care, productivity, and leisure) with total scores obtained for performance and satisfaction. Based on the Canadian Model of Occupational Performance	Canadian Association of Occupational Therapists, 110 Eglinton Ave. West, 3rd Floor, Toronto, Ontario, Canada M4R1A3

(continued)

Table 9–5. Psychosocial Assessment in Occupational Therapy: Cognitive and General Assessment *(continued)*

Test	Target Population	Purpose	Variables Assessed	Publisher
Cognitive Adaptive Skills Evaluation (CASE; Masagatani, 1994, 1999)	Clients with psychosocial dysfunction; can be used with adults and adolescents with developmental delays or cognitive dysfunction	Survey functional skills to examine individual's cognitive skills while performing a task and responding to interview questions	Performance summary using defined behavioral criteria based on analysis of task completion and responses to interview questions	Gladys Masagatani Eastern Kentucky University Department of Occupational Therapy Dizney 103 Richmond, KY 40475-3135
Devereaux Scales of Mental Disorders (Naglieri, LeBuffe, & Pfeiffer, 1994), and *Behavior Rating Scales–School Form* (Naglieri, LeBuffe, & Pfeiffer, 1992)	Children ages 3 through 18	Allows teachers and other professionals to evaluate and identify behavior in individuals perceived as having an emotional dysfunction	Behaviors associated with psychopathology, including conduct, attention, anxiety, depression, autism and acute problems	The Psychological Corporation, 555 Academic Court, San Antonio, TX 78204-2498
Functional Life Scale (FLS; Sarno, Sarno, & Levia, 1973; Dittmar & Gresham, 1997)	Adults in the community	Assessment of an individual's ability to participate in activities of daily living performed by most people	Forty-four items in five categories: • cognition • activities of daily living • activities in the home • outside activities • social interaction	In *Archives of Physical Medicine and Rehabilitation* (1973), *54,* 214–220.
Goal Attainment Scaling (GAS; Stolee, Rockwood, Fox, & Streiner,1992; Cot & Finch, 1991; Ottenbacher & Cusick, 1990)	Adolescents through adults	Assess changes in performance self-care goals	Range of change from expected change (0) to below average $(-2, -1)$ and above average $(+2, +1)$	In *Journal of the American Geriatrics Society* (1992), *4,* 575–578; *Physiotherapy Canada* (1991), *43,* 19–22; *American Journal of Occupational Therapy* (1990), *44,* 519–525.
Independent Living Behavior Checklist (ILBC; Walls, Zane, & Thveldt, 1979)	Adults with mental retardation or psychosocial disorder	Assess the ability for adults with disabilities to function in society	• mobility skills • self-care skills • home maintenance and safety skills • food skills • social and communication skills • functional academic skills.	West Virginia Research and Training Center; One Dunbar Plaza, Suite E, Dunbar, WV 25064

Table 9–6. Psychosocial Assessment of Independent Living Skills

Test	Target Population	Purpose	Variables Assessed	Publisher
Bay Area Functional Performance Evaluation (BaFPE; 2nd ed.; Williams & Bloomer, 1987; Klyczek, 1999)	Adults with psychosocial dysfunction	Assessment of cognitive, affective, and performance skills in daily living tasks and social interaction skills	Ten functional components and seven social interactions; communication and work skills within a group; positive and negative interactions between group members	Consulting Psychologists Press, 3803 East Bayshore Road, P.O. Box 10096, Palo Alto, CA 94303
Canadian Occupational Performance Measure (COPM; Law et al., 1991, 1994; Baptiste & Rochon, 1999)	Clients with disabilities; can be used with children as young as age 7	Outcome measure designed to detect changes in client's perception of occupational performance	Self-care, productivity, leisure, performance and satisfaction; based on the Canadian Model of Occupational Performance	Canadian Association of Occupational Therapists, 110 Eglinton Ave. West, 3rd Floor, Toronto, Ontario, Canada M4R1A3
Comprehensive Occupational Therapy Evaluation (COTE; Brayman, & Kirby, 1976; Kunz & Brayman, 1999)	Adults with acute psychosocial dysfunction who are hospitalized	Provides standard, objective means of rating behaviors of hospitalized patients on a frequent basis	General behavior; interpersonal behavior; task behaviors	In B. J. Hemphill- Pearson (1999), Assessments in occupational therapy mental health: An integrative approach (pp. 259–274). Thorofare, NJ: Slack.
Independent Living Skills Evaluation (ILSE; Johnson, Vinnicombe, & Merrill, 1980).	Adults (age 18 and above) with chronic psychosocial dysfunction who are living in independent living arrangements or living independently	Assess levels of living skills in areas necessary for independent community living	Ten major categories of independent living in home, community, and personal areas	Community Living Experiences, Inc., The Independent Living Project, 291 North Tenth Street, San Jose, CA, 95112

(continued)

Table 9–6. Psychosocial Assessment of Independent Living Skills (*continued*)

Test	Target Population	Purpose	Variables Assessed	Publisher
Kohlman Evaluation of Living Skills (KELS; 3rd ed.; McGourty, 1988; Thomson, 1992, 1999)	Clients with acute psychiatric disorders, elderly patients in acute care hospitals; adolescent through elderly; must be used cautiously with individuals hospitalized for more than 1 month	Quick assessment to provide information about a person's ability in everyday functioning in daily living skills, independent living, and work/leisure	Seventeen living skills in areas of self-care, safety/health, money management, transportation/telephone, work/leisure	American Occupational Therapy Association, 4720 Montgomery Lane, Bethesda, MD 20824-1220
Milwaukee Evaluation of Daily Living Skills (MEDLS; Leonardelli, 1988a, 1988b; Haertlein, 1999)	Adults with chronic mental illness who are inpatients or outpatients in a community mental health clinic (CMHC)	Assessment of behavior and skills needed for adequate functioning in the client's living situation	Twenty subtests measuring basic living skills, safety, communication, and transportation	Slack Inc., 6900 Grove Rd., Thorofare, NJ 08086
Performance Assessment of Self-Care Skills, version 3.1 (PASS; Rogers & Holm, 1999)	Adults	Assess the types of assistance needed to stay in or remain in the community	MOB, ADL, and IADL from perspectives of independence, safety, and task outcome	J. C. Rogers and M. B. Holm, WPIC #1237, 3811 O'Hara Street, Pittsburgh, PA 15213
Scorable Self-Care Evalution–Revised (Clark & Peters, 1993)	Adolescents and adults in acute and community settings	Comprehensive and brief measure of functional performance and identify difficulties in basic living skills	Four subscales, including personal care, housekeeping chores, work and leisure, and financial management	Therapy Skill Builders, a division of the Psychological Corporation, 555 Academic Court, San Antonio, TX 78204-2498
Street Survival Skills Questionnaire (SSSQ; Linkenhoker & McCarron, 1979, 1993)	Adolescents and adults with developmental disabilities, including psychosocial dysfunction	Assessment of specific aspects of adaptive behavior needed for independent living	Nine ares of adaptive behavior, including functional signs, tools, health and safety, time, and money	McCarron-Dial Systems, P. O. Box 45628, Dallas, TX 75245

Table 9–7. Assessment of Stress

Test	Target Population	Purpose	Variables Assessed	Publisher
Occupational Stress Inventory (OSI; Osipow & Spokane, 1987)	Employed adults	Assess occupational adjustment	Occupational adjustment, stress, psychological strain, and coping resources	Psychological Assessment Resources, Inc., P.O. Box 998, Odessa, FL 33556
Stress Audit Questionnaire (Miller & Smith, 1983; Miller, Smith, & Mehler, 1988)	Adults	Operationalization of biobehavioral model of stress into a self-report questionnaire	Situational stress, symptoms and vulnerability factors.	Biobehavioral Institute, 13309 Beacon Street, Suite 202, Brookline, MA 02146
Stress Management Questionnaire (SMQ; Stein, 1987; Stein, Bentley, & Natz, 1999; Stein & Cutler, 1998)	Typical adults and adults (18 and above) with disabilities	Assess symptoms precipitated by stress, stressors that cause a stress response, and coping activities used to manage stress	Symptoms of stress, stressors, and copers	Frank Stein, University of South Dakota, Department of Occupational Therapy, 414 E. Clark St., Vermillion, SD 57069
Survey of Recent Life Experiences (SLRE; Kohn & McDonald, 1992)	Adults	Measure of daily hassles in the lives of adults over the past month	Social and cultural difficulties; work; time pressure; finances; social acceptability; and social victimization.	*Journal of Behavioral Medicine* (1992), 15, 221–36.

Table 9–8. Psychosocial of Leisure Skills

Test	Target Population	Purpose	Variables Assessed	Publisher
Barth Time Construction (Barth, 1985)	Adults or adolescents with psychosocial dysfunction, although it may be used with any individual, adolescent through geriatric	Assess time-management skills	Qualitative summary of interests based on the Model of Human Occupation Frame of Reference	Available from Model of Human Occupation Clearinghouse, University of Illinois at Chicago, Dept.of OT (M/C 811), College of Associated Health Professions, 191 West Taylor St., Chicago, IL 60623-7250
Leisure Activities Finder (LAF; Holmberg, Rosen, & Holland, 1999)	Adults	Identify leisure time activities	Identification of leisure time activities using the self-directed search summary codes	Psychological Assessment Resources, Inc., P.O. Box 998, Odessa, FL 33556
NPI Interest Checklist (Matsutsuyu, 1967; Rogers, Weinstein, & Firone, 1978)	Adults with psychosocial dysfunction, adolescent through geriatric	Identify interest levels in leisure activities	Qualitative summary of interests based on the Model of Human Occupation frame of reference	Available from Model of Human Occupation Clearinghouse, University of Illinois at Chicago, Dept.of OT (M/C 811), College of Associated Health Professions, 191 West Taylor St., Chicago, IL 60623-7250
Occupational Performance History Interview (OPH-I; Kielhofner, Henry, & Walen, 1989; Henry & Mallinson, 1999)	Adolescents and adults with psychosocial or physical dysfunction	Gather history of work, play, and self-care performance	Five content areas of occupational performance, based on the Model of Human Occupation	American Occupational Therapy Association, 4720 Montgomery Lane, P.O. Box 31220, Bethesda, MD 20824-1220
Role Activity Performance Scale (RAPS; Good-Ellis, 1999)	Adults with acute or chronic psychiatric disorders	Measure range of past and present role functioning as basis for treatment planning	Twelve role domains in home, community, or interpersonal relationships up to an 18-month period	In B. J. Hemphill-Pearson (1999), *Assessments in occupational therapy mental health: An integrative approach*, pp. 206–226.
Role Checklist (Oakley, Kielhofner, Barris, & Reichler 1986; Oakley, F. M., 1988; Dickerson, 1999)	Adults, adolescents, and elderly people with psychosocial or physical dysfunction	Assess individual's perception of and identification with roles	Continuous, disrupted changes in past, present, and future roles, and the degree of value for each role	Frances Oakley, Occupational Therapy Service, National Institutes of Health, Building 10, Room 6S–235, 10 Center Drive, MSC 1604, Bethesda, MD 20892-1604

used in research studies of treatment outcome in psychiatry. The *Minnesota Multiphasic Personality Inventory* (MMPI), first published in 1942, is the most extensively used test for diagnosing psychological maladjustment. The researcher using objective personality tests should use caution in interpreting results. The methods of administering the tests and the subject's attitude toward the tests potentially can affect the results. Factors such as noise distractions, unmotivated and uncooperative subjects, and subject faking (sometimes referred to as *malingering*) are some of the problems encountered in personality testing. The ethical consideration in personality testing is another major consideration. The researcher should make efforts to ensure the anonymity and confidentiality of the subject. Most of the tests can only be given by evaluators trained in personality assessment. Some of the more common tests are described in the following paragraphs.

▶ *Minnesota Multiphasic Personality Inventory–2* (MMPI–2; Hathaway & McKinley, 1970) consists of 550 true-false items used for measuring adjustment on 10 psychiatric diagnostic scales. The test takes from 2 to 3 hours and is given to adults.

▶ *Million Adolescent Personality Inventory* (MAPI; Million, Green, & Meagher, 1982) is a personality test for adolescents ages 13 and up. The test is written in language understood by adolescents and is based on a model of personality development rather than clinical pathology. The paper-and-pencil test must be scored by computer through the National Computer Systems.

▶ *Edwards Personal Preference Schedule* (Edwards, 1959) has 225 paired forced choice items used to measure specific personality characteristics in adults. It is available through the Psychological Corporation.

▶ *Personality Inventory for Children–Revised* (PIC; Wirt, Lachar, Klinedinst, Seat, & Broen, 1998) is a questionnaire containing true-false items completed by an informant (usually the parent). The scale consists of three broad scales covering categories such as behaviors at home and school, family interactions, educational achievement, and possible diagnoses. Results can be compared with 12 clinical types for use in differential diagnosis. The scale can be used with children ages 3 through 16.

▶ *Children's Depression Inventory* (CDI; Kovacs, 1992), available through the Psychological Corporation, consists of 27 self-rating items in which the client must choose between one of three sentences that best describes his or her experience in the past 2 weeks. The test is sensitive to changes in mood and provides a valid severity level of depression. The test is designed for ages 7 to 17 and takes about 15 minutes to complete.

▶ *California Life Goals Evaluation Schedules* (Hahn, 1969) consists of 150 hypothetical questions that are rated to provide scores in 10 life goals. It is available through Western Psychological Services.

▶ *Sixteen Personality Factor Questionnaire* (5th ed.; 16PF; Cattell, Cattell, & Cattell, 1993) is a forced choice test used for measuring 16 independent factors of personality. It is designed for high school, college, and adult subjects and takes about an hour to administer. It is available through The Psychological Corporation.

▶ *California Psychological Inventory* (CPI; Gough, 1987) is available through The Psychological Corporation and is appropriate for individuals from age 14 through adulthood. It consists of 480 true-false items, which are used for measuring 18 personality traits.

9.9.2 Physical Dysfunction, Motor Control, Pain, and Independent Living

Tests of functional capacity, vocational aptitude, pain, and independent living assess the degree to which an individual can live and work independently in the community. They assess an individual's ability to perform physical movements as they relate to work, vocational activities, and activities of daily living. These measures are extremely important to rehabilitation research in determining whether an individual can return to work or live in independent housing.

Functional capacity evaluations are comprehensive and systematic approaches that measure the client's overall physical ability such as muscle strength, endurance, joint range of motion, ambulation, sitting, standing, and lifting. *Work samples* are well-defined activities that are similar to actual jobs. They can be used to assess an individual's vocational aptitudes, worker characteristics, and vocational interests. *Independent living measures* test the degree to which an individual can perform the activities of daily living. They include self-care, communication, leisure, shopping, mobility, and related areas. Table 9–9 summarizes information about each of these areas and gives examples of evaluation instruments.

Outcome Measures and Functional Assessment

There is a rising trend in health care to demonstrate effectiveness and client satisfaction. Outcome measures have been designed to evaluate the overall functional status of clients who have received treatment and rehabilitation services in hospitals, outpatient clinics, rehabilitation centers and home environments. These outcome measures (Keith, 1984) are usually designed for specific populations such as individuals with stroke, brain injury, spinal cord injury, low back pain, psychological diagnoses, and developmental disabilities. The outcome measures evaluate the client's ability to perform functional activities of daily living, the degree of pain intensity, ability to work, to engage in leisure activities, to have restful sleep, to drive, to be mobile in the community, to communicate, to ambulate, to academically achieve, and

to perform other activities related to functional abilities. Following is a list of some commonly used outcome measures for rehabilitation (also see Applegate, Blass, & Williams, 1990).

▶ *Levels of Rehabilitation Scale* (LORS–II; Carey & Posavac, 1980, 1982), designed to obtain functional ratings from individuals who are in hospital-based rehabilitation programs.

▶ *Katz Index of Independence in ADL* (Katz, Ford, Moskowitz, Jackson, & Jaffe, 1963), developed for use with rehabilitation in patients.

▶ *Functional Assessment Screening Questionnaire* (Granger & Wright, 1993), an instrument used with patients who have undergone rehabilitation.

▶ *Global Assessment of Functioning* (American Psychiatric Association, 1994), used with individuals with psychosocial diagnoses.

▶ *The Multilevel Assessment Instrument* (Lawton, Moss, Fulcomer, & Kleban, 1982), designed for older individuals.

▶ Unified ADL Evaluation form (Donaldson, Wagner, & Gresham, 1973)

▶ *Functional Life Scale* (Sarno, Sarno, & Levita, 1973)

▶ *Community Integration Questionnaire* (Willer, Ottenbacher, & Coad, 1994), used with individuals with traumatic brain injury

▶ *Barthel Index* (Mahoney & Barthel, 1965), designed to evaluate the degree of assistance required by an individual on 10 items of self-care and mobility

▶ The *Health Status Questionnaire* (Health Outcomes Institute, 1995), used to assess the functional status of adults with chronic illnesses.

▶ The *Sickness Impact Profile* (Bergner, Bobbitt, Carter, & Gilson, 1981; Gilson et al., 1975), used to assess a patient's function in such areas as sleep and rest, work, social interactions, leisure, and emotional behavior.

▶ *Functional Independence Measure* (Keith, Granger, Hamilton, & Sherwins, 1987),

Table 9–9. Functional Assessment of Physical Capacity, Motor Control, Pain, and Independent Living

	Functional Capacity Evaluations	Motor Control/Motor Skills	Pain	Independent Living Measures (Physical Disabilities)
Purpose	To evaluate a person's functional physical abilities as they relate to work performance (Lechner, Roth, & Straaton, 1991)	To evaluate a person's functional motor activities	To evaluate a client's pain to determine effectiveness of treatment (Ross & LaStayo, 1997)	To assess activities of daily living skills needed to function successfully in the community (Power, 2000)
Sample of Variables Assessed	• range of motion • muscle strength • coordination • manual dexterity • muscle endurance • position tolerance	• muscle tone • postural control • gross mobility • somatosensory function • functional hand skills • ambulation • balance	• pain intensity • pain tolerance • pain location	• social skills • self-care • safety and health • communication • transportation • money management • home making • leisure activities
Examples of Widely Used Instruments	Baltimore Therapeutic Equipment Work Stimulator (BTE; Baltimore Therapeutic Equipment,1992)	Assessment of Motor and Process Skills (AMPS; Fisher, 1994)	Descriptor Differential Scale (DDS; Gracely & Kwilosz, 1988)	Barthel Index (Mahoney & Barthel, 1965)
	Functional Capacities Evaluation (FCE; Smith, Cunningham, & Weinberg, 1986)	Bruininks-Oseretsky Test of Motor Proficiency (BOTMP; Bruinicks, 1978)	McGill Pain Questionnaire (MPQ; Melzack 1975)	Functional Autonomy Measuring System (SMAF; Hébert, Carrier, & Bilodeau, 1988)
	Grip Dynometer (Gilliam & Barstow, 1997)	Carr and Shepherd's Motor Assessment Scale for Stroke Patients (Carr, Shepherd, Nordholm, & Lynne, 1985)	Medical Rehabilitation Follow Along™ (MRFA instrument; Baker, Granger, & Fiedler, 1997)	Functional Independence Measure (FIMˢᴹ; Granger, Hamilton, Keith, Zielesky, & Sherwins, 1986; Keith, Granger, Hamilton, & Sherwins, 1987)
	Goniometric Range of Motion (Gilliam & Barstow, 1997)	Functional Test for the Hemiparetic Upper Extremity (Wilson, Baker, & Craddock, 1984)	Numerical Pain Rating Scale (Jensen, Karoly, & Braver, 1986)	Functional Status Index (FSI, Jette, 1980, 1987)

(continued)

Table 9–9. Functional Assessment of Physical Capacity, Motor Control, Pain, and Independent Living *(continued)*

Functional Capacity Evaluations	Motor Control/Motor Skills	Pain	Independent Living Measures (Physical Disabilities)
Isointertal Back Testing (Simmonds, 1997)	Fugl-Meyer Assessment (Fugl-Meyer; Jääskö, Leyman, Olsson, & Steglind, 1975)	Pain Discomfort Scale (PDS; Jensen, Karoly, & Harris, 1991)	Katz Index of Activities of Daily Living (KATZ-ADL; Katz, Ford, Moskowitz, Jackson, & Jaffe, 1963; Staff of the Benjamin Rose Hospital, 1959)
Jebsen Hand Function Test (Jebsen, Taylor, Trieschmann, Trotter, & Howard, 1969)	Rivermead Motor Assessment (Lincoln & Leadbitter, 1979)	Pain Drawing (Margolis, Tait, & Krause, 1986; Ransford, Cairns, & Mooney, 1976; Schwartz & DeGood, 1984)	Kenny Self-Care Evaluation (Schoening et al., 1965; Schoening & Iversen, 1968)
KEYMethod (Key, 1996). Available from Key Functional Assessments, Minneapolis, MN		Short-Form McGill Pain Questionnaire (SFMPQ; Melzack, R. 1987)	Klein-Bell Activities of Daily Living Scale (Klein-Bell ADL Scale; Klein & Bell, 1982, 1993)
Manual muscle tests (MMTs; Daniels & Worthingham, 1986; Kendall, McCreary, & Provance, 1993)		Verbal Rating Scale (Gracely, McGrath, & Dubner, 1978)	Level of Rehabilitation Scale (LORS-II; Carey & Posavac, 1980, 1982)
Medical Rehabilitation Follow Along™ (MRFA instrument; Baker, Granger, & Fiedler, 1997)		Visual Analog Scale (Carlsson, 1983)	Patient Evaluations Conference System (PECS®; Harvey, R. F., & Jellinek, H. M., 1981)
The Physical Work Performance Evaluation (Lechner; Jackson, Roth, & Straaton, 1994)			PULSES Profile (Moskowitz & McCann, 1957)
Pinch Meter (Available from Sammons Preston Inc., P.O. Box 5071, Bolingbrook, IL 60440-5071)			Safety Assessment of Function and the Environment for Rehabilitation (SAFER; Oliver, Bathwayt, Brackley, & Tamaki, 1993)
Work Capacity Evaluation (Matheson, 1988; Matheson & Ogden, 1987)			Structured Assessment of Independent Living Skills (SAILS; Mahurin, DeBettignies, & Pirozzolo, 1991)

designed as a tool to evaluate the patient's ability to complete activities of daily living.

9.9.3 Vocational and Prevocational

In assessing an individual's prevocational ability, an evaluator seeks information on basic ability levels required for specific occupations. Most prevocational tests involve some aspect of motor coordination. Such tests as the *Bennett Mechanical Comprehension Test* (Bennett, 1940), *Crawford Small Parts Dexterity Test* (Crawford & Crawford, 1956), *Stromberg Dexterity Test,* and *O'Conner Tweezer Dexterity Test* (see Table 9–10) require the subject to perform tasks using small tools in an assembly operation. Work samples are used to assess an individual's vocational aptitudes, worker characteristics, and vocational interests (Nadolsky, 1974) in areas of vocational potential in various fields, gross and fine manual dexterity, visual and tactile discrimination, and work habits. The tests purport to measure skill proficiencies related to industrial work. Tests have been devised, such as the *McCarron-Dial Systems* (1979) to evaluate work behavior at a sheltered workshop as indicative of vocational aptitude. Other work sampling tests include the *Micro Tower System of Vocational Evaluation* (IDC Rehabilitation and Research Center, NY, 1977) and the *VITAS: Vocational Interest, Temperament and Aptitude System* (Vocational Research Institute, n.d.). More elaborate methods for assessing vocational aptitude in various industrial occupations are available through the Valpar International Corporation (http://www.valparint.com) and Stout University.

There are many self-devised, unpublished, prevocational tests that are used in sheltered workshops, occupational therapy clinics, and special schools. Some of the more common prevocational tests are listed in Table 9–10, and Table 9–11 provides examples of the more common work sample systems and their addresses.

Vocational Interest Tests

Most investigators constructing vocational interest tests assume that

- ▶ Vocational interests are stable characteristics
- ▶ Vocational interests can be measured by paper-and-pencil tests
- ▶ Vocational interests are grouped around clusters of interest
- ▶ Individuals in occupations share common interests and characteristics
- ▶ There is a positive relationship between vocational interests and choice of occupation
- ▶ Job satisfaction is related to vocational interest and aptitude

The *Strong Vocational Interest Test* (SCII; Strong, Campbell, & Hansen, 1985) and the *Kuder Occupational Interest Survey* (Kuder, 1960) are the two tests most widely used by clinical psychologists and social researchers. Table 9–12 lists the most widely used tests available for measuring vocational interest.

9.9.4 Geriatrics

A number of tests have been developed specifically for the geriatric population. Many of these tests can be administered in a hospital, nursing home, or home setting. Table 9–13 describes some of the most commonly used tests administered by occupational therapists.

9.9.5 Pediatrics

The basic assumption underlying all child development scales is that development is vertical, sequential, and hierarchical. Arnold Gesell and associates in the Children's Development Laboratories at Yale University during the 1920s and 1930s used observational analysis of children's behavior to develop norms. Gesell provided the earliest data correlating age with task attainment in such areas as perceptual-motor,

Table 9-10. Vocational and Prevocational Tests

Test	Target Population	Purpose	Variables Assessed	Publisher
Bennett Mechanical Comprehension Test (Bennett, 1994)	Adolescents through adults	Paper-pencil test that measures the understanding of mechanical principles or general physical concepts in practical situations	• mechanical comprehension	The Psychological Corporation, 555 Academic Court, San Antonio, TX 78204-0952
Complete Minnesota Dexterity Test (n.d.)	Adolescents through adults	Measures simple hand-eye coordination and gross motor skills.	• placing • turning • displacing • one-hand turning and placing • two-hand turning and placing	Lafayette Instrument Company, P.O. Box 5729, Lafayette, IN 47903-5729
Crawford Small Parts Dexterity Test (Crawford & Crawford, 1956)	Adolescents through adults	Measure fine eye-hand coordination for vocational skills	• fine motor coordination • manual dexterity	The Psychological Corporation, 555 Academic Court, San Antonio, TX 78204-0952
Hand Tool Dexterity Test (Bennett, 1946)	Adolescents through adults	Assesses basic skills necessary for any job requiring hand tools	• fine motor coordination • manual dexterity	The Psychological Corporation, 555 Academic Court, San Antonio, TX, 78204-0952
Minnesota Rate of Manipulation (Employment Stabilization Research Institute, 1969)	Adolescents through adults	Assess arm, hand, and finger dexterity	• placing • turning • displacing • one-hand turning and placing • two-hand turning and placing	American Guidance Services, Publishers' Building, Circle Pines, MN 55014
O'Connor Finger Dexterity Test (O'Connor, circa 1920a)	Adolescents through adults	Assess rapid manipulation of small objects	• finger dexterity • speed	Lafayette Instrument Company, P.O. Box 5729, Lafayette, IN 47903-5729 or Stoelting Company, 620 Wheat Lane, Wood Dale, IL 60191

Table 9–10. Vocational and Prevocational Tests (continued)

Test	Target Population	Purpose	Variables Assessed	Publisher
O'Connor Tweezer Dexterity Test (O'Connor, circa 1920b)	Adolescents through adults	Assess aptitude for work involving precision with small tool usage	• fine motor coordination • speed	Lafayette Instrument Company, P.O. Box 5729, Lafayette, IN 47903-5729 or Stoelting Company, 620 Wheat Lane, Wood Dale, IL 60191
Purdue Pegboard (Tiffin, 1948)	Adults	Assess fine motor dexterity	• gross movements of hands, fingers, and arms • fingertip dexterity necessary for assembly tasks	Lafayette Instrument Company, P.O. Box 5729, Lafayette, IN 47903-5729 or London House, Inc., SRA Product Group, 9701 West Higgins Road, Rosemont, IL 60018
Roeder Manipulative Aptitude Test (Roeder, 1970)	Adults	Assess fine motor dexterity	• speed and accuracy for eye-hand coordination • finger dexterity	Lafayette Instrument Company, P.O. Box 5729, Lafayette, IN 47903-5729 or London House, Inc., SRA Product Group, 9701 West Higgins Road, Rosemont, IL 60018
Stromberg Dexterity Test (Stromberg, 1947)	Adolescents through adults	Measures manipulative skills for arm and hand movement	• speed and accuracy of arm movement • speed and accuracy of hand movement • sorting by color and sequence	The Psychological Corporation, 555 Academic Court, San Antonio, TX 78204-0952

Table 9–11. Examples of Work Sample Systems[1]

- *McCarron–Dial Systems, Inc.* Available from McCarron–Dial, P.O. Box 45628, Dallas, TX 75245 (http://www.mccarrondial.com)
  An assessment system that assesses strengths and weaknesses in verbal-cognitive-language, sensory, motor, emotional, and integration-coping. Information from these factors "may be used to estimate the appropriate program level for serving individuals in a preschool, transitional planning, prevocational or vocational setting" (McCarron-Dial, n. d., p. 1). Used with individuals ages 4 through adult.

- *Micro-Tower System of Vocational Education.* Available from the ICD Rehabilitation and Research Center, Micro Tower Research, 340 East 24th St., New York, NY 10010
  Work sample tests used to measure aptitudes (e.g., motor, clerical skill, spatial perception, verbal, and numerical) required for semiskilled and unskilled jobs. Appropriate for adolescents through adults.

- *Mobile Vocational Evaluation* (MVE; Hester,) Hester Evaluation Systems, Inc., 2410 Southwest Granthurst, Topeka, KS 66611-1274
  Composed of a number of tests used in vocational assessment (e.g., Minnesota Clerical Test, Ravens, Minnesota Dexterity Test) and designed to assist any individual with a disability to obtain a suitable vocation. For use with adolescents and adults in secondary and postsecondary schools, rehabilitation agencies, hospitals, and clinics.

- *Physical Work Capacity Fitness Evaluation System* (PWC-FES; Lafayette Instruments). Available through Lafayette Instrument Company, P.O. Box 5729, Lafayette, IN 47903-5729
  A comprehensive assessment system that allows objective worker baseline physical information for physically demanding jobs. Evaluation provides data to develop treatment protocols for clients in rehabilitation. The system requires application software for scoring and anlyzing results.

- *Talent Assessment Programs* (TAP; Nighswonger, 1981). Available from Talent Assessment, Inc., P.O. Box 5087, Jacksonville, FL 32207.
  Comprehensive assessment tool used for measuring production level capactities and vocational aptitudes of individuals in areas applicable for occupations in trade, industrial, technical and professional. Results from the test allow for integration of individuals' capabilities and interests, thereby providing aid in vocational counselling. The test is appropriately used with adolescents through adults.

- *Valpar Component Work Samples* (Valpar, 1973). Available from Valpar International Corporation, P. O. Box 5767 Tucson, AZ 85703 (http://www.valparint.com/)
  A comprehensive work evaluation system designed to assess vocational abilities through 23 different work samples. The original samples were developed in 1973, but have been updated as required. Tasks include mechanical, size, discrimination, range of motion and physical capacity, clerical abilities, assembly, coordination and motor dexterity, drafting skill, and electronic skills.

- *VIEWS: Vocational Information and Evaluations* (Vocational Research Institute, 1977). Available from Vocational Research Institute, 1528 Walnut Street, Suite 1502, Philadelphia, PA 19102 (http://www.vri.org/)
  This evaluation program for adults includes materials for 28 different work samples to assess aptitudes, vocational interests and work-related behaviors. Examples of samples include assembly activities (e.g., nut, bolt, and washer; grommet, belt, ladder), clerical (e.g., rubber stamping, filing, collating), and manufacturing (e.g., sign making, blouse making, vest making).

- *VITAS: Vocational Interest, Temperament and Aptitude System* (Vocational Research Institute, 1980). Available from Vocational Research Institute, 1528 Walnut Street, Suite 1502, Philadelphia, PA 19102 (http://www.vri.org/)
  VITAS was developed for individuals with mental retardation or who are educationally disadvantaged. Twenty-two job-like work samples in that represent work groups identified in the Guide for Occupational Exploration assess aptitudes, vocational interests, and work-related interests in skilled and unskilled vocations. Most work samples do not require any reading.

- *Wide Range Employability Sample Test* (WREST; Jastak & Jastak, 1980). Available through Jastak Associates, P.O. Box 3410,Wilmington, DE 19806
  Contains 10 clerical work tasks designed to evaluate individuals with disabilities and educationally disadvantaged in and out of residential settings. Test is nonverbal. Can be administered to adolescents through adults.

---

[1]Additional materials can be found through the Stout Vocational Rehabilitation Institute at the University of Wisconsin–Stout, http://www.chd.uwstout.edu/svri/, and *Vocational Educational Systems and Software: A Consumer's Guide* by C. Brown, R. McDaniel, R. Couch, & M. McClanahan (1994).

Table 9–12. Vocational Interest Tests

Test	Target Population	Purpose	Variables Assessed	Publisher
COPSystem (Knapp & Knapp, 1982; Knapp, L. & Knapp-Lee,1995; Knapp-Lee, Knapp, & Knapp, 1982)	Adolescents through adults	Identify occupational choices based on 14 occupational clusters through interests (COPS), abilities (CAPS), and values (COPES)	Self-administered inventory measures interests and values; paper-and-pencil tests is 8 abilities tests measures aptitude	Educational & Industrial Testing Service, (EdITS) P.O. Box 7234 San Diego, CA 92126
Geist Picture Interest Inventory-Revised (Geist, 1975)	Junior high school through adult	Identify vocational and avocational interests using a minimum of language	Picture selection test measures occupational interest. Spanish and deaf forms available	Western Psychological Services, Order Department, 12031 Wilshire Blvd, Los Angeles, CA 90025
Gordon Occupational Checklist II (Gordon, 1981)	Grade 8 through adults	Identify career interests of non-college bound individuals	Subject underlines preferred activities. Scoring identified major occupational areas of interest.	The Psychological Corporation, 555 Academic Court, San Antonio, TX 78204-0952.
Kuder Occupational Interest Survey (Form DD), (Kuder, 1979) Revision.	High school, adults	Assess vocational interests	Forced choice paper and pencil test measuring interest in specific occupations	Science Research Associates, 155 N. Wacker Drive, Chicago, IL 60606
Reading-Free Vocational Interest Inventory (Becker, 1981)	Adolescence and older who are earning disabled, mentally retarded, and disadvantaged	Measure vocational interests with special populations	Picture format measuring occupational interests. Specifically designed for individuals who can't read	Psychological Assessment Resources, Inc., P.O. Box 998, Odessa, FL 33556
Strong-Campbell Interest Inventory (SCII; Strong, Campbell, & Hansen, 1985)	Adolescents through adults	Assess occupational interests for individuals oriented toward college graduation and professional occupations	Self-record inventory containing 325 three-reponse items; computerized scoring required (disk available through CPP)	Consulting Psychologist Press (CPP), 3803 East Bayshort Rd., P.O. Box 10096, Palo Alto, CA 94303
Wide Range Interest-Opinion Test (Jastak & Jastak, 1979)	Junior high school through adult	Assess occupational interests	Picture format measuring occupational interest. Adaptations for individuals who are blind. Computer format is available, to take in two sessions.	Guidance Centre, The Ontario Institute of Studies in Education of the University of Toronto, 712 Gordon Baker Road, Toronto, Ontario, M2H 3R7

Table 9–13. Geriatric Scales

Test	Purpose	Variables Assessed	Format	Publisher
Cognitive Function				
Mini-Mental State (MMS; Folstein, Folstein, & McHugh, 1975)	Obtain a quantitative measure of cognitive performance for elderly with neurological dysfunction quickly	Five areas of cognition: • orientation • memory • attention and calculation • recall • following oral and written instructions	Oral questionnaire administered by examiner.	*Journal of Psychiatric Research* (1975), 12, 189–198.
Rivermead Behavioral Memory Test (RBMT; Wilson, Baddley, Cockburn, & Hioms, n.d.; Wilson, Cockburn, & Baddley, 1991)	Assess problems in memory and provide means for monitoring treatment outcomes	• immediate memory • short-delay • long-term memory • overall memory function	Visual or verbal presentation of questions with verbal response	National Rehabilitation Services, Northern Speech Service, Inc., 117 North Elm Stree, P. O. Box 1247, Gaylord, MI 49735
Short Portable Mental Status Questionnaire (SPMSQ; Pfeiffer, 1975)	Quick assessment of the degree of intellectual impairment in elderly patients in the home or in clinical setting	Level of intellectual functioning, taking into account educational level	Question and answer using pencil-and-paper	*Journal of the American Geriatrics Society* (1975), 23, 433–441.
Independent Living				
Assessment of Living Skills and Resources (ALSAR; Williams et al., 1991)	Assess the living skills and resources in a community-dwelling of elderly residents to determine treatment protocol and assist in problem-solving	Assesses areas of IADL including • use of community resources • leisure time • medication • finances • home management	Rating scale, with scores combined to determine risk	*Gerontologist* (1991), 31, 84–91 or Theresa Drinka; VA Madison GRECC (116), VAMC, 2500 Overlook Terrace, Madison, WI 53702
Functional Assessment Scale (FAS; Breines, 1988)	Scale designed to rate self-care function in patients who are in nursing homes or hospitals	Provides a single level of function, ranging from 1 "total care" to 10 "prepared to live independently"	Checklist-type rating scale	Geri-Rehab, Inc., 15 Hibbler Road, Lebanon, NJ 08833

Table 9–13. Geriatric Scales *(continued)*

Test	Purpose	Variables Assessed	Format	Publisher
Instrumental Activities of Daily Living (IADL Scale; Lawton & Brody, 1969)	Assess skills needed by elderly individuals to live independently	Eight categories of IADL (e.g., housekeeping, food preparation, finances) rated according to level of independence	Rating scale, with higher scores indicating need for more assistance	*Gerontologist* (1969), *9*, 179–186.
Maguire's Trilevel ADL Assessment (Maguire, 1995)	Assess ADL abilities in elderly clients in personal areas, home, or sheltered environment	• communication • food needs • dressing • hygiene • organization • mobility	Observation	In C. Lewis (1995), *Aging: The health care challenge: An interdisciplinary approach to assessment and rehabilitative management of the elderly* (pp. 61–71)
Older Adults Resources and Services (OARS; Duke University Center for the Study of Aging and Human Development, 1978)	Multidimensional instrument to obtain information in basic and instrumental activities of daily living for elderly clients living in the community	• social resources • economic resources • mental health • physical health • activities of daily living	Structured interview	Duke University Center for the Study of Aging and Human Development (1978)
Parachek Geriatric Rating Scale (3rd ed.; Parachek & King, 1986)	Screening tool to assist mental health workers in treatment planning for elderly patients	• level of physical capabilities • self-care skills • social interaction skills	Likert scale, rated by mental health workers or clinicians	Center for Neurodevelopmental Studies, 5340 West Glenn Drive, Glendale, AZ 85301
Rapid Disability Rating Scale (Linn, 1967; Linn, & Linn, 1982)	Assessment of functional disabilities in elderly clients	16 items grouped into • activities of daily life • sensory and communication • mental	Rating scale	*Journal of the American Geriatrics Society* (1982), *30*, 378–382.

(continued)

Table 9–13. Geriatric Scales (continued)

Test	Purpose	Variables Assessed	Format	Publisher
Geriatric Hopelessness Scale (Fry, 1984)	Assess attitudes of pessimism and futility in elderly clients towards themselves and their future.	Attitudes toward • physical and cognitive abilities • personal and interpersonal worth • spiritual faith • nurturance and respect	Rating scale	*Journal of Counseling Psychology* (1984), v31, 322–331
Quality of Life				
Life Satisfaction Index K (LSI-K; Koyano & Shibata, 1994)	Quick measure of one's self-perception of well-being in elderly clients	• cognitive/short-term • cognitive/long-term • emotional/short-term well-being	Self-administered paper-pencil test	*Facts and Research in Gerontology* (1994), Suppl. 2, 181–187.
Social Interaction				
Geriatric Depression Scale (Yesavage et al., 1983)	Easily administered survey used as screening instrument to evaluate depression.	Level of depression • normal • mild • severe	Paper-and-pencil survey test, completed by client or clinician.	*Journal of Psychiatric Research* (1983), 17, 37–49.
Geriatric Rating Scale (GRS; Plutchik et al., 1970)	Assessment of readiness of elderly patients to leave a hospital setting	• physical disability • apathy • communication failure • socially irritating behavior	Observational based behavioral rating scale	*Journal of the Geriatric Society* (1970), 18, 491–500.

language, and personal-social. Since Gesell, other developmental researchers have provided data demonstrating that the growth of human abilities are linked to a biological clock that determines when behavior unfolds at certain critical periods along an age continuum. Differences among child development tests are based on the factors identified and the methods used for assessment. These tests also vary in the time involved in administering a test and in the requirements needed to validly interpret results. For example, the *Denver Developmental Screening Test* (Frankenburg, Dodds, Archer, Shapiro, & Bresnick, 1990) takes about 15 minutes to administer by nonprofessional health aides, whereas the *Gesell Developmental Scale* requires at least 2 hours to administer by a professionally trained psychometrician. Examples of the most widely used child development scales are described below and are summarized in Table 9–14.

9.9.6 Special Populations

In addition to general tests in psychosocial function and physical disabilities, assessments have been developed for specific populations such as individuals with arthritis or stroke. These tests have been standardized with these specific populations and should not be used with typical individuals. Table 9–15 provides information about many of these tests.

9.9.7 Neuropsychological Batteries

Clinical neuropsychology is a relatively new field that attempts to relate behavior to brain functioning. Neuropsychological testing is requested by clinicians, therapists, and educators in special cases. For example, neuropsychological testing is usually requested when a client has sustained a traumatic or acquired brain injury. Neuropsychological testing may also be requested

when a more specific understanding of an individual's strengths and weaknesses is desired. Although individual neuropsychological tests can be given, frequently neuropsychologists use a specific battery of tests generated by their particular philosophical stance.

The *Halsted-Reitan Neuropsychological Test Battery* consists of up to 37 individual tests, each of which must be administered to obtain a complete profile of an individual's brain functioning. Diagnosis is dependent on (a) comparing the client's score with a comparison group, (b) comparing scores between individual tests, and (c) comparing differences between scores performed on the right or left side of the body. Based on the profile of scores, treatment for deficits are suggested.

Luria (1980) developed a second approach to neuropsychological testing by developing specific test items that would allow the clinician to identify the way in which a person approached a task. The *Luria-Nebraska Neuropsychological Battery* (LNNB; Golden, Purisch, & Hammeke, 1985) is an outgrowth of Luria's work. Although this battery is not frequently used, it does provide information for the clinician regarding brain–behavior relationships.

Edith Kaplan, using the philosophy and work of Luria, has proposed a third approach to neuropsychological testing: an evaluation should result in an understanding of the way in which a person approaches a task, regardless of which tests are used. This method, called the Boston process approach, relies less on specific instruments and more on observation of behavior during the evaluation. All neurological functioning (e.g., cognitive, perceptual, memory, language, organization, and personality) is evaluated in this approach. The *Wechsler Adult Intelligence Scale*–Revised–Neuropsychological Instrument (WAIS–R–NI; Kaplan, Fein, Morris, & Delis, 1991), developed by The Psychological Corporation, is an example of an instrument using the Boston process approach.

Table 9–14. Pediatric Assessments

Developmental	Behavior	Motor and Sensory Integration	Visual, Auditory, and Motor Processing	Play
Assessment of Preterm Infants' Behavior (ABIP; Als, 1984; Als, Duffy, & McAnulty, 1988a, 1988b).	Achenbach System of Empirically Based Assessment (ASEBA; Achenbach, 1991)	Alberta Infant Motor Scales (AIMS; Piper & Darrah, 1994)	Bender Visual Motor Gestalt Test (Bender, 1938; Koppitz, 1963, 1975)	Preschool Play Scale (PPS; Knox, 1974)
Bayley Scales for Infant Development–II (BSID-II; The Psychological Corporation, 1993)	Attention Deficit Disorders Evaluation Scale, School Version (ADDES; McCarney, 1996)	DeGangi-Berk Test of Sensory Integration (Berk & DeGangi, 1983)	Brunicks-Osteresky Motor Proficiency (BOMPT; Bruinicks, 1978)	Play History (Takata, 1969, 1974)
Denver Developmental Screening Test–II (DDST-II; Frankenburg, Dodds, Archer, Shapiro, & Bresnick, 1990)	Behavior Rating Profile–2 (2nd ed; BRP–2; Brown & Hammill, 1990)	Erhardt Developmental Prehension Assessment (Erhardt, 1989)	Developmental Test of Visual Perception (4th ed; VMI-4; Beery & Buketnica, 1996)	Play Observation (Kalverboer, 1977)
Early Intervention Developmental Profile (EIDP; Brown et al., 1981; Rogers & D'Eugenio, 1981)	Behavioral Assessment Scale of Oral Functions in Feeding (Stratton, 1981)	Miller Assessment for Preschoolers (Miller, 1988)	Motor-Free Visual Perception Test Revised (MVPT-R; Colarusso & Hammill, 1996)	Transdisciplinary Play-Based Assessment (Linder, 1990)

Table 9-14. Pediatric Assessments *(continued)*

Developmental	Behavior	Motor and Sensory Integration	Visual, Auditory, and Motor Processing	Play
McCarthy Scales of Children's Abilities (MSCA; McCarthy, 1972)	*Burks' Behavior Rating Scale* (Burks, 1968)	*Quality of Upper Extremity Skills Test* (QUEST; DeMatteo et al., 1993)	*Peabody Developmental Motor Scales* (PDMS; Folio & Fewell, 1983)	
Pediatric Evaluation of Disability Inventory (PEDI; Haley, Coster, Ludlow, Haltiwanger, & Andrellos, 1992)	*Children's Depression Inventory* (CDI; Kovacs, 1992)	*Sensory Integration and Praxis Tests* (SIPT; Ayres, 1989)	*Test of Visual-Motor Skills—Upper Level* (non-motor; TVPS-UL; Gardner, 1992)	
	Conners Teacher Rating Scale (CTRS; Conners, 1989b) and *Conners Parent Rating Scales* (CPRS; Conners, 1989a)	*Sensory Rating Scale for Infants and Young Children* (Provost & Oetter, 1993)	*Test of Visual Perceptual Skills* (nonmotor; TVPS; Gardner, 1982)	
	Devereaux Behavior Rating Scales—School Form (Naglieri, LeBuffe, & Pfeiffer, 1992)	*Toddler and Infant Motor Evaluation* (TIME; Miller & Roid, 1994)	*Test of Visual Perceptual Skills—Upper Level* (nonmotor; TVPS-UL; Gardner, 1992)	
	Personality Inventory for Children—Revised (Lachar, 1982)	*Touch Inventory for Elementary School* (TIE; Royeen, 1987a, 1990)		
	The Way I Feel About Myself: The Piers–Harris Self-Concept Scale (Piers & Harris, 1984)	*Touch Inventory for Preschoolers* (TIP; Royeen, 1987b)		

Table 9–15. Assessments for Special Populations

Arthritis	• *Impact Measurement Scales–2* (AIMS-2; Meenan, Mason, Anderson, Guccione, & Kazis, 1992). Available from Robert F. Meenan, M. D., Professor of Medicine, Dean of School of Public Health, Boston University, 80 East Concord Street, Boston, MA 02118-2394 • *Edinburgh Rehabilitation Status Scale* (ERSS; Affleck, Aitken, Hunter, McGuire, & Roy, 1988). Available from Rehabilitation Studies Unit, Princess Margaret Rose Hospital, Edinburgh, Scotland EH10 7ED • *Functional Status Index* (FSI; Jette, 1980, 1987). In *Archives of Physical Medicine and Rehabilitation* (1980), *61*, 395–401 • *Standardized Test of Patient Mobility* (Jebsen et al., 1970). In *Scandanavian Journal of Rehabilitation Medicine*, 7, 13–31
Low back pain	• *Oswestry Low Back Pain Disability Questionnaire* (Fairbank, Davies, Couper, & O'Brien, 1980). In *Physiotherapy* (1980), *66*, 271–273 • *Sickness Impact Profile™* (SIP; Bergner, Bobbit, Carter, & Gilson; 1981; Gilson, Gilson, Bergner, Bobbitt, Kressel, Pollard, & Vesselago, 1975). Available from Johns Hopkins University, School of Public Health, Department of Health Policy and Management, 624 N. Broadway, Room 647, Baltimore, MD 21205-1901
Spinal cord injury	• *Quadriplegic Index of Function* (QIF; Gresham et. al, 1986). In *Paraplegia* (1986), *24*, 38–44
Stroke	• *Frenchay Acitivities Index* (FAI; Holbrook & Skilbeck, 1983). In *Age and Ageing* (1983), *12*, 166–170 • *Fugl-Meyer Assessment* (Fugl-Meyer, Jääskö, Leyman, Olsson, & Steglind, 1975). In *Scandanavian Journal of Rehabilitation Medicine* (1975), *7*, 13–31 • *Time Care Profile* (Halstead & Hartley, 1975). In *Archives of Physical Medicine and Rehabilitation* (1975), *56*, 110–115
Traumatic brain injury	• *Agitated Behavior Scale* (ABS; Corrigan, 1989). Available from Dr. J. D. Corrigan, Department of Physical Medicine and Rehabilitation, The Ohio State University, 480 West 9th Avenue, Columbus, OH 43210 • *Community Integration Questionnaire* (Corrigan & Deming, 1995; Willer, Ottenbacher, & Coad, 1994). Available from Dr. B. Willer, Departments of Psychiatry and Rehabilitation Medicine, State University of New York, University at Buffalo, 3435 Main St., Buffalo, NY 14214 • *Disability Rating Scale* (Rappaport, Hall, Hopkins, Belleza, & Cope, 1982). In *Archives of Physical Medicine and Rehabilitation* (1982), *63*, 118–123 • *Rabideau Kitchen Evaluation-Revised: An Assessment of Meal Preparation Skill* (RKE-R; Neistadt, 1992). Available from University of New Hampshire Departments of Occupational Therapy, School of Health and Human Services, Durham, NH • *Rivermead Perceptual Assessment Battery* (RPAB; Bhavni, Cockburn, Lincoln, & Whiting, 1985). Published by NFER-NELSON Publishing Company Ltd. Available from Western Psychological Services, 12031 Wilshire Boulevard, Los Angeles, CA 90025-1251

Clinical researchers may not, at first, be involved in neuropsychological testing as part of their research. Nonetheless, information obtained from these tests, as well as use of pre- and posttest data can be useful as outcome measures in examining the relationship between changes in behavior and interventions.

9.10 Reviewing and Evaluating Tests

For the researcher, the selection of a valid and reliable instrument is critical. Knowledge in assessing the adequacy of a measuring instrument is extremely important in view of the literally thousands of tests that are published by test corporations. Before the clinical researcher chooses a test to use in research, the purpose for the test must be determined. Does the researcher need to screen participants for normal intelligence or average achievement? Is adaptive behavior a concern? If the purpose of the investigation is to evaluate the effect of a treatment on reducing low back pain, the researcher will want to make sure that all subjects have clinically significant low back pain (see Figure 9–4).

The next step in determining which test to use is to review the appropriate tests that are available, taking into account the psychometric properties, including the reliability, validity, and measurement scales of each test. If there are special qualifications in administering the test, the researcher must know who is able to administer the test and how long it will take to administer. The following outline and examples of reviews of tests will illustrate the manner in which tests are analyzed (Stein, 1988).

9.10.1 Outline for Reviewing Tests

1. Title
2. Date published, date revised
3. Authors
4. Publisher: Distributor of test or where test is available
5. Target Population: What was the original sample from which data were collected in terms of age, diagnostic group, and geographical location? Is there a specific target population for which the test is appropriate?
6. Variables Assessed: What are the specific areas of function, behavior, or personality that are being assessed? What are the major stated purposes of the test?
7. Measurement Scales: What is the level of measurement in the test?
   A. Qualitative (subjective judgment)
      i. Nominal scale of measurement refers to evaluating variables us-

ing independent categories such as *can* or *cannot perform a specific task.*
      ii. Ordinal scale of measurement refers to evaluating variables using magnitude and ranking such as *completely dependent in task, needs assistance,* or *independent functioning.* Variables can also be rated on a numerical scale from 1 to 5, for example, where 1 indicates *no self-care* and 5 *indicates cares for self independently.*
   B. Quantitative (objective evaluation)
      i. Interval scale of measurement refers to scoring variables on a continuous scale with equal distances between score values. Pulse rate, blood pressure, height, and weight are usually measured on interval scales using tests that produce mathematical data.
      ii. Ratio scale of measurement incorporates the concept of an absolute zero.
8. Administration of Instrument: Who administers the test and when is it administered? How long does it take to administer? Is there special training to administer the test? Are special materials or environments required?
9. Scoring and Interpretation of Results: Are there overall scores or subtest scores derived from the test results? Are there norms available to interpret raw scores? How are the results used in treatment planning, documentation of progress, and discharge recommendations?
10. Test Reliability and Validity
11. Other Comments: Included in this section are miscellaneous comments such as the theoretical orientation or conceptual framework of the test and its appropriateness for the clinical researcher.
12. References: Includes books, journals, test manuals, and other sources where the test has been published or critically evaluated.

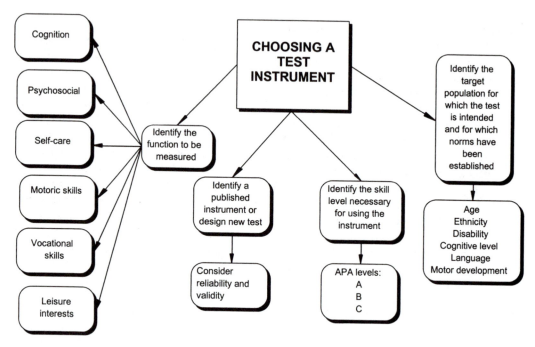

Figure 9–4. Factors in choosing a test instrument.

9.10.2 Example of Test Review

1. *Kohlman Evaluation of Living Skills* (KELS; Thompson, 1992)
2. Originally published in 1978, revised in 1992
3. Linda Kohlman Thomson, MOT, OTR, OT(C), FAOTA
4. American Occupational Therapy Association, 4720 Montgomery Lane, P.O. Box 31220, Bethesda, MD 20824-1220
5. Clients with acute psychiatric disorders, elderly patients in acute care hospitals; adolescent through elderly. Must be used cautiously with individuals hospitalized for more than 1 month.
6. Seventeen living skills categorized into five main domains: self-care, safety and health, money management, transportation and telephone, and work and leisure are measured.
7. Measurement Scales: Nominal and ordinal scales.
8. The test can be given by an occupational therapist or occupational thera-

pist assistant when supervised by the occupational therapist.
9. Each of the 17 living skills are scored for either "independent" or "needs assistance" with a score of 1 (½ for the work and leisure category) given if the client needs assistance. Items scored as independent are given a score of 0. Individuals obtaining an overall score of 5½ or less are considered able to live independently; scores above 5½ suggest the client needs assistance to live in the community.
10. Interrater reliability ranges from $r = .84$ to 1.00. Concurrent validity has been measured at $r = .78$ to $.89$ with Global Assessment Scale; $-.84$ with BaFPE. The test has successfully predicted which geriatric patients could live independently.
11. The test provides a quick assessment to provide information about a person's ability in everyday functioning in daily living skills, independent living, and work/leisure.

12. McGourty, L. K. (1988). Kohlman Evaluation of Living Skills (KELS). In B. J. Hemphill, *Mental health assessment in occupational therapy: A integrative approach to the evaluative process* (pp. 133–146). Thorofare, NJ: Slack.

Thompson, L. K. (1992). *The Kohlman Evaluation of Living Skills* (KELS, 3rd ed.). Rockville, MD: American Occupational Therapy Association.

Thompson, L. K. (1999). The Kohlman Evaluation of Living Skills. In B. J. Hemphill-Pearson, *Assessment in occupational therapy mental health: An integrative approach* (pp. 231–244). Thorofare, NJ: Slack.

9.11 Criterion-Referenced Tests and Normative-Referenced Tests

Until recently, most tests were normative-referenced tests, or NRTs. These tests, described previously, were developed to classify individuals into levels of instructional groups. The scores obtained by the normative sample on a norm-referenced test are distributed along a normal curve. Raw scores obtained by individuals taking a norm-referenced test are compared with the normative sample and can be converted into standard scores and percentiles.

There are several advantages to NRTs. Individuals taking the test are compared with the general population, thus the performance of a student or patient can be judged to be typical or atypical. Because NRTs are usually commercially published, psychometric characteristics such as reliability and item analysis are carefully considered in the development. Additionally, standardization of an NRT includes administering the test to large samples of individuals stratified across many socioeconomic groups, ages, ethnic backgrounds, and educational levels. In this way, raw scores obtained from a given individual can be compared to the raw score obtained by most of the population having the same characteristics.

At the same time, there are disadvantages to an NRT. Because the tests are broad measures of a subject and contain a limited number of items from many areas within that subject, they are often referred to as survey tests. It is not uncommon for an NRT designed to be used in grades 1 through 12 to include only 100 sight words. Because there is no national or state curriculum, the content found on the test may not match the curriculum of a particular school or community. Finally, because the number of items in each area is limited, the test results cannot be used to measure small gains in progress. Likewise, there is limited value for using the results of an NRT in determining an instructional or therapeutic program.

The purpose of NRTs is (a) to compare an individual's achievement or performance with other individuals of the same age, educational level, and socioeconomic status and (b) to obtain information regarding the normal population. When these tests are used with atypical populations, there may be a bias, which results in systematic error. In spite of these disadvantages, NRTs are useful in clinical research.

In testing circles during the last 20 years, there has been a growing interest in devising criterion-referenced tests in lieu of norm-referenced tests (Deno, 1985). Criterion-referenced tests (CRTs), first proposed by Glaser (1963), use content or curricular domains to set the standard of performance. They compare the performance of an individual with a specified level of mastery or achievement rather than with a normative population. Because the performance is compared with a criterion, performance on these tests allows the therapist or teacher to suggest specific classroom goals and objectives to use in program planning. Progress can be monitored more effectively and more discretely.

CRTs are based on a comprehensive theory that generates ideas for a specific content domain. In CRTs, items are selected systematically to represent the content domain. For example, if an investigator is interested in determining the visual perceptual skills of individuals, the first task would be to determine the dimensions of visual perception from the theoretical and experiential perspectives. The investigator would use the theoretical framework to guide the writing of test items, making sure that each aspect of the framework is covered by test items in the CRT. Operational performance standards, obtained by surveying a representational sample of the general population, are used in writing test items. For example, a survey of 10-year-olds would reveal that most of them have no difficulty with activities involving visual closure or visual figure ground. The operational performance standard, therefore, might be set at a criterion level of 90% accuracy for recognition of figures in tasks involving visual figure ground or visual closure.

One example of criterion-referenced testing occurs when measuring an individual's independent living skills. For instance, in the criteria of dressing completely, we might include the act of putting on all clothes right-side out and frontwards, tying shoes, and fastening all fasteners. The individual's ability to perform this activity is measured by a given standard. Until the individual has mastered the expected standard, the individual is not considered to have reached competency. Social skills and self-help skills are often evaluated by CRTs.

CRTs are sometimes referred to as curriculum based measures (CBMs) or curriculum-based assessments (CBAs). CBAs and CBMs establish a student's instructional needs in relationship to the requirements of the actual curriculum being used. Just as with CRTs, the CBAs and CBMs assess mastery of learning by providing an operational performance criterion as a necessary standard for passing. Although commercial CRTs are available, teachers and occupational therapists frequently develop the measurement instrument based on their own criteria.

In summary, a CRT is constructed to obtain measurements that can be interpreted in terms of specific criteria or performance standards. Scores obtained on NRTs, however, are interpreted in terms of comparison to a population. The choice of which test to use depends on the outcome desired. If a researcher is interested in the progress of a particular student over time, a CRT is more appropriate; however, if the researcher is interested in the differences between two groups of subjects, then an NRT may be more appropriate.

A summary of the differences between criterion- and norm-referenced tests is given in Table 9–16. This summary may help in deciding which type of test to use.

9.11.1 Applying Criterion-Referenced Concepts to Research

The major content areas for clinical researchers in evaluation include basic living skills, interests, work behavior, and skill attainment. If one uses a criterion-referenced approach to these areas, one should look for the following factors:

▶ The theory underlying these concepts is identified.
▶ Research evidence supporting any assumptions of the test are stated.
▶ The content domain of the test that considers a comprehensive view of skills, interests, and behavior is discussed.
▶ The specific target population is operationally defined in terms of age, intelligence, education, and degree of disability.
▶ The test items are generated by selecting representative samples of behavior.
▶ Performance standards in the test are based on systematically collected data from representative samples of the target population.
▶ Test items are pilot-tested for clarity and ease of administration.
▶ Scoring methods are devised that are operationally defined.
▶ Reliability and validity data are documented.

Table 9–16. Comparison of Criterion-Referenced Tests and Norm-Referenced Tests

Criterion-Referenced Tests	Norm-Referenced Tests
• absolute standards of competence or mastery are established based on theory	• relative standards are based on normal standards
• scores are derived from standards or behaviors or competency	• scores are compared to established norms
• scores are interpreted based on what the student can or cannot do and then used diagnostically	• scores are interpreted by percentile ranks, standard scores, and organized along a normal curve
• content or items are comprehensive of domain	• content of items are a sample of domain
• cut-off score for passing is based on minimal standards of competency	• cut-off score for passing is based on pre-established percentile rank
• theoretically all can pass or all can fail	• the number of failures is predicted before test is administered

▶ A test manual for administering, scoring, and interpreting data is provided.
▶ The degree of competency in the administration of the test is included in test descriptions.

9.12 Test Publishers

The development of new tests and measuring instruments is a relatively recent event in the occupational therapy professions. The clinical nature of these fields and the service-oriented process of treatment have led to the emphasis in the past on developing new treatment techniques rather than measuring outcome variables. However, as the need for accountability and validation for treatment continue on federal and state governmental levels (e.g., through laws such as Individuals with Disabilities Education Act [IDEA] and Americans with Disabilities Act [ADA]), the use of tests and measuring instruments to justify therapeutic and educational intervention has become more important. Many tests have been developed for use by occupational therapists in the past 10 years. In addition to publishing their own tests, most test corporations distribute the most widely used tests. Thus, in general, a researcher is not limited to one corporation to obtain a specific test.

The following list includes test publishers that are frequently used by occupational therapists and other clinicians.

▶ American Occupational Therapy Association (AOTA)
  http://www.aota.org./
▶ American Guidance Service, Inc.
  http://www.agsnet.com/
▶ California Test Bureau/McGraw-Hill
  http://www.mcgraw-hill.com/
▶ Consulting Psychologists Press, Inc.
  http://www.cpp-db.com
▶ Curriculum Associates, Inc.
  http://www.curriculumassociates.com
▶ Educational Testing Service
  http://www.ets.org
▶ Educational and Industrial Testing Service (EdITS) http://www.edits.net
▶ Flaghouse Rehabilitation
  http://www.flaghouse.com
▶ Institute for Personality and Ability Testing (IPAT) http://www.ipat.com/
▶ Lafayette Instrument
  http://www.lafayetteinstrument.com
▶ MHS
  http://www.mhs.com/
▶ PAR (Psychological Assessment Resources, Inc.) http://www.parinc.com/

▶ PRO-ED
http://www.proedinc.com/index.html
▶ Riverside Publishing
http://www.riverpub.com
▶ Stoelting Corporation
http://www.stoeltingco.com/index.htm
▶ Stout Vocational Rehabilitation Institute
http://www.rtc.uwstout.edu/
text_index.html
▶ The Psychological Corporation
http://www.hbtpc.com/
▶ Trace Research and Development Center
http://trace.wisc.edu/
▶ Valpar International Corporation
http://www.valparint.com/
▶ Western Psychological Services
http://www.wpspublish.com

9.13 Ethical Considerations in Testing

"Competence in test use is a combination of knowledge of psychometric principles, knowledge of the problem situation in which the testing is to be done, technical skill and some wisdom" (Davis, 1974, p. 6). This quote is from the Standards for Educational and Psychological Tests published by the American Psychological Association. To protect psychological tests from abuse, standards fall into three areas: guidelines for devising a new psychological test, qualifications for administering tests, and the guidelines for interpreting results. The following guidelines should be adhered to in using tests:

1. The researcher publishing a new test should provide reliability, validity, normative data, scoring procedure, and qualifications for using the test in an accompanying manual.

2. A standardized test procedure should be carefully followed by the tester.
3. Results should be reported that can be compared to specified populations.
4. The researcher using psychological tests should obtain informed consent for the subject and assure the subject's confidentiality.

9.14 Conclusion

In the last 10 years, literally hundreds of tests have been developed for use with individuals with disabilities. In this chapter, the authors have presented descriptions of tests that are the most commonly used in clinical practice. These tests are available to use by occupational therapists knowledgeable in the administration, scoring, and interpretation of test results. These tests can be used as outcome or descriptive measures in clinical research. The use of a specific test is a key component in the research process and could affect the results if the test selected is not sensitive to changes in individuals or is not reliable or valid; therefore, the researcher should have knowledge of reliability and validity of the test before using it. When using a test in research, the researcher must be aware of the level of qualification needed to administer it.

Because new tests are developed frequently, the researcher should keep informed of newly published tests. Annual catalogs obtained from the test publishers listed in Section 9.12 are helpful in locating new tests. Before developing a new test, occupational therapists should search the literature, references in testing, textbooks, publishers' catalogs, and Web sites for locating new tests.

CHAPTER

Scientific Writing and Thesis Preparation

> *Vigorous writing is concise. A sentence should contain no unnecessary words, a paragraph no unnecessary sentences, for the same reason that a drawing should have no unnecessary lines and a machine no unnecessary parts. This requires not that the writer make all his sentences short, or that he avoid all detail and treat his subjects only in outline, but that every word tell.*
>
> —W. Strunk Jr. and E. B. White, 1979,
> *The Elements of Style* (p. 23)

Operational Learning Objectives

By the end of this chapter, the learner will

1. State ways to prepare for writing a research paper
2. Name the important divisions of a research paper
3. Identify and correct sexist and racist language in the research paper
4. Use *people first* language
5. Recognize reasons for revising the original draft
6. Write a bibliography using American Psychological Association (APA) format
7. Proof for errors in language mechanics and style
8. Critically evaluate his or her own writing
9. Identify the major parts of the final format
10. Design a research proposal
11. Communicate results of research study

10.1 Preparation for Writing

It is as important to prepare oneself for writing as it is to complete the review of literature and collect the data for the research project. Prior to writing the research paper, many processes that facilitate writing should be taken into consideration.

One hindrance to the completion of the writing task is the failure to actually sit down and write, but allowing frequent interruptions during the actual writing period is equally problematic. The first task in the preparation for writing is to get oneself into the proper frame of mind. This includes taking care of as many "settling activities" that might lead to interruptions. This can be likened to an animal preparing to go to sleep: The animal roughs up the bed, circles the bed a number of times, grooms, and finally settles down. Similarly, settling activities for writers include planning a large block of time, getting one's coffee or drink, assembling all the materials needed, finding a quiet and comfortable place (preferably away from a phone), arranging for child care, putting the dog or cat outside, and taking care of any needed personal toiletries. Once one has completed those tasks and is settled, writing is made easier.

Effective writing is a skill that becomes more refined as it is practiced. Clear and simple language is the hallmark of good scientific writing, and its most important quality is objective self-criticism. For some individuals, a major block to the task of writing is the initial step of organizing their ideas on paper. The desire to write as if whatever one first put on paper is chipped forever in granite sometimes prevents the flow of ideas.

The place and time in which one writes are important initial considerations. Some individuals do their best writing during the morning in a quiet, sunny room with a large table where they can spread out reference books, scrap paper, and notes filed in manila folders. Others work better in the late evening. Some individuals can work 12–14 hours for several days, followed by several days of complete rest. Some students do their best work in a college library or cafeteria, despite visual and auditory distractions. Some can write using paper and pencil, while others prefer a computer or word processor. Whatever the method and place, one must be aware of the environment that best facilitates creative writing.

Another consideration for writers is a time schedule. Some writers report that they compose in spurts of creative inspira-

tion, while others work daily whether or not they feel inspired. Setting aside enough time is important, however, so that the writer does not feel rushed or under time constraints, allowing the writer to feel that something can be accomplished. Writing a research paper or article is unlike casual writing in which an individual can use spare minutes throughout the day to complete the task. Scientific writing takes mental energy and therefore requires concentrated effort.

A third consideration consists of assembling the materials to be used before beginning any writing task. Writing materials (e.g., pens, paper, computer), note cards prepared during the literature review, statistical analyses, and other references should be available and at hand. Just as one would not consider doing therapy without having all the tools and equipment available, one cannot expect to write adequately without having the proper tools and materials.

Writing a book, journal article, or thesis requires self-discipline. In a way, the individual should prepare for writing much as an athlete trains for a sporting event. A period of "conditioning" and mental rigor prior to writing is important. Some individuals take long walks, ride bicycles for miles, climb mountains, or take part in physical sports in preparation for writing. Others prepare mentally by playing chess, doing crossword puzzles, solving arithmetic problems, reading prolifically, or doing intricate manual work. Sleeping on an idea or letting it brew beneath the surface for a while also may be helpful. After the first draft, there will be ample time for revision, which in most cases will involve excision. For the author or research investigator, the completed document is analogous to giving birth. Writing is a continuous process with much editing and revision, but one should be careful not to abandon the initial efforts prematurely.

In Chapter 5, we talked about choosing a research topic. We stated that although the research topic must be meaningful to the researcher, the implications of the findings should lead to changes in the way the disability is viewed. These implications may affect evaluation or treatment of the disability or result in changes in administrative or educational practices. The purpose of the research paper includes an explanation of why the question was formulated and how the research methodology serves to answer the question. In the final project, that is, the research paper, the writer summarizes the literature, discusses the findings, and makes specific recommendations based on these findings. In this way, the final scientific paper becomes a part of the body of literature, placing the research findings within the context of previous works (Locke, Spirduso, & Silverman, 1997).

A well-conceived research paper requires active contemplation by the writer. The conceptual relationships between previous research and present findings must be considered. The hypothesis or guiding question(s) proposed by the researcher must be concisely and clearly stated and should cover all the points covered in the paper (Slade, Campbell, & Ballou, 1997). The summary and arguments used in the paper to advance one's theory must be compared with viewpoints held by established researchers. On the other hand, a researcher may present findings that are contradictory to accepted beliefs in the scientific community. Under attack, the researcher must be able to defend the validity of the research findings. For example, in spite of common belief that dyslexia is a result of visual-perceptual deficits, such as seeing and writing letters backwards, researchers such as Liberman (1973) and Kamhi and Catts (1998) have espoused the underlying deficit in dyslexia to be language related.

Another essential component for writing a research paper is to understand the literature encompassing the topic as fully as possible. This is accomplished by completing an exhaustive literature review as described in Chapter 6. The researcher will discover quickly, however, that much more literature has been reviewed than will be discussed in the paper. This fact does not

minimize the need for an extensive literature review; rather, it emphasizes the need for the researcher to understand and master the relationship of a specific literature within the context of a body of knowledge. For example, a cogent understanding of the methods used to teach students with dyslexia to read requires an examination of landmark studies directly related to the identification and diagnosis of this disability. It is not uncommon to revise the initial hypothesis or guiding question several times as one's knowledge base increases through reading and reviewing the literature.

Writing and reviewing literature is like an organic process that helps researchers to modify their thinking while extending their knowledge base. It is a creative process that allows one to be objective and self-critical. This process is sometimes referred to as cognitive dissonance (the state in which there is conflict between one's attitudes and one's behavior, generally resulting in changing one's thinking so that there is equilibrium between the two), reflective decision making (the process of making decisions by critically examining all sides of the issue), or the Socratic method of learning. All these methods rely on the individual's ability to question and rethink a body of knowledge.

10.2 Outlining the Research Study

The overall organization of the research study, outlined in Table 10–1, is dictated by tradition. Each of the major sections within the research paper contains specific issues and topics.

10.2.1 Introduction to the Research Paper

The first part of the research paper contains a brief introduction to the present study, including the purpose, the research or guiding question(s), and the significance when

Table 10–1. Major Parts of a Research Paper

I. Introduction to the Research Paper
  A. Statement of the Research Problem or Guiding Question
  B. Significance of the Research Problem
  C. Purposes of the Study
  D. Specific Definitions or Terms

II. Review of the Literature
  A. Major Studies
  B. Critical Analysis of Key Studies

III. Methodology
  A. Research Design
    1. Subjects (Number, Demographic Data)
    2. Procedures (Tests, Collection of Data)
    3. Statistical Analyses

IV. Results
  A. Presentation and Analysis of Data
  B. Relevant Tables and Figures

V. Discussion, Summary, Conclusions, and Implications of the Findings
  A. Limitations of the Study
  B. Significance of Study Related to Prior Research
  C. Future Research

VI. Reference List and Appendices

VII. Abstract (Placed after the Title Page)

examined beside findings from landmark studies (Best & Kahn, 1997). A pivotal part of this portion of the research paper, article, or manuscript is a clear statement of the hypotheses or guiding questions such that they are (a) well understood, (b) lead the reader to anticipate the major sections of the paper, and (c) indicate the direction or argument in which the paper will be written (Winkler & McCuen, 1998). Finally, this part of the research paper should include definitions for any terminology that are uncommon or might not be understood by the reader (Best & Kahn).

10.2.2 Review of the Literature

The second part of the research paper, which contains the literature review, is to some extent a measure of what the student knows about the subject (Best & Kahn,

1997; Krathwohl, 1988). In some papers, this section and the previous section are written as a single part. In a thesis or dissertation, this section is traditionally identified as Chapter 2 or, if written with the introduction, as Chapter 1.

The purpose of this section is to introduce further the reason for the study by reviewing previous research in the same area and by building a background for the study. Although it is not necessary to cite or review every article or book in the subject, as the researcher must presume that the reader has some knowledge in this area, the major studies must be discussed (American Psychological Association, 1994). For example, a student is interested in learning more about the relationship between cerebral damage and spasticity. In a preliminary literature review, the student will have read or identified many articles on the etiology and prognosis of a motor dysfunction plus some clinical descriptions of cerebral damage. A more in-depth review will yield studies regarding the relationship between specific types of cerebral damage as it relates to a motor dysfunction. A final review will examine those articles related to cerebral damage and spasticity. Although all these articles may be important, only the articles related directly to the research question will be discussed at length.

One way to outline this portion of the research paper is to organize the articles reviewed (described in Chapter 6). If the researcher used note cards, organization becomes a logical task of putting the note cards in the order in which they will be discussed. The selection of appropriate articles will be based both on the findings and on the relationship of the article to the research question. Some note cards will be put aside, because the articles will not be linked directly to the research question. Others will be mentioned only briefly as a means of presenting a background underlying the rationale behind the research question. Some articles will be especially important to build a strong argument for the research design, and a critical analysis of these articles will be an integral part of the literature review. Research literature and theory need to be reviewed and discussed objectively, citing both positive and negative research findings that relate to the present research question. In this way, one can avoid researcher bias, as shown in the following example from literature on treating depression.

A student is interested in the relationship between depression and use of cognitive-behavioral therapy. A review of literature identifies the following categories of studies involving the use of cognitive-behavioral therapy to treat individuals with depression: (a) those in which there was no improvement (e.g., Jacobson et al., 1996), (b) those in which there was improvement (e.g., Clarke, Rohde, Lewinsohn, Hops, & Seeley, 1999), and (c) those in which there was mixed success (e.g., Shapiro et al., 1996). Each of these articles should be critically analyzed and critiqued, with special attention given to the methodology used in the studies and the relationship of the findings to the present research question. The student should present studies in which both favorable and unfavorable results were found. In doing this, the student demonstrates objectivity in reviewing the literature and avoids research bias.

Once the note cards have been placed in a logical order, a formal outline should be written. There are many ways to write an outline. Some people prefer to use phrases or single words, while others prefer to use sentences for each level. Occasionally, a student may find it easier to jot down a paragraph describing and expanding on the topic. This paragraph becomes the outer edifice of the particular section. Regardless of the method that one chooses when organizing the topics, the outline facilitates the organization of the literature review.

An effective way to organize the outline and make it functional is to use parallel or grammatical structure. For example, a list written as:

a. planning a therapy session
b. obtaining materials
c. positioning the student

is easier to comprehend than one written as:

a. plan the therapy session
b. obtaining materials
c. to position the student

Use of parallel or grammatical structures in an outline is effective in clarifying one's writing. (Refer to the Section 10.6 [Format of a Paper] for further discussion regarding parallel construction.)

10.2.3 Methodology

The third section of the research paper includes a discussion of the methodology used in the study. This portion of the research paper should be written in a concise and succinct manner, with enough information available so that others can replicate the study.

Traditionally, there are three subdivisions in the methodology section: (a) subjects, (b) the apparatus or tests, and (c) the procedures used for data collection and analysis. Demographic information, such as the number of subjects, ages, gender, and ethnicity, is critical. Other additional demographic information that may be essential for the study might include education level, socioeconomic level, handedness, disabilities, prior testing, and previous need for therapies, especially occupational therapy. If a control group is used, the demographics of the control group must be contrasted with the experimental group. The manner in which subjects were chosen (e.g., stratified random sample, voluntary response to a newspaper ad) is also described in this section.

A description of the tests or apparatus includes the names of the tests or surveys used, any laboratory equipment needed, and any specific directions or adaptations to the test or procedure that might not be found in a test manual. For example, if only part of a perceptual motor test is used, one must name the subtests chosen and justify the modification. When a standardized test is used, the reliability and validity of the test (or test portions) used must be indicated. If a survey or questionnaire has been developed for the study, a copy is put into the appendix following the major divisions of the paper.

Finally, the researcher describes the methods of data collection and the statistical procedures used to analyze it (Best & Kahn, 1997). For example, did the researcher collect data alone, in person, or by telephone? Were others trained to collect the data? If a questionnaire was used, was it mailed or left in a public place for people to fill out as desired? Was a second letter sent as a follow-up? How long did data collection occur? Was it collected in one or two sessions? Was it collected by outcome measures (pre- and posttesting)? What types of statistical procedures were used to analyze the data?

10.2.4 Results

The fourth section of the research paper presents the results and statistical findings from the study without attempting to interpret them. Each hypothesis is discussed separately, with statistical interactions and main effects reported. Tables and figures depicting significant relationships between variables often make the text more understandable; however, they should be self-explanatory and add to the information in the text rather than add new information.

10.2.5 Summary, Discussion, and Implications of the Findings

In the final section, the writer summarizes the findings and attempts to interpret them in the context of previous studies in the same field. Conclusions regarding acceptance or rejection of hypotheses are stated in this section. Although statements of generalization can be made here, one must be careful not to overgeneralize or overstate the significance of the findings. The writer should be aware of the limitations of the study and state them, expressing any

cautions regarding generalization to populations not included in the sample. Implications for further research, present practice, or policy changes are advanced, along with the arguments for these changes. The internal and external validity of the study should be discussed.

According to Best and Kahn (1997), the discussion section of the research paper is the most difficult part to write. Inexperienced authors tend to over- or undergeneralize, thinking their results less or more important than the data would support (Winkler & McCuen, 1998). The discussion section should be a critical and analytical summary of the findings, rather than a superficial overview of the results. Because this part of the research paper is the most frequently read (Best & Kahn, 1997), it is crucial that the researchers summarize the results and critically review these findings in the context of prior studies. The usefulness of the research paper, despite the findings, can be determined by the way in which the discussion section is written.

10.2.6 Reference List and Appendices

In the last section of the research paper, the writer needs to list all of the cited references. The writer must be careful not to leave out any reference, to include all information in the citation, and to check for accuracy and correct spelling of information. There is nothing more frustrating than an incomplete or inaccurate citation when one wishes to obtain further information from the original article. (Refer to Section 10.5 [Bibliography] for further information.)

Sometimes a writer wishes to place a bibliography and a reference list into the research paper. A bibliography contains any article, book, or chapter that might be helpful in understanding the topic. A reference list, on the other hand, includes journal articles, books, or other sources used in the research and preparation of the paper and cited within the article (American Psychological Association, 1994). Any additional information (e.g., copy of the survey or test protocol, drawing of specific apparatus) can be placed in an appendix following the list of references.

10.2.7 Abstract

The abstract of a research study, which is written last and then placed at the beginning of the study, contains summary statements of each independent unit or section (i.e., the problem, literature review, research design, methodology, results, discussion, and conclusions). The abstract should contain enough information so that the reader will know the purposes of the study, the specific variables or groups investigated, the number of subjects, the measuring instruments used, the results, and the conclusions presented. An abstract of a research study is usually limited to between 150 and 300 words. When preparing an abstract, it is useful to extract key sentences from each part of the study and then integrate the sentences through transitional phrases. Abstracts are extremely important to investigators reviewing literature; therefore, it is vital to present as complete a summary of the total study as possible within the number of words permitted. Abstracts are not merely a summary or discussion of the results as perceived by some investigators. An abstract should be a complete statement representative of the total study. Whenever possible, key words or phrases should be identified by the author and placed below the abstract. These key words are used in data retrieval systems (see Chapter 6).

10.3 Writing the First Draft

Writers begin the first draft after completing the outline. As stated above, the outline aids in organizing the literature review, but the outline is not set in stone. After the first draft has been written, the organization may need to be revised. Nonetheless, having an outline allows the writer to have a

sense of the direction in which the paper is going.

Perhaps the hardest part of writing is putting initial thoughts on paper. Writers should compose these initial thoughts with the expectation of revising them later. There will be plenty of time for revision after the first draft has been written and writers should expect to revise their first work a number of times.

A difficult skill for inexperienced writers is the ability to use notes effectively. There is a tendency to quote extensively rather than paraphrase the author's words. Frequently, this is caused by a lack of understanding about what the author meant. If this is the case, researchers must do additional reading and studying until they completely understand the material. Although quotes from the original source can be an effective means of relating information, too many quotations make the research paper difficult to read and leave "the impression that students have done [no more than] 'cut and paste' from books and articles they have read" (Winkler & McCuen, 1979, p. 114). It is better to use quotations sparingly, intermixing the quotations with summaries and paraphrases of the original sources. When quoting or paraphrasing, one must document the source (see section on quotations).

The literary and scientific styles used for citations often are determined by a particular discipline. The four most commonly used systems are *The Chicago Manual of Style* (Turabian, 1996), the *Modern Language Association* (MLA; Gibaldi & Franklin, 1999), the *American Medical Association Manual of Style* (Iverson, 1997), and the *Publication Manual of the American Psychological Association* (APA, 1994). The latter style is used most frequently in psychology, education, and social and health sciences and will be discussed in this book.

The essential reference book for APA style is the fourth edition of the *Publication Manual of the American Psychological Association* (1994), generally available in university or college bookstores. If the university or local technical bookstore does not have one, it can be obtained from the American Psychological Association in Washington, D.C. Because of the extensiveness of the APA style, one will need to refer to this manual frequently. It is wise to get into the habit of referring to the APA Manual whenever there is a question about style, language mechanics, or format of the paper. Major highlights of the APA Manual will be discussed in the following sections of this chapter; however, because of space limitations, not all topics will be covered in detail.

10.4 Making Revisions

Once the research paper has been written, revisions will be necessary. Revising the research paper five or six times is not uncommon. Each time the writer reviews the research paper for accuracy and cohesiveness, he or she may discover additional ways for revision or clarity.

The function of revision is to make sure that specific editing requirements have been followed. These editing requirements are summarized in Table 10–2.

10.4.1 Gender or Ethnic Bias

First, the writer will want to make sure that no gender or ethnic bias has been introduced into the paper or into the study. Guidelines have been established by the APA for avoiding sexist and ethnic language in journal articles. Gender bias occurs when the writer uses the term *man* to mean the human race rather than using a less ambiguous term such as *person, people,* or *individual.* Additionally, use of specific gender words (e.g., his, her) or using terms that end in *man* or *men* (e.g., *postman, chairman, policemen*) must be avoided. Stereotyping (e.g., the psychologist . . . he; mothering) can be avoided by using specific language (e.g., boys enjoyed playing with Legos while girls enjoyed reading), by using parallel language (e.g., *men and women* rather than *men and girls*), or by

Table 10–2. Checklist for Proofing One's Article

1. Gender and Ethnic Bias
- Is the article free of language that might be ambiguous or stereotypical?

2. People First
- Is the manuscript written with the individual emphasized rather than the disability?
- Have all references to a disability been written in the form *individual with…*?

3. Grammar
- Are there run-on sentences or sentence fragments?
- Are there split infinitives, dangling modifiers, errors in verb-subject agreement?
- Is the writing in parallel structure?
- Are relative pronouns used appropriately?
- Has a grammar program been used to check the languge?

4. Spelling/Punctuation
- Has a spell check been used to check spelling?
- Has the article been reviewed for commas, quotation marks, hyphens, and apostrophes?

5. Abbreviations
- Is the abbreviation placed in parentheses following the full term the first time it is used?
- Are the Latin abbreviations used correctly and according to APA style?
- Are abbreviations invented by the author kept to a minimum?

6. Transitional Words, Phrases, and Sentences
- Are there transitional statements or words between ideas?
- Is there a sense of unity and integration in the paper?
- Do words such as "however," "although," or "nevertheless" need to be added?

7. Clarity
- Is the language clear and simple?
- Do any unusual terms need to be explained or defined?
- Would a figure or table help explain the information?

8. Organization
- Do the hypotheses or guiding question(s) drive the content of the research paper?
- Is there consistency between sections?
- Are unnecessary repetitions removed?
- Is the sequence of the research paper logical and coherent?

changing the term to a plural (e.g., *their* instead of *his* or *her*) (American Psychological Association, 1994).

Ethnic bias occurs when the writer attributes to a specific ethnic group something that has no supporting data (American Psychological Association, 1994). An example of this stereotyping occurs when someone writes "In general, all individuals with traumatic brain injury tend to have psychosocial difficulties." APA suggests that an informal test can be completed by substituting another group (e.g., your own) for the group being discussed. If the writer perceives offense in the revised statement, then bias is probably present.

10.4.2 *People First* Language

A *second reason* for revision is to make sure that the writing is in *People First* language. Because of the Individuals with Disabilities Education Act (1990), all references to disabilities must be written with the individual placed first. Thus, *child with autism* is correct, while the *autistic child* is incorrect. This convention emphasizes the value of the human being and delegates the disability to secondary importance.

The writer must distinguish also between the terms *handicap* and *disability*. A handicap can be thought of as a disadvantage imposed on an individual by the environment or by another person, whereas a disability is something that an individual is unable to do, a lack of a body part, or physical or psychosocial impairment. For example, an individual with a spinal cord injury may not be able to walk; the inability to walk is a disability. However, this disability becomes a handicap if there is no wheelchair access, or if the individual refuses to use a wheelchair. The presence of a disability does not make an individual handicapped.

10.4.3 Mechanics of Writing

Clear writing requires use of a formal writing style and using grammatically correct language. A *third reason* to revise the manuscript is to make sure that there are no grammatical errors. Errors such as subject-verb agreement (e.g., using *data is* rather than *data are*), punctuation and capitalization, run-on sentences, and sentence fragments are common for inexperienced writers. Run-on sentences and sentence fragments are an indication that either the writer is careless and has not proofread the research paper or that the writer needs help with writing skills. Other common errors include (a) failing to use parallel structure for grammatical units (e.g., using different parts of speech in a series or in connecting phrases), (b) having dangling modifiers (e.g., sentences in which the modifier is misplaced, such as "it is however believed," rather than "However, it is believed"), (c) splitting infinitives (e.g., "to swiftly complete the task" rather than "to complete the task swiftly"), (d) improperly using relative pronouns (e.g., "an individual must keep their head" rather than, "an individual must keep his head"), (e) using the passive tense rather than the active tense (e.g., "There were seven subjects" instead of "Seven subjects"), and (f) placing prepositions at the end of sentences ("ethical and legal obligations that occupational therapists are faced with" rather than "ethical and legal obligations that occupational therapists face"). If one is unsure about the proper grammatical structure, a basic grammar book is indispensable. Additional examples of these errors, as well as the correct usages are illustrated in Figure 10–1.

Following are many excellent references available to help writers avoid grammatical errors and improve their writing. Major references and computer software programs that are available to check spelling and grammar are listed also.

▶ Strunk, W., Jr., & White, E. B. (1999). *The elements of style* (4th ed.). Boston: Allyn & Bacon.
 A gold mine of writing ideas, including *rules of usage, principles of composition form, and writing style. The epitome of concise, effective writing.
▶ American Psychological Association (1994). *Publication manual of the American*

Type	Rules	Incorrect Example	Correct Usage
DANGLING OR MISPLACED MODIFIER OR PARTICIPLE	Modifiers and participles should be put as close as possible to the word they are to modify to prevent ambiguity or missing referents.	. . . would first determine. . . . . . local issues in that particular clinic that affect job satisfaction	. . . would determine first. . . . . . . local issues that affect job satisfaction in that particular clinic
SPLIT INFINITIVES	Place adverbs that modify the verb after the phase "to . . ." rather than between the "to" and the verb.	Occupational therapists need to carefully observe behaviors . . .	Occupational therapists need to observe carefully behaviors . . .
PARALLEL STRUCTURE	Expressions similar in function or content should be in the same grammatical construction.	(a) identification and clarification of . . . (b) assessing to . . . (c) determine whether . . .	(a) identification and clarification of . . . (b) assessment of . . . (c) determination of . . .
RELATIVE PRONOUNS	Use *that* with a restrictive clause (i.e., is essential to the passage).		The chimps that participated in the study were all kept unrestrained in an open testing area.
	Use *which* with an unrestrictive clause surrounded by commas (adds information, but is not essential to the sentence).		The glasses, which were on top of the container, belonged to the patient.

Figure 10–1. Common errors of writing style,

Type	Rules	Incorrect Example	Correct Usage
VOICE (ACTIVE/PASSIVE)	Use *who* in unrestrictive clauses in reference to people.		The students, who all had attention deficit disorder, won ribbons at the races.
	Use the active voice whenever possible.	The information examined by the authors' . . .	The authors examined . . .
POSSESSIVES	Place an apostrophe after the noun or pronoun to show possession. **Exception**: do not use an apostrophe after the word **it** when showing possession.	The subjects score . . .	The subject's score was . . .
		It's major strengths are . . .	The Wechsler has 12 subtests. Its first score is . . .
			But: It's cold (It is cold)
SERIATION	Place elements in a series in parallel form. (See Figure 10–2 for correct punctuation.)	. . . asked to read the directions, fill out the information, and then to turn in the form.	. . . to read the directions, fill out the information, and turn in the form.
	When the series of items is written in one sentence, use letters in parenthesis to separate each item. Use commas to separate the items, unless there are internal commas. Use semicolons to separate items of major categories.	The subjects were administered four tests: clinical observations, Stress Management Questionnaire, Crawford Small Parts Dexterity Test, and Strong Vocational Interest Test.	The subjects were administered four tests: (a) clinical observations, (b) Stress Management Questionnaire, (c) Crawford Small Parts Dexterity Test, and (d) Strong Vocational Interest Test.

Figure 10–1. (continued)

Type	Rules	Incorrect Example	Correct Usage
SERIATION (CON'T)	When each item in the series is placed into separate sentences or separate paragraphs, use numbers to separate the items.		The subjects were administered 3 outcome measures: 1. Stress Management Questionnaire to examine coping skills, 2. Crawford Small Parts Dexterity Test to assess dexterity, and 3. Strong Vocational Interest Test to determine interests.
PRONOUNS	Make sure that the referent for the pronoun is clear.	This was completed. Those were put over there.	This self-report scale was completed. Those books were put over there, on the bottom shelf.
	Make sure that the pronoun agrees in number with the noun it replaces and/or modifies the noun	His chart was placed in their folder. The group took their packages . . .	His chart was placed in his folder. The group took its packages . . .
SUBJECT-VERB AGREEMENT	Verbs must agree with the subject, regardless of intervening phrases and/or use of pronouns.	Data is; phenomena is The articles that were taken from a single journal was . . .	Data are; phenomena are The articles that were taken from a single journal were . . .
MISPLACED PREPOSITIONS	Prepositions should not be placed at the end of the sentences.	. . . the next area the clinicians were questioned in	. . . the next area in which the clinicians were questioned.

Figure 10–1. *(continued)*

Psychological Association (4th ed.). Washington, DC: Author.

An exhaustive guide to organizing a journal article for publication. Includes content areas such as headings, quotations, references, tables, figures and graphs, and other matters of style that can keep a writer up all night.

▶ Turabian, K. L. (1996). *A manual for writers of term papers, theses, and dissertations* (6th ed., Rev., ed. by J. Grossman & A. Bennett). Chicago: University of Chicago Press.

If the APA style manual is confusing on a question of style, Turabian is the final word.

▶ Slade, C., Campbell, W. G., & Ballou, S. V. (1997). *Form and style: Research papers, reports, theses* (10th ed.). Boston: Houghton Mifflin.

A well-written, up-to-date, guide for writing research papers. Focuses on the processes of writing and gives detailed coverage of *The Chicago Manual of Style*, Modern Language Association, and American Psychological Association styles. This text is helpful for the inexperienced writer, because there are many examples in the text.

▶ *Roget's International Thesaurus* (1993). New York: HarperCollins

An invaluable guide to the writer for selecting the most appropriate word. It is helpful both in locating a specific word and in varying one's language.

▶ Thomas, C. L. (Ed.). (1997). *Taber's cyclopedic medical dictionary* (18th ed.). Philadelphia: F. A. Davis. An essential guide for those researchers needing medical terms defined and clarified.

▶ Li, X., & Crane, N. B. (1996). *Electronic styles: A handbook for citing electronic information* (Rev. ed.). Medford, NJ: Information Today.

▶ *Merriam-Webster's Collegiate Dictionary* (10th ed.). (1993). Springfield, MA: Merriam-Webster.

▶ Weiss-Lambrou, R. (1989). *The health professional's guide to writing for publication.* Springfield, IL: Charles C. Thomas.

▶ The following Web site has information for citing electronic information in APA and MLD: http://www.uvm.edu/~ncrane/estyles/

A *fourth reason* for revision is to check for spelling and punctuation errors. It is critical to check one's spelling with a spell checker (available with most word-processing programs) to ensure that there are no errors. One must be careful, however, to read the article and proof for errors, rather than relying on the computerized speller to find all the errors. It cannot find errors when the words are spelled correctly but misused. For example, if the words *to* and *too* are used incorrectly, the speller will not identify the errors.

Punctuation errors must be found and corrected. Figure 10–2, adapted from the APA Manual (1994) and Slade, Campbell, and Ballou (1997), summarizes common punctuation rules. Reading the paper aloud is one method to revise the paper and find errors in punctuation and grammar.

In scientific articles, it is common practice to abbreviate terms used repeatedly (e.g., proprioceptive facilitation as [PF], neurodevelopmental therapy as [NDT], learning disability as [LD], perceptual-motor training as [PMT], and quality food index as [QFI]). Abbreviations invented by the writer should be kept to a minimum and used only for terms that are long and frequently repeated. Tables of statistical data containing abbreviations should contain a footnote defining the abbreviations.

Latin abbreviations are useful for shortening sentences. The following are the most commonly used abbreviations in scientific articles:

▶ ca. (circa): about a certain time, e.g., ca. BC 130
▶ e.g. (exempli grata): for example
▶ et al. (et alii): and others
▶ et seq. (et sequens): and the following
▶ ibid. (ibidem): in the same place

Type		Rule	Example
COMMA	**Seriation**	Use a comma after each word in a series of three or more items.	. . . equipment, apparatus, and tools. . .
	Parenthetical expression	Use a comma before and after a phrase that adds information but is not essential.	Collaboration can be an informal process, where two individuals meet to discuss a problem, or. . .
	Independent clause	Use a comma to separate independent clauses, but do not use to separate the two parts of a compound predicate.	Five of the participants were Black, and seven of the subjects were Anglo. (But notice: Six students were in seventh grade and were taking history.)
	Essential or restrictive clauses	Do not use a comma when the modifying phrase is used to identify, limit, or define a word and is essential to the meaning.	The subjects that were used for the control group included seven occupational therapists.
	Dependent clauses	Use a comma rather than a semicolon to separate a dependent and independent phrase.	Although the participants with developmental disabilities were separated from the rest of the participants, all the subjects were placed into a single group for evaluation.
SEMICOLON	**Independent clauses**	Use a semicolon when the independent clauses are not separated by a coordinating conjunction or when the clauses are separated by a conjunctive adverb.	The apparatus was put on the shelves; the writing materials were put into the desk. The client was interviewed . . ; however, . . .
	Seriation	Use a semicolon when there is a comma contained in any part of the seriation.	. . .: (a) red box, which contained 3 balls; (b) blue box, which contained 2 balls; and (c) yellow box, which contained 6 balls.
COLON	**References**	Use a colon after the place of publication and before the publisher	Boston, NY: Allyn and Bacon.
	Phrases	Use a colon before a phrase or example of explanatory material with an introductory phrase. If the example is a complete sentence, start it with a capital letter.	The recorded scores were in the following order: 37, 49, 24, 70. The material was made up of the following parts: Two blue boxes each contained 4 toys.

Figure 10–2. Common errors of punctuation. Adapted from the *Publication Manual of the American Psychological Association* (1994) and Slade, Campbell, & Ballou (1994).

Type		Rule	Example
QUOTATION MARKS	**Direct quotation**	Put quotation marks around any direct quote of 40 words or fewer. If the direct quote is more than 40 words, offset it in a paragraph, and indent on both right and left margins. Cite the reference with the author, date, and page or just the page in parentheses following the quote.	Locke, Spirduso, and Silverman (1987) caution that "[t]he problem in writing a proposal is essentially the same as in writing the final report" (p. 19). "The problem in writing a proposal is essentially the same as in writing the final report" (Locke, Spirduso, & Silverman, 1987, p. 19).
	Titles	Put quotation marks around any title of a chapter or article cited in the text. Do not put around any title in the reference list.	John's review discussed Chapter 2, "The Scientific Method."

	Terms	Use quotation marks when introducing a word or phrase used as slang, irony, or invented term. Do not use quotation marks when the word or phrase is used a second time. Do not use quotations (or italics) with commonly used foreign terms.	Ninja coined the term "normalization" . . .
			
			But:
			    per se
			    vis a vis

PARENTHESES	**Parenthetical information**	Use parentheses to set off material that is independent of the rest of the information. Put punctuation marks inside the parentheses if the material is a sentence and outside the parentheses if the material is a phrase.	The subjects (15 boys and 2 girls) were . . .
	References	Enclose citations with parentheses.	(Jones & Smith, 1994); Jones and Smith (1994)
	Abbreviations	Abbreviations should be put in parentheses the first time the full term is used. Thereafter, the abbreviation can be used instead of the full term.	Sensory integration therapy (SI). . . . . . .SI
	Seriation	Enclose the letters used in seriation in parentheses.	(a) . . ., (b) . . ., and (c) . . .
BRACKETS	**Parenthetical material**	Enclose parenthetical material that is within parentheses in brackets unless the use of commas will not confuse the reader.	(*Miller Assessment for Preschoolers* [MAP, 1988]) (Jones and Smith, 1990) denied this allegation.
	References	Enclose material inserted into a quotation with brackets.	". . .[the participants in the study] were asked to come . . ."

Figure 10–2. *(continued)*

► i.e. (id est): that is to say
► viz. (videlicet): namely, used to introduce lists.

Be sure to refer to the APA manual for the proper way to use abbreviations. For example, many abbreviations, (including *i.e.,* and, *e.g.*) must be used only within parentheses.

10.4.4 Transitional Words, Phrases, and Sentences

A *fifth reason* for revision is to make sure that transitional statements are present so that the flow of ideas is smooth. Writing a well-organized, integrated manuscript requires the use of words and phrases that connect ideas and summarize a section of a paper. In reviewing scientific literature, it is important to integrate the studies under topical areas and to develop a logical sequence. Writing should be coherent. The use of transitional words such as *however, although,* or *nevertheless,* can be used to make the transition smoother and the paper unified. (Note that many style guides frown on beginning a sentence with *however.*) In addition, sentences can be used to permit the smooth transition from one idea to another. The reader should have no difficulty following the train of thought or the arguments used to build a case. Additionally, reading the research paper as a whole will uncover any inconsistencies or repetitions between sections (Slade, Campbell, & Ballou, 1997). Often, having someone unacquainted with the topic read the work serves to ensure clarity, understanding, and consistency.

10.4.5 Clarity of Thought

The scientific writer should try to communicate ideas simply and rigorously. Some of the most profound ideas can be expressed in clear, direct language. It is not a sign of intellectual prowess to present ideas so that they are difficult to understand. Therefore, a *sixth reason* for revision is to ensure that the paper is written clearly. Scientific writing is particularly prone to abstruseness and ambiguity, especially in clinical areas where language is used loosely without precise operational definitions. One method of ensuring clarity is to include a conceptual or operational definition for unusual terms or for terms specific to a certain discipline. Even if the writer chooses not to create a glossary, uncommon terms must be defined operationally. Use of well-thought out charts, tables, or figures can facilitate the clarity of the research paper. It is not unusual for readers to look at charts, tables, or figures before reading the text, especially when these visual aids provide an overall summary of the principle finding.

10.4.6 Organization

Finally, the author should examine whether the background information is represented accurately, whether ideas unrelated to the topic have been introduced, and whether the hypothesis or guiding statement(s) have directed the writing (Slade, Campbell, & Ballou, 1997). Each statement of results should be supported by data. Differences or contradictions in findings compared with previous studies need to be discussed and, when possible, explained. The whole research paper should be reviewed for sequence of ideas. Eventually, even though additional changes are possible, the writer must accept the paper as it is.

> [T]he secret of good writing is to strip every sentence to its cleanest components. Every word that serves no function, every long word that could be a short word, every adverb which carries the same meaning that is already in the verb, every passive construction that leaves the reader unsure of who is doing what—these are the thousand and one adulterants that weaken the strength of a sentence. (Zinsser, 1990, pp. 7–8)

10.5 Quotations, Referenced Material, and Bibliographic Citations

Whenever one uses material written by another person, whether the material is directly quoted or only paraphrased, one must make reference to the original author(s). Failure to do so is plagiarism. Some authors (Winkler & McCuen, 1998) have suggested that plagiarism is common in everyday language. One might use in speech an example stated in a lecture by a professor and fail to give that professor the credit, for example. In another case one may use a proverb such as "A stitch in time saves nine" and fail to give Benjamin Franklin the credit. Although these examples are not routinely considered plagiarism and are generally acceptable in everyday speech, plagiarism is not accepted in a research or scholarly paper.

Plagiarism occurs when a researcher deliberately takes another person's ideas and incorporates them into his or her own writing without giving any credit to the original author. Examples of plagiarism include the following: (a) taking another's research ideas and submitting them as one's own, (b) paraphrasing an article without giving credit to the author, or (c) directly copying part of an article without citing the authors. Any copyright material used without giving credit to the original author is considered plagiarism (Winkler & McCuen, 1998).

If the material used is a direct quote from another author or authors, the writer must cite the author(s), year of publication, and page number of the quotation in the text. There must be no change in spelling, phrasing, capitalization, or punctuation from the original. The exception to this rule is when the first word of a quotation needs to be capitalized or placed in lower case to make the statement grammatically correct. When it is necessary to make changes (e.g., when a pronoun must be clarified or a word added to make the content more understandable), the change must be put in square brackets ([ ]). When a word is misspelled or the grammar is incorrect in the original, [*sic*] follows the misspelling or grammatical error to show that the quotation is reproduced exactly. For example, "The article was written by an england [*sic*] author."

A quote can be introduced as part of a grammatical sentence, or it may stand alone as a sentence. When material is omitted from the quotation, then an ellipsis (...) replaces the material that is left out. When the quote is more than 40 words, it should stand alone as a separate paragraph. In this case, the quoted material is punctuated, and the reference for the quoted material is placed after the paragraph, in parenthesis and with no punctuation. Examine the following:

> Slang, hackneyed or flippant phrases, and folksy style should be avoided. Since objectivity is the primary goal, there should be no element of exhortation or persuasion. The research report should describe and explain, rather than try to convince or move to action. In this respect, the research report differs from the essay or the feature article. (Best, 1977, p. 317)

When the material has fewer than 40 words, it is placed within the paragraph. The reference is placed in parentheses at the end of the quote. For example: According to Best (1977), "The research report should be presented in a style that is creative, clear, and concise" (p. 317).

When the writer wishes to paraphrase another author's material, then the writer must cite the author(s) and date of publication. Examine the following two examples:

1. Best & Kahn (1997) suggested that when writing a research article, one must be careful to write concisely and clearly.

> **2.** When writing a research article, one must be careful to write concisely and clearly (Best & Kahn, 1997; Winkler & McCuen, 1998).

Notice that no page numbers are used in either reference and that the author's name is put within parentheses at the end of the sentence if it has not been used as part of the sentence structure. Additional information regarding common citations of authors in the text is summarized in Figure 10–3.

Whether the writer has quoted the source directly or paraphrased the material, a complete reference must be placed in the reference list at the end of the research paper. Figure 10–4 summarizes the different styles for common reference citations, and Table 10–3 shows some examples of these citations. Further information regarding the appropriate style for dissertations, secondary sources, movies, or films can be found in the APA manual. Regardless of the type of publication, all citations must include enough information so that the reader can locate the original source.

10.6 Format of a Paper

The format of the research paper is dictated by the style of writing used. For journal publications using the APA style, the size of the margins, line spacing, and size of print are specified. Individual professors and non-APA style journals may have different requirements. In a thesis or dissertation, additional sections are required. A typical organization of the sequence for a thesis or dissertation is listed below.

1. Title page (see Figure 10–5)
2. Approval page indicating names and titles of thesis readers (required for a thesis or dissertation only)
3. Acknowledgments, including individuals who aided in the study and any grant support accepted
4. Table of contents, including chapter and section headings, appendix, and bibliography
5. List of statistical tables
6. List of illustrations, photographs, and figures
7. Abstract
8. The content of the text
   a. Introduction
   b. Review of the literature
   c. Methodology
   d. Results
   e. Discussion, including clinical implications of findings and limitations of study
   f. Conclusions and further research
9. Bibliography and references
10. Appendix
11. Vita, listing professional education, work history, and previous publications

A running title, consisting of three or four words, is placed in the upper right hand corner of each page. APA style dictates the position of page numbers (usually below the running title), the use of roman and arabic numbers, the type of paper, the levels of headings, spacing, and use of quotations.

10.6.1 Outline of a Research Proposal

1. Title of study
2. Investigator
3. Date
4. The research problem
   a. statement of problem in question form
   b. justification and need for the study
   c. implications of anticipated results in relation to clinical treatment, professional, education, or administrative problems
5. The literature review

	FIRST CITATION	ADDITIONAL CITATIONS IN THE TEXT
ONE AUTHOR	Last name, year, page (when applicable) Smith (1994) . . . (p. 94); (Smith, 1994, p. 94)	Last name, year, page, (when applicable) Smith (1994) or (Smith, 1994)
TWO AUTHORS	Last names, "and" or "&", year: Smith and Jones (1994); (Smith & Jones, 1994).	Last names and "and" or "&", year: Smith and Jones (1994); (Smith & Jones, 1994).
THREE TO SIX AUTHORS	Last names, separated by a comma, "and" or "&", year Smith, Jones, Johnson, and James (1994); (Smith, Jones, Johnson, & James, 1994)	Last name of first author, et al., year. Smith et al., (1994); (Smith et al., 1994)
SIX OR MORE AUTHORS	Last name of first author et al., year. Smith et al., (1994); (Smith et al., 1994)	Last name of first author, et al., year Smith et al., (1994)
TWO OR MORE CITATIONS	(James Smith & Johnson, 1994; Markley & Bennett, 1994)	(James et al., 1994; Markley & Bennett, 1994)

Figure 10–3. Writing citations using APA style. Authors are listed in alphabetical order in the citation. When the citation is used a second time in the same paragraph, leave out the date unless there are two citations by the same author or the citation can be confused with another citation.

	BOOK	JOURNAL	CHAPTER FROM A BOOK
AUTHOR(S)	Last name(s), initials, . . . & last name, initials; no additional punctuation at the end. **Jones, M. J., & Smith, J. C.**	Last name(s), initials, . . . & last name, initials; no additional punctuation at the end. **Jones, M. J., Johnson, P. G., & Smith, J. C.**	last name(s), initials, & last name, initials; no additional punctuation at the end. **Johnson, M. J., & James, P. G.**
YEAR	Place the year in parentheses, and put period after the parentheses. **(1994).**	Place year in parentheses and put period after the parentheses. For weekly issues, put the month, date, and year in parentheses. **(1977, October 15).**	Place year in parentheses and put period after the parentheses. **(1994).**
TITLE OF BOOK, ARTICLE, CHAPTER	Capitalize first word of the book and first word after a colon. End with a period unless there is an edition number. Underline the title of book or put it in italics. **Evaluation of therapeutic progress.**	Capitalize first word of the journal article and first word after a colon. End with a period. Do not underline the article title or put it in quotations. **Evaluation of classroom procedures.**	Capitalize first word of the chapter from a book and first word after a colon. End the chapter title with a period. **Evaluation of classroom procedures.**
TITLE OF JOURNAL		Capitalize important words in the journal title and underline it. Put a comma after the title. **Journal of Aging,**	

Figure 10–4. Common bibliographic references. Additional information regarding the appropriate style of dissertations, secondary sources, movies or films or other sources can be found in the APA manual. Adapted from the *Publication Manual of the American Psychological Association* (1994) and Slade, Campbell, & Ballou (1994).

	BOOK	JOURNAL	CHAPTER FROM A BOOK
EDITOR	Place the terms (Ed.). or (Eds.). before the title. Place a period at the end. **James, J. B., & Jones, J. J. (Eds.). <u>Evaluation procedures</u>**		Place the words term (Ed.) or (Eds.) before the title. Place a period at the end. **In J. C. Jones & M. C. Smith (Eds.), <u>Evaluation procedures</u>, pp. 779–891.**
EDITION	Put the edition number of the book in parentheses following title of the book. Place period at the end. **(2nd ed.).**		
VOLUME		Underline (or italize) the volume number and the comma placed after the number. <u>*17*</u> *17,*	
ISSUE		Only included the issue number if each issue begins with page 1. Place the issue number in parentheses after the volume number with no space between them. The issue number is not underlined or italized. <u>*17*</u>*(2),* *17(2),*	

Figure 10–4. *(continued)*

	BOOK	JOURNAL	CHAPTER FROM A BOOK
PAGE		Place the page number after the volume (or issue) number. Put a period after the page number. Don't use p. or pp. **79–95.**	Place the page numbers of the chapter inside parentheses after title of the book. Put a period after the parentheses. Use p. or pp. **(pp. 355–390).**
PLACE OF PUBLICATION	City, State: Publisher. Do not use state for major cities. Use the 2 letter abbreviation for states, when needed. **Boston: Allyn & Bacon** **Thorofare, NJ: Slack**		City, State: Publisher Do not use state for major cities. Use the 2 letter abbreviation for states, when needed. **Boston: Allyn & Bacon** **Thorofare, NJ: Slack**

Figure 10–4. (continued)

Table 10–3. Examples of Bibliographic References using APA Style

---

- **Book**

  Locke, L. F., Spirduso, W. W., & Silverman, S. J. (1997). *Proposals that work* (3rd ed.). Newbury Park: Sage.

- **Journal Article**

  Smith, J. C., & Jones, J. M. (1993). Reconstructing the facial features. *Journal of Paleontology, 17,* 339–431.

- **Chapter in a Book**

  Rutter, M., Chadwick, O., & Shaffer, D. (1983). Head injury. In M. Rutter (Ed.), *Developmental neuropsychiatry* (pp. 83–111). New York: Guilford.

- **Electronic sources**

  ClickArt 10,000. (No Date).[CD-ROM] Broderbund. Available: CLT844AE-CD. [1999, August 3]
  Crane, N. (1997). *Bibliographic Formats for Citing Electronic Information,* [On-Line]. Available: http://www.uvm.edu/~ncrane/estyles/

Note. Additional information regarding the appropriate style for dissertations, secondary sources, movies or films can be found in the APA manual.

Note. Adapted from the *Publication Manual of the American Psychological Association* (1994), Slade, Campbell, & Ballou (1994), and http://www.uvm.edu/~ncrane/estyles/.

  a. outline of major areas to be reviewed
  b. plan for search of related literature
  c. annotated bibliographical notation organized under major areas reviewed
6. Research design
  a. research model, (e.g., experimental, correlational, or methodological)
  b. operational definitions of variables
  c. statement of hypotheses or guiding questions
  d. identification of presumed independent or dependent variables
  e. theoretical explanation underlying study
7. Methodology
  a. procedure for selecting sample and screening criteria for subject inclusion
  b. setting for study and procedure for collecting data
  c. tests, questionnaires, or instruments applied to study

  d. methodological studies to include evaluation of
    - reliability
    - validity
  e. tentative time schedule for study
    - time period for literature review
    - collection of data: number of hours required
    - date for completion of research
  f. projected costs for study
    - clerical
    - instrumentation
    - other

10.7 Sample Proposal of a Graduate Research Project

An example of a graduate research project is on pages 443–463. The project has been reprinted by permission of the authors.

10.8 Preparation for Presentation

10.8.1 Poster Session

A poster display is an opportunity for researchers to present their research in an informal environment. At many conferences, a portion of the conference area is set aside for poster displays. Usually the researcher stays with the poster and discusses the data analysis and procedures with the conference participants. This is an opportunity for the participants to ask questions related to the research.

The poster should be presented in a clear and comprehensive manner. Components of the poster itself include (a) an abstract written in 25 to 50 words, (b) the purpose or aim of the study, (c) the methodology including subject selection, measurements, procedures or treatment techniques (d) results presented in graphic form, and (e) a summary of the conclusions. In addition to the poster, a handout is usually available that may include all the components, plus

Boston University

College of Allied Health Professions

The Effect of Biofeedback
on the
Hyperactivity of a 10-year-old Male Patient

by
Barbara Stein, B. S.

Submitted in partial fulfillment
of the
requirements for the degree of

Master of Science

September 1999

Figure 10–5. Example of a title page for a research paper, thesis, or dissertation.

a summary of literature review and a means of contacting the researchers.

Key Points in Preparing a Poster

▶ *Size of print:* The print size should be large enough for participants to read it at a distance of 4 feet, generally a font size 18- to 24-points.
▶ *Layout:* The layout is determined by the space provided at the conference and directions from the conference committee. Try different layouts designs. The material should be arranged to facilitate understanding of the material, generally top to bottom in a left-to-right sequence (see Figure 10–6).
▶ *Amount of information:* Information should be written in bullets (three-to-four word phrases) rather than in sentences. Include essential information about the design, procedure, and results. Figures, charts, and photographs are helpful in displaying results. Additional information can be included in the handout.
▶ *Color:* Use color in highlighting the results and conclusions. A light color (e.g.,

yellow) printed on a dark paper is frequently easier to read.
▶ *Background:* Use of contrasting color or border behind the individual components will make the poster visually attractive.

10.8.2 Conference Paper

Researchers are encouraged to present the results of their findings at local, state, national, and international conferences. A call for papers is issued in *OT Practice* and *Advance for Occupational Therapists*. When presenting a paper, it is important to recognize that those in attendance are adult learners with a heterogeneous knowledge base.

Key Points of Presenting a Paper

▶ Rehearse the presentation, considering time available for the presentation.
▶ Consider the number of people and the size of the room when preparing the paper. If a presenter has only 10 to 15 minutes, reading the paper verbatim is more feasible than if the presentation is a 90-minute workshop.

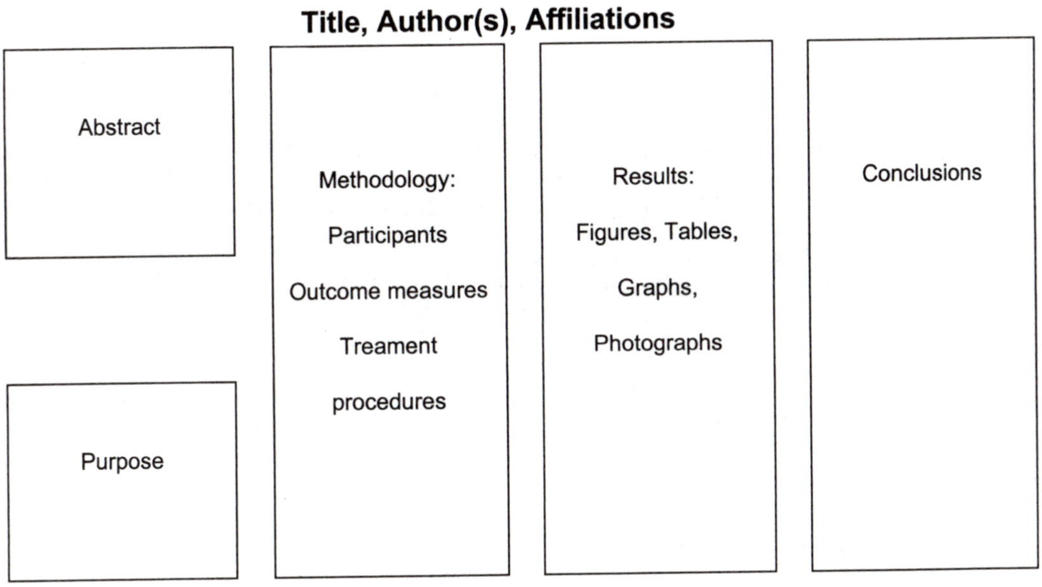

Figure 10–6. Sample of the layout of a poster session.

▶ Consider who will be in the audience (e.g., parents, professionals, new graduates, experienced clinicians) and plan your presentation accordingly.

▶ If the paper must be read verbatim, use conversational expression and eye contact with members of the audience.

▶ When presentations are more than 15 minutes long, prepare overheads or slides that can be used to discuss the paper rather than reading it verbatim.

▶ Use 3-by-5 cards to organize and remember the key points to present.

▶ Allow 5 to 10 minutes for questions from the audience.

▶ Speak loudly enough for everyone in the audience to hear.

▶ Prepare overheads and slides so that people in the last row can see them. If possible, provide handouts of the overheads (in smaller fonts).

▶ When preparing PowerPoint presentations, be sure that the print is large (fonts of 36 points or above) and that students have handouts of the presentations. A light print with a dark background (dark blue background with yellow print) is easier to read. A sans serif font (e.g., Ariel) is also preferable. Although adding animations can be entertaining, they may distract from the presentation.

▶ Be sure that equipment works prior to the presentation. Go to the room at least 10 minutes before the presentation and try out the equipment.

▶ Include a beginning, middle, and end in your presentation. The beginning should establish rapport and set the purpose of the presentation with the audience. The ending should summarize the presentation. Make your conclusion memorable.

▶ Generally, the audience will be adult learners. Adult learners are pragmatic, eager to apply what they learn, have a variety of experiences, and often challenge the presenter.

▶ Include a one-page handout with references.

Audiovisual Aids

▶ *Flip Charts:* Use dark-colored markers, write in large lettering, and place the easel on a platform above the audience so those in the back can see the chart.

▶ *Slides:* Arrange slides in a carousel and test prior to presentation. Use a dark background with highly contrasted and large lettering.

▶ *Overhead transparencies:* In general, prepare these with a word-processing program rather than free-hand print. Use color transparencies if possible. Pictures can be scanned into a document and printed. The print should be large enough for those in the back to see. Graphics should be clear without distracting material.

▶ *PowerPoint:* This is a useful tool for the organization of material. Individual points can be displayed as they are discussed, rather than all at once, as they would be on a transparency or slide. Sequencing and timing are easier than when using slides or overheads. Handouts should be used to help the audience follow the program. In addition, Speaker Notes can be scripted to remind the speaker of specific points. Because PowerPoint is updated frequently, the speaker should verify that the software and hardware are compatible.

10.8.3 Publication

Numerous opportunities exist for students and clinicians to publish their research in occupational therapy journals. The following outline lists the steps in selecting a journal and preparing the research study for publication. In addition, based on the first author's experience as an editor, questions used to evaluate a submitted manuscript to a referred journal have been included.

Selecting the Appropriate Journal

A more extensive list of all occupational therapy journals is found in Chapter 6. The major journals are listed here.

- American Journal of Occupational Therapy (AJOT) (http://www.aota.org/non members/area7/links/link3.html)
- Australian Occupational Therapy Journal (AOTJ) (http://www.blacksci.co.uk/products/journals/xajot.htm)
- British Journal of Occupational Therapy (BJOT) (http://www.iop.bpmf.ac.uk/home/trust/ot/otcot.htm 6-8)
- Canadian Journal of Occupational Therapy (CJOT) (http://www.caot.ca/pages/publications%26products/periodicals.html)
- Ergotherapie & Rehabilitation (http://www.ergotherapie-reha.de/Ergo/Ergo theraphie.html)
- The Israeli Journal of Occupational Therapy
- Journal D'Ergotherapie (http://www.bois-larris.com/centrdoc.html)
- Journal of Occupational Science (http://www.unisa.edu.au/ot/JOSA.htm)
- Journal of Occupational Therapy Students (http://www.aota.org/nonmem bers/area7/links/link4.html)
- Journal of Japanese Association of Occupational Therapists (JJAOT)
- Occupational Therapy in Health Care (OTHC) (http://web.spectra.net/~haworth/)
- Occupational Therapy in Mental Health (http://web.spectra.net/~haworth/)
- Occupational Therapy International (OTI) (http://www.allenpress.com/catalogue/index/occ_therapy_international/index.html)
- Physical and Occupational Therapy in Pediatrics (http://web.spectra.net/~haworth/)
- Physical and Occupational Therapy in Geriatrics (http://web.spectra.net/~haworth/)
- Occupational Therapy Journal of Research (OTJR) (http://www.slackinc.com/otpt/otjr/otjrhome.htm)
- Scandinavian Journal of Occupational Therapy (SJOT) (http://www.scup.no/journals/journals.html)
- South African Journal of Occupational Therapy (E-mail sajot cis.co.za)

The researcher should obtain the instructions for submission of a paper before submission. The style (e.g., APA, Turabian), margins, page length, manuscript length, number of copies, and the arrangement of the manuscript are specific to each journal. Most journals require work to be submitted on a disk.

Classifying the Manuscript

- Research paper, presenting original data (quantitative and qualitative)
- The position paper, (e.g., advocating change in health care system)
- Review article (integration of research studies)
- Description of clinical program
- Description of clinical device
- Book review
- Letter to the editor

Components of Manuscript

- *Title:* include variables, subjects, settings
- *Author(s):* include degrees, affiliation, E-mail address and corresponding address
- *Abstract:* 100–175 word summary of article
- *Key words:* 4–5 descriptive words (See MeSH as examples)
- *Literature review and introduction*
- *Methodology*
- *Results*
- *Discussion*
- *Conclusions*
- *Recommendations for further research and limitations of study*
- *Acknowledgments*
- *References*
- *Tables and Figures*

Process of Getting into Print

- Rewriting and multiple drafts are necessary
- Keep in mind that 30% of manuscripts are rejected

▶ The lag between submitting an article and seeing it in print is often up to 1 year

▶ Refereed journals: The types of decisions made include (a) accept with minor revisions, (b) accept with major revisions, (c) resubmit for additional review, and (d) reject.

The Journal Review Process (Questions Posed for the Reviewer)

▶ Is the title representative of the article?

▶ Is the abstract a summary of the main points of the study?

▶ Does the author justify the need and significance of research?

▶ Is the literature review comprehensive and up-to-date?

▶ Is the research design rigorous? (Internal validity)

▶ Is generalization to target population valid? (External validity)

▶ Does the investigator use the appropriate statistical tests?

▶ Are results consistent with statistical findings?

▶ Are the conclusions justified?

▶ Are the references up to date and from a variety of sources?

▶ Does the author recommend further research and state limitations of study?

▶ Are the figures and graphs labeled correctly?

▶ Do the figures and graphs add to the information presented?

10.9 Conclusion

One of the important purposes of this book is help the student and practitioner generate clinical research studies that validate practice. The authors have presented the research process in a systematic method. The research process presented incorporates both qualitative and quantitative research models. For the clinical researcher, these models can be used to validate practice. Research does not exist in a vacuum. There is a strong historical background for research that has led to the progress in medicine, rehabilitation, and habilitation. Occupational therapists are part of the behavioral medicine tradition that applies nonsurgical and nonpharmaceutical methods. Occupational therapists employing behavioral techniques and assistive technology, such as sensory integration therapy, neurodevelopmental theory, creative arts, relaxation therapy, splinting, and prescriptive exercise can use the clinical research methods described to establish evidence-based practice for the 21st century. It is the authors' intention that the development of treatment protocols can be useful in the establishment of a scientific foundation for occupational therapy.

The Needs of Alzheimer's Support Group Members

and

Occupational Therapy's Role

Completed by:

Jennifer Gill and Erin Larson

Submitted in partial fulfillment for

OCTH 725: Research Perspectives in Occupational Therapy

to Franklin Stein, Ph.D., OTR/L,

Submitted: April 21, 1999

Revised: August 19, 1999

TABLE OF CONTENTS

1.0 THE RESEARCH PROBLEM

1.1 Statement of Research Problem in Question Form

- What is Alzheimer's disease?

- What are the behavioral changes that accompany this disease?

- What are the stages that people with Alzheimer's disease progress through?

- How do caregivers cope with the progression of this disease?

- What are the psychological effects of the caregivers?

- How can occupational therapists educate support groups about our services?

- How many support groups are there in South Dakota?

- What do caregivers know about occupational therapy services?

- What activities are effective for use with people with Alzheimer's disease?

- Are there differences in the organization of support groups in this area?

- What are the differences in resources available to rural versus urban support groups?

- How do therapists help caregivers cope with this disease?

- What can therapists do for people with Alzheimer's disease and their caregivers?

- Who are the caregivers?

- How many people have Alzheimer's disease in South Dakota?

- What are the options available to caregivers?

- What do caregivers feel their needs are?

1.2 Justification and Need for Study

Alzheimer's disease affects an estimated 4 million middle-aged and older adults in the United States, according to the U.S. Department of Health and Human Services (1995). Alzheimer's disease is a progressive, irreversible disease of the brain (Elder Services of the Merrimack Valley, Inc., 1996). The National Alzheimer's Organization (1995) reported that it is the most common cause of dementia in older people. The nature of this disease requires a large amount of care. Most people with Alzheimer's disease require care for 9 to 15 years after the onset of the disease (Dhooper, 1991). Some people with Alzheimer's disease may live up to 30 years past the initial diagnosis; some caregivers face over a decade in the caregiver role (Martichuski, Knight, Karlin, & Bell, 1997).

Ninety percent of the long term care in the United States is provided by family members as reported in a study by Corcoran (1992). Caregivers are subject to problems such as family disruptions, psychological stress, physical fatigue, social isolation, financial problems and legal issues (Dhooper, 1991).

These caregivers may belong to support groups. Support groups are helpful to caregivers, offering emotional, social, and educational support (Martichuski et.al., 1997). There is little research done on occupational therapist's role in support groups. Occupational therapists can make a positive impact on the lives of caregivers of individuals with Alzheimer's disease. Occupational Therapists can teach caregivers coping strategies, time management skills, adaptation with ADLs, education about the disease, places to get help and a variety of other adaptive strategies (American Occupational Therapy Association [AOTA], 1994). Occupational therapy involves a continuous modification and adaptation of daily living tasks and the physical and social environments in which these tasks are performed. These adaptations help persons with dementia to use their abilities and retain as much control as possible over their lives (AOTA, 1994). Chung (1997) reported that although family carers assume a pivotal role in caring for relatives with dementia, few occupational therapy studies are directed toward them. "Through possessing this professional knowledge in dementia care, occupational therapists must work collaboratively with family carers to formulate realistic treatment programmes" (Chung, 1997, p. 75).

Occupational therapy intervention for caregivers also has financial implications for health care. The direct and indirect costs of care in the United States back in 1985 was estimated to be $88 billion, which will dramatically increase with the rising numbers of our elderly population (Bowlby, 1993). Though not specifically talking about occupational therapy, Mittelman, Ferris, Shulman, Steinberg, and Levin (1996) stated that family intervention can delay the nursing home placement of patients with Alzheimer's Disease. If nursing home placement could be delayed by one month for each patient with Alzheimer's Disease in the year 2020, it would result in an estimated savings of five billion dollars, a major consideration in attempts to contain costs of health care (Kawas & Morrison, 1997).

An understanding of Alzheimer's disease and its consequences is necessary for professionals who must intervene in the lives of those affected by Alzheimer's disease (Dhooper, 1991). Ghatak (1994) discussed the importance of caregiver intervention and emphasized that "this is an area that health care professionals need to focus on immediately"(p. 39). Therefore, we believe that more research should be done concerning occupational therapy's role in the lives of people with Alzheimer's disease and their caregivers. The purpose of this study is to identify the current role of occupational therapists in Alzheimer's support groups in the Midwest and to explore how that role can be expanded.

2.0 THE LITERATURE REVIEW

2.1 How the Literature Was Searched

- MEDLINE

- CINAHL

- ERIC

- PALS
- AOTA
- AOTF
- INTERNET SOURCES
- SUPPORT GROUPS

2.2 Underlying Theoretical Assumptions

- Caregiving is a stressful role (Walker, Pomeroy, McNeil, & Franklin, 1994).
- Occupational therapy can help caregivers by helping to reduce stress (Corcoran, 1992).
- The most effective care is given by caregivers that practice good stress management techniques (Corcoran, 1992).
- The nature of Alzheimer's disease requires caregiving (Alzheimer's Disease and Related Disorders Association, Inc., 1995).
- Occupational Therapists can teach caregivers coping strategies, time management skills, adaption with ADL's, education about the disease, places to get help and a variety of other adaptive strategies (AOTA, 1994).

2.3 Target Population

The researchers will send surveys to Alzheimer's Support Group members in the Midwest (Iowa, Nebraska, Minnesota, North Dakota, and South Dakota).

2.4 Literature Review Summary

Alzheimer's disease is a progressive, degenerative disease that attacks the brain and results in impaired memory, thinking and behavior (Alzheimer's Disease and Related Disorders Association, Inc., 1990). The disease begins slowly. Initially there are only mild symptoms. The Alzheimer's Disease and Related Disorders Association, Inc. (1996) reports possible symptoms such as (a) recent memory loss that affects job skills, (b) difficulty performing familiar tasks, (c) problems with language, (d) disorientation of time and place, (e) poor or decreased judgement, (f) problems with abstract thinking, (g) misplacing things, (h) changes in mood or behavior, (i) changes in personality, and (j) loss of initiative. The disease progresses until the symptoms begin causing problems in their daily lives, and continues until they can no longer function independently. Eventually, the brain no longer directs voluntary activities, and the person becomes totally dependent (Reisberg, 1984). Brain activity gradually diminishes until the person with Alzheimer's disease lapses into a coma and dies. The progression of these symptoms vary widely. The U.S. Department of Health and Human Services (1995) reported that some people may have the disease for 5 years, while others may have it for as many as 20 years. The cause of Alzheimer's disease is unknown, therefore, research is being conducted worldwide to explore possible factors. Some factors being explored are genetics, environment, and viruses (U.S. Department of Health and Human Services, 1995).

There are an estimated 4 million Americans adults that suffer from this disease (U.S. Department of Health and Human Services, 1995). It is the fourth leading cause of death among American adults (Alzheimer's Disease and Related Disorders Association, Inc., 1996). Alzheimer's disease is more likely to occur as a person gets older. Approximately 10% of people over age 65 are affected by Alzheimer's disease and this percentage rises to 47.2% in those age 85 or older (Alzheimer's Disease and Related Disorders Association, Inc., 1990). This is significant because the nation's entire aged population is increasing rapidly and it is estimated that by the year 2050, the U.S. will have 67.5 million people over the age 65 compared with 25.5 million today (Alzheimer's Disease and Related Disorders Association, Inc., 1990).

Seventy percent of the 4 million Americans with Alzheimer's disease are cared for at home (Alzheimer's Disease and Related Disorders Association, Inc., 1995). The nature of Alzheimer's disease requires large amounts of care. Caregivers of individuals with Alzheimer's disease spend an average of 70 to 100 hours per week tending to the needs of the person with Alzheimer's disease (Alzheimer's Disease and Related Disorders Association, Inc., 1996). According to Dhooper (1991) the tasks associated with caregiving have been classified into four groups :

• direct care of the patient

• intrapersonal tasks of the caregiver,

• interpersonal and familial tasks, and

• societal tasks.

The tasks that comprise direct care of the patient include (a) supervising prescribed treatment and recommendations, (b) performing the basic activities of daily living for the patient, (c) being available when needed, (d) providing structure to the patient's daily activities, (e) normalizing his/her routine within the bounds of impairment, and (f) coping with his/her upsetting behavior. The personal tasks faced by caregivers include (a) recovering personal time, (b) resolving guilt over negative feelings toward the patient and over ones' performance, (c) compensating for emotional drain from constant responsibility, (d) gaining knowledge about the disease and patient's condition, (e) avoiding severe drain on physical health, and (f) avoiding restrictions on future plans. The familial and societal tasks involve (a) managing feelings toward those family members that do not regularly help, (b) balancing the giving of assistance with responsibilities to other family members and (c) interacting with medical, health and social service professionals (Dhooper, 1991).

Providing this care can lead to stress on the part of the caregiver. Caregiver stress is frequently associated with a lack of knowledge about caregiving tasks, the amount of direct care provided, and lack of resources to provide care (Garity,

1997). This stress can lead to both physical and emotional strain. The Alzheimer's Disease and Related Disorders Association, Inc. (1995) reported that 80% of Alzheimer caregivers suffer from high levels of stress and nearly half suffer from depression. The signs of caregiver stress include: (a) denial, (b) anger, (c) social withdrawal, (d) anxiety, (e) depression, (f) exhaustion, (g) sleeplessness, (h) irritability, (i) lack of concentration, and (j) health problems (Alzheimer's Association, 1995).

In order to alleviate some of this stress, professionals offer many different services, including: educational programs, skills training and support groups, with support groups being the most common (Martichuski et.al., 1997). Studies have found support groups helpful in reducing the emotional impact and burden experienced by caregivers of Alzheimer's patients (Walker et al., 1994). Schmall (1984) divided support groups into four types, each differing in goals and approach: (a) education, (b) mutual/peer support, (c) education/mutual support, and (d) ventilation. The traditional support group typically focuses on a discussion of the emotional aspects of caregiving. Educational groups focus on the provision of information that will help the caregiver manage and plan for their loved one. Most of the groups are some combination of types (Walker et al., 1994). Some support groups meet the needs of individuals better than others, but small towns and rural areas are not likely to have more than one type (Martichuski et.al., 1997). The general structure of each support group and the elements surrounding the group influence each care provider's experience within the support group (Martichuski et al., 1997).

The issues addressed in support groups are also areas that occupational therapists can assist caregivers in managing on a day to day basis. Specialized treatment and care regimens maximize the self-esteem and functioning, and minimize the suffering and dependence of the millions of affected individuals during the long course of the illness (Bowlby, 1993) indicated that family, friends, and paid caregivers hve a reduced burden when treatment is provided.

Four main aspects of occupational therapy services are utilized in working with individuals with dementia. "The practice of intervention programmes is the most common practice" (Chung, 1997, p. 67). The specific type of occupational therapy intervention "depends on the stage of illness and the manner in which cognitive impairment is manifested in daily living activities" (AOTA, 1994, p. 1031).

The basic goals of intervention for persons with dementing illnesses are to (a) maintain, restore, or improve functional capacity, (b) promote participation in activities that optimize physical and mental health, and (c) to ease caregiving activities (AOTA, 1994). Bowlby (1993) indicated that interventions as reminiscence, sensory stimulation, purposeful activities, and environmental modifications are frequently used. Reminiscence is a structured group activity in which the group leader assists and guides the group members to recall previous life experiences and facilitates the group's affirmation of the value of these experiences. Sensory stimulation involves the use of meaningful smells, movements, sights, sounds, and tastes in a way that compensates for sensory deprivation sometimes experienced by those with Alzheimer's disease. Examples of purposeful activities that may be used include horticulture, religious activities, art and cooking (Pool, 1999). Environmental modifications change the surroundings in a way that simplifies the environment and provide prompts and cues for the person with Alzheimer's disease (Skolaski-Pellitteri, 1984).

The second aspect of occupational therapy practice focuses on assessments. Due to the fact that the abilities of individuals with dementia progressively deteriorate in the areas of cognition, behaviors, emotion, and personality, assessments are designed to assess these deficits in the following areas: activities of daily living, functional performance and process and motor ability (AOTA, 1994).

The third aspect occupational therapists are interested in is understanding the impairments of individuals with dementia. These impairments may have implications for occupational therapy, for instance, spatial disorientation and functional memory (Chung, 1997).

"The last and least noticeable aspect is home-based occupational therapy services for individuals with dementia and their family carers" (Chung, 1997, p. 67). This last aspect suggests that occupational therapists need to provide services for the caregivers as well as the person with dementia in order to provide optimal care. The literature suggest that occupational therapists must work with the caregivers in developing realistic treatment plans due to the fact that they are the most knowledgeable about the people that they are caring for and will be the ones to carry out the treatment plans (Chung, 1997). Occupational therapists can aid in caregivers' needs by addressing: environmental safety, behavior management, education on cognitive impairment of the client, the caregivers health (both physical and psychological) and community support available to them (Chung, 1997).

In summary, Alzheimer's disease is a progressive, degenerative illness that affects millions of people in the United States. The majority of people with Alzheimer's disease are cared for at home. The caregivers may experience stress caused by the large responsibility of caring for someone with Alzheimer's disease. Some caregivers may attend support groups as a way of coping with this stress. The best care is provided by caregivers that manage their stress. Occupational therapists can play a role in the education of caregivers in ways to manage the tasks associated with caregiving, thereby helping to alleviate some of the stress. In order for therapists to provide the best intervention, they must be aware of caregiver's needs. The purpose of this study is to explore the needs of caregivers attending Alzheimer's support groups and to identify the areas that occupational therapists can assist caregivers in reducing their stress and becoming more functional in helping the person with Alzheimer's disease.

3.0 RESEARCH DESIGN

3.1 Research Design Questions

- What states will we survey?

- How many Alzheimer's support groups are there in these states?

- How many support groups will we survey?
- How will we find these groups?
- How will we survey them?
- How will we test for reliability and validity of the survey?
- How many members are in these support groups?
- How will the data be collected?
- How will the data be analyzed?
- How will we increase response rate?

3.2 Guiding Question

What are the current and potential roles of occupational therapists in Alzheimer's support groups in the Midwest, and can that role be expanded?

3.3 Diagrammatical Relationship Between Variables

Target Populations:	Alzheimer's support group members in the Midwest
Representative Sample:	200 support group members in the Midwest
Statistic:	30% of sample
Method:	Mail questionnaires to support group leader
Test:	Data Analysis
Guiding question:	What are the current and potential roles of occupational therapists in Alzheimer's support groups in the Midwest, and can that role be expanded?
Statistical Tests:	Descriptive graphs

3.4 Possible Limitations of the Study

There are several possible limitations to this study. First, the sample population is small and cannot be generalized to represent the whole population of caregivers of people with Alzheimer's disease. A second limitation involves the collection procedure. Members may be unwilling to discuss personal issues with the researchers or they may give responses according to what they believe the researchers expect to hear. Researcher bias may influence the way in which the researchers perceive the information being presented to them. The third set of limitations involves the analysis of the data. The data collected is qualitative in nature, therefore it is subject to interpretation by the researchers and in this interpretation there may be errors.

4.0 METHODOLOGY

4.1 Screening Criteria for Target Populations

Participant must

- attend a support group
- be related to a person with Alzheimer's disease
- live in Iowa, Nebraska, Minnesota, North Dakota, or South Dakota

4.2 Data Collection Procedure

The researchers will attend three or more support groups and collect data based upon a custom designed observation form. This information will be used to support and contrast the information gathered in a survey designed by the researchers. The survey will be critiqued by a high school graduate, a survey expert, an occupational therapist, and a member of the Alzheimer's support group community. Support group leaders in Iowa, Nebraska, Minnesota, North Dakota, and South Dakota will be contacted to explain the survey that they will be receiving . The surveys will be mailed to support group leaders with a pre-addressed and postage paid envelopes with a one month time limit. A follow up postcard and/ or phone call will be given the day before the scheduled support group meeting is to occur. The group leaders will distribute surveys with cover letters to group members. The cover letter will serve the dual purpose of explaining the survey and acting as a consent form. Support group members will complete the survey and return it to the group leader to be placed in a manila envelope. Then the group leader will mail the survey back to us. Upon receiving the surveys, we will compile the data. We will send the findings to the support groups and provide information about occupational therapy at the support groups' request.

4.3 Projected Time Schedule for Completing Study

Selection of Topic	3 hours
Literature Review	50 hours
Research Proposal	45 hours
Contact Support Groups	5 hours
Create Survey	10 hours
Pretest Survey	8 hours
Travel	12 hours
Observation of Support Groups	6 hours
Develop Presentation	5 hours
Send Survey/Wait for Response	1 month

Alzheimer's Support Groups   11

Data Analysis .... 30 hours

Write Discussion .... 7 hours

Complete Research .... 5 hours

Total Time to Complete Study .... **Approximately 8 months**

4.4 Statistical Design for Analyzing Data

Descriptive statistics will be used to analyze the data gathered by the survey. The statistics will be summarized in the form of descriptive tables, graphs, and charts.

4.5 Projected Costs of Study

Travel $40

Telephone calls to obtain data $50

Data collection forms $30

Letter of informed consent $10

Collection of Literature Review $35

Presentation materials $5

Postage $150

Binder for study results $3

Total Cost of Study .... **Approximately $323**

4.6 Cover Letter

Dear Caregiver:

You are invited to participate in a research project entitled "The Needs of Alzheimer's Support Group Members and the Role of Occupational Therapy". The project is being conducted by Jennifer Gill and Erin Larson under the direction of the Occupational Therapy Department at the University of South Dakota for completion of their master's degree program.

The purpose of this project is to identify Alzheimer's support group members needs and to identify how occupational therapists can assist caregivers. You are asked to provide basic information about yourself, about the person with Alzheimer's and about the issues that you face as a caregiver.

Participation in this project is voluntary. If you consent to participate, you will be involved in the following process, which will take about 10 to 20 minutes of your time:

• fill out survey

• place and seal in envelope

• place in group leader's manila envelope

Your responses are strictly confidential. When the data are presented in the written report, you will not be linked to the data by your name, title or any other identifying item. There are no known risks to your participation in this study. However, some of the questions may be of a sensitive nature. If there are some questions that you do not feel comfortable answering, it is your right to skip that question. If issues arise upon filling out this questionnaire, we suggest speaking to your group leader.

There are no direct benefits upon completing this questionnaire. However, upon completing this project, we hope to educate occupational therapists about the needs of Alzheimer's support groups. In this way, we hope to better serve your needs.

If you have any questions, you may contact Jennifer Gill or Erin Larson. The information is provided below.

Thank you for your time and assistance.

Sincerely,

Erin Larson and Jennifer Gill

Erin Larson   Jennifer Gill

400 N. Plum 101   6 East Dartmouth St. 3

Vermillion, SD 57069   Vermillion, SD 57069

(605) 624-9195   (605) 624-3406

elarson@usd.edu   jlgill@usd.edu

4.7 Survey

Survey of Alzheimer's Support Group Members in the Midwest

Please answer the questions to the best of your knowledge. Place an X in the place provided. Thank you for your time.

1.   **Gender:**

   _____ Female   _____ Male

2.   **Age:**

   _____ 34 and under   _____ 65 - 79

   _____ 35 - 49   _____ 80 and above

   _____ 50 - 64

3.   What is your relationship to the person with Alzheimer's disease?

_____Spouse   _____Friend

_____Son / Daughter   _____Other _____

_____Granddaughter / Grandson

4.   How long (to the best of your knowledge) has the person been exhibiting symptoms of Alzheimer's disease? _____

5.   Do you consider yourself a caregiver? _____ Yes _____ No   If yes, answer the following two questions:

   a.   Indicate below what best describes your responsibilities.

   _____ live with the person and provide daily care

   _____ do not live with person but assist on a regular basis

   b.   How long have you been a caregiver? _____

6.   How long have you been attending this support group?

_____ less than 6 months   _____ 2-5 years

_____ 6 months to 1 year   _____ greater than 5 years

_____ 1-2 years

Please indicate the areas that are concerns for you in your role as a caregiver. Each term is defined on the last page of the survey. Indicate your level of concern in each area by circling the numbers from 1 to 5. Refer to the last page of this survey whenever necessary.

   1.   Never

   2.   Rarely

   3.   Sometimes

   4.   Almost always

   5.   Always

a.	Time Management	1	2	3	4	5
b.	Social Isolation	1	2	3	4	5
c.	Stress Management	1	2	3	4	5
d.	Outside Assistance with Care	1	2	3	4	5
e.	Depression	1	2	3	4	5
f.	Home Safety	1	2	3	4	5

g.	Physical Fatigue	1	2	3	4	5
h.	Financial Strain	1	2	3	4	5
i.	Family Stress	1	2	3	4	5
j.	Behavior Management	1	2	3	4	5
k.	Hygiene Care	1	2	3	4	5
l.	Dressing	1	2	3	4	5
m.	Cooking / Cleaning	1	2	3	4	5
n.	Schedule Planning	1	2	3	4	5
o.	Work Issues	1	2	3	4	5

Have you ever received occupational therapy services addressing the areas listed above ?

_____ Yes _____ No

If no, skip this question.

If yes, please complete the following:

Rank the effectiveness of these services on a scale of 1 to 3 with 1 being the least effective and 3 being the most effective by circling the number. Circle NA for not applicable if you have not encountered this service.

1. Not Effective

2. Somewhat Effective

3. Very Effective

NA Not Applicable

a.	Time Management	1	2	3	NA
b.	Social Isolation	1	2	3	NA
c.	Stress Management	1	2	3	NA
d.	Outside Assistance with Care	1	2	3	NA
e.	Depression	1	2	3	NA
f.	Home Safety	1	2	3	NA
g.	Physical Fatigue	1	2	3	NA
h.	Financial Strain	1	2	3	NA
i.	Family Stress	1	2	3	NA

Alzheimer's Support Groups   15

j.	Behavior Management	1	2	3	NA
k.	Hygiene Care	1	2	3	NA
l.	Dressing	1	2	3	NA
m.	Cooking / Cleaning	1	2	3	NA
n.	Schedule Planning	1	2	3	NA
o.	Work Issues	1	2	3	NA

Additional comments on your role as a caregiver:

_____

_____

_____

_____

4.7a Definition of terms.

<u>Definition of Terms</u>

Time Management: the use of time in a way that allows one to get things done

Social Isolation: the feeling of being alone

Stress Management: a way of dealing with stress in a healthy manner

Outside Assistance with Care: people outside of the home help either directly or indirectly

Depression: an overwhelming feeling of sadness

Home Safety: keeping oneself and others out of danger in the home

Physical Fatigue: the feeling of tiredness

Financial Strain: having to make the money stretch, difficulty paying bills

Family Stress: members of the family feel tension and/or pressure due to the caregiving situation

Hygiene Care: taking care of washing, bathing, and grooming

Dressing: putting clothes on

Cooking/Cleaning: making meals and taking care of the upkeep of the house

Schedule Planning: organizing the events and activities of oneself and the person with Alzheimer's disease

Work Issues: difficulty caused by things related to work, such as schedules, traveling, and wages

4.8 Evaluation of Survey

1. How long did it take you to complete the survey (minutes)? _____

2. Is the survey too long? Yes _____ No _____

3. Did you find the survey interesting? Yes _____ No _____

4. If not, please explain why:
   _____
   _____

5. Did you feel the survey will gather information applicable to occupational therapy's role in Alzheimer's support groups? Yes _____ No _____

6. Suggestions for improvement:

7. _____
   _____
   _____
   _____

8. Did you feel the questions were easily understood? Yes _____ No _____

   (Please indicate with a check mark those questions that were hard to understand and/or make corrections as you see fit.)

9. Did the questions flow in a logical sequence? Yes _____ No _____

10. Suggestions:
    _____
    _____
    _____

11. Please list any recommendations you may have that would improve our survey:
    _____
    _____
    _____
    _____
    _____

4.9 Support Group Observation Form

Observation of Support Group (to be completed by the researchers)

1. Name of Support Group: _____

2. Location/Address: _____
   _____

3. Number of Participants: _____

4. How often does the group meet? _____

Alzheimer's Support Groups   17

5. Purpose of Group:
    _____ Educational
    _____ Social Support
    _____ Combination

6. Symptoms of Alzheimer's disease discussed: _____
    _____
    _____
    _____
    _____

7. Possible stages of Alzheimer's disease discussed:
    _____ Early
    _____ Middle
    _____ Late

8. Issues Discussed   Caregiver   Alzheimer's disease
    _____ Time Management
    _____ Social Isolation
    _____ Stress Management
    _____ Outside Assistance with Care
    _____ Depression
    _____ Home Safety
    _____ Physical Fatigue
    _____ Financial Strain
    _____ Family Stress
    _____ Behavior Management
    _____ Hygiene Care
    _____ Dressing
    _____ Cooking / Cleaning
    _____ Schedule Planning
    _____ Work Issues

9. Role of Occupational Therapist
    _____ Active
    _____ Consultation
    _____ None

10.   Additional Comments: _____

_____

_____

_____

_____

5.0 REFERENCES

Alzheimer's Disease and Related Disorders Association, Inc. (1990). *Alzheimer's disease: An overview.* [Brochure]. Chicago, IL: Author.

Alzheimer's Disease and Related Disorders Association, Inc. (1996). Caregiving a labor of love. *Alzheimer's Association National Newsletter, 16*(4), 1–8.

Alzheimer's Disease and Related Disorders Association, Inc. (1995). *Caregiver stress: Signs to watch for . . . Steps to take.* [Brochure]. Chicago, IL: Author.

Alzheimer's Disease and Related Disorders Association, Inc. (1996). *Is it Alzheimer's?: Warning signs you should know.* (Brochure). Chicago, IL: Author.

American Occupational Therapy Association (1994). Statement: Occupational therapy services for persons with Alzheimer's Disease and other dementias. *The American Journal of Occupational Therapy, 48*(11), 1029–1031.

Bowlby, C. (1993). *Therapeutic activities with persons disabled by Alzheimer's disease and related disorders.* Gaithersburg, MD: Aspen.

Chung, J. (1997). Focus on family care givers for individuals with dementia: Implications for occupational therapy practice. *Occupational Therapy International, 4*(1), 66–80.

Corcoran, M. (1992). Gender differences in dementia management plans of spousal caregivers: Implications for occupational therapy. *The American Journal of Occupational Therapy, 46*(11), 1006–1011.

Dhooper, S. S. (1991). Caregivers of Alzheimer's disease patients: A review of the literature. *Journal of Gerontological Social Work, 18*(1/2), 19–36.

Elder Services of the Merrimack Valley, Inc. (1996). *Alzheimer's disease* [Online]. Available: http://goal.com/hope/alzheimr.htm.

Garity, J. (1997). Stress, learning style, resilience factors, and ways of coping in Alzheimer's family caregivers. *American Journal of Alzheimer's Disease, 12*(4), 171–178.

Ghatak, R. (1994). Effects of an intervention program on dementia patients and their caregivers. *Caring Magazine, 13*(8), 34–39.

Martichuski, D. K., Knight, B. J., Karlin, N. J., & Bell, P. A. (1997). Correlates of Alzheimer's disease caregivers' support group attendance. *Activities, Adaptation, and Aging, 21*(4), 27–40.

Mittelman, M. S., Ferris, S. H. Shulman, E., Steinberg, G., & Levin, B. (1996). A family intervention to delay nursing home placement of patients with Alzheimer disease. *Journal of the American Medical Association, 276*(21), 1725–1731.

National Alzheimer's Organization. (1995). *Alzheimer's disease fact sheet* [Online]. Available: http://www.alzheimers.org/adfact.html.

Pool, J. (1999). *The Pool Activity Level (PAL) Instrument: A practical resource for carers of people with dementia.* London, England: Jessica Kingsley Publishers Ltd.

Reisberg, B. (1984). Stages of cognitive decline. *American Journal of Nursing, 84*(2), 227.

Schmall, V.L. (1984). It doesn't just happen: What makes a support group good? *Generations, 9,* 64–67.

Skolaski-Pellitteri, T. (1984). Environmental adaptations which compensate for dementia. *Physical and Occupational Therapy in Geriatrics, 3*(1), 31–45.

Spaid, W. M. & Barusch, A. S. (1992). Social support and caregiver strain: types and sources of social contacts of elderly caregivers. *Journal of Gerontological Social Work, 18*(1/2), 151–161.

U.S. Department of Health and Human Services (1995). *Alzheimer's disease fact sheet.* [On-line]. Available: http://www.alzheimers.org/adfact.html

Walker, R. J., Pomeroy, E. C., McNeil, J. S., & Franklin, C. (1994). A psychoeducational model for caregivers of patients with Alzheimer's disease. *Journal of Gerontological Social Work, 22* (1/2), 75–90.

6.0 ANNOTATED BIBLIOGRAPHY

Chung, J. (1997). Focus on family care givers for individuals with dementia: Implications for occupational therapy practice. *Occupational Therapy International, 4*(1), 66—80.

Abstract: Family carers assume a pivotal role however, few occupational therapy studies are directed towards them. This qualitative study explores the feelings and experiences of family carers. The author describes four basic themes that emerged. These themes include: 1) hands on assistance, 2) carers devised caring strategies, 3) feelings were fluid and complex, and 4) negative experiences outweighed positive ones. The author urges occupational therapists to understand the unique needs of the family carers and include them in part of the treatment plan. Interventions are suggested including: collaborative work with family, support groups and education.

Corcoran, M. (1992). Gender differences in dementia management plans of spousal caregivers: Implications for occupational therapy. *The American Journal of Occupational Therapy, 46*(11), 1006-1011.

Abstract: The author of this article discuss an occupational therapy intervention designed specifically for family caregivers of persons with dementia. Use of the environment is the focus of this intervention. A case study is used to demonstrate this intervention.

Garity, J. (1997). Stress, learning style, resilience factors, and ways of coping in Alzheimer's family caregivers. *American Journal of Alzheimer's Disease, 12*(4), 171-178.

Abstract: This study investigated the relationship between stress level, learning, style, resilience factors and ways of coping in 76 participants from 11 support groups. The findings of the study show gender differences on burden and learning style, moderately high caregiver resilence, use of both problem-focused and emotion-focused coping and moderate correlations between levels of resilience and specific use of coping strategies.

Ghatak, R. (1994). Effects of an intervention program on dementia patients and their caregivers. *Caring Magazine, 13*(8), 34-39.

Abstract: This study was designed to test the hypothesis that better caregiver training will lead to positive outcomes in caregivers and patients with dementia. An intervention program called the Awareness Training Problem solving was used with 40 families. The scores revealed that the experimental groups had a positive outcome in patient orientation, patient behavior, and caregiver stress.

Martichuski, D. K., Knight, B. J., Karlin, N. J., & Bell, P. A. (1997). Correlates of Alzheimer's disease caregivers' support group attendance. *Activities, Adaptation, and Aging, 21*(4), 27-40.

Abstract: In order to help alleviate some of the burden experienced by caregivers, professional services may be offered, including: educational programs, skills training and support groups. Support groups are the most common, but often not attended. This study examined attendance statistics and caregiver perception of stress and support. 'Nevers' felt less stress and burden than 'currents'. This may be due to the different characteristics that people that do and do not attend support groups exhibit. Various reasons were given: logistical problems, personal, and social.

Mittelman, M. S., Ferris, S. H. Shulman, E., Steinberg, G., & Levin, B. (1996). A family intervention to delay nursing home placement of patients with Alzheimer disease. *Journal of the American Medical Association, 276*(21), 1725-1731.

Abstract: This study was designed to deterine the long-term effectiveness of comprehensive support and counseling for spouse-caregivers and families in postponing or preventing nursing home placement of patients with Alzheimer's disease. There were 206 volunteer participants. The intervention involved six caregiver counseling sessions. The results showed that the median time of postponement was 329 days longer in the treatment group than the control group.

Spaid, W. M. & Barusch, A. S. (1992). Social support and caregiver strain: types and sources of social contacts of elderly caregivers. *Journal of Gerontological Social Work, 18*(1/2), 151-161.

Abstract: In this study, the associations between sense of strain and three types of social support are described for a sample of 121 spouse caregivers. They found that adverse social contacts were associated with increased strain, while positive contacts were insignificant. The findings also emphasized the importance of interventions which include friends, neighbors and others.

APPENDIX

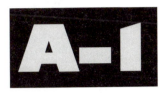

Web Addresses of Selected Professional Associations

► **American Academy of Medical Acupuncture**
http://www.medicalacupuncture.org/

► **American Academy of Physician Assistants**
http://www.aapa.org/

► **American Association for Respiratory Care Therapy**
http://www.aarc.org/

► **American Association of University Affiliated Programs (AAUAP)**
http://www.aauap.org/

► **American Association on Mental Retardation (AAMR)**
http://www.aamr.org/

► **American Chiropractic Association**
http://www.amerchiro.org/

► **American Dental Association**
http://www.ada.org/

► **American Dietetic Association**
http://www.eatright.org/

► **American Health Information Management Association (Medical Records)**
http://www.ahima.org/

► **American Hospital Association**
http://www.aha.org/

► **American Medical Association**
http://www.ama-assn.org

► **American Nurses Association**
http://www.nursingworld.org/

► **American Occupational Therapy Association (AOTA)**
http://www.aota.org/

► **American Optometric Association**
http://www.aoanet.org/

► **American Orthotic and Prosthetic Association**
http://www.oandp.com/organiza/aaop/no/aopa.htm

► **American Osteopathic Association**
http://www.aoa-net.org/

► **American Pharmaceutical Association**
http://www.aphanet.org/

► **American Physical Therapy Association**
http://www.apta.org/

► **American Podiatric Medical Association**
http://www.apma.org/

► **American Psychiatric Association**
http://www.appi.org/

► **American Psychological Association (APA)**
http://www.apa.org/

► **American Recreation Therapeutic Association (ARTA)**
http://www.atra-tr.org/

► **American Registry of Radiologic Technologists**
http://www.arrt.org/

▶ **American Speech–Language–Hearing Association (ASHA)**
http://www.asha.org/

▶ **American Society for Clinical Laboratory Science**
http://www.ascls.org/

▶ **Council for Exceptional Children (CEC; Special Education)**
http://www.cec.sped.org

▶ **National Association of School Psychologists (NASP)**
http://www.naspweb.org/

▶ **National Association of Social Workers**
http://www.naswdc.org/

▶ **National Rehabilitation Association (NRA)**
http://www.nationalrehab.org/website/index.html

▶ **Rehabilitation Engineering and Assistive Technology Society of North America (RESNA)**
http://www.resna.org/

APPENDIX

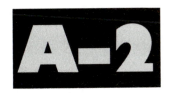

Selected List of Consumer Health Organizations

▶ **Alzheimer's Association**
http://www.alz.org/
▶ **American Cancer Society**
http://www.cancer.org/
index 4up.html
▶ **American Heart Association**
http://www.amhrt.org/
▶ **American Lung Association**
http://www.lungusa.org/
▶ **American Council of the Blind**
http://acb.org/
▶ **The Arc (Association for Retarded Citizens)**
http://theArc.org/
▶ **Arthritis Foundation**
http://www.arthritis.org/
▶ **Autism Society of America**
http://www.autism-society.org/
▶ **Brain Injury Association**
http://www.biausa.org/
▶ **Children with Attention Deficit Disorders (CHADD)**
http://chadd.org/
▶ **Cystic Fibrosis Foundation (CFF)**
http://www.cff.org/
▶ **Epilepsy Foundation of America**
http://www.efa.org/

▶ **Learning Disabilities Association**
http://www.ldanatl.org/
▶ **Muscular Dystrophy Association**
http://mdausa.org/
▶ **National Alliance for the Mentally Ill**
http://www.nami.org/
▶ **National Association of People with AIDS (NAPWA)**
http://www.napwa.org/
▶ **National Easter Seal Society (NESS)**
http://www.ness.org/
▶ **National Multiple Sclerosis Society**
http://www.nmss.org/
▶ **National Stroke Association**
http://www.stroke.org/
▶ **Spinal Injuries Associations**
http://www.spinal.co.uk/
▶ **Spina Bifida Association of America (SBAA)**
http://www.sbaa.org/
▶ **The Association for the Severely Handicapped (TASH)**
http://www.tash.org/
▶ **United Cerebral Palsy Association**
http://www.ucp.org

APPENDIX

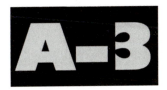

Commonly Used Medical Abbreviations

/d	per day	EEG	electroencephalogram
a	of each	EMG	electromyogram
a.c.	before a meal	ER	emergency room
ACTH	adrenocorticotropic hormone	FAS	fetal alcohol syndrome
ad lib.	freely	GBS	Guillain-Barre Syndrome
ADA	Americans with Disabilities Act	GI	gastrointestinal
ADD	attention deficit disorder	HIV	human immunodeficiency virus
ADHD	attention-deficit hyperactivity disorder	IDEA	Individuals with Disabilities Education Act of 1990
admov.	Apply	IEP	Individualized Education Plan
AIDS	acquired immuno deficiency syndrome	IFSP	Individualized Family Service Plan
ALS	amyotrophic lateral sclerosis	IM	intramuscular
alt.dieb	every other day	in d.	daily
ap	before dinner	IQ	intelligence quotient
b.i.d.	twice a day	ITP	Individualized Transition Plan
bib.	drink	IV	intravenous
bol.	pill	kg	kilogram
BP	blood pressure	lb	pound
c̄	with	MCP	metacarpophalangeal
CBC	complete blood count	MD	muscular dystrophy
CMC	carpometacarpal joint	MED	minimum effective dose
CNS	central nervous system	MMR	measles-mumps-rubella vaccine
CP	cerebral palsy	MR	mental retardation
CSF	cerebrospinal fluid	MS	multiple sclerosis
CVA	cerebro vascular accident	p	after
D and C	dilatation and curettage	p.c.	after meals
DIP	distal interphalangeal	PIP	proximal interphalangeal
Dx	diagnosis	p.r.n.	as needed
ECG	electrocardiogram	q.h.	every hour
ECT	electroconvulsive therapy	q.i.d.	four times a day
ED	emergency departure	quotid	everyday

RBC	red blood cells		sine	without
REM	rapid eye movement		SCI	spinal cord injury
RESNA	Rehabilitation Engineering and Assistive Technology Society of North America		STD	sexually transmitted disease
			t.i.d.	three times a day
			TBI	traumatic brain injury

APPENDIX

Landmarks in the History of Occupational Therapy

1752   Pennsylvania Hospital in Philadelphia established. Psychiatric patients were prescribed manual labor to counteract disease process.

1780   Clement-Joseph Tissot, a French physician in the cavalry, published a book prescribing the use of crafts and recreational activities for individuals with muscle and joint injuries.

1786   Philippe Pinel, a French psychiatrist in the Bicetre Asylum for the insane, prescribed humane treatment in the care of the mentally ill, including physical exercises, manual occupation, and music.

1803   Johanann Christian Reil, a German psychiatrist, advocated that activities such as swimming, dancing, gymnastics, arts and crafts, music, and theater be part of the everyday routine for patients.

1812   Benjamin Rush, the father of American psychiatry prescribed work, leisure activities, chess and other board games, exercise, and theatre for treatment of mental illness.

1813   Samuel Tuke, an English Quaker, founded the Retreat Asylum for the Insane in York, England. Tuke introduced the term *moral treatment* which was the application of humane practices—including exercise, recreation, arts and crafts, gardening, and regular employment—in the maintenance of the hospital.

1833   Samuel Woodard, a physician at the Worcester State Lunatic Hospital in Massachusetts, introduced the term *occupational therapy* as a therapeutic method to keep inmates active in varied tasks and leisure activities in regular routines. The therapeutic program was effective and produced a significant recovery rate.

1838   Jean Etienne Esquirol, a French psychiatrist, described the importance of corporal exercise, horseback riding, tennis, fencing, swimming, and travel for the treatment of depression.

1840   Francois Leuret, a French psychiatrist, advanced that moral treatment, including arts and crafts and work, are effective in treating individuals with mental illness and mental retardation.

1843   Dorothea Dix, a social reformer, worked diligently in the United States for humanistic care for individuals with mental illness, which included the use of therapeutic activities.

1854   Thomas Kirkbride, one of the founders of the American Psychiatric Association advocated a highly structured regimen for patients that included exercise, lectures, music, arts and crafts, and entertainment.

1895   William Rush Dunton, a psychiatrist and innovator in applying occupational therapy, used arts-and-crafts activities at Sheppard and Pratt Asylum in Baltimore.

1895/1922   Adolph Meyer, a strong advocate of occupation, believed in a holistic approach to treatment centering sleep habits, nutrition, work, play, and socialization.

1895   Mary Potter Meyer, a social worker and wife of Adolph Meyer, used arts and crafts activities in the State Hospital in Worcester, Massachusetts.

1904   Herbert Hall, a physician, prescribed occupation as a medicine to regulate the life and direct interests of the pa-

tient. He called this the "work cure."

1905   Susan Tracy, a nurse, applied occupational therapy activities in working with individuals with mental illness while she was director of the Training School for Nurses at the Adams Nervine Asylum in Boston.

1906   Herbert Hall was awarded a grant of $1,000 by Harvard University to study the application of activities and graded manual occupation in the treatment of psychiatric disorders.

1908   Training courses in occupations for hospital attendants were initiated at Chicago School of Civics and Philanthropy.

1909   Clifford Beers, founder of the National Committee for Mental Hygiene, described his emotional illness in the book, *A Mind that Found Itself* (1908). Beers reinforced the application of therapeutic activities in treating individuals with mental illness.

1910   Susan Tracy authored the first book on occupation studies, *Invalid Occupations: A Manual for Nurses and Attendants.*

1911   Susan Tracy initiated the first course on occupation in a general hospital at Massachusetts General Hospital in Boston.

1911   Eleanor Clark Slagle, a social worker, established an occupation department at Phipps Psychiatric Clinic at Johns Hopkins University in Baltimore.

1914   George Edward Barton, an architect who had contracted tuberculosis, introduced the term *occupational therapy* at a meeting in Boston of hospital workers.

1917   The National Society for the Promotion of Occupational Therapy was founded in Consolation House in Clifton Springs, New York. The charter members included George Barton, an architect; Eleanor Clark Slagle, a social worker at Hull House, Chicago; Thomas Kidner, vocational specialist from Canada; William Rush Dunton, a psychiatrist at Sheppard and Pratt Hospital in Baltimore; Susan Cox Johnson, an arts and crafts instructor from New York City; Isabel Newton; and Susan B. Tracy, a nurse at theAdams Nervine Asylum in Boston. This meeting led to the occupational therapy profession.

1917   Reconstruction aides were recruited to serve in army hospitals during World War I, applying arts and crafts and exercises in the treatment of physical and mental disorders.

1918   Educational training programs in occupational therapy were established at the Henry B. Favil School in Chicago, Teachers College of Columbia University, and the Boston School of Occupational Therapy.

1919   Bird T. Baldwin authored the *Army Manual on Occupational Therapy* that included information on evaluation and treatment procedures for the restoration of physical function.

1919   George Barton wrote the book *Teaching the Sick, A Manual of Occupational Therapy as Reeducation.*

1922   The Archives of Occupational Therapy was published and became the official journal of the American Association of Occupational Therapy.

1928   Six programs were available to prepare occupational therapists:

Boston School

Philadelphia School

St. Louis School

Milwaukee-Downer College

University of Minnesota

University of Toronto

1931   National registry for the American Occupational Therapy was established.

1933   The American Medical Association (AMA) began the accreditation of occupational therapy programs

1934   Essentials of an acceptable education in occupational therapy adopted by the Council on Medical Education and Hospitals.

1939   Among all AMA-approved hospitals, 13% employed occupational therapists.

1943   The Barden-LaFollette Vocational Rehabilitation Act was passed by Congress providing coverage of medical services including occupational therapy for individuals in vocational rehabilitation programs.

1945 — There were 18 approved programs in occupational therapy in the United States compared with 5 in 1940.

1947 — The first national registration examination for occupational therapists was given

1947 — Advanced master's degree in occupational therapy was offered at the University of Southern California and New York University.

1947 — Helen Willard and Clare S. Spackman, occupational therapy educators, authored the first textbook in occupational therapy.

1952 — The World Federation of Occupational Therapists was established. The founding member countries included Australia, Canada, Denmark, Great Britain, India, Israel, New Zealand, South Africa, Sweden, and the United States.

1964 — Certified occupational therapists assistants (COTAs) were certified in the United States.

1964 — The first entry-level master's program in occupational therapy was established at the University of Southern California. Shortly thereafter, basic master's programs were begun at Boston University and Virginia Commonwealth University.

1965 — The American Occupational Therapy Foundation (AOTF) was established as philanthropic organization for advancing the science of occupational therapy.

1973 — The Rehabilitation Act passed by Congress protecting the rights of persons with disabilities (Section 504).

1974 — New York University developed the first doctoral program in occupational therapy.

1975 — Education for All Handicapped Children Act (P.L. 94-142) facilitated free appropriate public education services for students with disabilities at all levels and provided funding for these services. The concept of least restrictive environment, inherent in the law, specifies that students with disabilities are educated with typical students "to the maximum extent possible."

1976 — Support was given to students for development of their organization on a national level, which was later named the American Student Occupational Therapy Alliance.

1979 — "Uniform Terminology System for Reporting Occupational Therapy Services" was developed and adopted by the Representative Assembly (RA).

1980 — AOTF published the *Occupational Therapy Journal of Research*.

1981 — Entry level Role Delineation for OTRs and COTAs adopted by RA.

1986 — Medicare amendments expanded coverage for occupational therapy services under Part B.

1990 — The Americans with Disabilities Act (ADA) was passed by Congress and signed by President Bush. The ADA guarantees equal opportunity for individuals with disabilities in employment, public accommodations, transportation, governmental services and telecommunications.

1990   P. L. 94-142 was reauthorized and renamed the Individuals with Disabilities Education Act (IDEA). This law continued federal funding from 94-142, and increased services by adding related services, transition from school to work, and parental involvement. Under this act, occupational therapy is considered a related service in helping students with disabilities in public schools.

1991   RA approved a physical agent modalities (PAMS) position paper that recommended the use of PAMS as an adjunct to purposeful activity to enhance occupational performance.

1994   *Occupational Therapy International* is founded as the first refereed journal publishing manuscripts by occupational therapists throughout the world

1997   The Balanced Budget Act PL 105-33 (BBA) significantly changed the procedures for payment of services for rehabilitation personnel affecting the quality of care, especially in home health.

1999   The RA passes a resolution to mandate that entry-level education in occupational therapy should be at the masters level.

APPENDIX

Statistical Tables

Table C–I Random Numbers

42633	85191	32547	32269	10908	35182	00284	99873	95254	40027
06209	88389	48024	95890	13292	16221	27782	09404	40189	48909
85898	48518	01214	37532	90850	17004	38953	45438	71640	84200
17400	40484	58975	03822	00198	62540	08208	82205	89763	44359
51364	07817	74822	95198	34819	25405	83700	05230	69497	61566
34213	08216	46959	13598	89666	28787	66484	82557	48150	81122
70400	43058	48979	96808	25443	34465	20115	42316	34080	41474
84299	66933	75092	83971	93540	05376	65480	75168	17532	63121
78898	16916	73510	63004	50028	20628	69911	83874	87816	79883
41147	30346	83101	00871	60805	91507	83296	18837	19083	77353
69188	42697	29250	11798	51714	62164	43985	70541	33481	30840
22989	80881	71584	41438	05866	37535	09563	42476	07407	91274
40099	81818	05353	98309	06652	34581	86018	52315	37575	79671
02452	17310	90430	14091	83717	99672	95237	79317	88585	80219
46530	90762	26018	96366	24901	16410	56321	00532	06681	12892
44577	11687	48201	99119	40613	09780	73211	22183	21860	24967
64872	97263	57319	39577	05130	36644	29826	94473	03378	10981
56857	78071	16266	99378	33372	14342	08779	49183	00800	07549
99752	05537	86961	06577	12200	05373	93315	11706	27400	01408
39304	76855	56687	29105	10115	23621	58117	65234	13430	36956
73023	80267	60894	25405	86174	77846	40441	04687	82391	67259
98011	28318	34823	05844	04665	24591	83957	90698	86199	36384
42788	15532	41566	31167	86497	93622	91529	32847	30910	43211
75472	52144	60842	11490	45700	03259	51719	03704	49174	37430
89811	97066	95603	16941	51187	08668	54111	91978	73757	93861
04777	69628	82825	68993	23145	77347	13748	29433	35462	99406
02313	39086	77605	25713	47946	13783	14899	41976	61464	83912
58476	04674	79654	75772	65232	56555	70766	18024	66966	52512
49864	49565	70584	31605	92906	39582	02907	25963	30476	47285
69315	87419	87510	51040	14911	03129	50254	79739	67229	14317
81086	71619	02829	13270	92828	65769	63155	29682	96185	41238
29540	79599	46241	19956	31435	44347	49646	44797	16704	10947
78091	53339	11535	79479	58427	81372	49797	68726	00013	55003
89736	90234	44334	88512	37652	31853	93140	50757	67760	65361
08245	09009	11510	84653	30109	33482	14014	20335	41614	78466

Source: The table was generated by Y. L. Lio, Department of Mathematics, University of South Dakota, using the software in IMSL statistical library.

Table C–2 Proportion of Areas Under the Normal Curve (Percentile Rank)

z	0.00	0.01	0.02	0.03	0.04	0.05	0.06	0.07	0.08	0.09
0.00	.5000	.5040	.5080	.5120	.5160	.5199	.5239	.5279	.5319	.5359
0.10	.5398	.5438	.5478	.5517	.5557	.5596	.5636	.5675	.5714	.5753
0.20	.5793	.5832	.5871	.5910	.5948	.5987	.6026	.6064	.6103	.6141
0.30	.6179	.6217	.6255	.6293	.6331	.6368	.6406	.6443	.6480	.6517
0.40	.6554	.6591	.6628	.6664	.6700	.6736	.6772	.6808	.6844	.6879
0.50	.6915	.6950	.6985	.7019	.7054	.7088	.7123	.7157	.7190	.7224
0.60	.7257	.7291	.7324	.7357	.7389	.7422	.7454	.7486	.7517	.7549
0.70	.7580	.7611	.7642	.7673	.7704	.7734	.7764	.7794	.7823	.7852
0.80	.7881	.7910	.7939	.7967	.7995	.8023	.8051	.8078	.8106	.8133
0.90	.8159	.8186	.8212	.8238	.8264	.8289	.8315	.8340	.8365	.8389
1.00	.8413	.8438	.8461	.8485	.8508	.8531	.8554	.8577	.8599	.8621
1.10	.8643	.8665	.8686	.8708	.8729	.8749	.8770	.8790	.8810	.8830
1.20	.8849	.8869	.8888	.8907	.8925	.8944	.8962	.8980	.8997	.9015
1.30	.9032	.9049	.9066	.9082	.9099	.9115	.9131	.9147	.9162	.9177
1.40	.9192	.9207	.9222	.9236	.9251	.9265	.9279	.9292	.9306	.9319
1.50	.9332	.9345	.9357	.9370	.9382	.9394	.9406	.9418	.9429	.9441
1.60	.9452	.9463	.9474	.9484	.9495	.9505	.9515	.9525	.9535	.9545
1.70	.9554	.9564	.9573	.9582	.9591	.9599	.9608	.9616	.9625	.9633
1.80	.9641	.9649	.9656	.9664	.9671	.9678	.9686	.9693	.9699	.9706
1.90	.9713	.9719	.9726	.9732	.9738	.9744	.9750	.9756	.9761	.9767
2.00	.9772	.9778	.9783	.9788	.9793	.9798	.9803	.9808	.9812	.9817
2.10	.9821	.9826	.9830	.9834	.9838	.9842	.9846	.9850	.9850	.9857
2.20	.9861	.9864	.9868	.9871	.9875	.9878	.9881	.9884	.9887	.9890
2.30	.9893	.9896	.9898	.9901	.9904	.9906	.9909	.9911	.9913	.9916
2.40	.9918	.9920	.9922	.9925	.9927	.9929	.9931	.9932	.9934	.9936
2.50	.9938	.9940	.9941	.9943	.9945	.9946	.9948	.9949	.9951	.9952
2.60	.9953	.9955	.9956	.9957	.9959	.9960	.9961	.9962	.9963	.9964
2.70	.9965	.9966	.9967	.9968	.9969	.9970	.9971	.9972	.9973	.9974
2.80	.9974	.9975	.9976	.9977	.9977	.9978	.9979	.9979	.9980	.9981
2.90	.9981	.9982	.9982	.9983	.9984	.9984	.9985	.9985	.9986	.9986
3.00	.9987	.9987	.9987	.9988	.9988	.9989	.9989	.9989	.9990	.9990
3.10	.9990	.9991	.9991	.9991	.9992	.9992	.9992	.9992	.9993	.9993
3.20	.9993	.9993	.9994	.9994	.9994	.9994	.9994	.9995	.9995	.9995
3.30	.9995	.9995	.9995	.9996	.9996	.9996	.9996	.9996	.9996	.9997
3.40	.9997	.9997	.9997	.9997	.9997	.9997	.9997	.9997	.9997	.9998
3.50	.9998	.9998	.9998	.9998	.9998	.9998	.9998	.9998	.9998	.9998
3.60	.9998	.9998	.9999	.9999	.9999	.9999	.9999	.9999	.9999	.9999
3.70	.9999	.9999	.9999	.9999	.9999	.9999	.9999	.9999	.9999	.9999
3.80	.9999	.9999	.9999	.9999	.9999	.9999	.9999	.9999	.9999	.9999

Note: z score values are given for two places after the decimal point. For example, a *z* score of 1.03 represents .8485 proportion of the normal curve or percentile rank.

Source: Adapted from Table 1.1 The Normal Distribution and Related Functions, *Handbook of Statistical Tables* (pp. 3–10), by D. B. Owen, 1962, Reading, MA: Addison-Wesley. Reprinted with permission of the publisher.

Table C–3 Critical Values for *t* Test

df	Level of significance for one-tailed test				
	.10	.05	.025	.01	.005
	Level of significance for two-tailed test				
	.20	.10	.05	.02	.01
1	3.0777	6.3138	12.7062	31.8207	63.6574
2	1.8856	2.9200	4.3027	6.9646	9.9248
3	1.6377	2.3534	3.1824	4.5407	5.8409
4	1.5332	2.1318	2.7764	3.7469	4.6041
5	1.4759	2.0150	2.5706	3.3649	4.0322
6	1.4398	1.9432	2.4469	3.1427	3.7074
7	1.4149	1.8946	2.3646	2.9980	3.4995
8	1.3968	1.8595	2.3060	2.8965	3.3554
9	1.3830	1.8331	2.2622	2.8214	3.2498
10	1.3722	1.8125	2.2281	2.7638	3.1693
11	1.3634	1.7959	2.2010	2.7181	3.1058
12	1.3562	1.7823	2.1788	2.6810	3.0545
13	1.3502	1.7709	2.1604	2.6503	3.0123
14	1.3450	1.7613	2.1448	2.6245	2.9768
15	1.3406	1.7531	2.1315	2.6025	2.9467
16	1.3368	1.7459	2.1199	2.5835	2.9208
17	1.3334	1.7396	2.1098	2.5669	2.8982
18	1.3304	1.7341	2.1009	2.5524	2.8784
19	1.3277	1.7291	2.0930	2.5395	2.8609
20	1.3253	1.7247	2.0860	2.5280	2.8453
21	1.3232	1.7207	2.0796	2.5177	2.8314
22	1.3212	1.7171	2.0739	2.5083	2.8188
23	1.3195	1.7139	2.0687	2.4999	2.8073
24	1.3178	1.7109	2.0639	2.4922	2.7969
25	1.3163	1.7081	2.0595	2.4851	2.7874
26	1.3150	1.7056	2.0555	2.4786	2.7787
27	1.3137	1.7033	2.0518	2.4727	2.7707
28	1.3125	1.7011	2.0484	2.4671	2.7633
29	1.3114	1.6991	2.0452	2.4620	2.7564
30	1.3104	1.6973	2.0423	2.4573	2.7500
40	1.3031	1.6839	2.0211	2.4233	2.7045
50	1.2987	1.6759	2.0086	2.4033	2.6778
60	1.2958	1.6706	2.0003	2.3901	2.6603
70	1.2938	1.6669	1.9944	2.3808	2.6479
90	1.2910	1.6620	1.9867	2.3685	2.6316
120	1.2886	1.6577	1.9799	2.3578	2.6174
—	1.2816	1.6449	1.9600	2.3263	2.5758

Source: Adapted from Table 2.1 Critical Values for Students t-Distribution, by D. B. Owen, 1962, *Handbook of Statistical Tables.* Reading, MA: Addison-Wesley. Reprinted with permission of the publisher.

Steps in Determining Critical Values for *t* for Table C–3.

1. Calculate the degrees of freedom (*df*):

- In one-sample *t* test it is number of cases of the sample minus 1
- In paired-data of correlated *t* test it is number of pairs minus 1
- In independent *t* test it is number of cases in $N_1 + N_2$ minus 2

2. Determine if hypothesis is one-tailed or two-tailed test.
3. Establish level of significance (.05 or .01)
4. Locate *t* critical (crit) value:

$$e.g., 10 \; df, \text{ two-tailed test, } .05 \text{ level}$$
$$t_{crit} = 2.28$$

5. Note that these critical values are the same for negative or positive numbers.
6. Calculate *t* observed (obs) from formulas for three *t* tests.
7. Decision rule:

- If t_{obs} is equal to or above t_{crit} then reject the null hypothesis.
- If t_{obs} is below t_{crit} then accept the null hypothesis.

Table C–4 Critical Values for F (Analysis of Variance, ANOVA)

df Associated with the Denominator		1	2	3	4	5	6	7	8	9
					df Associated with the Numerator					
1	5%	161	200	216	225	230	234	237	239	241
	1%	4052	5000	5403	5625	5764	5859	5928	5982	6022
2	5%	18.5	19.0	19.2	19.2	19.3	19.3	19.4	19.4	19.4
	1%	98.5	99.0	99.2	99.2	99.3	99.3	99.4	99.4	99.4
3	5%	10.1	9.55	9.28	9.12	9.01	8.94	8.89	8.85	8.81
	1%	34.1	30.8	29.5	28.7	28.2	27.9	27.7	27.5	27.3
4	5%	7.71	6.94	6.59	6.39	6.26	6.16	6.09	6.04	6.00
	1%	21.2	18.0	16.7	16.0	15.5	15.2	15.0	14.8	14.7
5	5%	6.61	5.79	5.41	5.19	5.05	4.95	4.88	4.82	4.77
	1%	16.3	13.3	12.1	11.4	11.0	10.7	10.5	10.3	10.2
6	5%	5.99	5.14	4.76	4.53	4.39	4.28	4.21	4.15	4.10
	1%	13.7	10.9	9.78	9.15	8.75	8.47	8.26	8.10	7.98
7	5%	5.59	4.74	4.35	4.12	3.97	3.87	3.79	3.73	3.68
	1%	12.2	9.55	8.45	7.85	7.46	7.19	6.99	6.84	6.72
8	5%	5.32	4.46	4.07	3.84	3.69	3.58	3.50	3.44	3.39
	1%	11.3	8.65	7.59	7.01	6.63	6.37	6.18	6.03	5.91
9	5%	5.12	4.26	3.86	3.63	3.48	3.37	3.29	3.23	3.18
	1%	10.6	8.02	6.99	6.42	6.06	5.80	5.61	5.47	5.35
10	5%	4.96	4.10	3.71	3.48	3.33	3.22	3.14	3.07	3.02
	1%	10.0	7.56	6.55	5.99	5.64	5.39	5.20	5.06	4.94
11	5%	4.84	3.98	3.49	3.26	3.11	3.00	2.91	2.85	2.80
	1%	9.65	7.21	6.22	5.67	5.32	5.07	4.89	4.74	4.63
12	5%	4.75	3.89	3.49	3.26	3.11	3.00	2.91	2.85	2.80
	1%	9.33	6.93	5.95	5.41	5.06	4.82	4.64	4.50	4.39
13	5%	4.67	3.81	3.41	3.18	3.03	2.92	2.83	2.77	2.71
	1%	9.07	6.70	5.74	5.21	4.86	4.62	4.44	4.30	4.19
14	5%	4.60	3.74	3.34	3.11	2.96	2.85	2.76	2.70	2.65
	1%	8.86	6.51	5.56	5.04	4.70	4.46	4.28	4.14	4.03
15	5%	4.54	3.68	3.29	3.06	2.90	2.79	2.71	2.64	2.59
	1%	8.68	6.36	5.42	4.89	4.56	4.32	4.14	4.00	3.89
16	5%	4.49	3.63	3.24	3.01	2.85	2.74	2.66	2.59	2.54
	1%	8.53	6.23	5.29	4.77	4.44	4.20	4.03	3.89	3.78
17	5%	4.45	3.59	3.20	2.96	2.81	2.70	2.61	2.55	2.49
	1%	8.40	6.11	5.18	4.67	4.34	4.10	3.93	3.79	3.68
18	5%	4.41	3.55	3.16	2.93	2.77	2.66	2.58	2.51	2.46
	1%	8.29	6.01	5.09	4.58	4.25	4.01	3.84	3.71	3.60
19	5%	4.38	3.52	3.13	2.90	2.74	2.63	2.54	2.48	2.42
	1%	8.18	5.93	5.01	4.50	4.17	3.94	3.77	3.63	3.52

(continued)

Table C–4 Critical Values for F (Analysis of Variance, ANOVA) *(continued)*

df Associated with the Denominator		df Associated with the Numerator								
		1	2	3	4	5	6	7	8	9
21	5%	4.32	3.47	3.07	2.84	2.68	2.57	2.49	2.42	2.37
	1%	8.02	5.78	4.87	4.37	4.04	3.81	3.64	3.51	3.40
22	5%	4.30	3.44	3.05	2.82	2.66	2.55	2.46	2.40	2.34
	1%	7.95	5.72	4.82	4.31	3.99	3.76	3.59	3.45	3.35
23	5%	4.28	3.42	3.03	2.80	2.64	2.53	2.44	2.37	2.32
	1%	7.88	5.66	4.76	4.26	3.94	3.71	3.54	3.41	3.30
24	5%	4.26	3.40	3.01	2.78	2.62	2.51	2.42	2.36	2.30
	1%	7.82	5.61	4.72	4.22	3.90	3.67	3.50	3.36	3.26
25	5%	4.24	3.39	2.99	2.76	2.60	2.49	2.40	2.34	2.28
	1%	7.77	5.57	4.68	4.18	3.86	3.63	3.46	3.32	3.22
26	5%	4.23	3.37	2.98	2.74	2.59	2.47	2.39	2.32	2.27
	1%	7.72	5.53	4.64	4.14	3.82	3.59	3.42	3.29	3.18
27	5%	4.21	3.35	2.96	2.73	2.57	2.46	2.37	2.31	2.25
	1%	7.68	5.49	4.60	4.11	3.78	3.56	3.39	3.26	3.15
28	5%	4.20	3.34	2.95	2.71	2.56	2.45	2.36	2.29	2.24
	1%	7.64	5.45	4.57	4.07	3.75	3.53	3.36	3.23	3.12
29	5%	4.18	3.33	2.93	2.70	2.55	2.43	2.35	2.28	2.22
	1%	7.60	5.42	4.54	4.04	3.73	3.50	3.33	3.20	3.09
30	5%	4.17	3.32	2.92	2.69	2.53	2.42	2.33	2.27	2.21
	1%	7.56	5.39	4.51	4.02	3.70	3.47	3.30	3.17	3.07
40	5%	4.08	3.23	2.84	2.61	2.45	2.34	2.25	2.18	2.12
	1%	7.31	5.18	4.31	3.83	3.51	3.29	3.12	2.99	2.89
60	5%	4.00	3.15	2.76	2.53	2.37	2.25	2.17	2.10	2.04
	1%	7.08	4.98	4.13	3.65	3.34	3.12	2.95	2.82	2.72
120	5%	3.92	3.07	2.68	2.45	2.29	2.18	2.09	2.02	1.96
	1%	6.85	4.79	3.95	3.48	3.17	2.96	2.79	2.66	2.56

Source: Adapted from "Tables of Percentage Points of the Inverted Beta (F) Distribution," by M. Merrington and C.M. Thompson, 1943, *Biometrika, 33,* pp. 73–88. Reprinted with permission of the publisher.

Steps in Determining Critical Values for *F* for Table C–4.

1. Calculate the degrees of freedom (*df*) for numerator and denominator:

- The *df* for numerator is derived from the number of groups in the study minus 1. For example, if three treatment methods are being compared, then *df* equals 3 minus 1, or 2 df, for numerator.
- The df for denominator is derived from the total number of subjects in all groups being compared minus the number of groups. For example for three treatment methods with 6 subjects in each group the df for the denominator will equal 18 minus 3, or 15 df.

2. Apply the level of significance, such as .05 or .01.
3. Locate critical value of F.

    e.g., *df* equals 2/15 at .05 level then $F_{crit} = 3.68$.

4. Calculate F_{obs} for data.
5. Decision rule:

    • If F_{obs} is equal to or above F_{crit} then reject the null hypothesis.
    • If F_{obs} is below F_{crit} accept the null hypothesis.

Table C–5 Critical Values for the Pearson Product–Moment Correlation Coefficient

	Level of significance for one-tailed test					
	.25	.10	.05	.025	.01	.005
	Level of significance for two-tailed test					
df	.50	.20	.10	.05	.02	.01
1	0.7071	0.9511	0.9877	0.9969	0.9995	0.9999
2	0.5000	0.8000	0.9000	0.9500	0.9800	0.9900
3	0.4040	0.6870	0.8054	0.8783	0.9343	0.9587
4	0.3473	0.6084	0.7293	0.8114	0.8822	0.9172
5	0.3091	0.5509	0.6694	0.7545	0.8329	0.8745
6	0.2811	0.5067	0.6215	0.7067	0.7887	0.8343
7	0.2596	0.4716	0.5822	0.6664	0.7498	0.7977
8	0.2423	0.4428	0.5493	0.6319	0.7155	0.7646
9	0.2281	0.4187	0.5214	0.6021	0.6851	0.7348
10	0.2161	0.3981	0.4973	0.5760	0.6581	0.7079
11	0.2058	0.3802	0.4762	0.5529	0.6339	0.6835
12	0.1968	0.3646	0.4575	0.5324	0.6120	0.6614
13	0.1890	0.3507	0.4409	0.5140	0.5923	0.6411
14	0.1820	0.3383	0.4259	0.4973	0.5742	0.6226
15	0.1757	0.3271	0.4124	0.4822	0.5577	0.6055
16	0.1700	0.3170	0.4000	0.4683	0.5426	0.5897
17	0.1649	0.3077	0.3887	0.4555	0.5285	0.5751
18	0.1602	0.2992	0.3783	0.4438	0.5155	0.5614
19	0.1558	0.2914	0.3687	0.4329	0.5034	0.5487
20	0.1518	0.2841	0.3598	0.4227	0.4921	0.5368
21	0.1481	0.2774	0.3515	0.4132	0.4815	0.5256
22	0.1447	0.2711	0.3438	0.4044	0.4716	0.5151
23	0.1415	0.2653	0.3365	0.3961	0.4622	0.5052
28	0.1281	0.2407	0.3061	0.3610	0.4226	0.4629
33	0.1179	0.2220	0.2826	0.3338	0.3916	0.4296
38	0.1098	0.2070	0.2638	0.3120	0.3665	0.4026
43	0.1032	0.1947	0.2483	0.2940	0.3457	0.3801
48	0.0976	0.1843	0.2353	0.2787	0.3281	0.3610
58	0.0888	0.1678	0.2144	0.2542	0.2997	0.3301
68	0.0820	0.1550	0.1982	0.2352	0.2776	0.3060
78	0.0765	0.1448	0.1852	0.2199	0.2597	0.2864
88	0.0720	0.1364	0.1745	0.2072	0.2449	0.2702
98	0.0682	0.1292	0.1654	0.1966	0.2324	0.2565

Source: Adapted from Table 19.1 Critical Values for the Product–Moment Correlation Coefficient, *Handbook of Statistical Tables*, (pp. 509–510), by D. B. Owen, 1962. Reading, MA: Addison-Wesley. Reprinted with permission of the publisher.

Steps in Determining Critical Values for Pearson *r* for Table C–5.

1. Determine the number of variables being correlated. For example if $x = 20$ and $y = 20$, then $n = 20$.
2. Determine if hypothesis calls for a one-tailed or two-tailed test. Usually a null hypothesis indicates a one-tailed test and a directional hypothesis indicates a two-tailed test of significance.
3. Apply level of significance, for example, .05 or .01.
4. Locate critical value of r from statistical table. For example, with $n = 20$, two-tailed test, .05 level, then $r_{crit} = .4438$ df = 18.
5. Calculate r_{obs} from data.
6. Decision Rule:

- If r_{obs} is equal to or greater then r_{crit}, then reject null hypothesis.
- If r_{obs} is below r_{crit} then accept null hypothesis.

Table C–6 Spearman Rank Order Correlation Coefficient

	Level of significance for one-tailed test			
	.05	**.025**	**.01**	**.005**
	Level of significance for two-tailed test			
n*	**.10**	**.05**	**.02**	**.01**
5	.900	1.000	1.000	—
5	.900	1.000	1.000	—
6	.829	.886	.943	1.000
7	.714	.786	.893	.929
8	.643	.738	.833	.881
9	.600	.683	.783	.833
10	.564	.648	.746	.794
12	.506	.591	.712	.777
14	.456	.544	.645	.715
16	.425	.506	.601	.665
18	.399	.475	.564	.625
20	.377	.450	.534	.591
22	.359	.428	.508	.562
24	.343	.409	.485	.537
26	.329	.392	.465	.515
28	.317	.377	.448	.496
30	.306	.364	.432	.478

*n = number of pairs

Source: Adapted from "The 5 percent significance levels of sums of squares of rank differences and a correction," by E. G. Olds, 1949, *Annals of Mathematical Statistics, 20,* pp. 117–118; and "Distribution of the sum of squares of rank differences for small numbers of individuals," by E. G. Olds, 1938, *Annals of Mathematical Statistics, 9,* pp. 133–148; and *Fundamentals of Behavioral Statistics,* by R. P. Runyon and A. Haber, 1967, Reading, MA: Addison-Wesley. Reprinted with permission of the publishers.

Steps in Determining Critical Values for Spearman r_s (formerly rho) for Table C–6.

1. Determine the number of pairs of variables being correlated.
2. Determine if hypothesis calls for a one-tailed or two-tailed test.
3. Apply level of significance, .05 or .01
4. Locate critical value of r_s from statistical table. For example, with n = 12, two-tailed test, .05 level, then r_s critical = .591.
5. Calculate $r_{s\text{-obs}}$ from data.
6. Decision Rule:

   • If $r_{s\text{-obs}}$ is equal to or greater then $r_{s\,crit}$, then reject the null hypothesis.
   • If $r_{s\text{-obs}}$ is below rs crit then accept the null hypothesis.

Table C–7A Critical Values for the Mann-Whitney U Test[a]

n_B \ n_A	1	2	3	4	5	6	7	8	9	10	11	12	13	14	15	16	17	18	19	20
1	—	—	—	—	—	—	—	—	—	—	—	—	—	—	—	—	—	—	—	—
2	—	—	—	—	—	—	—	0/16	0/18	0/20	0/22	1/23	1/25	1/27	1/29	1/31	2/32	2/34	2/36	2/38
3	—	—	—	—	0/15	1/17	1/20	2/22	2/25	3/27	3/30	4/32	4/35	5/37	5/40	6/42	6/45	7/47	7/50	8/52
4	—	—	—	0/16	1/19	2/22	3/25	4/28	4/32	5/35	6/38	7/41	8/44	9/47	10/50	11/53	11/57	12/60	13/63	13/67
5	—	—	0/15	1/19	2/23	3/27	5/30	6/34	7/38	8/42	9/46	11/49	12/53	13/57	14/61	15/65	17/68	18/72	19/76	20/80
6	—	—	1/17	2/22	3/27	5/31	6/36	8/40	10/44	11/49	13/53	14/58	16/62	17/67	19/71	21/75	22/80	24/84	25/89	27/93
7	—	—	1/20	3/25	5/30	6/36	8/41	10/46	12/51	14/56	16/61	18/66	20/71	22/76	24/81	26/86	28/91	30/96	32/101	34/106
8	—	0/16	2/22	4/28	6/34	8/40	10/46	13/51	15/57	17/63	19/69	22/74	24/80	26/86	29/91	31/97	34/102	36/108	38/111	41/119
9	—	0/18	2/25	4/32	7/38	10/44	12/51	15/57	17/64	20/70	23/76	26/82	28/89	31/95	34/101	37/107	39/114	42/120	45/126	48/132
10	—	0/20	3/27	5/35	8/42	11/49	14/56	17/63	20/70	23/77	26/84	29/91	33/97	36/104	39/111	42/118	45/125	48/132	52/138	55/145
11	—	0/22	3/30	6/38	9/46	13/53	16/61	19/69	23/76	26/84	30/91	33/99	37/106	40/114	44/121	47/129	51/136	55/143	58/151	62/158
12	—	1/23	4/32	7/41	11/49	14/58	18/66	22/74	26/82	29/91	33/99	37/107	41/115	45/123	49/131	53/139	57/147	61/155	65/163	69/171
13	—	1/25	4/35	8/44	12/53	16/62	20/71	24/80	28/89	33/97	37/106	41/115	45/124	50/132	54/141	59/149	63/158	67/167	72/175	76/184
14	—	1/27	5/37	9/47	13/57	17/67	22/76	26/86	31/95	36/104	40/114	45/123	50/132	55/141	59/151	64/160	67/171	74/178	78/188	83/197
15	—	1/29	5/40	10/50	14/61	19/71	24/81	29/91	34/101	39/111	44/121	49/131	54/141	59/151	64/161	70/170	75/180	80/190	85/200	90/210
16	—	1/31	6/42	11/53	15/65	21/75	26/86	31/97	37/107	42/118	47/129	53/139	59/149	64/160	70/170	75/181	81/191	86/202	92/212	98/222
17	—	2/32	6/45	11/57	17/68	22/80	28/91	34/102	39/114	45/125	51/136	57/147	63/158	67/171	75/180	81/191	87/202	93/213	99/224	105/235
18	—	2/34	7/47	12/60	18/72	24/84	30/96	36/108	42/120	48/132	55/143	61/155	67/167	74/178	80/190	86/202	93/213	99/225	106/236	112/248
19	—	2/36	7/50	13/63	19/76	25/89	32/101	38/114	45/126	52/138	58/151	65/163	72/175	78/188	85/200	92/212	99/224	106/236	113/248	119/261
20	—	2/38	8/52	13/67	20/80	27/93	34/106	41/119	48/132	55/145	62/158	69/171	76/184	83/197	90/210	98/222	105/235	112/248	119/261	127/273

[a] Test for a one-tailed test at .025 or a two-tailed test at .05. If the U_{obs} value falls within the two values in the table for n_A and n_B, do not reject the null hypothesis. If the U_{obs} is less than or equal to the lower value in the table or greater than or equal to the larger value in the table then reject the null hypothesis.

Source: "On a test of whether one of two random variables is stochastically larger than the other," by H. B. Mann and D. R. Whitney, 1947, *Annals of Mathematical Statistics,* (pp. 18, 52–54); Extended tables for the Mann-Whitney statistic, *Bulletin of the Institute of Educational Research at Indiana University,* 1, No. 2; and *Fundamentals of Behavioral Statistics,* by R. P. Runyon and A. Haber, 1967, Reading, MA: Addison-Wesley. Reprinted with permission of the publishers.

Table C–7B Critical Values for the Mann-Whitney U Test[b]

n_B \ n_A	1	2	3	4	5	6	7	8	9	10	11	12	13	14	15	16	17	18	19	20
1	—	—	—	—	—	—	—	—	—	—	—	—	—	—	—	—	—	—	0 / 19	0 / 20
2	—	—	—	—	0 / 10	0 / 12	0 / 14	1 / 15	1 / 17	1 / 19	1 / 21	2 / 22	2 / 24	2 / 26	3 / 27	3 / 29	3 / 31	4 / 32	4 / 34	4 / 36
3	—	—	0 / 9	0 / 12	1 / 14	2 / 16	2 / 19	3 / 21	3 / 24	4 / 26	5 / 28	5 / 31	6 / 33	7 / 35	7 / 38	8 / 40	9 / 42	9 / 45	10 / 47	11 / 49
4	—	—	0 / 12	1 / 15	2 / 18	3 / 21	4 / 24	5 / 27	6 / 30	7 / 33	8 / 36	9 / 39	10 / 42	11 / 45	12 / 48	14 / 50	15 / 53	16 / 56	17 / 59	18 / 62
5	—	0 / 10	1 / 14	2 / 18	4 / 21	5 / 25	6 / 29	8 / 32	9 / 36	11 / 39	12 / 43	13 / 47	15 / 50	16 / 54	18 / 57	19 / 61	20 / 65	22 / 68	23 / 72	25 / 75
6	—	0 / 12	2 / 16	3 / 21	5 / 25	7 / 29	8 / 34	10 / 38	12 / 42	14 / 46	16 / 50	17 / 55	19 / 59	21 / 63	23 / 67	25 / 71	26 / 76	28 / 80	30 / 84	32 / 88
7	—	0 / 14	2 / 19	4 / 24	6 / 29	8 / 34	11 / 38	13 / 43	15 / 48	17 / 53	19 / 58	21 / 63	24 / 67	26 / 72	28 / 77	30 / 82	33 / 86	35 / 91	37 / 96	39 / 101
8	—	1 / 15	3 / 21	5 / 27	8 / 32	10 / 38	13 / 43	15 / 49	18 / 54	20 / 60	23 / 65	26 / 70	28 / 76	31 / 81	33 / 87	36 / 92	39 / 97	41 / 103	44 / 108	47 / 113
9	—	1 / 17	3 / 24	6 / 30	9 / 36	12 / 42	15 / 48	18 / 54	21 / 60	24 / 66	27 / 72	30 / 78	33 / 84	36 / 90	39 / 96	42 / 102	45 / 108	48 / 114	51 / 120	54 / 126
10	—	1 / 19	4 / 26	7 / 33	11 / 39	14 / 46	17 / 53	20 / 60	24 / 66	27 / 73	31 / 79	34 / 86	37 / 93	41 / 99	44 / 106	48 / 112	51 / 119	55 / 125	58 / 132	62 / 138
11	—	1 / 21	5 / 28	8 / 36	12 / 43	16 / 50	19 / 58	23 / 65	27 / 72	31 / 79	34 / 87	38 / 94	42 / 101	46 / 108	50 / 115	54 / 122	57 / 130	61 / 137	65 / 144	69 / 151
12	—	2 / 22	5 / 31	9 / 39	13 / 47	17 / 55	21 / 63	26 / 70	30 / 78	34 / 86	38 / 94	42 / 102	47 / 109	51 / 117	55 / 125	60 / 132	64 / 140	68 / 148	72 / 156	77 / 163
13	—	2 / 24	6 / 33	10 / 42	15 / 50	19 / 59	24 / 67	28 / 76	33 / 84	37 / 93	42 / 101	47 / 109	51 / 118	56 / 126	61 / 134	65 / 143	70 / 151	75 / 159	80 / 167	84 / 176
14	—	2 / 26	7 / 35	11 / 45	16 / f54	21 / 63	26 / 72	31 / 81	36 / 90	41 / 99	46 / 108	51 / 117	56 / 126	61 / 135	66 / 144	71 / 153	77 / 161	82 / 170	87 / 179	92 / 188
15	—	3 / 27	7 / 38	12 / 48	18 / 57	23 / 67	28 / 77	33 / 87	39 / 96	44 / 106	50 / 115	55 / 125	61 / 134	66 / 144	72 / 153	77 / 163	83 / 172	88 / 182	94 / 191	100 / 200
16	—	3 / 29	8 / 40	14 / 50	19 / 61	25 / 71	30 / 82	36 / 92	42 / 102	48 / 112	54 / 122	60 / 132	65 / 143	71 / 153	77 / 163	83 / 173	89 / 183	95 / 193	101 / 203	107 / 213
17	—	3 / 31	9 / 42	15 / 53	20 / 65	26 / 76	33 / 86	39 / 97	45 / 108	51 / 119	57 / 130	64 / 140	70 / 151	77 / 161	83 / 172	89 / 183	96 / 193	102 / 204	109 / 214	115 / 225
18	—	4 / 32	9 / 45	16 / 56	22 / 68	28 / 80	35 / 91	41 / 103	48 / 114	55 / 123	61 / 137	68 / 148	75 / 159	82 / 170	88 / 182	95 / 193	102 / 204	109 / 215	116 / 226	123 / 237
19	0 / 19	4 / 34	10 / 47	17 / 59	23 / 72	30 / 84	37 / 96	44 / 108	51 / 120	58 / 132	65 / 144	72 / 156	80 / 167	87 / 179	94 / 191	101 / 203	109 / 214	116 / 226	123 / 238	130 / 250
20	0 / 20	4 / 36	11 / 49	18 / 62	25 / 75	32 / 88	39 / 101	47 / 113	54 / 126	62 / 138	69 / 151	77 / 163	84 / 176	92 / 188	100 / 200	107 / 213	115 / 225	123 / 237	130 / 250	138 / 262

[b]Test for a one-tailed test at .05 or a two-tailed test at .10. If the U_{obs} value falls within the two values in the table for n_A and n_B, do not reject the null hypothesis. If the U_{obs} is less than or equal to the lower value in the table or greater than or equal to the larger value in the table then reject the null hypothesis.

Table C–7C Critical Values for the Mann-Whitney U Test[c]

n_B \ n_A	1	2	3	4	5	6	7	8	9	10	11	12	13	14	15	16	17	18	19	20
1	—	—	—	—	—	—	—	—	—	—	—	—	—	—	—	—	—	—	—	—
2	—	—	—	—	—	—	—	—	—	—	—	—	0	0	0	0	0	0	1	1
													26	28	30	32	34	36	37	39
3	—	—	—	—	—	—	0	0	1	1	1	2	2	2	3	3	4	4	4	5
							21	24	26	29	32	34	37	40	42	45	47	50	52	55
4	—	—	—	—	0	1	1	2	3	3	4	5	5	6	7	7	8	9	9	10
					20	23	27	30	33	37	40	43	47	50	53	57	60	63	67	70
5	—	—	—	0	1	2	3	4	5	6	7	8	9	10	11	12	13	14	15	16
				20	24	28	32	36	40	44	48	52	56	60	64	68	72	76	80	84
6	—	—	—	1	2	3	4	6	7	8	9	11	12	13	15	16	18	19	20	22
				23	28	33	38	42	47	52	57	61	66	71	75	80	84	89	94	93
7	—	—	0	1	3	4	6	7	9	11'	12	14	16	17	19	21	23	24	26	28
			21	27	32	38	43	49	54	59	65	70	75	81	86	91	96	102	107	112
8	—	—	0	2	4	6	7	9	11	13	15	17	20	22	24	26	28	30	32	34
			24	30	36	42	49	55	61	67	73	79	84	90	96	102	108	114	120	126
9	—	—	1	3	5	7	9	11	14	16	18	21	23	26	28	31	33	36	38	40
			26	33	40	47	54	61	67	74	81	87	94	100	107	113	120	126	133	140
10	—	—	1	3	6	8	11	13	16	19	22	24	27	30	33	36	38	41	44	47
			29	37	44	52	59	67	74	81	88	96	103	110	117	124	132	139	146	153
11	—	—	1	4	7	9	12	15	18	22	25	28	31	34	37	41	44	47	50	53
			32	40	48	57	65	73	81	88	96	104	112	120	128	135	143	151	159	167
12	—	—	2	5	8	11	14	17	21	24	28	31	35	38	42	46	49	53	56	60
			34	43	52	61	70	79	87	96	104	113	121	130	138	146	155	163	172	180
13	—	0	2	5	9	12	16	20	23	27	31	35	39	43	47	51	55	59	63	67
		26	37	47	56	66	75	84	94	103	112	121	130	139	148	157	166	175	184	193
14	—	0	2	6	10	13	17	22	26	30	34	38	43	47	51	56	60	65	69	73
		28	40	50	60	71	81	90	100	110	120	130	139	149	159	168	178	187	197	207
15	—	0	3	7	11	15	19	24	28	33	37	42	47	51	56	61	66	70	75	80
		30	42	53	64	75	86	96	107	117	128	138	148	159	169	179	189	200	210	220
16	—	0	3	7	12	16	21	26	31	36	41	46	51	56	61	66	71	76	82	87
		32	45	57	68	80	91	102	113	124	135	146	157	168	179	190	201	212	222	233
17	—	0	4	8	13	18	23	28	33	38	44	49	55	60	66	712	77	82	88	93
		34	47	60	72	84	96	108	120	132	143	155	166	178	189	201	212	224	234	247
18	—	0	4	9	14	19	24	30	36	41	47	53	59	65	70	76	82	88	94	100
		36	50	63	76	89	102	114	126	139	151	163	175	187	200	212	224	236	248	260
19	—	1	4	9	15	20	26	32	38	44	50	56	63	69	75	82	88	94	101	107
		37	53	67	80	94	107	120	133	146	159	172	184	197	210	222	235	248	260	273
20	—	1	5	10	16	22	28	34	40	47	53	60	76	73	80	87	93	100	107	114
		39	55	70	84	98	112	126	140	153	167	180	193	207	220	233	247	260	273	286

[c]Test for a one-tailed test at .01 or a two-tailed test at .02. If the U_{obs} value falls within the two values in the table for n_A and n_B, do not reject the null hypothesis. If the U_{obs} is less than or equal to the lower value in the table or greater than or equal to the larger value in the table then reject the null hypothesis.

Source: Adapted from "On a Test of Whether One of Two Random Variables Is Stochastically Larger Than the Other," by H. B. Mann and D. R. Whitney, 1947, *Annals of Mathematical Statistics,* (pp. 18, 52–54); Extended tables for the Mann-Whitney statistic, *Bulletin of the Institute of Educational Research at Indiana University, 1,* No. 2; and *Fundamentals of Behavioral Statistics,* by R. P. Runyon and A. Haber, 1967. © 1967 by Addison-Wesley Publishing Company, Inc. Reprinted by permission of Addison-Wesley Publishing Company, Inc.

Table C–8 Critical Values of *T* for Wilcoxon's Signed Ranks Test[a]

	Level of significance for one-tailed test					Level of significance for one-tailed test			
	.05	.025	.01	.005		.05	.025	.01	.005
	Level of significance for two-tailed test					Level of significance for two-tailed test			
N	.10	.05	.02	.01	**N**	.10	.05	.02	.01
5	0	—	—	—	28	130	116	101	91
6	2	0	—	—	29	140	126	110	100
7	3	2	0	—	30	151	137	120	109
8	5	3	1	0	31	163	147	130	118
9	8	5	3	1	32	175	159	140	128
10	10	8	5	3	33	187	170	151	138
11	13	10	7	5	34	200	182	162	148
12	17	13	9	7	35	213	195	173	159
13	21	17	12	9	36	227	208	185	171
14	25	21	15	12	37	241	221	198	182
15	30	25	19	15	38	256	235	211	194
16	35	29	23	19	39	271	249	224	207
17	41	34	27	23	40	286	264	238	220
18	47	40	32	27	41	302	279	252	233
19	53	46	37	32	42	319	294	266	247
20	60	52	43	37	43	336	310	281	261
21	67	58	49	42	44	353	327	296	276
22	75	65	55	48	45	371	343	312	291
23	83	73	62	54	46	389	361	328	307
24	91	81	69	61	47	407	378	345	322
25	100	89	76	68	48	426	396	362	339
26	110	98	84	75	49	446	415	379	355
27	119	107	92	83	50	466	434	397	373

[a]The T_{crit} value indicates the smaller sum of ranks associated with differences that are all of the same sign. For any given N (number of ranked differences), the T_{obs} is significant at a given level if it is equal to or less than the critical value in the table.

Source: Handbook of Statistical Tables (pp. 325–362), by D. B. Owen, 1962, Reading, MA: Addison-Wesley Publishing, and adapted from *Fundamentals of Behavioral Statistics* (p. 266), by R. P. Runyon and A. Haber, 1967, Reading, MA: Addison-Wesley. Reprinted with permission of the publisher. We acknowledge the assistance of Y. L. Lio, Mathematics Department, University of South Dakota, in interpreting the tables.

Table C–9 Student Range Statistic for Tukey's Honestly Significantly Difference Test (HSD)

df for Error Term	\(k = \) Number of Treatments										
	2	3	4	5	6	7	8	9	10	11	12
5	3.64	4.60	5.22	5.67	6.03	6.33	6.58	6.80	6.99	7.17	7.32
	5.70	**6.98**	**7.80**	**8.42**	**8.91**	**9.32**	**9.67**	**9.97**	**10.24**	**10.48**	**10.70**
6	3.46	4.34	4.90	5.30	5.63	5.90	6.12	6.32	6.49	6.65	6.79
	5.24	**6.33**	**7.03**	**7.56**	**7.97**	**8.32**	**8.61**	**8.87**	**9.10**	**9.30**	**9.48**
7	3.34	4.16	4.68	5.06	5.36	5.61	5.82	6.00	6.16	6.30	6.43
	4.95	**5.92**	**6.54**	**7.01**	**7.37**	**7.68**	**7.94**	**8.17**	**8.37**	**8.55**	**8.71**
8	3.26	4.04	4.53	4.89	5.17	5.40	5.60	5.77	5.92	6.05	6.18
	4.75	**5.64**	**6.20**	**6.62**	**6.96**	**7.24**	**7.47**	**7.68**	**7.86**	**8.03**	**8.18**
9	3.20	3.95	4.41	4.76	5.02	5.24	5.43	5.59	5.74	5.87	5.98
	4.60	**5.43**	**5.96**	**6.35**	**6.66**	**6.91**	**7.13**	**7.33**	**7.49**	**7.65**	**7.78**
10	3.15	3.88	4.33	4.65	4.91	5.12	5.30	5.46	5.60	5.72	5.83
	4.48	**5.27**	**5.77**	**6.14**	**6.43**	**6.67**	**6.87**	**7.05**	**7.21**	**7.36**	**7.49**
11	3.11	3.82	4.26	4.57	4.82	5.03	5.20	5.35	5.49	5.61	5.71
	4.39	**5.15**	**5.62**	**5.97**	**6.25**	**6.48**	**6.67**	**6.84**	**6.99**	**7.13**	**7.25**
12	3.08	3.77	4.20	4.51	4.75	4.95	5.12	5.27	5.39	5.51	5.61
	4.32	**5.05**	**5.50**	**5.84**	**6.10**	**6.32**	**6.51**	**6.67**	**6.81**	**6.94**	**7.06**
13	3.06	3.73	4.15	4.45	4.69	4.88	5.05	5.19	5.32	5.43	5.53
	4.26	**4.96**	**5.40**	**5.73**	**5.98**	**6.19**	**6.37**	**6.53**	**6.67**	**6.79**	**6.90**
14	3.03	3.70	4.11	4.41	4.64	4.83	4.99	5.13	5.25	5.36	5.46
	4.21	**4.89**	**5.32**	**5.63**	**5.88**	**6.08**	**6.26**	**6.41**	**6.54**	**6.66**	**6.77**
15	3.01	3.67	4.08	4.37	4.59	4.78	4.94	5.08	5.20	5.31	5.40
	4.17	**4.84**	**5.25**	**5.56**	**5.80**	**5.99**	**6.16**	**6.31**	**6.44**	**6.55**	**6.66**
16	3.00	3.65	4.05	4.33	4.56	4.74	4.90	5.03	5.15	5.26	5.35
	4.13	**4.79**	**5.19**	**5.49**	**5.72**	**5.92**	**6.08**	**6.22**	**6.35**	**6.46**	**6.56**
17	2.98	3.63	4.02	4.30	4.52	4.70	4.86	4.99	5.11	5.21	5.31
	4.10	**4.74**	**5.14**	**5.43**	**5.66**	**5.85**	**6.01**	**6.15**	**6.27**	**6.38**	**6.48**
18	2.97	3.61	4.00	4.28	4.49	4.67	4.82	4.96	5.07	5.17	5.27
	4.07	**4.70**	**5.09**	**5.38**	**5.60**	**5.79**	**5.94**	**6.08**	**6.20**	**6.31**	**6.41**
19	2.96	3.59	3.98	4.25	4.47	4.65	4.79	4.92	5.04	5.14	5.23
	4.05	**4.67**	**5.05**	**5.33**	**5.55**	**5.73**	**5.89**	**6.02**	**6.14**	**6.25**	**6.34**
20	2.95	3.58	3.96	4.23	4.45	4.62	4.77	4.90	5.01	5.11	5.20
	4.02	**4.64**	**5.02**	**5.29**	**5.51**	**5.69**	**5.84**	**5.97**	**6.09**	**6.19**	**6.28**
24	2.92	3.53	3.90	4.17	4.37	4.54	4.68	4.81	4.92	5.01	5.10
	3.96	**4.55**	**4.91**	**5.17**	**5.37**	**5.54**	**5.69**	**5.81**	**5.92**	**6.02**	**6.11**
30	2.89	3.49	3.85	4.10	4.30	4.46	4.60	4.72	4.82	4.92	5.00
	3.89	**4.45**	**4.80**	**5.05**	**5.24**	**5.40**	**5.54**	**5.65**	**5.76**	**5.85**	**5.93**
40	2.86	3.44	3.79	4.04	4.23	4.39	4.52	4.63	4.73	4.82	4.90
	3.82	**4.37**	**4.70**	**4.93**	**5.11**	**5.26**	**5.39**	**5.50**	**5.60**	**5.69**	**5.76**
60	2.83	3.40	3.74	3.98	4.16	4.31	4.44	4.55	4.65	4.73	4.81
	3.76	**4.28**	**4.59**	**4.82**	**4.99**	**5.13**	**5.25**	**5.36**	**5.45**	**5.53**	**5.60**

(continued)

Table C–9 Student Range Statistic for Tukey's Honestly Significantly Difference Test (HSD) *(continued)*

df for Error Term	*k = Number of Treatments*										
	2	**3**	**4**	**5**	**6**	**7**	**8**	**9**	**10**	**11**	**12**
120	2.80	3.36	3.68	3.92	4.10	4.24	4.36	4.47	4.56	4.64	4.71
	3.70	**4.20**	**4.50**	**4.71**	**4.87**	**5.01**	**5.12**	**5.21**	**5.30**	**5.37**	**5.44**
∞	2.77	3.31	3.63	3.86	4.03	4.17	4.29	4.39	4.47	4.55	4.62
	3.64	**4.12**	**4.40**	**4.60**	**4.76**	**4.88**	**4.99**	**5.08**	**5.16**	**5.23**	**5.29**

Note that critical values in the table for (q) the boldface type represents values at the $p = .01$ level and the regular type represents values at the $p = .05$ level.

Source: Biometrika Tables for Statisticians (3rd ed.), by E. Pearson and H. Hartley, 1966, New York: Cambridge University Press, and *Statistics for the Behavioral Sciences* (pp. A–35, 36), by F. J. Gravetter and L. B. Wallnau, 1985, St. Paul: West. Reprinted with permission of the publishers.

Table C–10 Critical Values for the Chi-Square Distribution

df	.25	.10	.05	.025	.01	.005
1	1.323	2.706	3.841	5.024	6.635	7.879
2	2.773	4.605	5.991	7.378	9.210	10.597
3	4.108	6.251	7.815	9.348	11.345	12.838
4	5.385	7.779	9.488	11.143	11.277	14.860
5	6.626	9.236	11.071	12.833	15.086	16.750
6	7.841	10.645	12.592	14.449	16.812	18.548
7	9.037	12.017	14.067	16.013	18.475	20.278
8	10.219	13.362	15.507	17.535	20.090	21.955
9	11.389	14.684	16.919	19.023	21.666	23.589
10	12.549	15.987	18.307	20.483	23.209	25.188
11	13.701	17.275	19.675	21.920	24.725	26.757
12	14.845	18.549	21.026	23.337	26.217	28.299
13	15.984	19.812	22.362	24.736	27.688	29.819
14	17.117	21.064	23.685	26.119	29.141	31.319
15	18.245	22.307	24.996	27.488	30.578	32.801
16	19.369	23.542	26.296	28.845	32.000	34.267
17	20.489	24.769	27.587	30.191	33.409	35.718
18	21.605	25.989	28.869	31.526	34.805	37.156
19	22.718	27.204	30.144	32.852	36.191	38.582
20	23.828	28.412	31.410	34.170	37.566	39.997
21	24.935	29.615	32.671	35.479	38.932	41.401
22	26.039	30.813	33.924	36.781	40.289	42.796
23	27.141	32.007	35.172	38.076	41.638	44.181
24	28.241	33.196	36.415	39.364	42.980	45.559
25	29.339	34.382	37.652	40.646	44.314	46.928
26	30.435	35.563	38.885	41.923	45.642	48.290
27	31.528	36.741	40.113	43.194	46.963	49.645
28	32.620	37.916	41.337	44.461	48.278	50.993
29	33.711	39.087	42.557	45.722	49.588	52.336
30	34.800	40.256	43.773	46.979	50.892	53.672
31	35.887	41.422	44.985	48.232	52.191	55.003
32	36.973	42.585	46.194	49.480	53.486	56.328
33	38.058	43.745	47.400	50.725	54.776	57.648
34	39.141	44.903	48.602	51.966	56.061	58.964
35	40.223	46.059	49.802	53.203	57.342	60.275
36	41.304	47.212	50.998	54.437	58.619	61.581
37	42.383	48.363	52.192	55.668	59.892	62.883
38	43.462	49.513	53.384	56.896	61.162	64.181
39	44.539	50.660	54.572	58.120	62.428	65.476
40	45.616	51.805	55.758	59.342	63.691	66.766
41	46.692	52.949	56.942	60.561	64.950	68.053
42	47.766	54.090	58.124	61.777	66.206	69.336
43	48.840	55.230	59.304	62.990	67.459	70.616
44	49.913	56.369	60.481	64.201	68.710	71.893
45	50.985	57.505	61.656	65.410	69.957	73.166

Source: Adapted from Table 3.1 Critical Values for the Chi-square Distribution, *Handbook of Statistical Tables* (pp. 49–55), by D. B. Owen, 1962, Reading, MA: Addison-Wesley. Reprinted with permission of the publisher.

Steps in Determining Critical Values for Chi-Square for Table C–10

1. Calculate the degrees of freedom (df). The formula is $df = (r - 1)(c - 1)$. r = number of rows in the matrix and c = number of columns in the matrix. For example, in a 2×3 matrix, 2 rows and 3 columns, $df = (2 - 1)(3 - 1) = 2\ df$.

2. Apply level of significance such as .05 or .01.

3. Locate critical value for chi-square from statistical table. For example, $df = 2$, .05 level, chi-square $_{crit}$ = 5.99.

4. Calculate chi-square $_{obs}$ from data.

5. Decision rule:

- If chi-square $_{obs}$ is equal to or above chi-square $_{crit}$ reject the null hypothesis.
- If chi-square $_{obs}$ is below chi-square $_{crit}$ accept the null hypothesis.

Glossary

a priori: reasoning from cause to effect. *A priori* criteria are criteria that an investigator states before collecting data.

A-B research design: single subject research where the A phase represents the collection of baseline data and the B phase represents the treatment phase. Variations of this include A-B-A, A-B-A-B, and other related research designs. *See also* case study

abscissa: the horizontal coordinate or *x* axis in a distribution.

abstract: a summary of a published article (150 to 300 words) that contains the important points of each section, including purpose of study, literature review, methodology, results, limitations of research design, and recommendations for further research.

action research: application of research to a site-specific environment using a problem-solving approach. It is an outgrowth of both qualitative and quantitative research. For example, an occupational therapist is interested in finding the best splint to use with a client who has a cumulative trauma injury. The results of this research may be applied to another individual in similar circumstances.

alpha: the probability of a Type I error in research. It is usually defined as .05 or .01 in the social sciences. It is also referred to as significance level and *p* value.

alternative hypothesis (H_1): the hypothesis that is the opposite of the stated hypothesis and is not predicted to be true.

analysis of covariance (**ANCOVA**): a statistical test arising from an analysis of variance that adjusts for a priori differences in comparable groups.

analysis of variance (**ANOVA**): an inferential statistical test that is applied to data when comparing two or more independent group means. An *F* score is derived. The formula for *F* in a one-way ANOVA is:

$$F = \frac{\text{Variance between group means}}{\text{Variance within groups}}$$

annotated bibliography: includes the bibliographical citation and the abstract.

applied research: the direct application of research to improving the quality of life in areas such as reduction of work injuries, prevention of alcoholism, and evaluation of clinical treatment methods. *See also* problem-oriented research.

aptitude: inherent, natural ability of individual; underlying capacity to learn or perform in a specific area.

artifact: an unexplained result in an experiment not caused by the independent variable.

associational relationship: degree of correlation between two variables.

attitude scale: a measure of an individual's feeling, belief, or opinion toward a subject or topic.

bar graph: a histogram with unattached bars.

baseline data: the results of initial testing of a subject before intervention.

basic research: investigations in areas related to processes, functions, and attributes that can lead to applied research. An example of basic research is examining how serotonin, a neurochemical transmitter, operates in the brain. The results of basic research often have important significance for clinical researchers.

before-and-after design: an experimental research design in which performance or characteristics are measured before and after a treatment intervention.

beta: the probability of a Type II error in research.

bias: any prejudicial factor in the researcher or methodology that may distort results.

biased sample: a sample that is not representative of a target population from which it is drawn. It does not reflect the major characteristics of the target population, and therefore results from a biased sample cannot be generalized.

bibliographical citation: the exact reference for a journal, book, or article referred to in the research paper or manuscript. The citation includes the author; title of article, journal, or book; volume and page numbers, and in books; the place of publication and the publisher.

bimodal: a frequency distribution showing two highest points.

box and whisker plots, box plots, box graphs: descriptive figures that displays the maximum and minimum scores and the median and quartiles in a rectangular box. Useful in demonstrating graphically the degree of skewness of data.

case study: intensive study of individual either through an experimental prospective design or through retrospective research.

central tendency: a summary measure of a distribution indicated by the mean, median, or mode. Frequently referred to as measures of central tendency.

chi-square: a nonparametric statistical technique that tests the probability between observed and expected frequencies using nominal level measurement.

clinical observation research: the systematic and objective investigation in normal development, course of a disease, cultural ethnography, field studies, and naturalistic observations.

clinical trial: in experimental medical research, a clinical trial refers to large-scale research studies exploring the effectiveness of drugs or vaccines on populations. For example, the Salk vaccine was used in a clinical trial during the 1950s to examine its effectiveness in preventing polio.

closed-ended questions: questions that can be answered by either *yes* or *no*. This type of question is not considered useful in survey research. The opposite of a closed-ended question is an open-ended question.

cohort: a study population that has common characteristics, such as the residents of a community or an occupational group.

concurrent validity: a measure of a test's correlation with an established instrument to test its accuracy in measuring a variable. For example, a new test for intelligence frequently will be correlated with the Wechsler Intelligence Scales because it has a high reliability and established validity. New tests are developed to include updated concepts and improved administration, cost, and time considerations.

confidence interval: the area in a distribution that contains a population parameter. The confidence interval is related to the level of statistical confidence in results.

confounding variable: the effect of extraneous variables on research results. For example, test anxiety, fatigue, and lack of control are confounding variables.

content validity: the most elementary type of validity. It is determined by a logical analysis of test items to see whether the items are consistent and measure what they purport to measure. Sometimes referred to as face validity.

contingency table: a table of values that includes observed and expected frequencies such as in a chi-square table.

continuous variable: a quantitative value that has infinite number of measures between any two points. Examples of continuous variables are height, weight, and heart rate.

control group: a comparative included in a study group to control for the Hawthorne effect and other extraneous variables. Both the experimental and comparative groups receive equal time or attention.

convenience sample: a sample selected that is readily available. For example, a researcher will select participants who are in a hospital where the researcher is employed.

correlation coefficient: a statistical value that indicates the degree of relationship between two variables. It can range from +1.00 to 0 to −1.00.

correlation matrix: a statistical table describing the degree of correlation between two variables. The correlation matrix indicates the correlation coefficient index for each pair of correlates.

correlational research: retrospective investigations into the relationship between variables. Variables are not manipulated by the researcher, as they would be in experimental research.

credibility: in qualitative research, the authenticity of the results based on acceptance of the conclusions from the phenomenological evidence. Triangulation (e.g., obtaining data from different perspectives) increases the credibility of the research.

criterion: standard of performance that is the basis or yardstick for comparisons.

criterion-referenced test: a test based on a standard of performance, competence, or mastery, rather than on a comparison with a normative group. For example, for an individual to pass a test in driver competency, he or she would have to demonstrate mastery of a specific set of criteria. The determination of the criteria is not based on the bell-shaped curve but is based on minimal standards for performance.

critical value: the statistical value displayed in tables that is used to accept or reject the null hypothesis.

cross-validation: a method to measure test validity by extending testing from the initial target population to other groups.

culture-free test: a test that is not culturally biased and can be administered across cultures.

data: the numerical results of a study. The term is always plural (e.g., data are . . .).

decile: a point in a distribution where 10% of the cases fall at or below that point.

deductive reasoning: inference to particulars from a general principle. For example, proposing a theory and then hypothesizing specific results from an experiment.

degrees of freedom (df): a mathematically derived value that is used in reading statistical tables.

demographic variables: related to the statistical characteristics of a target population such as distribution of ages, gender, income, presence of disease (morbidity), death rates (mortality), occupation, accident and injury rates, health status, and nutritional input.

demography: the application of statistical methods to describe human populations regarding, for example, mortality, morbidity, birth and marriage rates, gender differences, physical and intellectual characteristics, socioeconomic status, and religious beliefs. In general, demography can be defined as the statistical study of human populations regarding their size, their structure, and development (United Nations, 1958).

dependent variable: resultant effect of the independent variable. In clinical research, the dependent variable represents the desired outcome, such as decrease in anxiety, increase in range of motion, or increase in reading achievement.

descriptive statistics: statistical tests or procedures to describe a population, sample, or variable. Examples of descriptive statistics include measures of central tendency, measures of variability, frequency distribution, vital statistics, scatter diagram, polygons, and histograms.

developmental test: a measure of a child's performance in age-related tasks such as language, perceptual-motor, social, emotional, and ambulation.

"devil effect": a negative prejudgment of a subject's performance based on the rater's bias.

directional hypothesis: a statement by the researcher predicting that there will be a statistically significant difference or relationship between variables. For example, a clinical researcher states, "Aerobic exercise is more effective than antidepressive medication in reducing anxiety in individuals with clinical depression."

discourse analysis: the study of language as communication through the forms and mechanisms of verbal interaction.

discrete variable: a variable that is distinct and does not have an infinite number of values between categories. Examples of discrete variables are gender, diagnostic categories, or eye color.

double-blind control: a research design in which neither the researcher nor the subjects know whether the subjects are in the experimental or control group.

effect size: the degree of differences between two means or the degree of relationship between two variables in the results of a study. Effect size index is related to statistical power, which is the probability of not making a Type II error (e.g., accepting the null hypothesis when it should be rejected). (See Cohen, 1977, for a further discussion of effect size and statistical power.)

empiricism: the philosophy that advocates knowledge based on controlled observation and experiment.

error variance: the presence of error factors in the subject, researcher, test instrument, and environment that threatens internal validity. These factors include poor motivation, fatigue, and test anxiety in the subject; researcher bias; unreliability of the test instrument; and a distracting or noisy testing environment.

ethnoscience: the study of the characteristics of language as culture in terms of lexical or semantic relations.

evaluation research: the qualitative and systematic evaluation of systems and organizations such as hospitals and educational programs by applying a priori criteria or standards.

evidence-based practice: the application of research studies to justify treatment. The occupational therapists uses the results of research design treatment protocols.

experimental group: the group identified that is manipulated by the researcher, for example, the experimental group receives an innovative method of teaching.

experimental research: a prospective study in which the investigator seeks to discover cause-and-effect relationships by manipulating the independent variable and observing the effects on the dependent variable.

ex post facto design: a retrospective study in which the investigator examines the relationships of variables that have already occurred.

external validity: the degree to which the results of a study can be generalized to a target population. External validity depends on the representativeness of a sample and the rigor of an experiment. Replication of a study producing consistent results increases the external validity.

extraneous historical factors: threats to internal validity when unexpected events take place during an experiment that affect the results. These unpredictable events in the subject are extraneous variables.

extraneous variable: a variable other than the independent variable that can potentially affect the results of a study. Extraneous variables can include such factors as gender, intelligence, severity of disability, or socioeconomic status. These variables, if they are uncontrolled, can threaten the internal validity of a study.

factor analysis: a statistical method to categorize data into identifiable factors. The procedure is an extension of a correlation matrix where a set of variables are correlated with each other.

factorial design: a research study exploring the interaction between variables, such as a two-factor analysis of variance.

feasible research study: a study in which the investigator has examined in detail and provided solutions for the practical aspects of implementing a research study, such as costs, time, setting, availability of subjects, human ethics, selection of outcome measures, and procedure for collecting data.

forced choice test items: items that require participants to make a choice when completing a questionnaire, rating scale, or attitude inventory. Participants select items generated by the researcher.

frequency distribution table: a descriptive statistic summarizing data by showing the number of times each score value occurs in a set category or interval.

frequency polygon: a line graph depicting the number of cases that fall into designated categories. It is composed of an X and a Y axis.

functional capacity evaluation (FCA): a comprehensive and systematic approach that measures the client's overall physical capacity such as muscle strength and endurance. Examples are the Isernhagen Work Systems and BTE.

grounded theory analysis: referring to qualitative research, the search for regularities by constantly comparing and contrasting similarities and differences in incidents to form categories or themes with distinctive properties and conceptual relationships.

Guttman scale: a cumulative attitude scale that indicates an individual's feelings toward a specific issue. The respondent usually answers *yes* or *no* to a statement.

"halo effect": A carry-over effect from previous knowledge of an individual, resulting in a bias on the part of a tester or rater. Halo effects typically occur when raters positively prejudge a subject's performance based on the rater's previous experience with him or her. It is a bias in testing.

Hawthorne effect: a confounding variable that creates a positive result that is not caused by the independent variable. The Hawthorne effect is eliminated by introducing a control group or by using the subject as one's own control.

hermeneutics: the study and interpretation of text in which each event is understood by reference to the whole of which it is a part, especially the broader historical context.

heterogeneous: of different origin or characteristic, such as male and female or mixed ages.

heuristic research: investigations that seek to discover relationships between variables through pilot studies and factor analysis.

The major purpose is to generate further research.

histogram: a descriptive statistic describing a frequency distribution using attached bars.

historical research: the systematic and objective investigation, through primary sources, into the events and people that shaped history.

homogeneous: of like characteristic such as age, gender, or intelligence.

honeymoon effect: a confounding variable that produces a short-term beneficial effect. It is created by the initial optimism of the researcher desiring to show the positive effects of a specific treatment method and the patient or subject wanting the treatment method to work. The subject rejects the initial effects of treatment and disregards side effects or negative results. It is controlled by long-term follow-up and reducing researcher bias.

hypothesis: a statement that predicts results and can be testable. An example of a hypothesis is aerobic exercise lowers blood pressure in middle-aged, sedentary men. A hypothesis can be stated in a null or directional form.

idiographic approach: intensive study of an individual or dynamic case study.

incidence rate: the rate of the initial occurrence or new cases of a disease over a period of time. For example, the incidence of AIDS in the United States for the year 2000 includes all the new cases of AIDS diagnosed during 2000.

independent living evaluation: an assessment tool used to measure a client's ability to perform the activities of daily living. An example is the Barthel Self Care Index.

independent variable: a variable manipulated by the researcher. In clinical research, it represents the treatment method, such as sensory integration therapy, or cognitive-behavioral therapy.

inductive reasoning: inferences from particulars or experiments to the general. For example, integrating the results of research studies to a general theory or conclusion.

inferential statistics: statistical tests of procedures for making inferences from sample and populations based on objectively derived data. They include t tests, analysis of variance, chi-square, correlation coefficients, factor analysis, and multiple regression.

information retrieval systems: automated system for storing and retrieving information. In the health fields, examples include MedLine, CINAHL, HealthStar, and OT BIBSys.

informed consent form: a voluntary consensual agreement between the investigator and the subject detailing the procedures in the study and the possible psychological and physical risks that could result in harm to the subject.

institutional review board: An interdisciplinary committee established in a university, hospital, or private industry to protect the rights of human subjects from possible harm that could occur by participating in a research study. It is recommended that all research with human subjects be approved for ethical consideration before data are collected or the research is initiated.

internal validity: the degree of rigor in an experiment in controlling for extraneous variables and error variance. Potential sources of internal validity have been identified as extraneous historical factors, maturation, instrumentation, and lack of random sampling. Internal validity is an indication of the trustworthiness of the results. Well-designed studies with good control of variables that can potentially distort the results have high internal validity. The quality of a research study is increased by eliminating the threats to internal validity.

interrater reliability: the degree of agreement and consistency between two independent raters in measuring a variable.

interval scale of measurement: quantification of a variable in which there are infinite points between each measurement, as well as equal intervals. Examples include the measurement of systolic blood pressure and intelligence scores as measured by the Wechsler scales. An absolute zero is not assumed in measuring a variable, nor are comparative statements such as X is twice as large as Y assumed.

intrarater reliability: the degree of consistency within a single rater.

kappa test (k): a statistical procedure to detect the degree of interrater agreement based on probability.

key word: an important word or concept in a study that is identified by the researcher. It is used to retrieve a study when it is part of a database.

Kruskal-Wallis test: a nonparametric test that is an alternative to the one-way ANOVA for comparing significant differences between several groups.

Likert scale: a measurement scale used in questionnaires to assess a subject's agreement or disagreement with a statement. Likert scales usually include five to seven descriptors, such as totally agree, agree, neutral, disagree, or totally disagree.

logical positivism: a philosophical approach to verifying reality. Logical positivists assert that reality is a result of sensory data.

MANCOVA: multiple analysis of covariance is a statistical technique that is based on the analysis of variance where multiple variables are being analyzed and corrected for differences in initial scores.

Mann-Whitney test: a nonparametric test that is an alternative to the independent t test when testing significant differences between two independent means. The normality assumptions and equal variances assumptions need not be satisfied when applying the Mann-Whitney test.

matched group: a control group selected to use as a comparable group to experimental group. Variables matched typically include age, gender, intelligence, socioeconomic status, and degree of disability.

maturation: a threat to internal validity that occurs when the researcher does not account for the subject's maturity during an experiment. For example, in testing children, the researcher must consider the age variable in measuring changes from pre- to posttest evaluation. Maturation can also refer to a practice effect and development in the subject during the experiment.

mean: the arithmetic average derived from all scores in a distribution.

measures of central tendency: mean, mode, and median.

measures of variability: range, variance, and standard deviation.

median: the score at the 50th percentile or midpoint where all the cases in a distribution are divided in half.

meta-analysis: a quantitative or qualitative analysis of a group of related research studies to determine if the results of the study are consistent and therefore lend support to their conclusions. Meta-analysis is based on the effect size estimation. (See Rosenthal and Rosnow, 1991, for a detailed discussion of meta-analysis.)

methodological research: objective and systematic investigation for designing instruments, tests, procedures, curriculum, software programs, and treatment programs.

mode: the most frequent score or numerical value in a frequency distribution.

multiple regression: a statistical method that is used to predict the individual effects of independent variables on a designated dependent variable. Multiple regression has been used in medical research to identify the multiple risk factors in a certain disease such as cardiovascular disease, stroke, or emphysema. For example, multiple regression is used to predict the effect of designated risk factors (presumed independent variables) on a dependent variable (such as heart disease).

nominal scale of measurement: classification of variables into discrete categories, such as diagnostic groups, professions, or gender. There is no specific order in the categories; no category is more important than any other category. Likewise, each category is mutually exclusive from any other category.

nomothetic approach: research leading to general laws in science or universal knowledge.

nonparametric statistical tests: inferential statistical procedures that calculate data from samples that are distribution-free and not based on the normal curve. These tests include Mann-Whitney, Kruskall-Wallis, chi-square, Spearman correlational coefficient, and Wilcoxon.

normal curve: a bell-shaped polygon that describes a mathematical probability distribution of a variable where most scores cluster around the mean.

norm-referenced test: a test used to assess the degree of achievement, aptitude, capacity, interest, or attitude compared to established norms or standard scores based on population.

null hypothesis (H_0): a statement by the researcher that predicts no statistically significant differences or relationships between variables. For example, a clinical researcher states, "There is no statistically significant difference between exercise and splinting in reducing spasticity in children with cerebral palsy."

objective psychological test: standardized test that contains comparative norms for interpreting individual raw scores.

observed statistical value: the value obtained from applying a statistical formula to statistical results. These values such as t or F observed are compared to the critical value that is derived from a statistical table to accept or reject the null hypothesis.

open-ended questions: used in survey research. The investigator elicits attitudes, beliefs, and emotions from subjects by asking nonobjective questions, or questions that cannot be answered by *yes* or *no*. The opposite of an open-ended question is a closed-ended question.

operational definition of variable: specific test, procedure, or set of criteria that defines independent or dependent variables and target population. This factor is important in replicating a study or in evaluating a group of studies such as through a meta-analysis.

ordinal scale of measurement: classification of variables into rank order, such as the degree of anxiety, or academic achievement, or grade level. The classification defines which group is first, second, third, an so forth; however, it does not define the distance between classifications.

outcome measure: the specific test or procedure to measure the dependent variable. For example an outcome measure for pain is the *McGill-Melzack Pain Inventory*.

outlier: a test result or score outside the normal range of values.

p value: the risk of making a Type I error, or the level of significance. In the social sciences, it is usually established at the $p < .05$ or $p < .01$ level.

parameter: a descriptive value assigned to a condition or population. Parameters are constant, such as the characteristics of a specified population.

parametric statistical tests: inferential statistics that are based on certain assumptions, such as the normally distributed population variable, random selection of subjects, homogeneity of variance and independence of samples.

Pearson product-moment correlation coefficient: an inferential test used to test whether there is a statistically significant relationship between two variables. An *r* score is derived: *r* can range from +1.00 (a perfect correlation), to 0.00 (no correlation), to −1.00 (a perfect negative or inverse correlation). A computational formula is used in calculating *r*.

percentage: the number of cases per hundred.

percentile: a point in a distribution that defines where a given percentage of the cases fall. For example the 80th percentile is the point where 80% of the cases are at that point or below.

performance test: a test of an individual's skill or capacity, such as grip strength, range of motion, manual dexterity, or driving skills.

personal equation in measurement: the affect of the presence of the tester on the subject's performance. The tester, as the evaluator is a variable in the test situation, and if uncontrolled, can distort the test results.

pilot study: a research study usually with a small number of subjects, that is innovative but that does not control for all extraneous variables. The primary advantage of a pilot study is that it generates further research.

placebo effect: a confounding variable that occurs when the subject shows signs of improvement or the reduction of symptoms that is not caused by a treatment effect. It is instead caused by the subject's belief that a treatment method is causing improvement even though the subject is receiving a "dummy" or "sham" treatment. The placebo effect was initially observed in drug studies where an experimental drug was compared to a placebo or nonactive drug. Researchers observed that some of the subjects receiving a placebo improved. The current explanation of the placebo effect is that the subject produces a psychophysiologic response that results in more relaxed and less stressed individual. In a way, the subject wills himself or herself to health in a placebo effect. The placebo effect is controlled by comparing baseline measures with posttreatments in the experimental and control groups.

positive correlation: a relationship between two variables when scores on both variables tend to be in the same direction such as high values for cholesterol and obesity.

posttesting: the results of testing after the intervention has taken place.

postulate: a principle or hypothesis presented without supporting evidence.

predictive validity: the degree to which a test or measuring instrument can predict future performance, functioning. or behavior. For example, the Scholastic Aptitude Test (SAT) is tested for predictive validity in its ability to predict academic success in college.

pretesting: the results of testing before intervening with an independent variable or treatment.

prevalence rate: the number of individuals with a disability or disease divided by the total individuals in a population. For example the prevalence rate of spinal cord injury in the United States in 1994 is the number of individuals with spinal cord injury living in the United States in 1994 divided by the total population in the United States in 1994.

primary prevention: the prevention of the initial onset of a disease, such as the prevention of polio with a vaccination.

primary source: published articles or conference proceedings that include original data, such as a research study or theoretical paper.

probability: the mathematical or statistical likelihood that an event will occur.

problem-oriented research: applied research initiated by the investigator identifying a significant problem, such as a rapid increase in attention deficit disorders in children, or the dramatic rise of homeless men in urban areas. The research design addresses the problem directly.

"Procrustean Bed": applying a treatment method such as a panacea to all patients regardless of individual differences and needs. For example, applying a treatment procedure to all patients with arthritis, as well as to all patients with cancer, without regard to the individual and specific needs of the patient. In this method, the patient is fitted to the treatment method rather than, as in good treatment, being given the best and most effective treatment method.

prospective study: research that is future oriented and attempts to discover causes-and-effect relationships between variables. In prospective studies the investigator manipulates or observes an independent variable that is predicted to affect function or performance and then collects data. Experimental or longitudinal research are examples of prospective designs.

qualitative research: study of people and events in their natural setting. This type of research uses multimodal methods in a naturalistic setting. The researcher using qualitative research methods seeks to explore perceptions and experiences to understand phenomena in terms of the meanings that people bring to them.

quantitative research: the application of the scientific method to test hypotheses. The quantitative researcher begins with a testable hypothesis, collects data, and uses statistical analyses to decide whether to accept or reject the hypothesis. Objectivity of the researcher, operational definitions of the variables, and control of extraneous factors are the key points in quantitative research.

quartile: a point in a distribution where 25% of the cases fall at or below that point.

quasi-experimental designs: a term defined by Campbell and Stanley (1963) to identify research studies in which subjects are not randomly assigned to equivalent groups or in which single case studies are employed. In general, most clinical research studies are within the quasi-experimental model because it is almost impossible to truly select a random sample from a target population or to have truly equivalent experimental and control groups.

random assignment: assigning subjects to experimental or control groups with every subject having an equal chance of being selected.

random errors: the effect of uncontrolled variables in an experiment, such as unexpected events, test procedural errors, and anxiety within the subject. These errors are unpredictable and unsystematic.

random sample: an unbiased portion of a target population that has been selected by chance such as through random numbers.

range: a measure of variability that is the difference between the highest and lowest values in a distribution of scores.

rank order variables: examples of ordinal scale measurement in which ranks are assigned in measuring a variable. Most personality tests such as the Minnesota Multiphasic Personality Inventory (MMPI) measure rank order variables.

rating scale: an individual's appraisal regarding such variables as competence, nonacademic qualities in students, or patient behavior in a psychiatric hospital.

ratio scale of measurement: quantification of a variable that includes equal intervals and an absolute zero point, such as in measuring heart rate, height, and weight. Comparative statements using "twice as" or "half" are possible with ratio scales.

referral source: a database that lists journal articles and books, such as Psychological Abstracts, Index Medicus, and information retrieval systems accessed by computer (e.g., PsychLit, ERIC, MedLine), as well as E-mail and news lists.

regression line: a figure that best describes the linear relationship between the X and Y variables. In a high correlation, the researcher is able to predict the unknown value of Y from the known value of X.

regression to the mean: the observation by statisticians that outlier scores will affect the value of the mean disproportionately especially when there are small numbers of cases. It is also apparent when one remeasures a variable and finds that the initial score was unexpectedly very high or very low as compared with the group mean. On the second measure, the score usually comes closer to the group mean.

reliability: a measure of the consistency of a test instrument. For example, a test has high reliability if it produces consistent results when measuring a variable. Threats to test reliability include ambiguity in the questions and poor test procedures. Reliability is indicated by the correlation coefficient (r). An acceptable test reliability is usually an r of .7 or above.

repeated measures designs: the replication of observations of the effects of treatment methods over a period of time, for example, measuring the effects of biofeedback in reducing anxiety after meditation or exercise.

replicate a research design: to carry out a research design for the second time by replicating the research methodology. The purpose is to strengthen generalizability of the findings and to insure internal validity.

representative sample: an unbiased portion of a target population that is representative in terms of demographic characteristics.

research: the systematic and objective investigation into a topic by stating a hypothesis or guiding question and collecting primary data. It includes quantitative and qualitative designs.

response rate: the number and proportion of responses to a researcher's questionnaire or survey.

retrospective study: research based on causative factors that have already occurred. For example, in a correlational study the researcher may want to examine the relationship between the onset of emphysema and previous smoking behavior. Both variables have already occurred. The researcher tries to reconstruct events and to hypothesize regarding a presumed cause-and-effect relationship. Retrospective research can be used to generate experimental designs to further investigate cause-and-effect relationships.

risk-benefit ratio: The estimation by the investigator of the possible risks to the research subject and the benefits accrued for the study. The researcher reveals the potential risks and benefits to the subject taking part in the study through an informed consent form.

sampling error: the error that results from estimating a population value from a sample.

scales of measurement: the level at which a test or instrument measures a specific variable such as intelligence, behavior, personality, muscle strength, or academic achievement. Traditionally, scales of measurement are classified into four levels: nominal, ordinal, interval, and ratio.

scattergram/scatter diagram/scatterplot: a figure describing the relationship between the X and Y variables.

scientific law: consistent and uniform occurrences that are predictable. Mendelian law of genetic determination predicts characteristics of offspring when genetic traits of parents are known.

scientific method: objective systematic investigation into a subject by stating a hypothesis and collecting empirical data.

secondary prevention: the prevention of the recurrence of a disease, such as preventing a second stroke in an individual.

secondary source: a published article or book that reviews primary sources, such as a literature review.

self-evaluation method: subjects in a clinical research study assess their own progress. Self-evaluation is an important factor in assessing treatment effectiveness. Other factors used in assessing treatment effectiveness include objective tests, psychophysiological measures, and mechanical procedures.

self-fulfilling prophecy: the expectation by the researcher or rater that a subject will perform at a certain level based on prejudice or bias towards the group to which the subject belongs.

semantic differential: an attitude scale in which the respondent rates concepts such as good-bad, fast-slow, and hard-soft.

significance level: in testing a hypothesis, it is the critical level between accepting or rejecting the null hypothesis.

single-subject or case-study design: *See* case study

skewness: an indication in a frequency polygon of the asymmetry of a distribution. A distribution can be skewed to the right side or left side of the polygon.

slope: the linear direction and angle of a line. It is calculated in the regression line.

Spearman rank correlation coefficient (formerly rho [ρ]): a nonparametric test measured by ordinal scales used in determining the degree of relationship between two variables. It is an alternative to the Pearson product-moment coefficient (r).

split-half reliability: a method to estimate the degree of consistency in a test by correlating one half of the test items, such as even number items, with the other half of the test, such as the odd number items.

standard deviation (SD): a statistical measure of the variability of scores from the mean.

standard error of the mean (Se$_m$): a pooled standard deviation of samples of group means drawn randomly from a target population.

standard error of measurement (SEM): a statistical value that indicates the band of error surrounding a test score. For example, a raw score of 90 with a SEM of 4 represents a score ranging from 86 to 94.

standardized test: a test that has been administered to a target population and for which norms are available.

statistical assumptions: conditions in research required for a specific statistical test. These assumptions relate to randomness, scale of measurement, sample size, and independence of samples.

statistical pie: a descriptive statistic using the circumference of a circle to describe the percentage of cases for each category within a frequency distribution.

statistical sample: a portion of a target population comprising a specific variable such as gender, age, geographical location, income, or occupation.

statistical significance: the statistical evidence that an observed value is equal to or more than the critical value derived from a statistical table in rejecting the null hypothesis.

stem and leaf display: descriptive figure that displays raw scores from high to low values, organizing scores into leading digits (stems) and secondary digits (leaves). Useful in displaying trends or patterns in data.

survey research: a systematic and objective investigation into the characteristics, attitudes, opinions, and behaviors of target populations through questionnaires and interviews.

t tests: inferential statistics that are used to determine whether the difference between two means are statistically significant or are attributable to chance. They include one-sample *t* test, independent *t* test, and correlated or paired-data *t* test. For testing two independent groups with approximately the same variance, the formula is:

$$t = \frac{\text{Mean}_1 - \text{Mean}_2}{\text{Standard error of the differences between the means}}$$

target population: an identified group in which a representative or random sample of subjects are selected.

tertiary prevention: the prevention of secondary problems that can result from a disability, such as preventing decubiti in individuals with spinal cord injury.

test battery: a group of tests selected to comprehensively measure an individual's capacity, such as in performance, vocational interests, attitudes, and intelligence.

test-retest reliability: a method to estimate the degree of consistency of a test. In this method a test is administered to the same group of subjects over a short period of time. Maturation and changes in the subjects can affect the results and must be controlled by the investigator.

theory: a comprehensive body of writings that attempts to explain, for example, how individuals contract and resist disease, learn motoric tasks, and develop cognitive and language functions.

time series research: in experimental research, time series research indicates the measurement of the dependent variable over time intervals, such as 2 weeks or 3 months. Its purpose is to evaluate the effect of a number of interventions or treatment techniques with the same subject or group.

transformational research: the use of research as a personal-political activity whereby the research participants become empowered by active engagement in the research process.

treatment effects: in experimental research, the application of independent variable in producing a desired or predicted outcome. For example, the use of sensory integration therapy in reducing inattention.

treatment protocols: operational definitions of the methods used by clinicians.

They are described in enough detail so that replication is possible. Treatment protocols are generated through research and are used in evidence-based practice.

triangulation: the use of multiple approaches in collecting data and measuring variables. For example, in measuring a variable such as functional independence, the investigator would use a standardized ADL scale, use a functional capacity evaluation, and apply a self-report measure where the patient evaluates his or her performance in self-care activities.

Type I error: rejection of the null hypothesis when it should be accepted. Analogous to a false positive in medicine when a physician detects a disease when no disease is present.

Type II error: acceptance of the null hypothesis when it should be rejected. Analogous to a false negative in medicine when a physician fails to detect a disease when a disease is present.

unobtrusive methodology: a research method in which the investigator collects data from indirect sources, such as patient records, historical documents, letters, and relics.

validity: as pertaining to measurement, it refers to the degree to which a test or measuring instrument actually measures what it purports to measure. Validity can also refer to the rigor of an experiment in controlling extraneous variables and the generalizability of the results of a study to a target population.

variability: *See* measures of variability.

variables: characteristics, factors, or attributes that can be measured qualitatively or quantitatively. Variables can be homogeneous groups, such as physical therapy students, individuals with stroke, or hospital administrators. Variables can also be treatment methods such as exercise or biofeedback or outcomes such as muscle strength, spasticity, functional capacity, or academic achievement.

variance: the average of each score's deviation from the mean. Variance is an intermediate value that is used in calculating the standard deviation. The variance is the square of the standard deviation.

vocational interest test: a measure of an individual's preferences toward occupation-related tasks or jobs.

Wilcoxon signed rank test for correlated samples: a nonparametric test and an alternative to the correlated *t* test when comparing matched subjects or two sets of scores from the same subjects. Before-and-after studies are examples of correlated groups.

work samples: well-defined activities that are similar to an actual job. Examples include Valpar and Micro-Tower.

z score: a score based on standard deviation units from the mean, for example, a z score of +1 is one standard deviation unit above the mean.

References

Achenbach, T. M. (1991). *Achenbach System of Empirically Based Assessment* (ASEBA). Burlington, VT: University Medical Educational Association. (Available from the University of Vermont College of Education, Room 6436, 1 South Prospect St., Burlington, VT; http://www.uvm.edu/~cbcl/) [2000, January 14].

Ackoff, R. L., & Rivett, P. (1963). *A manager's guide to operation research.* New York: Wiley.

Adger, C. (1994). Enhancing the delivery of services to Black special education students from non-standard English backgrounds. Final Report. College Park: Maryland University, College Park Institute for the Study of Exceptional Children and Youth. (ERIC Document Reproduction Service No ED 370-377)

Adler, P. A., & Adler, P. (1994). Observational techniques. In N. K. Denzin & Y. S. Lincoln (Eds.), *Handbook of qualitative research* (pp. 377–392). Thousand Oaks, CA: Sage.

Affleck, J. W., Aitken, R. C., Hunter, J. A., McGuire, R. J., & Roy, C. W. (1988). Rehabilitation status: A measure of medicosocial dysfunction. *The Lancet, 1,* 230–233.

Allen, C. K. (1985). *Occupational therapy for psychiatric diseases: Measurement and management of cognitive disabilities.* Boston: Little, Brown.

Allen, C. K. (1992). Cognitive disabilities. In N. Katz (Ed.), *Cognitive rehabilitation: Models for intervention in occupational therapy* (pp. 1–21). Boston: Andover Medical.

Allen, C. K., Earhart, C. A., & Blue, T. (1992). *Occupational therapy treatment goals for the physically and cognitively disabled.* Rockville, MD: American Occupational Therapy Association.

Als, H. (1984). *Manual for the naturalistic observation of newborn behavior (preterm and full term infants).* Boston: Children's Hospital.

Als, H., Duffy, F. H., & McAnulty, G. B. (1988a). The APIB, an assessment of functional competence in preterm and full-term newborns regardless of gestational age at birth: II. *Infant Behavior and Development, 11,* 319–331.

Als, H., Duffy, F. H., & McAnulty, G. B. (1988b). Behavioral differences between preterm and full-term newborns as measured with the APIB system scores: I. *Infant Behavior and Development, 11,* 305–318.

American Occupational Therapy Association. (1999). *OT BibSys,* [On-Line]. Available: http://www.aotf.org/html/ot_bibsys.html [1999, October 5].

American Psychiatric Association. (1994). *Diagnostic and statistical manual* (4th ed.). Washington, DC: Author.

American Psychological Association. (1994). *Publication manual of the American Psychological Association,* (4th ed.). Washington, DC: Author.

Americans with Disabilities Act [ADA] of 1990, Pub. L. No. 101–336, § 2, 104 Stat. 328 (1991).

Anastasi, A. (1988). *Psychological testing* (6th ed.). New York: Macmillan.

Anastasi, A., & Urbina, S. (1997). *Psychological testing* (7th ed.). Englewood Cliffs, NJ: Prentice Hall.

Anderson, G. M., & Lomas, J. L. (1988). Monitoring the diffusion of technology: Coronary artery bypass surgery in Ontario. *American Journal of Public Health, 78,* 251–254.

Anderson, M. H., Bechtol, C. O., & Sollars, R. E. (1959). *Clinical prosthetics for physicians and therapists.* Springfield: IL: Charles C. Thomas.

Applegate, W., Blass, J., & Williams, F. (1990). Instruments for the functional assessment of older patients. *New England Journal of Medicine, 322,* 1207–1214.

Armstrong, C. J. (Ed.). (1993). *World databases in medicine.* London: Bowker-Saur.

Arthur, G. (1949). The Arthur Adaptation of the International Performance Scale. *Journal of Clinical Psychology, 5,* 345–349.

Åsberg, M., Perris, C., Schalling, D., & Sedval, G. (1987). The CPRS—Development and applications of a psychiatric rating scale. *Acta Psychiatrica Scandinavia, 271*(Suppl.), 1–27.

Asher, I. E. (1996). *Occupational therapy assessment tools: An annotated index* (2nd ed.). Rockville, MD: American Occupational Therapy Association.

Atwater, E. C. (1973). The medical profession in a new society, Rochester, York (1811–60). *Bulletin of the History of Medicine, 47,* 221–235.

Auble, D. (1953). Extended tables for the Mann-Whitney statistic. *Bulletin of the Institute of Educational Research at Indiana University, 1,* No. 2.

Ayres, A. J. (1976). *Interpreting the Southern California Sensory Integration Tests.* Los Angeles: Western Psychological Services.

Ayres, A. J. (1989). *Sensory Integration and Praxis Tests* (SIPT). Los Angeles: Western Psychological Association.

Baltimore Therapeutic Equipment Company. (1992). *Clinical application model: A clinically oriented reference model for users of the BTE work simulator.* Baltimore: Author.

Baker, J. G., Granger, C. V., & Fiedler, R. C. (1997). A brief outpatient functional assessment measure: Validity using Rasch measures. *American Journal of Physical Medicine and Rehabilitation, 76,* 8–13.

Baptiste, S., & Rochon, S. (1999). Client-centered assessment: The Canadian Occupational Performance Measure. In B. J. Hemphill-Pearson (Ed.), *Assessments in occupational therapy mental health: An integrative approach* (pp. 41–58). Thorofare, NJ: Slack.

Barnhard, C. L. (Ed.). (1948). *American college dictionary.* New York: Random House.

Barth, T. (1985). *Barth time construction.* New York: Health Related Consulting Services.

Barzun, J. (1974). *Clio and the doctors: Psycho-history, quanto-history and history.* Chicago: University of Chicago Press.

Barzun, J., & Graff, H. (1970). *The modern researcher.* New York: Harcourt, Brace and World.

Bayley, N. (1993). *Bayley Scales of Infant Development—II* (BSID-II). San Antonio, TX: The Psychological Corporation.

Beck, A. T., Ward, C. H., Mendelson, M., Mock, J., & Erbaugh, J. (1961). An inventory for measuring depression. *Archives of General Psychiatry, 4,* 561–571.

Becker, R. L. (1981). *Reading-Free Vocational Interest Inventory.* Columbus, OH: Elbern.

Beers, C. A. (1908). *A mind that found itself.* New York: Doubleday.

Beery, K. E., & Buketnica, N. A. (1996). *The Developmental Test of Visual-Motor Integration* (4th ed.; VMI-4). Austin, TX: Pro-Ed.

Bender, L. (1938). A visual motor Gestalt test and its clinical use. *American Orthopsychiatric Association Research Monograph,* No. 3.

Benison, S. (1972). The history of polio research in the United States: Appraisal and lessons. In G. Holton (Ed.), *The twentieth-century sciences: Studies in the biography of ideas* (pp. 308–343). New York: W. W. Norton.

Bennett, G. K. (1946). *Hand Tool Dexterity Test.* San Antonio, TX: The Psychological Corporation.

Bennett, G. K. (1994). *Bennett Mechanical Comprehension Test.* San Antonio, TX: The Psychological Corporation.

Bergner, M., Bobbitt, R. A., Carter, W. B., & Gilson, B. S. (1981). The Sickness Impact Profile: Development and final revision of a health status measure. *Medical Care, 19,* 787–805.

Bernard, C. (1957). *An introduction to the study of experimental medicine* (H. C. Greene, Trans.). New York: Dover. (Original work published 1865)

Best, J. W. (1979). *Research in education* (3rd ed.). Englewood Cliffs, NJ: Prentice Hall.

Best, J. W., & Kahn, J. V. (1997). *Research in education* (8th ed.). Boston: Allyn & Bacon.

Bettelheim, B. (1967). *The empty fortress: Infantile autism and the birth of the self.* New York: The Free Press.

Bettelheim, B. (1969). *Children of the dream.* New York: Macmillan.

Binet, A. (1899/1912). *The psychology of reasoning: Based on experimental researches in hypnotism* (2nd ed.). (A. G. Whyte, Trans.). Chicago: Open Court.

Black, M. K. (1991). *Standardization of instructions and test–retest reliability of a manual dexterity and work skills assessment tool.* Unpublished master's thesis, Virginia Commonwealth University, Richmond.

Black, M. K., Nelson, C. E., Maurere, P. A., & Bauer, D. F. (1993). Test–retest reliability of the Work Box® : A work sample with standard instructions. *Work: A Journal of Prevention and Rehabilitation, 3*(4), 26–34.

Black, M. M. (1976). Adolescent role assessment. *American Journal of Occupational Therapy, 30,* 73–79.

Blake, J. B., & Roos, C. (Eds.). (1967). *Medical reference works 1679–1966: A selected bibliography.* Chicago: Medical Library Assoc.

Blankenship, K. (1984). *Individual rehabilitation: Procedure manual.* Mason, GA: American Therapeutics.

Blue, F. R. (1979). Aerobic running as a treatment for moderate depression. *Perceptual and Motor Skills, 48,* 228.

Blumberg, D. F. (1972). The city as a system. In J. Beishon & G. Peters (Eds.), *Systems behavior.* New York: Harper and Row.

Blumstein, J. F. (1997). The Oregon experiment: The role of cost-benefit analysis in the allocation of Medicaid funds. *Social Science & Medicine, 45,* 545–554.

Booth, T., & Booth, W. (1994). The use of depth interviewing with vulnerable subjects: Lessons from a research study of parents with learning difficulties. *Social Science and Medicine, 39,* 415–424.

Borowitz, G. H., Costello, J., & Hirsch, J. G. (1971). Clinical observation of ghetto 4-year-olds: Organization, involvement, interpersonal responsiveness and psychosexual content of play. *Journal of Youth and Adolescence, 1,* 59–71.

Bosscher, R. J. (1993). Running and mixed physical exercises with depressed psychiatric patients. *International Journal of Sport Psychology, 24,* 170–184.

Botterbusch, K. F. (1980). *A comparison of commercial vocational evaluations systems.* Menomonie, WI: Stout Vocational Rehabilitation Institute.

Bowker Company. (1995). *Medical and health care books and serials in print: An index to literature in the health sciences.* New York: Author.

Bowling, A. (1999). *Measuring health: A review of quality of life measurement scales* (2nd ed.). Buckingham, Great Britain: Open University Press.

Brayman, S. J., & Kirby, T. (1976). Comprehensive Occupational Therapy Evaluation. *American Journal of Occupational Therapy, 30,* 94–100.

Breines, E. (1988). The Functional Assessment Scale as an instrument for measuring changes in levels of function for nursing home residents following occupational therapy. *Canadian Journal of Occupational Therapy, 55,* 135–140.

Brollier, C., Hamrick, N., & Jackson, B. (1994). Aerobic exercise: A potential occupational therapy modality for adolescents with depression. *Occupational Therapy in Mental Health, 12,* 19–29.

Brown, C., McDaniel, R., Couch, R., & McClanahan, M. (1994). *Vocational educational systems and software: A consumer's guide.* Menomonie, WI: Stout Vocational Rehabilitation Institute, University of Wisconsin-Stout.

Brown, G. T., & Rodger, S. (1999). Research utilization models: Frameworks for implementing evidence-based occupational therapy practice. *Occupational Therapy International, 6,* 1–23.

Brown, L., & Hammill, D. D. (1990). *Behavior Rating Profile—2.* Austin, TX: Pro-Ed.

Brown, S. L., D'Eugenio, D. B., Drews, J. E., Haskin, B. S., Lynch, E. W., Moersch, M. S., & Rogers, S. J. (1981). Preschool assessment: An application. In D. B. D'Eugenio & M. Moersch (Eds.), *Developmental programming for infants and young children* (Vol. 4). Ann Arbor: University of Michigan Press.

Bruininks, R. H. (1978). *Bruininks–Oseretsky Test of Motor Proficiency.* Circle Pines, MN: American Guidance Service.

Bryman, A., & Burgess, R. G. (Eds.). (1994). *Analyzing qualitative data.* London: Routledge.

Bulgren, J. A., Schumaker, J. B., & Deshler, D. D. (1994). The effects of a recall enhancement routine on the test performance of secondary students with and without learning disabilities. *Learning Disabilities Research, 9,* 1–11.

Bulmer, M. (Ed.). (1982). *Social research ethics.* London: Macmillan.

Burks, H. (1968). *Burks' Behavior Rating Scales.* Los Angeles: Western Psychological Services.

Callinan, N. J., & Mathiowetz, V. (1996). Soft versus hard resting hand splints in rheumatoid arthritis: Pain relief, preference, and compliance. *American Journal of Occupational Therapy, 50,* 347–353.

Campbell, D. T., & Stanley, J. (1963). *Experimental and quasi-experimental design for Research.* Chicago: Rand-McNally.

Campione, J. C., & Brown, A. L. (1978). Toward a theory of intelligence: Contributions from research with retarded children. *Intelligence, 2,* 279–304.

Cannon, W. B. (1932). *The wisdom of the body.* New York: W. W. Norton.

Carey, R. G., & Posavac, E. J. (1980). *Manual for the Level of Rehabilitation Scale II.* Park Ridge, IL: Lutheran General Hospital.

Carey, R. G., & Posavac, E. J. (1982). Rehabilitation program evaluation using a revised level of rehabilitation scale (LORS-II). *Archives of Physical Medicine and Rehabilitation, 63,* 367–370.

Carlsson, A. M. (1983). Assessment of chronic pain, Part I: Aspects of the reliability and validity of the visual analogue scale. *Pain, 16,* 87–101.

Carr, J. H., Shepherd, R. B., Nordholm, L., & Lynne, D. (1985). Investigation of a new motor assessment scale for stroke patients. *Physical Therapy, 65,* 175–178.

Cattell, R. B. (1950). *Culture Fair Intelligence Test.* Champaign, IL: Institute for Personality and Ability Testing.

Cattell, R. B. (1963). Theory of fluid and crystalized intelligence: A critical experiment. *Journal of Educational Psychology, 54,* 615–618.

Cattell, R. B., Cattell, A. K., & Cattell, H. E. P. (1993). *Sixteen Personality Factor Questionnaire* (5th ed.). San Antonio, TX: The Psychological Corporation.

Center for Functional Assessment Research. (1993). *Functional Independent Measure.* Buffalo, NY: State University of New York.

Centers for Disease Control and Prevention, National Center for Health Statistics. (1996, February 29). Advance report of final mortality statistics, 1993. *Monthly Vital Statistics Report, 44*(Suppl. 7), pp. 1–83. Available: http://www.cdc.gov/nchs/data/mvs44_7s.pdf [1999, October 2].

Centers for Disease Control and Prevention. (1997, October 7). Mortality Patterns—1997. *Morbidity and Mortality Weekly Report (MMWR), 47*(4), 664–680. Available: http://www.cdc.gov/nchs/data/47_4t17.pdf [1999, October 2].

Centers for Disease Control and Prevention, National Center for Health Statistics. (1998, March). Ambulatory and inpatient procedures in the United States, 1995. *Vital Health Statistics, 13*(135), 1–124. Available: http://www.cdc.gov/nchswww/data/sr13_135.pdf [1999, October 2].

Centers for Disease Control and Prevention, National Center for Health Statistics. (1998, Nov. 20). Summary of Notifiable Diseases, United States, 1997. *Morbidity and Mortal-ity Weekly Report (MMWR), 46*(54) 1–14. Available: http://www2.cdc.gov/mmwr/mmwr_wk.html or ftp://ftp.cdc.gov/pub/Publications/mmwr/wk/mm4654.pdf [1999, October 2].

Centers for Disease Control and Prevention, National Center for Health Statistics. (1999, June 30). Deaths: Final data for 1997. *National Vital Statistics Report, 47*(19), 1–108. Available: http://www.cdc.gov/nchs/data/nvs47_19.pdf [1999, October 2].

Cheng, T. C. E. (1993). Operations research and high education administration. *Journal of Educational Administration, 31,* 77–99.

CHID Technical Director. (n.d.). *Welcome to the combined health information database* [On-Line]. Available: http://chid.nih.gov/welcome/welcome.html [1999, August 16].

Cinahl Information Systems. (1997). *Cumulative index to nursing and allied health (CINAHL) database.* Available: http://www.biomedsearch.lib.umn.edu/ovidweb/fldguide/nursing.htm [1999, August 16].

Clandinin, D. J., & Connelly, F. M. (1994). Personal experience methods. In N. K. Denzin & Y. S. Lincoln (Eds.), *Handbook of qualitative research* (pp. 413–427). Thousand Oaks, CA: Sage.

Clark, E. N. (1999). Build a city: A projective task concept. In B. J. Hemphill-Pearson (Ed.), *Assessments in occupational therapy mental health: An integrative approach* (pp. 156–169). Thorofare, NJ: Slack.

Clark, E. N., & Peters, M. (1993). *Scorable self-care evaluation* (rev. ed.). San Antonio, TX: Therapy Skill Builders/The Psychological Corporation.

Clark F., Azen, S. P., Zemke R., Jackson, J., Carlson, M., Mandel, D., Hay, J., Josephson, K., Cherry, B., Hessel, C., Palmer, J., & Lipson, L. (1997). Occupational therapy for independent-living older adults. A randomized controlled trial. *The Journal of the American Medical Association, 278,* 1321–1326.

Clark, J., Koch, B. A., & Nichols, R. C. (1965). A factor analytically derived scale: For rating psychiatric patients in occupational therapy. *American Journal of Occupational Therapy, 19,* 14–18.

Clarke, G. N., Rohde, P., Lewinsohn, P. M., Hops, H., & Seeley, J. R. (1999). Cognitive-behavioral treatment of adolescent depression: Efficacy of acute group treatment and booster sessions. *Journal of the American Academy of Child and Adolescent Psychiatry, 38,* 272–279.

Clifford, C. (1990). *Nursing and health care research; A skills-based introduction* (2nd ed.). London: Prentice Hall.

Clifton, D. W., & Burcham, M. (1997). Utilization review: Disability duration tables: Borders or barriers? Part I. *P. T.—Magazine of Physical Therapy, 5*(9), 3–38.

Cohen, J. (1960). A coefficient of agreement for nominal scales. *Educational and Psychological Measurement, 20,* 37–46.

Cohen, J. (1977). *Statistical power analysis for the behavioral sciences* (Rev. ed.). New York: Academic Press.

Colarusso, R. P., & Hammill, D. D. (1996). *Motor-Free Visual Perception Test—Revised* (MFVPT-R). Novato, CA: Academic Therapy Publications.

Cole, B., Finch, E., Gowland, C., & Mayo, N. (1994). *Physical rehabilitation outcome measures.* Toronto, Ontario: Canadian Physiotherapy Association.

Collins, J. G. (1997). *Vital and health statistics, prevalence of selected chronic conditions: United States, 1990–1992,* Series 10, No. 194. Centers for Disease Control and Prevention, National Centers for Health Statistics. Available: http://www.cdc.gov/nchs/products/pubs/pubd/series/sr10/199-190/se10_194.htm [1999, December 26].

Colton, T. (1974). *Statistics in medicine.* Boston: Little, Brown.

Conant, J. B. (1951). *Science and common sense.* New Haven, CT: Yale University Press.

Conners, C. K. (1989a). *Conners Parent Rating Scales.* North Tonawanda, NY: Multi-Health Systems.

Conners, C. K. (1989b). *Conners Teacher Rating Scales.* North Tonawanda, NY: Multi Health Systems.

Conoley, J. C., & Impara, J. C. (Eds.). (1995). *The twelfth mental measurements yearbook* (12th ed.). Lincoln, NE: Buros Institute of Mental Measurements. Available: http://www.unl.edu/buros/catalog.html#mmy [1999, October 29].

Conoley, J. C., Kramer, J. J., & Murphy, L. I. (1992). *The mental measurements yearbook* (11th ed.), *mental measurements supplement, or tests in print,* Lincoln: NE: The University of Nebraska Press.

Copi, I. (1953). *Introduction to logic.* New York: Macmillan.

Corcoran, K., & Fischer, J. (1987). *Measures for clinical practice: A source book.* New York: The Free Press.

Corrigan, J. D. (1989). Development of a scale for assessment of agitation following traumatic brain injury. *Journal of Clinical and Experimental Neuropsychology, 11,* 261–277.

Corrigan, J. D., & Deming, R. (1995). Psychometric characteristics of the community integration questionnaire: Replication and extension. *Journal of Head Trauma Rehabilitation, 10,* 41–53.

Cot, C., & Finch, E. (1991). Goal setting in physical therapy practise. *Physiotherapy Canada, 43,* 19–22.

Crawford, J. E., & Crawford, D. M. (1975). *The Crawford Small Parts Dexterity Test.* San Antonio, TX: The Psychological Corporation.

Creighton, C., Dijkers, M., Bennett, N., & Brown, K. (1995). Reasoning and the art of therapy for spinal cord injury. *American Journal of Occupational Therapy, 49,* 311–317.

Creswell, J. W. (1998). *Qualitative inquiry and research design: Choosing among five traditions.* Thousand Oaks, CA: Sage.

Cronbach, L. J. (1984). *Essentials of psychological testing* (4th ed.). New York: Harper and Row.

Crowther, J. G., & Whiddington, R. (1948). *Science at war.* New York: Philosophical Library.

Crump, A. (1997). Room to remember. *Elderly Care, 9,* 8–10.

Cunningham, P. H., & Bartuska, T. (1989). The relationship between stress and leisure satisfaction among therapeutic recreation personnel. *Therapeutic Recreation Journal 23,* 65–70.

Cutler, S. K. (1992). *Executive functioning in middle school students who have learning disabilities.* Unpublished doctoral dissertation. University of New Mexico, Albuquerque.

Cutler, S. K., Keyes, D. W., & Urquhart, M. (1993). [Effects of teaching methods on understanding collaboration concepts.] Unpublished raw data.

Daniels, L., Williams, M., & Worthingham, C. (1956). *Muscle testing: Techniques of manual examination* (2nd ed.). Philadelphia: W. B. Saunders.

Daniels, L., & Worthingham, C. (1986). *Muscle testing: Techniques of manual examination* (5th ed.). Philadelphia: W. B. Saunders.

Das, J. P., Kirby, J., & Jarman, R. (1975). An alternative model for cognitive abilities. *Psychological Bulletin, 82,* 87–103.

Davis, F. B. (Chair). (1974). *Standards for education and psychological tests.* Prepared by a joint committee of the American Psychological Association, American Educational Research Association, and National Council on Measurement in Education. Washington, DC: American Psychological Association.

Dawber, T. R., Meaders, G. F., & Moore, F. E., Jr. (1951). Epidemiological approaches to heart disease: The Framingham study. *American Journal of Public Health, 41,* 279–286.

Dean, C., & Gadd, E. M. (1990). Home treatment for acute psychiatric illness. *British Medical Journal, 301,* 1021–1023.

DeGangi, R. A., & Berk, G. A. (1983). *DeGangi-Berk Test of Sensory Integration.* Los Angeles: Western Psychological Services.

Delaney-Black, V., Covington, C., Templin, T., Ager, J., Martier, S., Compton, S., & Sokol, R. (1998). Prenatal coke: What's behind the smoke? Prenatal cocaine/alcohol exposure and school-age outcomes: The SCHOO-BE experience. *Annals of the New York Academy of Science, 846,* 277–288.

DeMatteo, C., Law, M., Russell, D., Pollack, N., Rosenbaum, P., & Walter, S. (1993). The reliability and validity of the Quality of Upper Extremity Skills Test. *Physical and Occupational Therapy in Pediatrics, 13*(2), 1–18.

Deno, S. L. (1985). Curriculum-based assessment: The emerging alternative. *Exceptional Children, 52,* 219–232.

Denzin, N. K., & Lincoln, Y. S. (Eds.). (1994a). *Handbook of qualitative research.* Thousand Oaks, CA: Sage.

Denzin, N. K., & Lincoln, Y. S. (1994b). Introduction: Entering the field of qualitative research. In N. K. Denzin & Y. S. Lincoln (Eds.), *Handbook of qualitative research* (pp. 1–17). Thousand Oaks, CA: Sage.

Dewey, J. (1933). *How we think.* Boston: D. C. Heath.

Dickerson, A. E. (1999). The Role Checklist. In B. Hemphill-Pearson (Ed.), *Assessments in occupational therapy mental health: An integrative approach* (pp. 175–182). Thorofare, NJ: Slack.

Dittmar, S. S., & Gresham, G. E. (1997). *Functional assessment and outcome measures for the rehabilitation health professional.* Gaithersburg, MD: Aspen.

Donaldson, S. W., Wagner, C. C., & Gresham, G. E. (1973). Unified ADL evaluation form. *Archives of Physical Medicine and Rehabilitation, 54,* 175–179, 185.

Downer, A. H. (1970). *Physical therapy techniques.* Springfield, IL: Charles C. Thomas.

Doyne, E. J., Chambless, D. L., & Beutler, L. E. (1983). Aerobic exercise as a treatment for depression in women. *Behavior Therapy, 14,* 434–440.

Doyne, E. J., Ossip-Klein, D. J., Bowman, E. D., Osborn, D. M., McDougall-Wilson, I. B., & Neimeyer, R. A. (1987). Running versus weight lifting in the treatment of depression. *Journal of Consulting Clinical Psychology, 55,* 748–754.

Duke University Center for the Study of Aging and Human Development. (1978). *Functional assessment: The OARS methodology.* Durham, NC: Duke University.

Dukes, W. F. (1965). $N = 1$. *Psychological Bulletin, 64,* 73–79.

Dunn, L. M. (1968). Special education for the mildly retarded—Is much of it justifiable? *Exceptional Children, 35,* 5–22.

Dunn, W. (1990). A comparison of service provision models in school-based occupational therapy services: A pilot study. *Occupational Therapy Journal of Research, 10,* 300–320.

Earhart, C. A., & Allen, C. A. (1988). *Cognitive disabilities: Expanded activity analysis.* Los Angeles County: University of Southern California Medical Center.

Easton, D. (1961). *A framework for political analysis.* Englewood Cliffs, NJ: Prentice-Hall.

Edgerton, R. B., & Langness, L. L. (1978). Observing mentally retarded persons in community settings: An anthropological perspective. In G. P. Sackett (Ed.), *Observing behavior. Theory and applications in mental retardation* (pp. 335–348). Baltimore: University Park Press.

Education for All Handicapped Children Act of 1974 [EAHCA; Pub. L. 94-142] U.S.C., Title 20, Sections 1400 et seq. (1975).

Education for All Handicapped Children Act of 1986 [Pub. L. 101-476] U.S.C., 1988, Title 20, Sections 1400 et seq. (1987).

Edwards, A. L. (1959). *Edwards Personal Preference Schedule.* San Antonio, TX: The Psychological Corporation.

Edwards, D. R., & Bristol, M. M. (1991). Autism: Early identification and management in family practice. *AFP, 44,* 1755–1764.

Emerson, H., Cook, J., Polatajko, H., & Segal, R. (1998). Enjoyment experiences as described by persons with schizophrenia: A qualitative study. *Canadian Journal of Occupational Therapy, 65,* 183–192.

Employment Stabilization Research Institute, University of Minnesota. (1969). *Minnesota Rate of Manipulation Tests.* Circle Pines, MN: American Guidance Service.

Enders, A., & Hall, M. (Eds.). (1990). *Assistive technology sourcebook.* Washington, DC: RESNA Press.

Englehart, M. D. (1972). *Methods of educational research*. Chicago: Rand McNally.

Epps, S., & Tindall, G. (1987). The effectiveness of differential programming in serving students with mild handicaps: Placement options and instructional programming. In M. C. Wang, M. C. Reynolds, & H. J. Walberg (Eds.), *Handbook of special education: Research and practice*. (Vol. 1, pp. 213–248). Oxford, England: Pergamon Press.

Erhardt, R. (1989). *Erhardt Developmental Prehension Assessment*. Tucson, AZ: Therapy Skill Builders/The Psychological Corporation.

Ernst, A. A., Houry, D., & Weiss, S. J. (1997). Research funding in the four major emergency medicine journals. *American Journal of Emergency Medicine, 15*, 268–270.

Fairbank, J. C. T., Davies, J. B., Couper, J., & O'Brien, J. P. (1980). The Oswestry Low Back Pain Disability Questionnaire. *Physiotherapy, 66*, 271–273.

Falk-Ross, F. (1996, Feb.). *Classroom-based language remediation programs: Roles, routines, and reflections*. Paper presented at the 36th Annual Convention of the Illinois Speech-Language-Hearing Association. (ERIC Document Reproduction Service No. ED417-539)

Feden, S. D. (1993). *Test-retest reliability of the Work Box® with nondisabled female subjects*. Unpublished research project, Virginia Commonwealth University, Richmond.

Feigin, G., An, C., Connors, D., & Crawford, I. (1996, April). Shape up, ship out, [On-Line]. *ORMS Today, 23*(2), 1–7. Available: www. lionhrtpub.com/orms/orms-4-96/ibm.html [1999, May 2].

Feldman, P. A. (1990). Upper extremity casting and splinting. In M. D. Glenn & J. Whyte (Eds.), *The practical management of spasticity in children and adults*. Malvern, PA: Lea & Febiger.

Ferber, R., & Verdoorn, P. J. (1962). *Research methods in economics and business*. New York: Macmillan.

Ferguson, P. M., Ferguson, D. L., & Taylor, S. J. (Eds.). (1992). *Interpreting disability. A qualitative reader*. New York: Teachers College Press.

Festinger, L., & Katz, O. (1953). *Research methods in the behavioral sciences*. New York: Holt, Rinehart and Winston.

Finley, T. W. (1989). Research in physical medicine and rehabilitation: II. The conceptual review of the literature or how to read more articles than you ever want to see in your entire life. *American Journal of Physical Medicine & Rehabilitation, 68*, 97–102.

Fischer, J., & Corcoran, K. (1995). *Measures for clinical practice: A sourcebook* (2nd ed.). New York: Free Press.

Fisher, A. (1994). *Assessment of motor and process skills* (AMPS). Unpublished manual. (Available from A. Fisher, Department of Occupational Therapy, University of Illinois at Chicago)

Fitzgerald, M. H., Mullavey-O'Byrne, C., & Clemson, L. (1997). *Australian Occupational Therapy Journal, 44*, 1–21.

Fleischman, D. A., & Gabriele, J. D. (1998). Repetition priming in normal aging and Alzheimer's disease: A review of findings and theories. *Psychology and Aging, 13*, 88–119.

Flexner, A. (1910). *Medical education in the United States and Canada: A report to the Carnegie Foundation for the Advancement of Teaching* (Bulletin No. 4). New York City: Carnegie Foundation.

Flood, J. F., & Morley, J. E. (1998). Learning and memory in the SAMP8 mouse. *Neuroscience & Biobehavioral Reviews, 22*, 1–20.

Folio, M. R., & Fewell, R. R. (1983). *Peabody Developmental Motor Scales*. Allen, TX: DLM Teaching Resources.

Folstein, M. F., Folstein, S. E., & McHugh, P. R. (1975). Mini-mental state: A practical method for grading the cognitive state of patients for the clinician. *Journal of Psychiatric Research, 12*, 189–198.

Fontana, A., & Frey, J. H. (1994). Interviewing: The art of science. In N. K. Denzin & Y. S. Lincoln (Eds.), *Handbook of qualitative research* (pp. 361–376). Thousand Oaks, CA: Sage.

Forness, S. R., & Kavale, K. A. (1984). Education of the mentally retarded: A note on policy. *Education and Training of the Mentally Retarded, 19*, 239–245.

Fraenkel, J. R., & Wallen, N. E. (1990). *How to design and evaluate research in education*. New York: McGraw.

Frank, G. (1996). Life histories in occupational therapy clinical practice. *American Journal of Occupational Therapy, 50*, 251–264.

Frank, G., Bernardo, C. S., Tropper, S., Noguchi, F., Lipman, C., Maulhardt, B., & Weitze, L. (1997). Jewish spirituality through actions in time: Daily occupations of young orthodox Jewish couples in Los Angeles. *American Journal of Occupational Therapy, 51*, 199–206.

Frankenburg, W. K., Dodds, J. B., Archer, P., Shapiro, H., & Bresnick, B. (1990). *Denver Devel-*

opmental Screening Test—II. Denver: Denver Developmental Materials.

Frederick, M. (1928). *Thrasher, the gang: A study of 1,313 gangs in Chicago.* Chicago: University of Chicago Press.

French, S. (Ed.). (1994). *On equal terms. Working with disabled people.* Oxford: Butterworth/ Heinemann.

Frey, J. J., & Fontana, A. (1995). *The group interview.* Newbury Park, CA: Sage.

Fry, P. S. (1984). Development of a geriatric scale of hopelessness: Implications for counseling and intervention with the depressed elderly *Journal of Counseling Psychology, 31,* 322–331.

Friedman, G. D. (1980). *Primer of epidemiology.* New York: McGraw-Hill.

Fruchter, B. (1954). *Introduction to factor analysis.* Princeton, NJ: D. Van Nostrand.

Fugl-Meyer, A. R., Jääskö, L., Leyman, I., Olsson, S., & Steglind, S. (1975). The poststroke hemiplegic patient I. A method for evaluation of physical performance. *Scandinavian Journal of Rehabilitation Medicine, 7,* 13–31.

Fukutani, Y., Sasaki, K., Mukai, M., Matsubara, R., Isaki, K., & Cairns, N. J. (1997). Neurons and extracellular neurofibrillary tangles in the hippocampal subdivisions in early-onset familial Alzheimer's disease: A case study. *Psychiatry & Clinical Neurosciences, 51,* 227–231.

Gale Group. (1999). *Encyclopedia of associations: International organizations. An associations unlimited reference* (34th ed.). Detroit: Gale Group.

Galen, C. (1971). *On the natural faculties.* In W. P. D. Wightman (Ed.), *The emergence of scientific medicine.* Edinburgh: Oliver and Boyd. (Original work published ca. 192 A.D.)

Gardner, H. (1983). *Frames of mind: Theories of multiple intelligences.* New York: Basic Books.

Gardner, M. F. (1982). *Test of Visual Perceptual Skills (non-motor).* Burlingame, CA: Psychological and Educational Publications.

Gardner, M. F. (1992). *Test of Visual-Motor Skills— Upper Level* (TVMS-UL). Burlingame, CA: Psychological and Educational Publications.

Gee, W. (1950). *Social science research methods.* New York: Appleton-Century-Crofts.

Gesell, A. (1928). *Infancy and human growth.* New York: McGraw-Hill.

Gesell, A., & Thompson, H. (1923). *Infant behavior: Its genesis and growth.* New York: McGraw-Hill.

Gibaldi, J., & Franklin, P. (1999). *MLA handbook for writers of research papers* (5th ed.). New York: Modern Language Association.

Gilliam, J., & Barstow, I. K. (1997). Joint range of motion. In J. Van Deusen & D. Brunt (Eds.), *Assessment in occupational therapy and physical therapy* (pp. 49–77). Philadelphia: W. B. Saunders.

Gilson, B. S., Gilson, J. S., Bergner, M., Bobbitt, R. A., Kressel, S., Pollard, W. E., & Vesselago, M. (1975). The Sickness Impact Profile: Development of an outcome measure of health care. *American Journal of Public Health, 65,* 1304–1310.

Glaser, B. G., & Strauss, A. L. (1967). *The discovery of grounded theory: Strategies for qualitative research.* Chicago: Aldine.

Glaser, R. (1963). Instructional technology and the measurement of learning outcomes. *American Psychologist, 18,* 510–522.

Gleason, J. J. (1990). Meaning of play: interpreting patterns in behavior of persons with severe developmental disabilities. *Anthropology and Education Quarterly, 21,* 59–77.

Glesne, C., & Peshkin, A. (1992). *Becoming qualitative researchers: An introduction.* New York: Longman.

Goffman, E. (1961). *Asylums: Essays on the social situation of mental patients and other inmates.* Garden City, NJ: Anchor Books.

Gold, R. L. (1958). Roles in sociological field observations. *Social Forces, 36,* 217–223.

Goldberg, R. T. (1974). Rehabilitation research, new directions. *Journal of Rehabilitation, 40*(3), 12–14.

Golden, C. J., Purisch, A. D., & Hammeke, T. A. (1985). *Luria–Nebraska Neuropsychological Battery: Forms I and II* (Manual). Los Angeles: Western Psychological Services.

Good-Ellis, M. A. (1999). The Role Activity Performance Scale. In B. Hemphill-Pearson (Ed.), *Assessments in occupational therapy mental health: An integrative approach* (pp. 206–226). Thorofare, NJ: Slack.

Gordon, E. E. (1968). A view of the target population. In A. J. Tannenbaum (Ed.), *Special education programs for disadvantaged children and youth* (pp. 5–18). Washington, DC: The Council for Exceptional Children.

Gordon, L. V. (1981). *Gordon Occupational Check List II.* San Antonio: The Psychological Corporation.

Gough, H. G. (1987) *California Psychological Inventory.* New York: Consulting Psychologists Press.

Gould, J., & Kolb, J. G. (Eds.). (1964). *A dictionary of the social sciences.* (Compiled under the auspices of the United Nations Educational,

Scientific and Cultural Organizations.) New York: The Free Press.

Gould, S. J. (1996). *The mismeasure of man* (Rev. ed.). New York: Norton.

Gracely, R. H., & Kwilosz, D. M. (1988). The Descriptor Differential Scale: Applying psychophysical principles to clinical pain assessment. *Pain, 35,* 279–288.

Gracely, R. H., McGrath, P., & Dubner, R. (1978). Validity and sensitivity of ratio scales of sensory and affective verbal pain descriptors: Manipulation of affect by diazepam. *Pain, 5,* 19–29.

Granger, C. V., & Greer, D. S. (1976). Functional status measurement and medical rehabilitation outcomes. *Archives of Physical Medicine and Rehabilitation, 57,* 103–109.

Granger, C. V., Hamilton, B. B., Keith, R. A., Zielesky, M., & Sherwins, F. S. (1986). Advances in functional assessment for medical rehabilitation. *Topics in Geriatric Rehabilitation, 1,* 59–74.

Granger, C. V., & Wright, B. (1993). Looking ahead to the use of functional assessment in ambulatory physiatric and primary care. *Physical Medicine and Rehabilitation Clinics of North America, 4*(3), 1–11.

Gravette, F. J., & Wellnau, L. B. (1985). *Statistics for the behavioral sciences.* St. Paul, MN: West.

Greist, J. H., Klein, M. H., Eischens, R. R., Faris, J., Gurman, A. S., & Morgan, W. P. (1979). Running as treatment for depression. *Comprehensive Psychiatry, 20,* 41–54.

Guba, E. G. (1990). Carrying on the dialog. In E. G. Guba (Ed.), *The paradigm dialog* (pp. 368–378). Newbury Park, CA: Sage.

Guilford, J. P. (1967). *The nature of human intelligence.* New York: McGraw-Hill.

Haertlein, C. L. (1999). The Milwaukee Evaluation of Daily Living Skills (MEDLS). In B. J. Hemphill-Pearson (Ed.), *Assessments in occupational therapy mental health: An integrative approach* (pp. 245–258). Thorofare, NJ: Slack.

Hahn, M. E. (1969). *California Life Goals Evaluation Schedules.* Los Angeles: Western Psychological Services.

Haley, S. M., Coster, W. J., Ludlow, L. H., Haltiwanger, J. T., & Andrellos, P. J. (1992). *Pediatric Evaluation of Disability Inventory* (PEDI). (Available from PEDI Research Group, Department of Rehabilitation Medicine, New England Medical Center Hospital, #75K/R, 750 Washington Street, Boston, MA 02111-2901)

Hall, E. T. (1966). *The hidden dimension.* New York: Doubleday.

Hallahan, D. P., & Kauffman, J. M. (1993). *Exceptional children: Introduction to special education* (6th ed.). Boston: Allyn and Bacon.

Halstead, L. & Hartley, R. B. (1975). Time Care Profile: An evaluation of a new method of assessing ADL dependence. *Archives of Physical Medicine and Rehabilitation, 56,* 110–115.

Hamilton, M. (1960). A rating scale for depression. *Journal of Neurology, Neurosurgery, and Psychiatry, 23,* 468–477.

Harper, D. (1989). Visual sociology: Expanding sociological vision. In G. Blank et al. (Eds.), *New technology in sociology: Practical applications in research and work* (pp. 81–97). New Brunswick, NJ: Transaction Books.

Harvard Medical School. (1991). *Guidelines for investigators in scientific research.* (Available from the Office for Research Issues, Harvard Medical School, 25 Shattuck Street, Boston, MA 02115)

Harvard Medical School. (1996). *Guidelines for investigators in clinical research,* [On-Line] Available: http://www.hms.harvard.edu/integrity/clinical.html [1999, December 29].

Harvey, W. (1938). *On the motion of the heart and blood in animals* (R. Willis, Trans.). In C. W. Eliot (Ed.), *The Harvard classics scientific papers.* New York: P. E. Collier and Sons. (Original work published 1628)

Harvey, W. (1952). An anatomical disquisition on the motion of the heart and blood in animals. In R. M. Hutchins (Ed.), & R. Willis (Trans.), *Great books of the western world* (Vol. 28, pp. 267–304). Chicago: Encyclopedia Britannica. (Original work published ca. 1628.)

Harvey, R. F., & Jellinek, H. M. (1981). Functional performance assessment: A program approach. *Archives of Physical Medicine and Rehabilitation, 62,* 456–460.

Hasselkus, B. R., & Dickie, V. A. (1993). Doing occupational therapy: Dimensions of satisfaction and dissatisfaction. *American Journal of Occupational Therapy, 48*(2), 145–154.

Hatch, M. C., Wallenstein, S., Beyen, J., Nieves, J. W., & Susser, M. (1991). Cancer rates after the Three Mile Island nuclear accident and proximity of residents to the plan. *American Journal of Public Health, 81,* 719–724.

Hathaway, S., & McKinley, C. (1970). *Minnesota Multiphasic Personality Inventory.* Minneapolis, MI: National Computer Systems.

Havighurst, R. J. (1952). *Developmental tasks and education.* New York: Longmans, Green.

Haynes, M. C., & Jenkins, J. R. (1986). Reading instruction in special education resource room. *American Educational Research Journal,* 23, 161–190.

Health Outcomes Institute. (1995). *Health Status Questionnaire* (HSQ-12, version 2.0). (Available from Health Outcomes Institute, 2901 Metro Drive, Suite 400, Bloomington, MN, 55425)

Hébert, R., Carrier, R., & Bildeau, A. (1988). The functional autonomy measurement system (SMAF): Description and validation of an instrument for the measurement of handicaps. *Age and Aging,* 17, 2933–3302.

Hemphill, B. J. (Ed.). (1982). *The evaluative process in psychiatric occupational therapy.* Thorofare, NJ: Slack.

Hemphill, B. J. (Ed.). (1988). *Mental health assessment in occupational therapy: An integrative approach to the evaluative process.* Thorofare, NJ: Slack.

Hemphill-Pearson, B. J. (1999a). How to use the BH battery. In B. J. Hemphill-Pearson (Ed.), *Assessments in occupational therapy mental health: An integrative approach* (pp. 140–155). Thorofare, NJ: Slack.

Hemphill-Pearson, B. J. (Ed.). (1999b). *Assessments in occupational therapy mental health: An integrative approach.* Thorofare, NJ: Slack.

Henry, A. D., & Mallinson, T. (1999). The Occupational Performance History Interview. In B. J. Hemphill-Pearson (Ed.), *Assessments in occupational therapy mental health: An integrative approach* (pp. 59–72). Thorofare, NJ: Slack.

Henry, J. (1971). *Pathways to madness.* New York: Random House.

Hester, P. H. (1994, November). *A contextual analysis of classroom interaction at the university level: An operations research approach.* Paper presented at the Annual Meeting of the Mid-South Educational Research Association, Nashville, TN. (ERIC Document Reproduction Service Number ED 382-139)

Hewitt, N. G. (1997). Manipulating the environment—Intensive care versus specialist neurosurgical care. *Australasian Journal of Neuroscience,* 10, 10–12.

Higgs, J. (Ed.). (1997). *Qualitative research: Discourse on methodologies.* Sydney, Australia: Hampden.

Higgs, J. (Ed.). (1998). *Writing qualitative research.* Sydney, Australia: Hampden.

Hill, A. B. (1971). *Principles of medical statistics.* London: Lancet.

Hinshelwood, J. (1917). *Congenital word blindness.* London: Lewis.

Hippocratic writings. (1952). *On the articulations.* In R. M. Hutchins (Ed.), & F. Adams (Trans.), *Great books for the western world* (Vol. 10, pp. 91–121). Chicago: Encyclopedia Britannica. (Original work published ca. 5th century).

Hoaglin, C. C., Mosteller, F., & Tukey, J. N. (1991). *Fundamentals of exploratory analysis of variance.* New York: Wiley.

Hoehn, T. P., & Baumeister, A. A. (1994). A critique of the application of sensory integration therapy to children with learning disabilities. *Journal of Learning Disabilities,* 27, 338–350.

Holbrook, M., & Skilbeck, C. E. (1983). *An activities index for use with stroke patients. Age and Ageing* 12, 166–170.

Holm, M. B., & Rogers, J. C. (1999). Performance assessment of self-care skills. In B. Hemphill-Pearson (Ed.), *Assessments in occupational therapy mental health: An integrative approach* (pp. 117–124). Thorofare, NJ: Slack. (Available from Holm & Rogers at SPIC # 1237, 3811 O'Hara Street, Pittsburgh, PA 15213)

Holmberg, K., Rosen, D., & Holland, J. L. (1999). *The Leisure Activities Finder™* (LAF). Odessa, FL: Psychological Assessment Resources.

Holstein, J. A., & Gubrium, J. F. (1995). *The active interview.* Thousand Oaks, CA: Sage.

Hoppes, S. (1997). Can play increase standing tolerance? A pilot-study. *Physical and Occupational Therapy in Geriatrics,* 15, 65–73.

Horn, J. L. (1968). Organization of abilities and the development of intelligence. *Psychological Review,* 75, 242–259.

Howland, D. S., Trusko, S. P., Savage, M. J., Reaume, A. G., Lange, D. M., Hirsch, J. D., Maeda, N., Siman, R., Greenberg, B. D., Scott, R. W., & Flood, D. G. (1998). Modulation of secreted beta-amyloid precursor protein and amyloid beta-peptide in brain by cholesterol. *Journal of Biological Chemistry,* 273, 16576–16582.

Huberman, A. M., & Miles, M. B. (1994). Data management and analysis methods. In N. K. Denzin & Y. S. Lincoln (Eds.), *Handbook of qualitative research* (pp. 428–444). Thousand Oaks, CA: Sage.

Huezo, C. (1997). Factors to address when periodic abstinence is offered by multi-method family planning programs. *Advances in Contraception,* 13, 261–267.

Hunt, N., & Marshall, K. (1994). *Exceptional children and youth.* Geneva, IL: Houghton Mifflin.

ICD Rehabilitation and Research Center, NY.

(1977). *Micro Tower System of Vocational Evaluation.* New York, NY: Author. (Available from ICD Rehabilitation & Research Center, 340 East 24th St., New York, NY 10010)

Iliff, A., & Lee, V. A. (1952). Pulse rate, respiratory rate and body temperature of children between two months and eighteen years of age. *Child Development, 23,* 237–245.

Illingworth, W. H. (1910). *History of the education of the blind.* London: Marston.

Impara, J. C., & Plake, B. S. (Eds.). (1998). *The thirteenth mental measurements yearbook.* Lincoln: NE: The University of Nebraska Press.

Individuals with Disabilities Education Act Amendments of 1997 [IDEA], PL. 105-17. 20 U.S.C. § 1400 et seq.

Iverson C. (Ed.). (1997). *American Medical Association manual of style: A guide for authors and editors* (8th ed.). Philadelphia: Lippincott, Williams and Wilkins.

Jacobson, M. L., Mercer, M. A., Miller, L. K., & Simpson, T. W. (1987). Tuberculosis risk among migrant farm workers on the Relmarva Peninsula. *American Journal of Public Health, 77,* 29–32.

Jacobson, N. S., Dobson, K. S., Traux, P. A., Addis, M. E., Koerner, K., Gollan, J. K., Gortner, E., & Prince, S. E. (1996). A component analysis of cognitive-behavioral treatment for depression. *Journal of Consulting and Clinical Psychology, 64,* 295–304.

Jahoda, M., Deutsch, M., & Cook, S. W. (1951). *Research methods in social relations.* New York: Dryden Press.

Jastak, J. F., & Jastak, S. (1979). *Wide Range Interest-Opinion Test* (WRIOT). Wilmington, DE: Jastak Associates. (Available from Guidance Centre, The Ontario Institute of Studies in Education of the University of Toronto, 712 Gordon Baker Road, Toronto, Ontario, M2H 3R7)

Jastak, J. F., & Jastak, S. (1980). *Wide Range Employability Sample Test* (WREST). Wilmington, DE: Jastak Associates.

Jebsen, R. H., Taylor, N., Trieschmann, R. B., Trotter, M. J., & Howard, L. A. (1969). An objective and standardized test of hand function. *Archives of Physical Medicine and Rehabilitation, 50,* 311–319.

Jebsen, R. H., Trieschmann, R. B., Mikuli, M. A., Hartley, R. B., McMillan, J. A., & Snook, M. E. (1970). *Archives of Physical Medicine and Rehabilitation, 50,* 311–319.

Jensen, M. P., Karoly, P., & Braver, S. (1986). The measurement of clinical pain intensity: A comparison of six methods. *Pain, 27,* 117–126.

Jensen, M. P., Karoly, P., & Harris, P. (1991). Assessment of the affective component of chronic pain: Development of the Pain Discomfort Scale. *Journal of Psychosomatic Research, 35,* 149–154.

Jessor, R., Colby, A., & Shweder, R. A. (Eds.). (1996). *Ethnography and human development: Context and meaning in social inquiry.* Chicago: University of Chicago.

Jette, A. M. (1980). Functional Status Index: Reliability of a chronic disease evaluation instrument. *Archives of Physical Medicine and Rehabilitation, 61,* 395–401.

Jette, A. M. (1987). The Functional Status Index: Reliability and validity of a self-report functional disability measure. *Journal of Rheumatology, 14*(Suppl. 15), 573–580.

Joint Commissions on Accreditation of Health Care Organizations. (1998). *Glossary of terms for performance measurement systems,* [On-Line]. Available: http://wwwb.jcaho.org/perfmeas/glossry.html [1999, December 29].

Johnson, K. (1998). *Deinstitutionalising women: An ethnographic study of institutional closure.* Cambridge, England: Cambridge University Press.

Johnson, T. P., Vinnicombe, B. J., & Merrill, G. W. (1980). The independent living skills evaluation. *Occupational Therapy in Mental Health, 1*(2), 5–18.

Jonsson, H. (1998). Ernst Westerlund—A Swedish doctor of occupation. *Occupational Therapy International 5*(2), 155–171.

Jung, B., & Tryssenaar, J. (1998). Supervising students: Exploring the experience through reflective journals. *Occupational Therapy International, 5*(1), 35–48.

Juul, D. (1981). Special education in Europe. In J. M. Kauffman & D. P. Hallahan (Eds.), *Handbook of special education.* Englewood Cliffs, NJ: Prentice Hall.

Kalverboer, A. (1977). A measurement of play: Clinical applications. In B. Tizard & D. Harvey (Eds.), *Biology of play.* Philadelphia: Lippincott.

Kamhi, A., & Catts, H. (Eds.). (1998). *Language and reading disabilities.* Boston: Allyn & Bacon.

Kaplan, E., Fein, D., Morris, R., & Delis, D. C. (1991). *WAIS–R as a neuropsychological instrument.* San Antonio, TX: The Psychological Corporation.

Kaplan, K., Mendelson, L. B., & Dubroff, M. P. (1983). The effect of a jogging program on psychiatric inpatients with symptoms of depression. *The Occupational Therapy Journal of Research, 3,* 173–175.

Katz, M. M., & Lyerly, S. B. (1963). Methods for measuring adjustment and social behavior in the community: I. Rationale, description, discriminative validity and scale development. *Psychological Reports, 13,* 503–535.

Katz, S., Ford, R. Q., Moskowitz, R. W., Jackson, B. A., & Jaffe, M. W. (1963). Studies of illness in the aged, the index of ADL: A standardized measure of biological and psychosocial functions. *Journal of the American Medical Association, 185,* 914–918.

Kaufman, A. S., & Kaufman, N. L. (1993). *Kaufman Adolescent and Adult Intelligence Test.* Circle Pines, MN: American Guidance Service.

Kazdin, A. E. (1992). *Research design in clinical psychology* (2nd ed.). Boston: Allyn & Bacon.

Keith, R. A. (1984). Functional assessment measures in medical rehabilitation: Current status. *Archives of Physical Medicine and Rehabilitation, 65,* 74–78.

Keith, R. A., Granger, C. V., Hamilton, B. B., & Sherwins, F. S. (1987). The functional independence measure. *Advances in Clinical Rehabilitation, 1,* 6–18.

Keller, S., & Hayes, R. (1997). The relationship between the Allen Cognitive Level Test and the Life Skills Profile. *The American Journal of Occupational Therapy, 52,* 851–856.

Kendall, F. P., McCreary, E. K, & Provance, P. G. (1993). *Muscle testing and function* (4th ed.). Baltimore: Williams and Wilkins.

Kendall, H. O., & Kendall, F. M. P. (1949). *Muscles, testing and function.* Baltimore: Williams and Wilkins.

Kenig, S. (1992). *Who Plays?, Who Pays?, Who Cares?: A Case Study in Applied Sociology, Political Economy and the Community Mental Health Centers Movement.* Amityville, NY: Baywood.

Kerlinger, F. N. (1986). *Foundations of behavioral research* (3rd ed.). New York: Holt, Rinehart, and Winston.

Key, G. (Ed.). (1996). *Industrial therapy.* St. Louis, MO: Mosby.

Kielhofner, G., Henry, A. D., & Walens, D. (1989). *A user's guide to the Occupational Performance History Interview.* Rockville, MD: American Occupational Therapy Association.

Kinosian, B., Glick, H., & Garland, G. (1994). Cholesterol and coronary heart disease: Predicting risks by levels and ratios. *Annals of Internal Medicine, 121,* 641–647.

Kirk, J., & Miller, M. L. (1986). *Reliability and validity in qualitative research.* Thousand Oaks, CA: Sage.

Kirk, S. A. (April, 1963). Behavioral diagnosis and remediation of learning disabilities. In *Proceedings of the conference on exploration into the problems of the perceptually handicapped child: First Annual Meeting, Vol. 1.* Chicago, IL: Association for Children with Learning Disabilities.

Kirk, S. A., & Gallagher, J. J. (1989). *Educating exceptional children* (5th ed.). Boston: Houghton Mifflin.

Klein, R. M., & Bell, B. (1982). Self-care skills: Behavior measurements with the Klein-Bell ADL Scale. *Archives of Physical Medicine and Rehabilitation, 63,* 335–338.

Klein, R. M., & Bell, B. (1993). *Klein-Bell Activities of Daily Living Scales.* (Available from Health Sciences Center for Educational Resources, University of Washington, T-281 Health Sciences Building, Box 357161, Seattle, WA)

Kliebsch, U., Sturmer, T., Siebert, H., & Brenner, H. (1998). Risk factors of institutionalization in an elderly disabled population. *European Journal of Public Health, 8,* 106–112.

Klyczek, J. P. (1999). The Bay Area Functional Performance Evaluation. In B. J. Hemphill-Pearson (Ed.), *Assessments in occupational therapy mental health: An integrative approach* (pp. 87–109). Thorofare, NJ: Slack.

Knapp, L. F., & Knapp, R. R. (1982). *CAPS.* San Diego: Educational & Industrial Testing Service.

Knapp, R. B., & Knapp-Lee, L. (1995). *COPSystem Interest Inventory* (Rev. ed.). San Diego: Educational & Industrial Testing Service.

Knapp-Lee, L, Knapp, R. R., & Knapp, L. F. (1982). *COPES.* San Diego: Educational & Industrial Testing Service.

Knox, S. H. (1974). In M. Reilly (Ed.), *Play as exploratory learning* (pp. 247–266). Thorofare, NJ: Slack.

Kohn, P. M., & MacDonald, J. E. (1992). A survey of recent life experiences: A decontaminated hassles scale for adults. *Journal of Behavioral Medicine, 15,* 221–236.

Kohs, S. (1923). *Intelligence measurements.* New York: Macmillan.

Kopolow, M. S., & Jensen, B. M. (1975). *Psychosocial adjustment to quadriplegia: A double case study.* Unpublished master's thesis, Sargent College, Boston University, Massachusetts.

Koppitz, E. M. (1963). *The Bender Gestalt Test for Young Children.* New York: Grune & Stratton.

Koppitz, E. M. (1975). *The Bender Gestalt Test for Young Children: Volume II: Research and application, 1963–1973.* New York: Grune & Stratton.

Kovacs, M. (1992). *Children's Depression Inventory.* San Antonio: The Psychological Corporation.

Koyano, W., & Shibata, H. (1994). Development of a measure of subjective well-being in Japan: Construct validity and reliability of the Life Satisfaction K. *Facts and Research in Gerontology, Suppl. 2,* 181–187.

Kozak, L. J., & Owings, M. F. (1998). *Vital and Health Statistics, Ambulatory and Inpatient Procedures in the United States, 1995,* Series 13: Data from the National Health Care Survey No. 135. Government Publication Office: U.S. Department of Health and Human Services, Centers for Disease Control and Prevention, National Centers for Health Statistics. Available: http://www.cdc.gov/nchswww/data/sr13_135.pdf [1999, October 29].

Krathwohl, D. R. (1988). *How to prepare a research proposal: Guidelines for funding and dissertations in the social and behavioral sciences* (3rd ed.). Syracuse, NY: Syracuse University Press.

Kuder, F. (1979). *Kuder Occupational Interest Survey—Form DD* (Rev.). Chicago: Science Research Associates.

Kunz, K. R., & Brayman, S. J. (1999). The comprehensive occupational therapy evaluation. In B. J. Hemphill-Pearson (Ed.), *Assessments in occupational therapy mental health: An integrative approach* (pp. 259–274). Thorofare, NJ: Slack.

Kuzma, J. W. (1984). *Basic statistics for the health sciences.* Palo Alto, CA: Mayfield.

Lachar, D. (1982). *Personality Inventory for Children—Revised.* Los Angeles: Western Psychological Services.

Lane, H. (1976). *The wild boy of Aveyron.* Cambridge, MA: Harvard University Press.

Lang, C. E. (1998). Comparison of 6- and 7-day physical therapy coverage on length of stay and discharge outcome for individuals with total hip and knee arthroplasty. *Journal of Orthopaedic & Sports Physical Therapy, 28,* 15–22.

Larson, R. J. (1975). *Statistics for the allied health sciences.* Columbus, OH: Merrill.

Laszlo, J. I. (1990). Child perceptuo-motor development: Normal and abnormal development of skilled behaviour. In C. A. Hauert (Ed.), *Developmental psychology: Cognitive,* perceptuo-motor and neuropsychological perspectives (pp. 278–308). Amsterdam: Elsevier Science.

Lau, A., Chi, I., & McKenna, K. (1998). Self-perceived quality of life of Chinese elderly people in Hong Kong. *Occupational Therapy International, 5,* 118–139.

Laver, A., & Powell, G. (1995). *The Structured Observational Test of Function.* Windsor Brookshire, England: NFER-Nelson Publishing Company.

Law, M., Baptiste, S., Carswell-Opzoomer, A., McColl, M., Polatajko, H., & Pollock, N. (1991). *Canadian Occupational Performance Measure manual.* Toronto, Ontario: Canadian Association of Occupational Therapists.

Law, M., Baptiste, S., Carswell, A., McColl, M. A., Polatajko, H., & Pollock, N. (1994). *Canadian Occupational Performance Measure* [COPM] (2nd ed.). Toronto, Ontario: Canadian Association of Occupational Therapists.

Lawton, E. B. (1956). *Activities of daily living.* New York: New York Institute of Physical Medicine and Rehabilitation, NYU-Bellevue Medical Center.

Lawton, M. P., & Brody, E. M. (1969). Assessment of older people: Self-maintaining and instrumental activities of daily living. *Gerontologist, 9,* 179–186.

Lawton, M. P., Moss, M., Fulcomer, M., & Kleban, M. H. (1982). A research and service orientated multilevel assessment instrument. *Journal of Gerontology, 37,* 91–99.

Lechner, D. E., Jackson, J. R., Roth, D. L., & Straaton, K. V. (1994). Reliability and validity of a newly developed test of physical work performance. *Journal of Occupational Medicine, 36,* 997–1004.

Lechner, D. E., Roth, D., & Straaton, K. (1991). Functional capacity evaluation in work disability. *Work, 1,* 37–47.

Leiter, R. G. (1948). *Leiter International Performance Scale.* Chicago: Stoelting.

Leonardelli, C. A. (1988a). The Milwaukee Evaluation of Daily Living Skills: Evaluation in long-term psychiatric care. In B. J. Hemphill (Ed.), *Mental health assessment in occupational therapy: A integrative approach to the evaluative process* (pp. 151–162). Thorofare, NJ: Slack.

Leonardelli, C. A. (1988b). *The Milwaukee Evaluation of Daily Living Skills* (MEDLS). Thorofare, NJ: Slack.

Lerner, C. J. (1982). Magazine Picture Collage. In B. J. Hemphill (Ed.), *The evaluative process in psychiatric occupational therapy* (pp. 139–154, 361–362). Thorofare, NJ: Slack.

Lerner, C. J., & Ross, G. (1977). The Magazine Picture Collage: Development of an objective scoring system. *American Journal of Occupational Therapy, 31,* 156–161.

Levy, D., Wilson P. W., Anderson, K. M., & Castelli, W. P. (1990). Stratifying the patient at risk from coronary disease: New insights from the Framingham Heart Study. *American Heart Journal, 119,* 712–717.

Lewin, K. (1939). Field theory and experiment in social psychology: Concepts and methods. *American Journal of Sociology, 44,* 868–897.

Lewis, C. B., & McNerney, T. (1994). *The functional tool box: Clinical measures of functional outcomes.* Washington, DC: Learn.

Lewis, O. (1965). *La vida.* New York: Random House.

Lezak, M. (1984). *Neuropsychological assessment* (2nd ed.). New York: Oxford University Press.

Lezak, M. (1995). *Neuropsychological assessment* (3rd ed.). New York: Oxford University Press.

Li, X., & Crane, N. B. (1996). *Electronic styles: A handbook for citing electronic information* (Rev. ed.). Medford, NJ: Information Today, 143 Old Marlton Pike, Medford, NJ 08055-9912.

Liberman, I. Y. (1973). Segmentation of the spoken word and reading acquisition. *Bulletin of the Orton Dyslexia Society, 23,* 65–77.

Lincoln, N., & Leadbitter, D. (1979). Assessment of motor function in stroke patients. *Physiotherapy, 65,* 51–58.

Lincoln, Y. S., & Guba, E. G. (1985). *Naturalistic inquiry.* Beverly Hills, CA: Sage.

Linder, T. W. (1990). *Transdisciplinary play-based assessment.* Baltimore, MD: P. H. Brookes.

Linkenhoker, D., & McCarron, L. T. (1979). *Adaptive behaviors: Street Survival Skills Questionnaire (SSSQ).* (Available from McCarron-Dial Systems, P.O. Box 45628, Dallas, TX 75245)

Linkenhoker, D., & McCarron, L. T. (1993). *Adaptive behaviors: Street Survival Skills Questionnaire (SSSQ; Rev. ed.).* (Available from McCarron-Dial Systems, P.O. Box 45628, Dallas, TX 75245)

Linn, M. W. (1967). A rapid disability rating scale. *Journal of the American Geriatrics Society, 15,* 211–214.

Linn, M. W., & Linn, B. S. (1982). The Rapid Disability Rating Scale-2. *Journal of the American Geriatrics Society, 30,* 378–382.

Liu, L., Gauthier, L., & Gauthier, S. (1991). Spatial disorientation in persons with early senile dementia of the Alzheimer type. *The American Journal of Occupational Therapy, 45,* 67–74.

Llewellyn, G. (1995). Qualitative research with people with intellectual disability. *Occupational Therapy International, 2,* 108–127.

Llewellyn, G., Sullivan, G., & Minichiello, V. (1999). Sampling in qualitative research. In V. Minichiello, R. Axford, K. Greenwood, & G. Sullivan (Eds.), *Handbook of research methods in health.* Melbourne, Australia: Addison, Wesley, Longman.

Lloyd, C. (1995). Trends in forensic psychiatry. *British Journal of Occupational Therapy, 58,* 209–213.

Lo, J., & Zemke, R. (1997). The relationship between affective experiences during daily occupations and subjective well-being measures: A pilot study. *Occupational Therapy in Mental Health, 13,* 1–21.

Locke, L. F., Spirduso, W. W., & Silverman, S. J. (1987). *Proposals that work: A guide for planning dissertations and grant proposals* (2nd ed.). Newbury Park, CA: Sage.

Locke, L. F., Spirduso, W. W., & Silverman, S.J. (1997). *Proposals that work: A guide for planning dissertations and grant proposals* (3rd ed.). Newbury Park, CA: Sage.

Lofquist, L. H. (1957). *Vocational counseling with the physically handicapped.* New York: Appleton-Century-Crofts.

Longmore, D. (1970). *Machines in medicine.* New York: Doubleday.

Lubin, B. (1981). Additional data on the reliability and validity of the brief lists of the depression adjective check lists. *Journal of Clinical Psychology, 37,* 809–811.

Luera, M. (1994). *Understanding family uniqueness through cultural diversity. Project ta-kos.* Albuquerque, NM: Alta Mira Specialized Family Services, Inc. (ERIC Document Reproduction Service No. ED 379-839)

Luria, A. R. (1961). *The role of speech in the regulation of normal and abnormal behavior.* London: Pergaman.

Luria, A. R. (1980). *Higher cortical functions in man* (2nd ed.; B. Haigh, Trans.). New York: Basic Books.

Luria, A. R., & Yudovich, F. I (1959). *Speech and the development of mental process in the child.* London: Staples Press.

Macdonald, K. C., Epstein, C. F., & Vastano, S. (1986). Roles and functions of occupational therapy in adult day-care. *American Journal of Occupational Therapy, 40,* 817–821.

Maguire, G. H. (1995). Activities of daily living. In C. B. Lewis (Ed.), *Aging, the health care challenge: An interdisciplinary approach to assessment and rehabilitative management of the elderly* (3rd ed.; pp. 61–71). Philadelphia: F. A. Davis Company.

Maher, B. A. (1978). A reader's, writer's, and reviewer's guide to assessing research reports in clinical psychology. *Journal of Consulting and Clinical Psychology, 46,* 835–838.

Mahoney, F. I., & Barthel, D. W. (1965). Functional evaluation: Barthel Index. *Maryland State Medical Journal, 14,* 61–65.

Mahurin, R. K., DeBettignies, B. H., & Pirozzolo, F. J. (1991). Structured Assessment of Independent Living Skills: Preliminary report of performance measure of functional abilities in dementia. *Journal of Gerontology, 46,* 58–66.

Malave, L. M., & Duquette, G. (1991). *Language, culture and cognition: A collection of studies in first and second language acquisition* (Vol. 69, Multilingual Matters). (Available from Multilingual Matters Ltd., 1900 Frost Road, Suite 101, Bristol, PA 19007.) (ERIC Document Reproduction Service No. ED 386-929)

Mann, H. B., & Whitney, D. R. (1947). On a test of whether one of two random variables is stochastically larger than the other. *Annals of Mathematical Statistics, 18,* 52–54.

Margolis, R. B., Tait, R. C., & Krause, S. J. (1986). A rating system for use with patient pain drawings. *Pain, 3,* 49–51.

Marti-Ibanez, F. (1962). *The epic of medicine.* New York: Bramhall House.

Martin, R. P., Hooper, S., & Snow, J. (1986). Behavior rating scale approaches to personality assessment in children and adolescents. In H. M. Knoff (Ed.), *The assessment of child and adolescent personality* (pp. 309–351). New York: Guilford.

Martinsen, E. W., Medhus, A., & Sandvik, L. (1985). Effects of aerobic exercise on depression: A controlled study. *British Medical Journal, 291,* 109.

Martinsen, E. W., Medhus, A., & Solberg, O. (1989). Comparing aerobic with nonaerobic forms of exercise in the treatment of clinical depression: A randomized trial. *Comprehensive Psychiatry, 30,* 324–331.

Masagatani, G. N. (1994). *Cognitive Adaptive Skills Evaluation manual* (Rev. ed.). Unpublished manuscript. (Available from Gladys Masagatani, Eastern Kentucky University, Department of Occupational Therapy, Dizney 103, Richmond, KY 40475-3135)

Masagatani, G. N. (1999). The Cognitive Adaptive Skills Evaluation. In B. J. Hemphill-Pearson (Ed.), *Assessments in occupational therapy mental health: An integrative approach* (pp. 279–288). Thorofare, NJ: Slack.

Maslow, A. H. (1954). *Motivation and personality.* New York: Harper.

Matheson, L. (1988). *Work Capacity Evaluation* (procedure manual). Anaheim, CA: Employment and Rehabilitation Institute of California.

Matheson, L., & Ogden, L. (1987). *Work Capacity Evaluation.* Anaheim, CA: Employment and Rehabilitation Institute of Southern California.

Matsutsuyu, J. (1967). The Interest Checklist. *American Journal of Occupational Therapy, 11,* 179–181.

Matter, S., Weltman, A., & Stamford, B. A. (1980). Body fat content and serum lipid levels. *Journal of the American Dietetic Association, 77,* 149–152.

McCall, R. B. (1986). *Fundamental statistics for behavioral sciences* (4th ed.). San Diego: Harcourt Brace Jovanovich.

McCarney, S. B. (1995). *Attention Deficit Disorders Evaluation Scale—School version* (ADDES; 2nd ed.). Columbia, MO: Hawthorne Educational Services.

McCarron-Dial Systems, Inc. (n.d.). *Home-page,* [On-Line]. Available: http://www.mccarron dial.com [2000, January 12].

McCarthy, D. A. (1972). *McCarthy Scales of Children's Abilities.* San Antonio: The Psychological Corporation.

McColl, M. A., & Peterson, J. (1997). A descriptive framework for community-based rehabilitation. *Canadian Journal of Rehabilitation, 10,* 297–306.

McConnell, D. B. (1994). Clinical observations and developmental coordination disorder: Is there a relationship? *Occupational Therapy International, 1,* 278–291.

McFall, S. A., Deitz, J. C., & Crowe, T. K. (1993). Test-retest reliability of the test of visual perceptual skills with children with learning disabilities. *The American Journal of Occupational Therapy, 47,* 819–824.

McGourty, L. K. (1988). Kohlman Evaluation of Living Skills (KELS). In B. J. Hemphill (Ed.), *Mental health assessment in occupational therapy: A integrative approach to the evaluative process* (pp. 133–146). Thorofare, NJ: Slack.

McGowan, J. F. (Ed.). (1960). *An introduction to the vocational rehabilitation services* (Series no. 555; guidance, training and placement bulletin no. 3). Washington, DC: Office of Vocational Rehabilitation, U.S. Government Printing Office.

McKinney, M., & Leary, K. (1999). Integrating quantitative and qualitative methods to study multifetal pregnancy reduction. *Journal of Women's Health, 8,* 259–268.

Mead, M. (1928). *Coming of age in Samoa.* New York: Blue Ribbon Books.

Meenan, R. B., Mason, J. H., Anderson, J. J., Guccione, A. A., & Kazis, L. E. (1992). AIMS-2: The content and properties of a revised and expanded Arthritis Impact Measurement Scales Health Questionnaire. *Arthritis and Rheumatism, 35,* 1–10.

Melzack, R. (1975). The McGill Pain Questionnaire: Major properties and scoring methods. *Pain, 1,* 277–299.

Melzack, R. (1987). The short-form McGill Pain Questionnaire. *Pain, 30,* 191–197.

Mental Measurements Yearbook, Mental Measurements Supplement, or Tests in Print, published by The University of Nebraska Press. Available: http://www.unl.edu/buros/ [2000 January 1].

Mercer, C. (1983). *Students with learning disabilities* (2nd ed.). Columbus, OH: Merrill.

Merriam-Webster's Collegiate Dictionary. (10th ed.). (1993). Springfield, MA: Merriam-Webster.

Merrington, M., & Thompson, C. M. (1943). Tables of percentage points of the inverted beta *(F)* distribution. *Biometrica, 33,* 73–88.

Meyen, E. L., & Skrtic, T. M. (1988). *Exceptional children and youth* (3rd ed.). Aspen, CO: Love.

Miles, M. B., & Huberman, A. M. (1994). *Qualitative data analysis. An expanded sourcebook* (2nd ed.). Thousand Oaks, CA: Sage.

Miller, E. R., & Parachek, J. F. (1974). Validation and standardization of a goal-oriented, quick-screening geriatric scale. *Journal of the American Geriatrics Society, 22,* 278–283.

Miller, L. H., & Smith, A. D. (1983). Stress Audit Questionnaire. *Your Life and Health, 98,* 20–30.

Miller, L. H., Smith, A. D., & Mehler, B. L. (1988). *The Stress Audit manual.* Brookline, MA: Biobehavioral Institute.

Miller, L. J. (1988). *Miller Assessment for Preschoolers.* San Antonio, TX: The Psychological Corporation.

Miller, L. J., & Roid, G. H. (1994). *Toddler and Infant Motor Evaluation* (TIME). Tucson, AZ: Therapy Skill Builders/The Psychological Corporation.

Miller, M. (1990). Ethnographic interviews for information about classrooms: An invitation. *Teacher Education and Special Education, 13,* 233–234.

Miller, N. E. (1969). Learning of visceral and glandular responses. *Science, 163,* 434–445.

Million, T., Green, C. J., & Meagher, R. B., Jr. (1982). *Million Adolescent Personality Inventory.* Minneapolis, MN: National Computer Services, Inc.

Mills v. Board of Education of the District of Columbia, 348 F. Supp. 866 (1972).

Minichiello, V., Aroni, R., Timewell, E., & Alexander, L. (1995). *In-depth interviewing: Principles, techniques, & analysis* (2nd ed.). Melbourne, Australia: Longman Cheshire.

Montessori, M. (1912). *The Montessori method* (A. E. George, Trans.). New York: Frederick A. Stokes.

Montgomery, S. A., & Åsberg, M. (1979). A new depression scale designed to be sensitive to change. *British Journal of Psychiatry, 134,* 382–389.

Morris, W. (Ed.). (1973). *The American Heritage dictionary of the English language.* Boston: Houghton Mifflin.

Morse, J. M. (Ed.). (1994). *Critical issues in qualitative research methods.* Thousand Oaks, CA: Sage.

Morton, T., & Godholt, S. (Eds.). (1993). *Information sources in the medical sciences* (4th ed.). London: Bowker-Saur.

Moustakas, C. (1994). *Phenomenological research methods.* Thousands Oaks, CA: Sage.

Moskowitz, E., & McCann, C. B. (1957). Classification of disability in the chronically ill and aging. *Journal of Chronic Disease, 5,* 342–346.

Muhr, T. (1991). ATLAS/Ti. A prototype for the support of text interpretation. *Qualitative Sociology, 14,* 349–371.

Nadolsky, J. M. (1974). The work sample in vocational evaluation: A consistent rationale. *Vocational Evaluation and Work Adjustment Bulletin, 7,* 2–5.

Naglieri, J. A., LeBuffe, P. A., & Pfeiffer, S. I. (1992). *Devereaux behavior rating scales—School form.* San Antonio, TX: The Psychological Corporation.

Naglieri, J. A., LeBuffe, P. A., & Pfeiffer, S. I. (1994). *Devereaux scales of mental disorders.* San Antonio, TX: The Psychological Corporation.

National Center for Health Studies (1974). *Inpatient health facilities as reported from the 1971 MFI Survey. Data on national health resources*

(Series 14, Number 12), DHEW Publication No. (HRA) 74-1807.

National Information Center on Health Services Research & Health Care Technology Fact Sheet (26Apr94). Available E-mail: nichsr@nlm.nih.gov or National Information Center on Health Services Research and Health Care Technology (NICHSR), National Library of Medicine.

National Institute on Disability and Rehabilitation Data. (n.d.). *What is ABLEDATA?* [On-Line]. Available: http://www.abledata.com/Site_2/project.htm [1999, August 16].

National Institutes of Health Consensus Development Panel on Triglyceride, High-Density Lipoprotein and Coronary Heart Disease (1993). *Journal of the American Medical Association, 269*, 505–510.

National Library of Medicine. (1999a). *Fact sheet: Internet Grateful Med®,* [On-Line]. Available: http://www.nlm.nih.gov/pubs/factsheets/igm.html [1999, August 19].

National Library of Medicine. (1999b). *Fact sheet: Medline®* [On-Line]. Available: http://www.nlm.nih.gov/pubs/factsheets/medline.html [1999, August 19].

National Library of Medicine. (1999c). *Fact sheet: Medical subject headings (MeSH®)* [On-Line]. Available: http://www.nlm.nih.gov/pubs/factsheets/mesh.html [1999, August 19].

National Library of Medicine. (1999d). *Fact sheet: National Information Center on Health Services Research and Health Care Technology (NICHSR),* [On-Line]. Available: http://www.nlm.nih.gov/pubs/factsheets/nichsr_fs.html [1999, August 19].

National Rehabilitation Information Center. (n.d.). *Welcome to NARIC,* [On-Line]. Available: http://www.naric.com/ [1999, August 19].

Neistadt, M. E. (1992). *Rabideau Kitchen Evaluation—Revised* (RKE-R). (Available from University of New Hampshire Departments of Occupational Therapy, School of Health and Human Services, Durham, NH.)

Nighswonger, W. E. (1981). *Talent Assessment Programs.* Jacksonville, FL: Talent Assessment, Inc. (Available from Talent Assessment, Inc.; P.O. Box 5087; Jacksonville, FL 32207)

Northrop, F. S. C. (1931). *Science and first principles.* New York: Macmillan.

Oakley, F. M. (1988). *Role Checklist–Revised.* (Available from Frances Oakley, Occupational Therapy Service, National Institutes of Health, Building 10, Room 6S-235, 10 Center Drive MSC 1604, Bethesda, MD, 20892-1604)

Oakley, F. M., Kielhofner, G., Barris, R., & Reichler, R. K. (1986). The role checklist: Development and empirical assessment of reliability. *Occupational Therapy Journal of Research, 6,* 157–170.

O'Connor, J. (circa 1920a). *O'Connor Finger Dexterity Test.* Wood Dale, IL: Stoelting Company.

O'Connor, J. (circa 1920b). *O'Connor Tweezer Dexterity Test.* Wood Dale, IL: Stoelting Company.

Olds, E. G. (1938). Distribution of the sums of squares of rank differences for small numbers of individuals. *Annals of Mathematical Statistics, 9,* 133–148.

Olds, E. G. (1949). The 5 percent significant levels of sums of squares of rank differences and a correction. *Annals of Mathematical Statistics, 20,* 117–118.

Oliver, M. (Ed.). (1991). *Social work: Disabled people and disabling environments.* London: Jessica Kingsley.

Oliver, R., Blathwayt, J., Brackley, C., & Tamaki, T. (1993). Development of the safety assessment of function in the environment for rehabilitation (Safer tool). *Canadian Journal of Occupational Therapy, 60,* 78–82.

Osipow, S. H., & Spokane, A. R. (1987) *Occupational Stress Inventory manual: Research version.* Odessa, FL: Psychological Assessment Resources.

Ottenbacher, K. J. (1992). Confusion in occupational therapy research: Does the end justify the method? *American Journal of Occupational Therapy, 46,* 871–874.

Ottenbacher, K. J., & Barrett, K. A. (1990). Statistical conclusion validity in rehabilitation research. *American Journal of Physical Medicine and Rehabilitation, 69,* 102–107.

Ottenbacher, K. J., & Cusick, A. (1990). Goal attainment scaling as a method of clinical service evaluation. *American Journal of Occupational Therapy, 44,* 519–525.

Owen. D. B. (1962). *Handbook of statistical tables.* Reading MA: Addison-Wesley.

Palmer, M. (1989). Mobilization following lumbar discectomy: A comparison of two methods of bed transfer. *Physiotherapy Canada, 41,* 146–152.

Paracelsus. (1971). *Paragranum.* In W. P. D. Wightman (Ed.), *The emergence of scientific medicine.* Edinburgh, Scotland: Oliver and Boyd. (Original work published 1528)

Parachek, J. F., & King, L. J. (1986). *Parachek Geriatric Rating Scale* (3rd ed.). (Available from Center for Neurodevelopmental Studies, 5340 West Glenn Drive, Glendale, AZ 85301)

Parker, G., & Hadzi-Pavlovic, D. (1995). The capacity of a measure of disability (the LSP) to predict hospital readmission in those with schizophrenia. *Psychological Medicine, 25,* 157–163.

Parsons, T. (1939). The professions and social structure. *Social Forces, 17,* 457–467.

Parsons, T. (Ed.). (1964). *Max Weber: The theory of social and economic organization.* New York: Free Press.

Patterson, C. H. (1958). *Counseling the emotionally disturbed.* New York: Harper and Brothers.

Patton, M. Q. (1990). *Qualitative evaluation and research methods* (2nd ed.). Newbury Park, CA: Sage.

Pavlov, I. P. (1927). *Conditioned reflexes.* London: Oxford University Press.

Pearson, E., & Hartley, H. (1966). *Biometricka tables for statisticians* (3rd ed.). New York: Cambridge University Press.

Pennsylvania Association of Retarded Citizens (PARC) v. Commonwealth of Pennsylvania, 343 F. Suppl. 279 (E. D. Pa., 1972).

Penny, N. H., Mueser, K. T., & North, C. T. (1995). The Allen Cognitive Level test and social competence in adult psychiatric patients. *American Journal of Occupational Therapy, 49,* 420–427.

Perls, F. (1969). *Gestalt therapy verbatim.* Lafayette, CA: Real People Press.

Pfeiffer, E. (1975). A short portable mental status questionnaire for the assessment of organic brain deficit in elderly patients. *Journal of the American Geriatrics Society, 23,* 433–441.

Piaget, J. (1926). *The language and thought of the child* (M. Gabain & R. Gabain, Trans.). London: K. Paul, Trench, Trubner.

Piers, E. V., & Harris, D. B. (1984). *The Piers–Harris Children's Self-Concept Scale: Revised manual.* Los Angeles: Western Psychological Services.

Piper, M. C., & Darrah, J. (1994). *Alberta Infant Motor Scales* (AIMS). Philadelphia: W. W. Saunders.

Plutchik, R., Conte, H., Lieberman, M., Baker, M., Grossman, J., & Lehrman, N. (1970). Reliability and validity of a scale for assessing the functioning of geriatric patients. *Journal of the Geriatric Society, 18,* 491–500.

Polatajko, H. J., Kaplan, B. J., & Wilson, B. N. (1992). Sensory integration treatment for children with learning disabilities: Its status 20 years later. *The Occupational Therapy Journal of Research, 12,* 323–341.

Power, P. (1991). *A guide to vocational assessment* (2nd ed.). Austin, TX: Pro–Ed.

Power, P. (2000). *A guide to vocational assessment* (3rd ed.). Austin, TX: Pro–Ed.

Powers, R. K., Marder-Meyer, J., & Rymer, W. Z. (1988). Quantitative relations between hypertonia and stretch reflex threshold in spastic hemiparesis. *Annals of Neurology, 23,* 115–124.

Poynter, N. (1971). *Medicine and man.* Middlesex, England: Penguin Books.

Pribram, K. (1958). Comparative neurology and the evolution of behavior. In A. Roe & G. G. Simpson (Eds.), *Behavior and evolution* (pp. 140–164). New Haven, CT: Yale University.

Prince, F., Winter, D. A., Sjonnensen, G., Powell, C., & Wheeldon, R. K. (1998). Mechanical efficiency during gait of adults with transtibial amputation: A pilot study comparing the SACH, Seattle, and Golden-Ankle. *Journal of Rehabilitation Research & Development, 35,* 177–185.

Provost, B., & Oetter, P. (1993). The Sensory Rating Scale for Infants and Young Children: Development and reliability. *Physical and Occupational Therapy in Pediatrics, 13*(4), 15–35.

Rankin, J. (1957). Cerebral vascular accidents in patients over the age of 60. II. Prognosis. *Scottish Medical Journal, 2,* 200–215.

Ransford, A. O., Cairnes, D., & Mooney, V. (1976). The pain drawing as an aid to the psychologic evaluation of patients with low-back pain. *Spine, 1,* 127–134.

Rape, R. N. (1987). Running and depression. *Perceptual Motor Skills, 64,* 1303–1310.

Rappaport, M., Hall, K. M., Hopkins, K., Belleza, T., & Cope, D. N. (1982). *Disability Rating Scale for severe head trauma patients: Coma to community.* Archives of Physical Medicine and Rehabilitation, 63, 118–123.

Reason, P. (Ed.). (1988). *Human inquiry in action: Developments in new paradigm research.* London: Sage.

Rehabilitation Engineering and Assistive Technology Society of North America [RESNA]. (n.d.). *Membership,* [On-Line]. Available: http://www.resna.org/resna/resmem.html [1999, August 16].

Reid, D. T., & Jutai, J. (1997). A pilot study of perceived clinical usefulness of a new computer-based tool for assessment of visual perception in occupational therapy practice. *Occupational Therapy International, 4,* 81–98.

Reid, W. M., Seavor, C., & Taylor, R. G. (1991). Application of a computer-based zero-one methodology to the assignment of nurses to a clinical rotation schedule. *Computers in Nursing, 9,* 219–223.

Reish, W. T. (Ed.). (1998). *Encyclopedia of bioethics.* New York: Macmillan Library Reference, Simon and Schuster.

Reynolds, M., & Walberg, H. J. (Eds.). (1987). *Handbook of special education: Research and practice, Volume I: Learning characteristics and adaptive education* (pp. 213–248). Oxford: Pergamon.

Reynolds, W. M., & Kobak, K. A. (1995). *Hamilton Depression Inventory (HDI), professional manual.* Odessa, FL: Psychological Assessment Resources.

Richards, T., & Richards, L. (1997). *NUD.IST 4.* Melbourne, Australia: QSR.

Richards, T., & Richards, L. (1999). *NVIVO.* Melbourne, Australia: QSR.

Richardson, G. A. (1998). Prenatal cocaine exposure. A longitudinal study of development. *Annals of the New York Academic of Science, 846,* 144–152.

Richardson, G. M., Kline, F. M., & Huber, T. (1996). Development of self-management in an individual with mental retardation: A qualitative case study. Journal of Special Education, 30, 278–304.

Roeder, E. W. (1970). *Roeder Manipulative Aptitude Test.* Lafayette. IN: Lafayette Instruments.

Rogers, J. C., & Holm, M. B. (1999). *Performance Assessment of Self-Care Skills, version 3.1* (PASS). (Available from J. C. Rogers and M. B. Holm, WPIC # 1237, 3811 O'Hara Street, Pittsburgh, PA 15213)

Rogers, J. C., Weinstein, J., & Firone, J. (1978). The Interest Checklist: An empirical assessment. *American Journal of Occupational Therapy, 32,* 628–630.

Rogers, R. J., & D'Eugenio, D. B. (1981). Assessment and application. In D. B. D'Eugenio & M. Moersch (Eds.), *Developmental programming for infants and young children* (Vol. 4). Ann Arbor: University of Michigan Press.

Roget's International Thesaurus. (1993). New York: HarperCollins.

Ronald and Nancy Reagan Research Institute of the Alzheimer's Association and the National Institute on Aging Working Group. (1998). Consensus report of the Working Group on "Molecular and biochemical markers of Alzheimer's disease." *Neurobiology of Aging, 19,* 109–116.

Roper, F. W., & Boorkman, J. A. (1994). *Introduction to reference sources in the health sciences* (3rd ed.). Metuchen, NJ: Scarecrow.

Rosenblatt, R. A. (1991). Summary and reactions: Rural health manpower research. In H. Hibbard et al. (Eds.), *Primary care research: Theory and methods. Conference proceedings.* Washington DC: United States Department of Health & Human Services Publications.

Rosenthal, R., & Rosnow, R. (1991). *Essentials of behavioral research: Methods and data analysis* (2nd ed.). New York: McGraw-Hill.

Ross, R. G., & LaStayo, P. C. (1997). Clinical assessment of pain. In J. Van Deusen & D. Brunt (Eds.), *Assessment in occupational therapy and physical therapy* (pp. 123–133). Philadephia: W. B. Saunders.

Rousseau, J. J. (1883). *Emile: Or, concerning education* (J. Steeg, Ed.; E. Worthington, Trans.) Boston: D. C. Heath & Co. (Original work published 1762)

Royeen, C. B. (1987a). Test-retest reliability of a touch scale for tactile defensiveness. *Physical and Occupational Therapy in Pediatrics, 7*(3), 45–52.

Royeen, C. B. (1987b). TIP–Touch Inventory for Preschoolers: A pilot study. *Physical and Occupational Therapy in Pediatrics, 7*(1), 29–40.

Royeen, C. B. (1990). Touch inventory for elementary-school-aged children. *American Journal of Occupational Therapy, 44,* 155–159.

Runyon, R. (1977). *Nonparametric statistics.* Reading, MA: Addison-Wesley.

Runyon, R. P., & Haber, A. (1967). *Fundamentals of behavior statistics.* Reading, MA: Addison-Wesley.

Rushmer, R. F. (1972). *Medical engineering: Projections for health care delivery.* New York: Academic Press.

Rusk, H. A. (1971). *Rehabilitation medicine.* St. Louis, MO: Mosby.

Russell, B. (1928). *Sceptical essays.* London: Allen and Unwin.

Sachs, D., & Linn, R. (1997). Client advocacy in action: Professional and environmental factors affecting Israeli occupational therapists' behaviour. *Canadian Journal of Occupational Therapy, 64,* 207–215.

Sachs, D., & Sussman, N. (1995). Historical research: The first decade of occupational therapy in Israel: 1946–1956). *Occupational Therapy International, 2,* 241–256.

Sailor, W. (1991). Special education in the restructured school. *Remedial and Special Education, 12*(6), 8–22.

Saint-John, L. M., & White, M. A. (1988). The effect of coloured transparencies on the reading performance of reading disabled children. *Australian Journal of Psychology, 40,* 403–411.

Sand, R. (1952). *The advance to social medicine.* London: Staples Press.

Sarlov, A. R., Ware, J. E., Greenfield, S., Nelson, E. C., Perrin, E., & Zubkoff, M. (1989). The medical outcomes study: An application of methods for monitoring the results of medical care. *Journal of the American Medical Association, 262,* 925–930.

Sarno, J. E., Sarno, M. R., & Levita, E. (1973). Functional Life Scale. *Archives of Physical Medicine and Rehabilitation, 54,* 214–220.

Sattler, J. M. (1988). *Assessment of children* (3rd ed.). San Diego: Sattler.

Sattler, J. M. (1992). *Assessment of children* (3rd ed., Rev.). San Diego: Sattler.

Schatzman, L., & Strauss, A. L. (1973). *Field research. Strategies for a natural sociology.* Englewood Cliffs, NJ: Prentice-Hall.

Schoening, H. A., Anderegg, L., Bergstrom, D., Fonda, M., Steinke, N., & Ulrich, P. (1964). Numerical scoring of self-care status of patients. *Archives of Physical Medicine and Rehabilitation, 46,* 689–697.

Schoening, H. A., & Iversen, I. (1968). Numerical scoring of self-care status: A study of the Kenny Self-care Evaluation. *Archives of Physical Medicine and Rehabilitation, 49,* 221–229.

Schwandt, T. A., & Halpern, E. S. (1988). *Linking auditing and metaevaluation: Enhancing quality in applied research.* Newbury Park, CA: Sage.

Schwartz, C. A., & Turner, R. L. (1995). *Encyclopedia of associations* (3rd ed.). Detroit: Gale Research.

Schwartz, D. P., & DeGood, D. E. (1984). Global appropriateness of pain drawings. Blind ratings predict patterns of psychological distress and litigation status. *Pain, 19,* 383–388.

Schwartz, H., & Jacobs, J. (1979). *Qualitative sociology. A method to the madness.* New York: Free Press.

Seidel, J. (1989). *The ethnograph.* Littleton, CO: Qualis Research Associates.

Seidman, L. J., Biederman, J., Faraone, S. V., Weber, W., Mennin, D., & Jones, J. (1997). A pilot study of neuropsychological function in girls with ADHD. *Journal of the American Academic of Child & Adolescent Psychiatry, 36,* 366–373.

Selye, H. (1956). *Stress of life.* New York: McGraw-Hill Book.

Shaffir, W. B., & Stebbins, R. A. (Eds.). (1991). *Experiencing fieldwork. An inside view of qualitative research.* Newbury Park, CA: Sage.

Shalik, L. D. (1990). The level 1 fieldwork process. *American Journal of Occupational Therapy, 44,* 700–707.

Shapiro, D. A., Barkhma, M., Rees, A., Hardy, G. E., Reynolds, S., & Startup, M. (1996). Effects of treatment duration and severity of depression on the effectiveness of cognitive-behavioral and psychodynamic-interpersonal psychotherapy. *Journal of Consulting and Clinical Psychology, 64,* 1079–1085.

Shaw, G. B. (1919). Annajanska, the Bolshevik princess. In G. B. Shaw, *Collection of plays, heartbreak house, Great Catherine and playets of war.* London: Comfortable.

Shea, T. M., & Bauer, A. M. (1994). *Learners with disabilities: A social systems perspective of special education.* Madison, WI: Brown and Benchmark.

Sibley, L., & Armbruster, D. (1997). Public health perspectives. Obstetric first aid in the community—Partners in safe motherhood: A strategy for reducing material mortality. *Journal of Nurse-Midwifery, 42,* 117–121.

Sigmon, S. B. (1987). *Radical analysis of special education: Focus on historical development and learning disabilities.* London: Falmer Press.

Simmonds, M. J. (1997). Muscle strength. In J. Van Deusen & D. Brunt (Eds.), *Assessment in occupational therapy and physical therapy* (pp. 27–48). Philadelphia: W. B. Saunders.

Simmons, L., & Wolff, H. G. (1954). *Social science in medicine.* New York: Russell Sage Foundation.

Skinner, B. F. (1953). *Science and human behavior.* New York: Macmillan.

Slade, C., Campbell, W. G., & Ballou, S. V. (1997). *Form and style: Research papers, reports, theses* (10th ed.). Boston: Houghton Mifflin.

Smith, D. D. (1998). *Introduction to special education* (3rd ed.) Boston: Allyn and Bacon.

Smith, L. M. (1994). Biographical method. In N. K. Denzin & Y. S. Lincoln (Eds.), *Handbook of qualitative research* (pp. 286–305). Thousand Oaks, CA: Sage.

Smith, N. R., Kielhofner, G., & Watts, S. J. H. (1986). The relationships between volition, activity pattern, and life satisfaction in the elderly. *American Journal of Occupational Therapy, 40,* 278–283.

Smith, S. L., Cunningham, S., & Weinberg, R. (1986). The predictive validity of the functional capacities evaluation. *American Journal of Occupational Therapy, 40,* 564–567.

Smyth, T. R. (1991). Abnormal clumsiness in children: A defect of motor programming? *Child: Care, Health and Development, 17,* 283–293.

Snow, C. P. (1964). *The two cultures and a second look.* Cambridge, England: Cambridge University Press.

Soderback, I., & Paulsson, E. H. (1997). A needs assessment for referral to occupational therapy: Nurses' judgment in acute cancer care. *Cancer Nursing, 20,* 267–273.

Sparrow, S., Balla, D., & Ciocchetti, D. (1984). *Vineland Adaptive Behavior Scales.* Circle Pines, MN: American Guidance Service.

Spearman, C. E. (1927). *The abilities of man.* New York: Macmillan.

Speller, L., Trollinger, J. A., Maurer, P. A., Nelson, C. E., & Bauer, D. F. (1997). Comparison of the test-retest reliability of the Work Box® using three administrative methods. *The American Journal of Occupational Therapy, 51,* 516–522.

Spence, K. V. (1948) The postulates and methods of "behaviorism." *Psychological Review, 55,* 67–68.

Spielberger, C. D. (1983). *Manual for the State-Trait Anxiety Inventory.* Palo Alto, CA: Consulting Psychologists Press.

Spielberger, C. D. (1985). Assessment of state and trait anxiety: Conceptual and methodological issues. *The Southern Psychologist, 2,* 6–16.

Spradley, J. P. (1979). *The ethnographic interview.* Fort Worth, TX: Holt, Rinehart and Winston.

Staff of the Benjamin Rose Hospital. (1959). Multidisciplinary studies of illness in aged persons: II. A new classification of functional status in activities of daily living. *Journal of Chronic Disability, 9,* 55–62.

Stainback, S., & Stainback, W. (Eds.). (1992). *Controversial issues confronting special education.* Boston: Allyn & Bacon.

Stanton, A. H., & Schwartz, M. S. (1954). *The mental hospital: A study of institutional participation in psychiatric illness and treatment.* New York: Basic Books.

Statistical analysis. (1999). [On-Line]. Available: http://www.sas.com/software/industry/healthcare.html. [1999, August 16].

Stefanyshyn, D. J., Engsberg, J. R., Tedford, K. G., & Harder, J. A. (1994). A pilot study to test the influence of specific prosthetic fea-tures in preventing trans-tibial amputees from walking like able-bodied subjects. *Prosthetics & Orthotics International, 18,* 180–190.

Stein, F. (1989). *Anatomy of clinical research: An introduction to scientific inquiry in medicine, rehabilitation, and related health professions* (Rev. ed.). Thorofare, NJ: Slack.

Stein, F. (1987). *Stress Management Questionnaire.* Unpublished questionnaire. (Available from F. Stein, Department of Occupational Therapy, University of South Dakota, 414 E. Clark Street, Vermillion, SD 57069)

Stein, F. (1988). Research analysis of O.T. assessments used in mental health. In B. J. Hemphill (Ed.), *The mental health assessment in occupational therapy: An integrative approach to the evaluative process* (pp. 225–247). Thorofare, NJ: Slack.

Stein, F., Bentley, D. E., & Natz, M. (1999). Computerized assessment: The Stress Management Questionnaire. In B. J. Hemphill-Pearson (Ed.), *Assessments in occupational therapy mental health: An integrative approach* (pp. 321–337). Thorofare, NJ: Slack.

Stein, F., & Cutler, S. K. (1998). *Psychosocial occupational therapy: A holistic approach.* San Diego: Singular Publishing Group.

Stein, F., & Nikolic, S. (1989). Teaching stress management techniques to a schizophrenic patient. *American Journal of Occupational Therapy, 43,* 162–169.

Stein, F., & Smith, J. (1989). Short-term stress management programme with acutely depressed in-patients. *Canadian Journal of Occupational Therapy, 56,* 185–192.

Stevens, S. (1951). *Measurement and psychophysics.* New York: Wiley.

Stolee, P., Rockwood, K., Fox, R. A., & Streiner, D. L. (1992). The use of goal attainment scaling in a geriatric care setting. *Journal of the American Geriatrics Society, 4,* 575–578.

Stonefelt, L. L., & Stein, F. (1998). Sensory integrative techniques applied to children with learning disabilities: An outcome study. *Occupational Therapy International, 5,* 252–272.

Strauss, A. A., & Kephart, N. C. (1940). Behavior differences in mentally retarded children measured by a new behavior rating scale. *American Journal of Psychiatry, 96,* 1117–1123.

Stratton, M. (1981). Behavioral Assessment of Oral Functions in Feeding. *The American Journal of Occupational Therapy, 35,* 719–721.

Strauss, A. A., & Lehtinen, L. L. (1947). *Psychopathology of the brain-injured child.* New York: Grune & Stratton.

Strauss, A. A., & Werner, H. (1941). The mental organization of the brain-injured mentally defective child. *American Journal of Psychiatry, 97,* 1194–1202.

Strauss, A. A., & Werner, H. (1943). Comparative psychopathology of the brain-injured child and the traumatic brain-injured adult. *American Journal of Psychiatry, 99,* 835.

Strauss, A. L., & Corbin, J. (1994). Grounded theory methodology: An overview. In N. K. Denzin & Y. S. Lincoln (Eds.), *Handbook of qualitative research* (pp. 273–285). Thousand Oaks, CA: Sage.

Strauss, A. L., & Corbin, J. (1998). *Basics of qualitative research: Techniques and procedures for developing grounded theory.* Newbury Park, CA: Sage.

Stromberg, E. L. (1947). *The Stromberg Dexterity Test.* San Antonio, TX: The Psychological Corporation.

Strong, K. E., Campbell, D. P., & Hansen, J. (1985). *The Strong-Campbell Interest Inventory.* Minneapolis, MN: National Computer Systems.

Strunk, W., & White, E. B. (1979). *The elements of style* (3rd ed.). New York: Macmillan.

Strunk, W., & White, E. B. (1999). *The elements of style* (4th ed.). Boston: Allyn & Bacon.

Suchman, E. A. (1967). *Evaluative research: Principles and practice in public service and social action programs.* New York: Russell Sage Foundation.

Swanson, H. L., & Watson, B. L. (1989). *Educational and psychological assessment of exceptional children: Theories, strategies, and applications* (2nd ed.). Columbus, OH: Merrill.

Takata, N. (1969). The play history. *American Journal of Occupational Therapy, 23,* 314–318.

Takata, N. (1974). Play as a prescription. In M. Reilly (Ed.), *Play as exploratory learning* (pp. 209–246.) Beverly Hills, CA: Sage.

Taylor M. L., & Marks M. (1955). *Aphasic rehabilitation: Manual and workbook.* New York: Rehabilitation, NYU-Bellevue Medical Center.

Terman, L. (1916). *The measurement of intelligence.* Boston: Houghton Mifflin.

Terman, L., & Merrill, M. (1973). *Stanford–Binet Intelligence Scale.* Boston: Houghton Mifflin.

Tesch, R. (1990). *Qualitative research: Analysis types and software tools.* New York: Falmer.

Thomas, C. L. (Ed.). (1997). *Taber's cyclopedic medical dictionary* (18th ed.). Philadelphia: F. A. Davis.

Thomson, L. K. (1992). *The Kohlman Evaluation of Living Skills* (3rd ed.). Rockland, MD: American Occupational Therapy Association.

Thomson, L. K. (1999). The Kohlman Evaluation of Living Skills. In B. J. Hemphill-Pearson (Ed.), *Assessment in occupational therapy mental health: An integrative approach* (pp. 231–244). Thorofare, NJ: Slack.

Thorndike, E. (1927). *The measurement of intelligence.* New York: Teachers College Press.

Thorndike, R., Hagen, E., & Sattler, J. (1985). *Stanford-Binet Intelligence Scale: Fourth Edition (SB:FE).* Chicago: Riverside.

Thornwald, J. (1963). *Science and secrets of early medicine.* New York: Harcourt, Brace and World.

Thurstone, L. L. (1938). Primary mental abilities. *Psychometric Monographs, No. 1.*

Tiffin, J. (1948). *Purdue Pegboard.* Rosemont, IL: London House.

Timpka, T., Leijon, M., Karlsson, G., Svensson, L., & Bjurulf, P. (1997). Long-term economic effects of team-based clinical case management of patients with chronic minor disease and long-term absence from working life. *Scandinavian Journal of Social Medicine, 25,* 229–237.

Tona, J. L., & Schneck, C. M. (1993). The efficacy of upper extremity inhibiting casting: A single subject pilot study. *The American Journal of Occupational Therapy, 47,* 901–910.

Townsend, E. (1996). Institutional ethnography: A method for showing how the context shapes practice. *Occupational Therapy Journal of Research, 16,* 179–199.

Tukey, J. W. (1977). *Exploratory data analysis.* Reading, MA: Addison-Wesley.

Turabian, K. L. (1996). *A manual for writers of term papers, theses, and dissertations* (6th ed.; rev. by J. Grossman & A. Bennett). Chicago: University of Chicago Press.

Turnbull, H. R., III. (1998). *Free appropriate public education: The law and children with disabilities* (5th ed.). Aspen, CO: Love.

Underwood, R. J., Duncan, C. P., Taylor, J. A., & Cotton, J. W. (1954). *Elementary statistics.* New York: Appleton-Century-Crofts.

Unistat for Windows: Key Features. (1999). [On-Line]. Available: http://www.unistat.com/features.htm [1999, August 14].

United Nations. (1958). *Population studies* (Number 29). New York: Author.

United States Department of Defense, Joint Services Steering Committee. (1963). *Human engineering guide to equipment design.* (Morgan, C. T., et al., Eds.). New York: McGraw-Hill.

United States Department of Education. (1990). *Individuals with Disabilities Education Act.* Washington, DC: Office of Special Education and Rehabilitation Services.

United States Department of Education. (1993). *To assure the free appropriate public education of all children with disabilities: Fifteenth Annual Report to Congress on the Implementation of the Education of the Handicapped Act.* Washington, DC: U.S. Government Printing Office.

United States Department of Education. (1998). *To assure the free appropriate public education of all children with disabilities: Twentieth annual report to Congress on the implementation of the Individuals With Disabilities Education Act.* Washington, DC: U.S. Government Printing Office.

United States Department of Health and Human Services, Health Care Financing Administration. (n.d.). *Your guide to choosing a nursing home* [On-Line]. Washington, DC: U.S. Government Printing Office. Available: http://www.medicare.gov/nursing.htm.l [1999, October 16].

United States Department of Health and Human Services, National Institutes of Health, Office for Protection from Research Risks. (1991). *Code of federal regulations. Title 45: Public welfare; Part 46: Protection of human subjects,* [On-Line]. *Washington, DC: U.S. Government* Printing Office. Available: http://www.fas.harvard.edu/~research/45CFR46.html#¤46.115 [1999, October 16].

United States Department of Labor. (1951, 1972–73, 1988–89, 1992–93, 1998–99). *Occupational outlook handbook.* Washington, DC: U.S. Government Printing Office. Available: http://stats.bls.gov/ocohome.htm [2000, January 11].

United States Department of Labor. (1991). *Dictionary of occupational titles* (4th ed.). Washington, DC: U.S. Government Printing Office. Available: http://www.wave.net/upg/immigration/dot index.html [2000, January 11].

University of Minnesota Libraries. (1998). *Description of Indexes—Science Citation Index Expanded,* [On-Line]. Available: http://www.lib.umn.edu/index/about/a-scie.html [1999, August 16].

Valpar International Corporation. (1973). *Valpar component work samples.* Tucson, AZ: Author.

(Available from Valpar International Corporation, P. O. Box 5767 Tucson, AZ 85703; http://www.valparint.com/)

Van Deusen, J., & Brunk, D. (1997). *Assessment in occupational therapy and physical therapy.* Philadelphia: Saunders.

Van Manen, M. (1990). *Researching lived experience: Human science for an action sensitive pedagogy.* London, Ontario: State University of New York.

Velligan, D. I., True, J. E., Lefton, R. S., Moore, T. C., & Flores, C. V. (1995). Validity of the Allen Cognitive Levels assessment: A tri-ethnic comparison. *Psychiatry Research, 56,* 101–109.

Vergason, G. A., & Anderegg, M. L. (1992). Preserving the least restrictive environment. In S. Stainback & W. Stainback (Eds.), *Controversial issues confronting special education* (pp. 45–54). Boston: Allyn & Bacon.

Vidich, A. J., & Lyman, S. M. (1994). Qualitative methods: Their history in sociology and anthropology. In N. K. Denzin & Y. S. Lincoln (Eds.), *Handbook of qualitative research* (pp. 23–59). Thousand Oaks, CA: Sage.

Vocational Rehabilitation Act of 1973, 29 U.S.C. § 794 (§504).

Vocational Research Institute. (1977). *VIEWS: Vocational Information and Evaluations.* (Available from Vocational Research Institute, 1528 Walnut Street, Suite 1502; Philadelphia, PA 19102; http://www.vri.org/)

Vocational Research Institute. (1980). *VITAS: Vocational Interest, Temperament and Aptitude System.* (Available from Vocational Research Institute, 1528 Walnut Street, Suite 1502; Philadelphia, PA 19102; http://www.vri.org/)

Vygotsky, L. S. (1962). *Thought and language.* (E. Hanfmann & G. Vaka, Eds. & Trans.). Cambridge, MA: MIT Press. (Original work published 1934)

Walker, J. E., & Howland, J. (1991). Falls and fear of falling among elderly persons living in the community. *American Journal of Occupational Therapy, 45,* 119–122.

Wallas, G. (1926). *The art of thought.* New York: Harcourt, Brace.

Wallis, W. A., & Roberts, H. V. (1962). *The nature of statistics.* New York: Free Press.

Walls, R. T., Zane, T., & Thveldt, J. E. 1979. *Independent Living Behavior Checklist.* Dunbar: West Virginia Research and Training Center.

Walters, L. (Ed.). (1998). *Bibliography of bioethics* (Vol. 24). Washington, DC: Georgetown University, Kennedy Institute.

Walters, L., & Kahn, T. J. (Eds.). (1990). *Bibliography of bioethics* (Vol. 16). Washington, DC: Georgetown University, Kennedy Institute.

Watson, J. D. (1968). *The double helix.* New York: Atheneum.

Weaver, W. (1947). *The scientists speak.* New York: Boni and Gaar.

Weiss, C. H. (1972). *Evaluation research: Methods for assessing program effectiveness.* Englewood Cliffs, NJ: Prentice-Hall.

Weiss-Lambrou, R. (1989). *The health professional's guide to writing for publication.* Springfield, IL: Charles C. Thomas

Weitzman, E. A., & Miles, M. B. (1995). *Computer programs for qualitative analysis.* Thousand Oaks, CA: Sage.

Welch, J., & King, T. A. (1985). *Searching the medical literature: A guide to printed and online sources.* London: Chapman and Hall.

Welkowitz, J., Ewen, R. B., & Cohen, J. (1971). *Introductory statistics for the behavioral sciences.* New York: Academic Press.

What people do with SPSS. (1999), [On-Line]. Available: http://www.spss.com/software/spss/cando.htm#he [1999, August 14].

White, R. W. (1952). *Lives in progress.* New York: Rinehart and Winston.

Whiteford, G. E. (1995). Other worlds and other lives: A study of occupational therapy student perceptions of cultural difference. *Occupational Therapy International, 2,* 291–313.

Wiener, N. (1948). *Cybernetics: Or, control and communication in the animal and the machine.* New York: Wiley.

Wightman, W. P. D. (1971). *The emergence of scientific medicine.* Edinburgh, Scotland: Oliver and Boyd.

Will, M. (1986). Educating children with learning problems: A shared responsibility. *Exceptional Children, 52,* 411–415.

Willard, H. S., & Spackman, C. S. (1971). *Occupational therapy* (4th ed.). Philadelphia: J. B. Lippincott.

Willer, B., Ottenbacher, K. J., & Coad, M. L. (1994). The community integration questionnaire: A comparative examination. *American Journal of Physical Medicine & Rehabilitation, 73,* 103–111.

Williams, J. H., Drinka, T. J., Greenberg, J. R., Farrell-Holtan, J. Euhardy, R., & Schram, M. (1991). Development and testing of the assessment of living skills and resources (ALSAR) in elderly community-dwelling veterans. *Gerontologist, 31,* 84–91.

Williams, S., & Bloomer, J. (1987). *Bay Area Functional Performance Evaluation* (2nd ed.). Palo Alto, CA: Consulting Psychologists Press.

Wilson, B., Baddley, A., Cockburn, J., & Hiorns, R. (n.d.). *The Rivermead Behavioural Memory Test. Supplement 2: Validation study.* Titchfield, Hants, England: Thames Valley Test Company.

Wilson, B., Cockburn, J., & Baddley, A. (1991). *The Rivermead Behavioural Memory Test.* Edmunds, England: Thames Valley Test Company.

Wilson, B. N., & Kaplan, B. J. (1994). Follow-up assessment of children receiving sensory integration treatment. *The Occupational Therapy Journal of Research, 14,* 244–266.

Wilson, B. N., Pollock, N., Kaplan, B. J., Low, M., & Faris, P. (1992). Reliability and construct validity of the Clinical Observations of Motor and Postural Skills. *American Journal of Occupational Therapy, 46,* 775–783.

Wilson, D. J., Baker, L. L., & Craddock, J. A. (1984). Functional test for the hemiparetic upper extremity. *American Journal of Occupational Therapy, 38,* 159–164.

Wilson, E. B. (1984). Occupational therapy for children with minimal handicaps. Unpublished manual.

Winkler, A. C., & McCuen, J. R. (1979). *Writing the research paper: A handbook.* New York: Harcourt, Brace, & Jovanovich.

Winkler, A. C., & McCuen, J. R. (1998). *Writing the research paper: A handbook* (5th ed.). New York: Harcourt, Brace, & Jovanovich.

Winnie, A. J. (1912). *History and handbook of day schools for the deaf and blind.* Madison, WI: State Department of Education.

Wirt, R. D., Lachar, D., Klinesinst, J. E., Seat, P. D., & Broen, W. E. (1998). *Personality Inventory for Children* (Rev. ed.). Los Angeles: Western Psychological Services.

Wolfensberger, W. (1972). *The principle of normalization in human services.* Toronto, Ontario: National Institution on Mental Retardation.

Wolpe, J. (1969). *The practice of behavior therapy.* New York: Pergamon.

Woods, K., Karrison, T., Koshy, M., Patel, A., Friedmann, P., & Cassel, C. (1997). Hospital utilization patterns and costs for adult sickle cell patients in Illinois. *Public Health Reports, 112,* 44–51.

World Health Organization. (1998). *Fifty facts from the world health report 1998: Global health situation and trends 1955–2025,* [On-Line].

Available: http://www.who.int/whr/1998/factse.htm [1999, February 27].

World Medical Association. (1997). *Handbook of declarations,* [On-Line]. Ferney- Voltaire, France: Author. Available: http://bioscience.igh.cnrs.fr//guides/declhels.htm [1999, October 16].

Xakellis, G. C., Frantz, R. A., Lewis, A., & Harvey, P. (1998). Cost-effectiveness of an intensive pressure ulcer prevention protocol in long-term care. *Advances in Wound Care: The Journal for Prevention & Healing, 11,* 22–29.

Yasakawa, A. (1990). Case report–Upper extremity casting: Adjunct treatment for a child with cerebral palsy hemiplegia. *American Journal of Occupational Therapy, 44,* 840–846.

Yau, M. K-S (1997). The impact of refugee resettlement on southeast Asian adolescents and young adults: Implications for occupational therapist. *Occupational Therapy International, 4,* 1–16.

Yesavage, J. A., Brink, T. A., Rose, T. L., Lum, O., Huang, V., Adey, M., & Leire, V. O. (1983). Development and validation of a geriatric depression screening scale: A preliminary report. *Journal of Psychiatric Research, 17,* 37–49.

Zinsser, W. (1990). *On writing well: An informal guide to writing nonfiction* (4th ed.). New York: HarperCollins.

Zung, W. K. (1965). A self-rating depression scale. *Archives of General Psychiatry, 12,* 63–75.

Index

A

ABLEDATA, 207
Abstract, 421
Allied health professionals, evolution of, 17–18
Allied health treatment technologies, 18, 20–21
American Medical Association Manual of Style,
    421
American Statistical Index, 212–213
Analysis of variance (ANOVA), 345–351
    one-way, 345–346
    post hoc analysis, examples, 351
    stepwise procedure for, 347–351
    two-factor, 346
Analyzing data, 172–176
    credibility in, 174–176
    principles, 173–174
    practice, 174
Anatomy and physiology, growth of, 3–5
Annual Reviews Inc., 211
Appendices and referenced list, 420–421
Assessment instruments, 86–87
Assisted living (nonmedical), definition of, 227
Associational relationships between variables,
    112
Assumptions in clinical evaluation, 380
    stating, 228
Attentive listening, 168–169
Audiovisual aids, 440

B

Bar graphs, 291–292
    constructing, 291
Bibliographic citations, use of in writing,
    431–432

Bibliographic indexes and abstracting
    periodicals, 208–211
    Annual Reviews, Inc., 211
    Biological Abstracts and Biology Digest, 210
    Cumulative Index Medicus, 209
    Cumulative Index to Nursing and Allied
        Health Literature (CINAHL), 209
    Current contents, 210–211
    Dissertation Abstracts, 210
    Ergo Werb, 209
    Excerpta Medica Abstract Journals, 209
    Health Education Research, 209
    Hospital and Health Administration Index,
        209–210
    Index Medicus, 209
    Mental Health, 209
    NIH Office of Extramural Research, 211
    Psychological Abstracts, 210
    Science Citation Index, 210
    Social Work Research and Abstracts, 210
    Sociological Abstracts, 210
Bibliographic references, common, 434–436
Bibliographic sources for testing, 383–384
Binet tests
    tests, alternative to, 374–375
    influence of on IQ testing, 374
Biography of Bioethics, 214
Biological Abstracts and Biology Digest, 210
Biological description of medical research,
        stage I
    Galen, 6–7
    growth of scientific anatomy and physiology,
        3–5
    Harvey, 8–9
    Hippocratic writings, 5–6
    Paracelsius, medical chemist, 8

Occupational therapy (OT)
  assessment, tests used in, 385
  history, landmarks in, 471–475(app)
  literature search in, 199
  questions examined in, 160
  and special education, definition and
    purposes of, 2–3
Occupational therapy, application of survey
    research to, 122–125
  distribution of health care, 122
  educational planning, 123–124
  occupational health planning, 124
  planning therapeutic services, 123
  preventive programs in schools and
    communities, 124–125
One-sample problems, model II, 279–280,
    327–331
Operational learning objectives, 1, 39, 63, 133,
    177, 193, 223, 269, 371, 415
Operational procedure of observed versus
    expected frequencies (chi-square),
    360–363
Operationally defining variable, 224–228
Operations research, 142–147
  example of, 145–146
Ordinal scale data, 246–247, 248
Organization, writing, 430
OT BibSys, 205–206
Outline
  of overall evaluative process of testing,
    377–378
  of research proposal, 432, 437
  for tests, 409–410
Outlining literature review section, 217,
    219–222
Outlining research study, 417–421
  abstract, 421
  introducing research paper, 417–418
  methodology, 419–420
  reference list and appendices, 420–421
  results, 420
  reviewing of literature, 418–419

P

Pain, tests to measure, 393–397
Paired data sample, 341
Paired data sample, model IV, 281
  correlated *t* tests, 339–343
  Wilcoxon test for paired data samples,
    343–345
Paracelsius, 8
Participants for research, selection of, 239–244
  convenience sample and volunteers, 243–244
  external validity, 241–242

random sampling, 242–243
Pearson Product-Moment correlation
    coefficient, critical values for, 485–486
  steps in determining, 486
Pediatric assessment, 406–407
Pediatrics tests, 397–405
People first language, 423
Percentages, table of, 282–283
Perceptual spatial orientation tasks,
    comparison, 332
Perseverance, as quality in research, 51
Physical dysfunction tests, 393–397
Physical evaluation techniques and treatment
    hardware, 90
Physical medicine and rehabilitation, 18
Physiology and anatomy, growth of, 3–5
Pilot studies in heuristic research, application
    of, 99, 102
Poster, key points in preparing, 439
Poster session, 437, 439
Predictive validity, 252
Preparation for presentation, 437–442
  conference paper, 439–440
  poster session, 437, 439
  publication, 440–442
Preparation for writing, 415–417
Prevention in medicine, stage IV, 13–14
Preventive programs in schools and
    communities, 124–125
Prevocational tests, 397
Principle survey methods, relative merits of,
    118
Printing, process of, 441–442
Problem-oriented research in health
    professions, need for, 177–178
Professional education, identifying significant
    issues in, 181–182
Professional associations, selected, web
    addresses of, 465–466(app)
Professional programs in OT, methodology and
    content of, 182
Proofing an article, checklist for, 422
Proportion of areas under normal curve, 479
Psychiatric rehabilitation, 21–22
PsychoINFO, 207
Psychological Abstracts, 210
Psychological blocks in selection of research
    problems, 186–187
Psychosocial assessment in OT, 386–390
Psychosocial tests, 384–393
  behavior rating scales, 384
  objective personality tests, 384
Publication of article, 440–442
  classifying manuscript, 441
  components of manuscript, 442

Y

Z